COMPREHENSIVE PERIODONTICS
FOR THE DENTAL HYGIENIST

THIRD EDITION

COMPREHENSIVE PERIODONTICS FOR THE DENTAL HYGIENIST

Mea A. Weinberg, D.M.D., M.S.D., R.Ph.
Cheryl Westphal, R.D.H., M.S.
Stuart J. Froum, D.D.S.
Milton Palat, D.D.S., J.D.
Robert S. Schoor, D.D.S.

New York University College of Dentistry
New York, New York

Pearson

Boston   Columbus   Indianapolis   New York   San Francisco
Upper Saddle River   Amsterdam   Cape Town   Dubai   London
Madrid   Milan   Munich   Paris   Montreal   Toronto   Delhi
Mexico City   Sao Paulo   Sydney   Hong Kong   Seoul   Singapore
Taipei   Tokyo

Library of Congress Cataloging-in-Publication Data

Comprehensive periodontics for the dental hygienist /
Mea A. Weinberg ... [et al.]— 3rd ed.
   p. ; cm.
  Includes bibliographical references and index.
  ISBN-13: 978-0-13-501542-1
  ISBN-10: 0-13-501542-1
  1. Periodontics. 2. Dental hygiene. I. Weinberg, Mea A.
[DNLM: 1. Periodontal Diseases. WU 240 C737 2010]
RK361.C58 2010
617.6´32—dc22

        2008053848

Notice:
The authors and the publisher of this volume have taken care that the information and technical recommendations contained herein are based on research and expert consultation, and are accurate and compatible with the standards generally accepted at the time of publication. Nevertheless, as new information becomes available, changes in clinical and technical practices become necessary. The reader is advised to carefully consult manufacturers' instructions and information material for all supplies and equipment before use, and to consult with a health care professional as necessary. This advice is especially important when using new supplies or equipment for clinical purposes. The authors and publisher disclaim all responsibility for any liability, loss, injury, or damage incurred as a consequence, directly or indirectly, of the use and application of any of the contents of this volume.

Publisher: Julie Levin Alexander
Assistant to Publisher: Regina Bruno
Editor-in-Chief: Mark Cohen
Development Editor: Melissa Kerian
Assistant Editor: Nicole Ragonese
Senior Media Editor: Amy Peltier
Managing Production Editor: Patrick Walsh
Production Liaison: Christina Zingone
Production Editor: Bruce Hobart, Pine Tree Composition
Manufacturing Manager: Ilene Sanford
Manufacturing Buyer: Pat Brown
Art Director: Kenny Beck
Cover and Interior Designer: LCI Design

Director of Marketing: Karen Allman
Executive Marketing Manager: Katrin Beacom
Marketing Specialist: Michael Sirinides
Marketing Assistant: Judy Noh
Media Project Manager: Lorena Cerisano
Manager, Rights and Permissions: Zina Arabia
Manager, Visual Research: Beth Brenzel
Manager, Cover Visual Research & Permissions: Karen Sanatar
Image Permission Coordinator: Fran Toepfer
Composition: Pine Tree Composition, Inc.
Printer/Binder: CJ Krehbiel
Cover Printer: Lehigh/Phoenix Color Corporation
Cover Image: Belle Media/Shutterstock

10 9 8 7 6 5 4 3 2 1

www.pearsonhighered.com

ISBN-10:   0-13-501542-1
ISBN-13:   978-0-13-501542-1

Contents

Foreword   vii

Preface   ix

Contributors   xi

Reviewers   xiii

PART I

Periodontal Diseases: Introduction and Background   1

1 Anatomy of the Periodontal Structures: The Healthy State   2

2 Epidemiology of Periodontal Diseases   25

3 Dental Biofilms: Microbiology of Periodontal Diseases   51

4 Bacteria–Host Response: Inflammatory and Immunology Fundamentals   65

5 Local Contributory Factors for Periodontal Diseases   81

6 Oral-Systemic Disease Connection   93

PART II

Periodontal Diseases: Classification   111

7 Gingival Diseases   112

8 Periodontitis and Other Periodontal Conditions   128

9 Necrotizing Periodontal Diseases   147

10 Occlusal Trauma   153

11 Abscesses of the Periodontium   170

PART III

Periodontal Diseases: The Assessment Phase   177

12 Dental Hygiene Process of Care for the Patient with Periodontal Disease   178

13 Patient History   182

14 Clinical Examination: Extraoral/Intraoral Examination and Dental Evaluation   187

15 Clinical Examination: Gingival Assessment   198

16 Clinical Examination: Periodontal Assessment   209

17 Radiographic Assessment   233

18 Advances in Detecting and Monitoring the Periodontal Diseases   249

v

PART IV

Periodontal Diseases: Treatment Planning, Implementation, and Evaluation Phase 257

19 Problem/Evidence-Based Treatment Planning   258

20 Oral Hygiene for the Periodontal Patient: Beyond the Basics   285

21 Topical Drug Delivery Systems: Oral Rinses and Irrigation   320

22 Systemic and Local Drug Delivery Systems: Systemic Antibiotics, Local Drug Devices, and Enzyme Suppression Therapy   332

23 Healing After Nonsurgical Periodontal Therapy   348

24 Principles of Periodontal Surgery: Gingivectomy, Osseous Resection, and Periodontal Plastic Surgery   362

25 Principles of Periodontal Surgery: Periodontal Regeneration   394

26 Implantology   413

27 Periodontal Emergencies   438

28 Periodontal Maintenance Therapy   445

Appendices   460

A Periodontal Information Resources   461

B Reading the Literature   464

C Antibiotic Prophylaxis   467

Case Studies   469

Case Study I   469

Case Study II   475

Case Study III   481

Case Study IV   486

Glossary   493

Answers to Self-Quiz Questions   507

Index   509

Foreword

There is no subject of greater importance to the practice of dental hygiene than periodontology. *Comprehensive Periodontics for the Dental Hygienist* by Weinberg and colleagues offers an exceptional opportunity to learn this pivotal aspect of clinical practice at its best. This text accomplishes several important goals in thoughtful and compelling ways: It fosters an evidence-based approach—one that has become central to all clinical disciplines. It cultivates in the practitioner an identity as a person of science—that is, as a sophisticated *consumer* of research. While scientists are assigned the responsibility of generating new knowledge, every practitioner must see him- or herself as a consumer of such information, capable of assessing and critiquing it for him- or herself. The text also underscores the interrelationship between oral disease and systemic health while helping prepare the dental hygienist to cope with increasingly complex technologies and innovations.

The attentive student has much to gain from the text's format, including the convenient use of outlines, goals, statements of educational objectives, inclusion of key words, reference to relevant websites, and use of self-assessment quizzes. Extraordinary knowledge of the field is available to the student of dental hygiene who is willing to invest time and effort exploiting the opportunities this text affords.

Periodontology is a discipline with a strong scientific base. A flavor of the richness of the underlying literature is reflected in the citations at the end of each chapter. Thus students and practitioners have at their disposal the means to secure a more in depth treatment of specific topic areas by accessing the foundational literature upon which the text is based. Those who do so can become adept at interpreting that literature for themselves, developing in the process the tools they will need to think independently and to remain current in their discipline with the passage of time.

Charles N. Bertolami
Professor and Herman Robert Fox Dean
College of Dentistry
New York University

Preface

There is a significant body of knowledge about the risk factors, pathogenesis, treatment, and prevention of periodontal diseases. This knowledge is rarely applied as an evidence-based approach to the difficult problem of deciding when specific treatments or examination methods are appropriate. Classic and current references are included in each chapter, along with applicable websites so the reader can supplement information in the textbook with information from other sources.

This basic text has been written in an attempt to make the professions' understanding of periodontal diseases accessible to the dental hygiene student, the practicing dental hygienist, and the dentist needing to update their knowledge through a concise synopsis of clinical periodontics.

Part I deals with the anatomy of the periodontium, risk (markers) factors (e.g., dental biofilms, smoking, and diabetes mellitus) for periodontal diseases, and periodontal disease as a potential risk factor for systemic conditions (the periodontal/medicine relationship) such as stroke, cardiovascular disease, emphysema, and premature low-birth-weight babies. This interrelationship between medicine and periodontology has opened new insights into the concept of oral health being an integral part of the overall general and systemic health of an individual. Oral and intravenous bisphosphonates is discussed as it relates to osteonecrosis of the jaw (ONJ).

Part II discusses in detail the different periodontal diseases according to the 1999 Classification System of the Periodontal Diseases (American Academy of Periodontology).

Part III deals with the clinical assessment phase of the dental hygiene process of care. This part discusses the various assessment tools that are required to be performed on a patient for the development of a dental hygiene diagnosis.

Part IV discusses the treatment planning, implementation, and evaluation process of dental hygiene care. Nonsurgical and surgical therapy through problem-based learning (PBL) are discussed in detail. A problem-based system with basic concepts of treatment planning will be introduced to the student. A comprehensive review of halitosis is presented. In this section is an extensive review of drugs used in periodontal therapy including various controlled-release drug devices (e.g., PerioChip™, Atridox®, Arestin®) and enzyme suppression drugs (e.g., doxycycline 20 mg). An expanded section on surgery and implants is included with many color images. The appendices include a comprehensive listing of periodontic informatics, and how to critically assess the periodontal literature. Following Chapter 28 are four problem-oriented, evidence-based case studies. Each case details the problem, followed by a discussion of the questions and answers to the problem. "Rapid Dental Hints" remind students about key information or a task that should be performed related to the topic discussed. Additionally, there are "Did you know?" found within all chapters that provide whimsical information on the topic at hand.

We hope this book will serve as a helpful text for all dental practitioners.

Mea A. Weinberg, D.M.D., M.S.D., R.Ph.

Contributors

Mary Elizabeth Aichelmann-Reidy, D.D.S.
Assistant Professor, Department of Periodontics
University of Maryland
Baltimore, Maryland

Khalid Almas, B.D.S., M.Sc.
Associate Professor, Division of Periodontology,
School of Dental Medicine, University of Connecticut,
Farmington, Connecticut

Denise Estafan, D.D.S, M.S.
Associate Professor and Director of Clinical Esthetics
Division of Reconstructive and Comprehensive Care
New York University College of Dentistry
New York, New York

James Burke Fine, D.M.D
Associate Dean of Postgraduate Studies
Associate Professor of Clinical Dentistry
Director of Postgraduate Periodontics
Columbia University College of Dental Medicine
New York, New York

Suzanne K. Farrar, B.S., R.D.H., H.C.M.
Assistant Professor, Department of Periodontics
Louisiana State University School of Dentistry
New Orleans, Louisiana

Cynthia Fong, R.D.H., M.S.
Lecturer/Instructor in Periodontics Department of
Dental Hygiene
Pierce College
Tacoma, Washington

Herbert Frommer, D.D.S.
Professor and Director of Radiology
New York University College of Dentistry
New York, New York

Stuart J. Froum, D.D.S.
Clinical Professor, Director of Research
Department of Periodontology and Implant Dentistry
New York University College of Dentistry
New York, New York

Ann M. Goodwin, R.D.H., M.S.
Former Clinical Associate Professor, Dental Hygiene
Program
New York University College of Dentistry
New York, New York

Rosemary DeRosa Hays, R.D.H., M.S.
Clinical Associate Professor, Dental Hygiene Program
New York University College of Dentistry
New York, New York

Judith Kreismann, R.D.H., B.S., M.S.
Clinical Associate Professor, Dental Hygiene Program
New York University College of Dentistry
New York, New York

Eva M. Lupovici, R.D.H., M.S.
Clinical Associate Professor, Dental Hygiene Program
New York University College of Dentistry
New York, New York

John D. Mason, B.A., D.D.S.
Associate Professor, Department of Periodontics
Louisiana State University School of Dentistry
New Orleans, Louisiana

Trisha E. O'Hehir, R.D.H., B.S.
Editor of Perio Reports
Senior Consulting Editor, RHD Magazine
Vice President, Perio-Data™ Company
Assistant Visiting Professor Northern Arizona
University
Flagstaff, Arizona

Jill Rethman, R.D.H., B.A.
Visiting Clinical Instructor, Department of Dental Hygiene
University of Pittsburgh
Pittsburgh, Pennsylvania

Michael P. Rethman, D.D.S., M.S.
Past President of the American Academy of Periodontology
Former Chief of Periodontics
Tripler Medical Center
Honolulu, Hawaii

Robert S. Schoor, D.D.S.
Past President of the American Academy of Periodontology
Associate Professor and Director of Postgraduate Periodontics
Department of Periodontolgy and Implant Dentistry
Division of Diagnostics, Infectious Diseases and Health Promotion
New York University College of Dentistry
New York, New York

Surendra Singh, D.D.S., M.S.
Professor Department of Periodontics
University of Medicine and Dentistry of New Jersey School of Dentistry
Newark, New Jersey

Jeanne St. Germain, B.S., R.D.H.
Clinical Instructor, Department of Periodontics
Louisiana State University School of Dentistry
New Orleans, Louisiana

Mea A. Weinberg, D.M.D., M.S.D., R.Ph.
Clinical Associate Professor and Director of Second Year Periodontics
Department of Periodontology and Implant Dentistry
New York University College of Dentistry
New York, New York

Cheryl Westphal, R.D.H., M.S.
Clinical Associate Professor and Assistant Dean for Allied Health Programs
Director, Dental Hygiene Program
New York University College of Dentistry
New York, New York

Raymond A. Yukna, D.M.D., M.S.
Professor, Directory Periodontic Residency Program
University of Colorado

Selected Illustrations by Jesse Doscher, D.D.S.

Selected Photographs Courtesy of Dr. John Eum, Dr. James Fine, Dr. Xiu Yan Li, Dr. Jacqueline Plemmons, Dr. Jesse Sorrentino, Dr. Michael Turner, and Dr. Harvey Wishe

Reviewers

Lisa Bilich, R.D.H., M.S.
Assistant Professor, Dental Hygiene
Eastern Washington University
Spokane, Washington

Phebe Blitz, R.D.H., M.S.
Program Director, Dental Hygiene
Mesa Community College-Red Mountain
Mesa, Arizona

Barbara C. Bush, R.D.H., M.S.Ed.
Associate Professor, Allied Health
Western Kentucky University
Bowling Green, Kentucky

Connie Clark, M.Ed., R.D.H.
Clinical Coordinator, Dental Hygiene
Columbus State Community College
Columbus, Ohio

Shaunda L. Clark, C.D.A., R.D.H., M.Ed.
Program Director, Dental Hygiene
Kirkwood Community College
Cedar Rapids, Iowa

Mary Emmons, R.D.H., M.Ed.
Professor Emeritus, Dental Hygiene
Parkland College
Champaign, Illinois

Diane H. Estes, R.D.H., B.S., M.Ed.
Instructor/Clinical Coordinator, Dental Hygiene
Athens Technical College
Athens, Georgia

Deborah A. Graeff, R.D.H., M.S.
Professor, Dental Hygiene
Erie Community College
Williamsville, New York

Barbara Jarrett, C.D.A., R.D.H., M.S.
Program Coordinator, Dental Services
Trident Technical College
Charleston, South Carolina

Susan Jenkins, M.S., R.D.H.
Assistant Professor, Dental Hygiene
Massachusetts College of Pharmacy & Health Sciences
Boston, Massachusetts

Leah MacPherson, R.D.H., B.S., M.H.P.
Professor, Dental Hygiene
Middlesex Community College
Lowell, Massachusetts

Laura Mueller-Joseph, R.D.H., M.S., Ed.D.
Professor & Chair, Dental Hygiene
Farmingdale State College
Farmingdale, New York

Debbie Kelly, R.D.H., M.S.Ed.
Professor, Dental Hygiene
Bluegrass Community & Technical College
Lexington, Kentucky

Jean Kulbeth, R.D.H., M.S.
Academic Chair, Dental Hygiene
Fresno City College
Fresno, California

LeeAnn Simmons, R.D.H., M.S.
Instructor, Dental Hygiene
Delaware Technical and Community College
Wilmington, Delaware

Deborah Trunk, R.D.H., B.S.D.H., M.A.
Professor, Dental Hygiene
St. Louis Community College at Forest Park
St. Louis, Missouri

Sarah A. Turner, R.D.H., M.A.E.
Professor & Chair, Health Sciences
Chair, Dental Hygiene
Hawkeye Community College
Waterloo, Iowa

COMPREHENSIVE PERIODONTICS
FOR THE DENTAL HYGIENIST

Part I

Periodontal Diseases: Introduction and Background

Chapter **1**
Anatomy of the Periodontal Structures:
The Healthy State

Chapter **2**
Epidemiology of Periodontal Diseases

Chapter **3**
Dental Biofilms: Microbiology of Periodontal Diseases

Chapter **4**
Bacteria–Host Response: Inflammatory
and Immunology Fundamentals

Chapter **5**
Local Contributory Factors for Periodontal Diseases

Chapter **6**
The Oral-Systemic Disease Connection

Anatomy of the Periodontal Structures: The Healthy State

Mea A. Weinberg

OUTLINE

Clinical Anatomy of the Gingival Unit
Microscopic Anatomy of the Gingival Unit
Attachment Apparatus
Physiology of the Periodontium
Changes with Aging
Dental Hygiene Notes
Key Points
Self-Quiz
References

EDUCATIONAL OBJECTIVES

Upon completion of this chapter, the reader should be able to:

- Illustrate and discuss the clinical anatomy of the periodontium.
- Illustrate and describe the microscopic anatomy of the periodontium.
- List and describe the functions of the periodontium.
- Discuss the importance of the dentogingival unit.
- Describe the lymphatic, blood, and nerve supply to the gingiva and the attachment apparatus.

GOAL: To provide knowledge of the structures and functions of the periodontium in health.

KEY WORDS

attachment apparatus 3
biologic width 14
col 7
connective tissue attachment 12
dentogingival unit 13
gingiva 3
gingival crevice 4
oral epithelium 8
junctional epithelium 10
periodontium 3
sulcular epithelium 10

INTRODUCTION

The **periodontium**, translated in Latin to mean "around the tooth," consists of the **gingiva**, periodontal ligament, cementum, and alveolar and supporting bone of the teeth (Figure 1–1a ■). The **attachment apparatus** consists of periodontal tissues involved in the attachment and support of the root in the tooth socket, specifically the periodontal ligament, cementum, and alveolar bone (Hassell, 1993). A working knowledge of the ultrastructural anatomy and biology of the periodontal tissues is an important prerequisite for practitioners to recognize and treat periodontal diseases.

In order to understand the different stages of diseases in the periodontium, it is necessary to recognize the structures and functions of the periodontium in health (Bartold, 2006). This chapter describes the clinical and microscopic features of the periodontium in health and will be the foundation for ensuing discussions in this text.

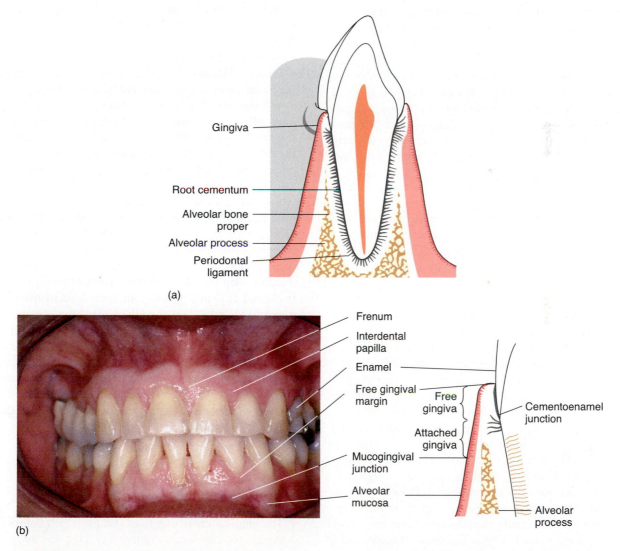

(a)

(b)

■ **FIGURE 1–1**   (a) Schematic drawing of a tooth with its periodontium. (b) Landmarks of the gingival unit. (*Left*) The gingiva is salmon pink, while the alveolar mucosa is thinner and redder in color. (*Right*) Schematic drawing of a cross-section of the periodontium. (Adapted from J. Lindhe and T. Karring, Anatomy of the periodontium, in *Clinical periodontology and implant dentistry,* ed. J. Lindhe. Copenhagen: Munksgaard, © 2003.)

CLINICAL ANATOMY OF THE GINGIVAL UNIT

The oral mucosa is divided into three types: (1) masticatory mucosa, which includes the gingiva and hard palate; (2) lining mucosa, which consists of the alveolar mucosa, soft palate, lining of lips, cheeks, and sublingual area; and (3) specialized mucosa, which is found on the dorsum of the tongue.

Masticatory Mucosa (Gingiva)

The gingiva forms a protective covering over the other components of the periodontium and is well adapted to protect against mechanical insults (e.g., toothbrushing and chewing). The gingiva encircles the cervical portion of the teeth and covers the alveolar process. Anatomically, the gingiva is subdivided into the free gingiva, attached gingiva, and interdental gingiva or papilla (Figure 1–1b). The outer surface of the gingiva consists of stratified squamous epithelium. Underneath the epithelium is gingival connective tissue, which is termed the lamina propria.

Free Gingiva (Marginal Gingiva)

The free gingiva or marginal gingiva surrounds the neck of the tooth. Its boundaries are, coronally, the free gingival margin; apically, the free gingival groove; and laterally, the gingival crevice and the tooth (see Figure 1–1b). The free gingiva is approximately 1.5 mm wide and has a smooth surface. The free gingiva lies on and adapts to the enamel and can be separated from the tooth with a periodontal instrument (Schroeder & Listgarten, 1997).

In health, the free gingival margin is the edge or the most coronal part of the free gingiva and in a fully erupted tooth is located on the enamel approximately 0.5 to 2 mm coronal to the cementoenamel junction (CEJ). In health and if teeth contact in the anterior region, the free gingival margin usually has a scalloped outline following the contour of the cementoenamel junction (see Figure 1–1b). If there is an open contact, the free gingival margin becomes blunted. In the posterior region, the architecture becomes less scalloped. Prior to the completed eruption of permanent teeth in children, the free gingival margin usually remains located on the cervical bulge of the enamel. This is a normal situation, and as the tooth erupts the free gingival margin will ultimately move apically.

Gingival Crevice   The **gingival crevice** is the space between the free gingiva and the tooth surface and is lined by nonkeratinized stratified squamous epithelium. In gingival health, the gingival crevice is termed a sulcus; once inflamed, it is termed a pocket. Healthy gingiva sulcular depth is approximately 1 to 3 mm when measured with a periodontal probe. Only in experimental conditions with germ-free animals can the sulcular depth be zero.

Gingival crevicular fluid (GCF) fills the sulcus, originates from blood vessels within the underlying connective tissue (lamina propria), and flows through the tissue into the gingival crevice. The rate of passage of this fluid is dependent upon the absence or presence of inflammation in the connective tissue of the gingiva. The flow is minimal to absent in health, but increases due to inflammation from accumulation of plaque in the gingival crevice (Alfano, 1974). Components of GCF resemble blood serum components and include elements such as calcium, sodium, potassium, and phosphorus, along with cells and bacteria. The role of GCF is both protective and destructive. While crevicular fluid flow cleanses the sulcus, it is also a source of nutrients for subgingival bacteria and supports subgingival calculus formation (Mukherjee, 1985). Certain antibiotics, including tetracyclines used in the treatment of periodontal diseases, have been found to concentrate in higher levels locally in the GCF (pocket area) than in the serum (Gordon, Walker, Murphy, Goodson, & Socransky, 1981).

Free Gingival Groove   The free gingival groove, a shallow depression on the outer surface of the gingiva, is about 1 to 2 mm apical from the margin of the gingiva and is slightly apical to the level of the cementoenamel junction. This groove separates the free gingiva from the attached gingiva. The free gingival groove is present in about 30 to 40% of adults and occurs most frequently in the mandibular premolar and incisor areas. It is more pronounced on the facial than on the lingual regions. Its absence or presence is not related to the health of the gingiva.

Did You Know?

The gingival crevicular fluid (GCF), which bathes the gingival crevice subgingivally, contains many minerals and substances. Subgingival calculus is usually a dark color, such as black, due to the influence of GCF.

Rapid Dental Hint

It is important to transpose the patient's free gingival margin and mucogingival junction to the periodontal chart because this will help you determine if there is a soft tissue defect present and to monitor the attachment level and gingival recession.

Attached Gingiva

The attached gingiva is continuous with the free gingiva and is firmly attached to the underlying cementum and periosteum (connective tissue) covering the alveolar process. It extends apically from the free gingival groove to the mucogingival junction (MGJ). If the free gingival groove is not present, then the landmark is at a horizontal plane placed at the level of the CEJ. The mucogingival junction joins the attached gingiva to the alveolar mucosa (see Figure 1–1b) except on the palate because the attached gingiva runs into the palatal mucosa. The width of the free gingiva and the attached gingiva consists of the total width of gingiva.

Attached gingiva is not movable, being bound down to the bone and cementum by connective tissue fibers, making it capable of withstanding forces from toothbrushing and chewing. The width of the attached gingiva varies in different areas of the mouth and between individuals (Figure 1–2 ■). On the facial aspect, the attached gingiva is widest in the incisor region and narrowest in the first premolar area. On the lingual aspect, the attached gingiva is widest in the molar region and narrowest in the incisor region.

The color of the gingiva is normally salmon pink with slight variations. The gingiva shows varying degrees of brownish-black color depending on ethnic variation (Figure 1–3 ■), which is considered to be normal gingival coloring and is referred to as melanin pigmentation.

Stippling   Clinically, the outer surface of the attached gingiva has an appearance similar to an orange

Did You Know?

Dogs, cats, and other animals also have gingiva, just like us.

(a)

(b)

■ **FIGURE 1–3**   (a) Physiological gingival pigmentation varies: light pigmentation. (b) darker, more pronounced pigmentation.

■ **FIGURE 1–2**   Varying amounts of attached gingiva; the narrowest width is on the mandibular premolars and the widest is on the maxillary incisors.

■ **FIGURE 1–4**   Surface stippling of the attached gingiva and the interdental gingiva. Note the dimpling or depressions on the surface. The surface of the free gingiva is not stippled.

peel with shallow depressions between elevations. The free gingiva has a smooth surface and is not stippled (Figure 1–4 ■). A histologic description of stippling is discussed in the following section.

Stippling may be present in health or disease. The absence of stippling does not necessarily indicate the presence of disease. On the other hand, the presence of inflammation with the loss of stippling can be consid-

ered part of the disease process, assuming stippling was present initially.

Stippling is present in only about 40% of adults and varies in different individuals, ages, and sexes. Stippling of the attached gingiva is absent in children under 5 years of age and may be more evident in men than women. It is more prominent in the anterior than the posterior region and may even be absent in the molar areas. The facial gingiva shows more prominent stippling than the lingual.

Interdental Gingiva (Interdental Papilla)

In health the interdental gingiva tightly fills the gingival embrasure, which is the space between the contact point and alveolar bone of two adjacent teeth. The margin and lateral borders of the interdental gingiva are an extension of the free gingiva, whereas the remaining parts are attached gingiva (Figure 1–5a ■).

The size and shape of the papillae are determined by tooth-to-tooth contact, the curvature of the cemen-

Rapid Dental Hint

Remember that anterior teeth may have a small col or it may not be detectable.

(a)

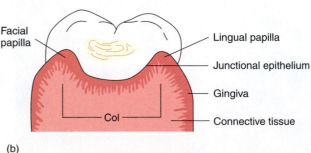

(b)

■ **FIGURE 1–5**   Features of the interdental gingiva. (a) In health the interdental gingiva fills the gingival embrasure (G). (b) The col is directly under the contact point of the teeth. (From P. F. Fedi, Jr., and A. R. Vernino, *The Periodontic Syllabus.* Copyright © 2000 by Lippincott Williams & Wilkins.)

toenamel junction, and the width (faciolingually) of the interproximal tooth surfaces. When teeth are crowded, often seen in mandibular incisors, the papillae may be slender and narrow. Anterior papillae are pyramidal in shape while posterior papillae are rounder and slightly flatter. An anterior papilla forms a single pyramidal structure because there is only one papilla. The papillae of posterior teeth (premolars and molars) are wedge shaped, with one vestibular (facial) and one oral (lingual) papilla connected by a concave area called the **col** (Fig. 1–5b). The col is directly apical to the contact area, representing the fusion of the interproximal junctional epithelia of two adjacent teeth. While an anterior papilla can form a col shape, it is more prominent in posterior papillae. When a diastema (loss of contact between two adjacent teeth) is present, the interdental papilla is absent, and there is no col. Since the shape of a col is concave and may not be keratinized, it may predispose the interproximal area to the accumulation of dental plaque.

Lining Mucosa

Alveolar Mucosa

Although not actually part of the periodontium, the alveolar mucosa is an important periodontal structure and deserves discussion. The alveolar mucosa extends apically from the mucogingival junction to the mucous membrane of the cheek, lip, and floor of the mouth (see Figure 1–1b). In comparison to the attached gingiva, alveolar mucosa is thinner and redder in color, has a smooth surface, is movable, and is not keratinized.

Frenum Attachments

Frenum (plural: frena) attachments are folds of alveolar mucosa. They are not concentrations of muscle, having no more muscle fibers than alveolar mucosa. The function of a frenum is to attach lips and cheeks to the maxillary and mandibular mucosa and to limit the movement of the lips and cheeks. There are usually seven frena located in the canine/premolar area, be-

> **Did You Know?**
>
> Gingiva is salmon pink in color due to keratin. Keratin is a protein that is also involved in forming hair, skin, and fingernails.

tween the central incisors and in the mandibular anterior lingual area.

Specialized Mucosa

The mucosa of the dorsum of the tongue contains numerous papillae of three types: filiform, fungiform, and circumvallate. The circumvallate papillae are located along the V-shaped groove on the back of the tongue. Each papilla is surrounded by a circular groove. The taste buds are located mainly on the sides of these papillae. The filiform papillae are slender ones and the most abundant, covering the entire top or dorsal surface of the tongue. No taste buds are associated with these papillae; they respond only to heat and mechanical stimuli. The fungiform papillae, which are broad and flat, are found chiefly at the edges of the tongue and are provided with taste buds.

MICROSCOPIC ANATOMY OF THE GINGIVAL UNIT

Gingival Epithelium

The gingiva is covered by a layer of stratified squamous epithelium with an underlying core of connective tissue called the lamina propria (Figure 1–6 ■). The gingival epithelium exists as structurally different forms specific to certain areas of the teeth. Thus, the gingival epithelium can be divided into (Figure 1–7 ■) the following elements:

- The oral epithelium (OE)
- The sulcular or crevicular epithelium (SE)
- The junctional epithelium (JE)

The gingival epithelium is avascular and relies upon the underlying lamina propria for its blood supply and nutrients. The epithelium found in the oral cavity consists of several layers of cells (see Figure 1–7):

- Stratum basale or stratum germinativum (basal cell layer); deepest layer next to the lamina propria.
- Stratum spinosum (spinous cell layer).
- Stratum granulosum (granular layer).
- Stratum corneum (keratinized/cornified cell layer; also called the superficial cell layer); this outermost layer serves as a barrier membrane protecting the underlying periodontal tissues from invasion by foreign substances.

Gingival crevice

Free gingiva

Gingival connective tissue

Gingival epithelium

Attached gingiva

Alveolar process

Cementum

■ **FIGURE 1-6**
Photomicrograph of the gingival epithelium. (Courtesy of Dr. Harvey Wishe, New York University College of Dentistry)

Cell Renewal

Just like the epithelium of the skin, the gingival epithelium is also subject to considerable insult and thus must have a means of regular renewal. The epithelium achieves this renewal by producing a pool of cells that migrate from the basal layer to the oral environment. This process by which epithelial cells differentiate or mature is called keratinization. The type of differentiation reflects the functional demands or stimulus placed on the tissue. During keratinization, the entire thickness of the epithelium is replaced. The time it takes for this replacement or cell renewal is called the turnover time. This time differs with the various types of epithelium. Such differences become important during tissue healing after periodontal surgery or tissue damage.

The keratinization process occurs as follows (Moss-Salentijn & Hendricks-Klyvert, 1990):

- Basal cells in the basal cell layer divide and produce new cells.
- The "older" basal cells travel or move into the next layer, the spinous cell layer, on their way to the most outer epithelial cell layer.
- Once in the spinous cell layer, the basal cells become keratinocytes. On their way to the outer surface, the keratinocytes synthesize or produce keratin.

- Keratin is a protein that contributes to the mechanical toughness of the outer surface of the epithelium.
- When the keratinocytes reach the outer epithelial surface, they are shed from the surface into the oral cavity.

Three grades of keratinization or maturation are identified according to the completeness of the transition of the keratinocyte from the basal cell layer to the outermost, superficial cell layer. Consequently, epithelium can be (ortho) keratinized, parakeratinized, or nonkeratinized. Keratinized epithelium is composed of all four layers and is primarily seen in the skin. Fully keratinized cells form keratin and lose their nuclei by the time they migrate to the outer surface. Findings show that 76% of the gingival exhibit parakeratin cells which retain their nuclei but show some signs of being keratinized. The stratum granulosum is usually difficult to recognize and a surface parakeratinized outer layer is present. Epithelial cells found in the junctional epithelium and alveolar mucosas are nonkeratinized and do not undergo keratinization.

Oral Epithelium

The **oral epithelium** faces the oral cavity on the outer surface of the free and attached gingivae extending from

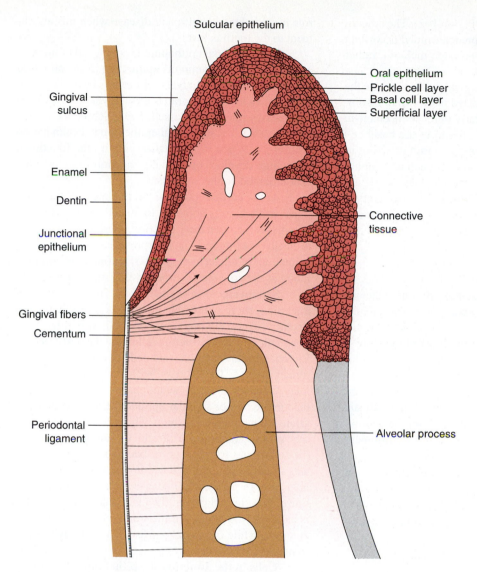

■ **FIGURE 1–7** Diagram of the layers of the gingival epithelium. Underlying the epithelium is the gingival connective tissue (lamina propria).

the free gingival margin to the mucogingival junction. The gingiva is usually composed of parakeratinized stratified squamous epithelium.

The gingiva has an epithelial turnover time of approximately ten days as demonstrated in an animal model (Schroeder & Listgarten, 1997), while in the skin it is approximately 28 days.

Cells in the Oral Epithelium   The function of the oral epithelium is to protect the underlying structures and act as a mechanical barrier. The oral epithelium contains the following types of cells:

• Keratinocytes
• Nonkeratinocytes (also called clear cells)

• Melanocytes
• Langerhans cells
• Merkel cells
• Inflammatory cells (e.g., neutrophils)

Keratinocytes make up the majority of oral epithelial cells. Keratinocytes function to synthesize keratin, which contributes to the mechanical toughness of the outer surface of the oral epithelium and relative impermeability to fluids and cells. It is also responsible for the salmon pink color of the gingiva.

Melanocytes located in the basal cell layer secrete melanin, which is responsible for the brownish pigmentation in the gingiva. Pigmentation is more prominent in darker-skinned individuals (see Figure 1–3). The amount of pigmentation is genetically predetermined according to the potential of the cells to produce melanin, rather than to the number of cells present.

Other cell types in the gingival epithelium are the Langerhans cells, which are located in the stratum spinosum and are involved in the early defense mechanism of the gingiva. Merkel cells are found in the basal cell layer and are associated with nerve endings acting as touch-sensory cells. White blood cells such as lymphocytes and neutrophils or polymorphonuclear leukocytes (PMNs) are transiently found in the epithelial layers in health but increase in numbers in periodontal disease, functioning to defend the body against bacteria and other invaders.

Sulcular Epithelium

The **sulcular epithelum** is structurally similar to the oral epithelium except that it is less keratinized. The sulcular epithelium exhibits good resistance to mechanical forces and is relatively impermeable (resistant) to the flow of fluids and cells. The sulcular epithelium has epithelial ridges, or rete pegs, as does the oral epithelium but to a lesser extent. Sulcular or crevicular epithelium lines the gingival sulcus without being attached to the tooth surface. It is generally nonkeratinized and thin but can become parakeratinized if exposed to the oral environment. The sulcular epithelium exhibits two or three cell layers but a definitive and continuous cornified layer is absent. At the free gingival margin, the sulcular epithelium is continuous with the oral epithelium. Apically, it overlaps the coronal surface of the junctional epithelium (see Figure 1–7).

Junctional Epithelium

The **junctional epithelium** is a band of epithelial cells that surrounds the tooth and creates a "seal" at the gingival crevice to hold it firmly in place. It is continuous with the free gingiva and provides the contact between the gingiva and the tooth. The junctional epithelium can be regarded as a downgrowth of the squamous epithelium of the gingiva and is continuous with the sulcular epithelium, extending from the bottom of the crevice to the cementoenamel junction in health and in gingivitis; there is no loss of attachment. It forms a collar around the neck of the tooth on the cervical part of the enamel.

The junctional epithelium, through the epithelial attachment, contributes to the direct attachment of the gingiva to the tooth surface and thus serves a significant role in periodontal health and disease when this attachment to the tooth is lost.

The junctional epithelium is composed of nonkeratinized stratified squamous epithelium. It is composed of only two epithelial layers, either an active basal cell layer and an inactive suprabasal cell layer or a basal cell and spinous cell layer (Hassell, 1993; Schroeder & Listgarten, 1997). The junctional epithelium in health has no rete ridges. When inflammation sets in, the junctional epithelium develops epithelial projections into the adjacent inflamed connective tissue.

At the coronal portion, the thickness of the junctional epithelium is about 15 to 30 cells, while apically, near the cementoenamel junction, there may be only 1 to 2 cells (see Figure 1–7). Interproximally, the junctional epithelium of adjacent teeth fuses coronally to form the lining of the col area (Schroeder & Listgarten, 1997).

Semipermeable Membrane   The junctional epithelium is more permeable than the oral or sulcular epithelium. Thus, the junctional epithelium is referred to as a semipermeable structure, allowing the movement of bacterial products, fluids, and cells of certain sizes (Kornman, Page, & Tonetti, 1997). There are fewer intercellular junctions and thus wider spaces between the cells than in the oral or sulcular epithelium, and the cells are arranged in a parallel fashion. This allows for easy passage of cells and tissue fluid from the lamina propria into the sulcus and for passage of bacteria and its by-products from the gingival sulcus into the lamina propria. It is also more permeable because the cells do not keratinize. The coronal part of the junctional epithelium that is closest to the bottom of the sulcus is the most permeable part, while the apical part is where cell division for tissue renewal occurs.

Cells in the Junctional Epithelium   In addition to keratinocytes, the junctional epithelium may contain clear cells. In health, small numbers of PMNs are transiently seen in the junctional epithelium (Tonetti, Imboden, Gerber, & Lang, 1995). They will usually pass through the junctional epithelium into the gingival sulcus,

---

Did You Know?

The junctional epithelium is only three to four layers thick in early life but its thickness increases with age. The length of junctional epithelium is only about 0.25 to 1.35 mm. Just think about this — only about 1 mm long!

where they play a role in the defense of the host (body) against bacteria and other microorganisms.

Cellular Turnover   A unique characteristic of the junctional epithelium is its high rate of cellular turnover. As demonstrated in an animal model, the cells of the junctional epithelium undergo constant turnover every four to seven days, whereby the basal cells migrate coronally out through the sulcus where the old cells are shed into the oral cavity.

Alveolar Mucosa

The alveolar mucosa is compressible and movable due to the presence of a submucosa between the thin lamina propria and the underlying tissue, usually muscle. The presence of elastic fibers, and an underlying loose connective tissue that is attached to the underlying periosteum of the alveolar process, also allows for movement.

The epithelium of the alveolar mucosa has about the same thickness as that of the gingiva, but its structure is completely different (Schroeder, 1991; Schroeder & Listgarten, 1997). A granular layer is not present and the superficial layer does not histologically stain, as does the surface of parakeratinized epithelium (Squier & Hill, 1998). The epithelium contains melanocytes, Langerhans cells, Merkel cells, and small lymphocytes.

Epithelial ridges are usually not present; if present, they are indistinct because they are shorter and wider than in the gingiva, giving a smoother surface texture. The color is darker red than the gingiva because of its highly vascular underlying connective tissue. The point where there is a marked increase in elastic fibers within the underlying connective tissue demarcates the mucogingival junction.

Gingival Connective Tissue

Underlying the stratified squamous epithelium and encircling the tooth is the gingival connective tissue or lamina propria (Nanci & Bosshardt, 2006)

Connective Tissue/Epithelium Interface

The interface between the connective tissue and oral epithelium is through connecting epithelial ridges that extend into the connective tissue (Figure 1–8 ■). At the intersection of epithelial ridges are pits or depressions that contain connective tissue extensions called connective tissue papillae. Clinically, these depressions may be evident on the surface of the gingiva, creating a stippled appearance. Stippling is established at the areas of fusion between adjacent epithelial ridges. In periodontal health the epithelial ridges are absent from the junctional epithelium and are not well developed in the sulcular epithelium. The main purposes of stippling are to aid in the increased strength between the epithelium and connective tissue and to enable the epithelium to obtain its blood supply from the connective tissue papillae in the shortest distance possible (Nanci & Bosshardt, 2006).

Gingival Connective Tissue

The main component of the gingival connective tissue, as with all connective tissue, is collagen fibers, accounting for about 60% of the total volume. Collagen is a protein composed of amino acids. There are many different types of collagen, with Types I (95%) and III (5%) found in gingival connective tissues. Type I collagen fibers give the gingiva its firmness and resiliency. The lamina pro-

Connective tissue papillae

Connective tissue

Oral epithelium

Epithelial ridges

■ **FIGURE 1–8**   A photomicrograph of the gingival oral epithelium/connective tissue interface. Note prominent epithelial ridges. Intersections between the epithelial ridges under the epithelial surface correspond to depressions seen on the surface of the gingiva. Fingerlike projections termed connective tissue papillae extend into the depressions on the undersurface of the epithelium. This produces the characteristic stippled appearance of the attached gingiva. (Courtesy of Dr. Harvey Wishe, New York University College of Dentistry) pria provides mechanical support and nutrients for the avascular epithelium. The remainder of gingival connective tissue consists of ground substance, which is composed of proteins termed proteoglycans, in which the collagen fibers, cells (5%), nerves, and blood vessels (65%) are embedded. Proteoglycans have a protein core with carbohydrate side chains (glycosaminoglycans) of chondroitin sulphate, heparin sulphate, and hyaluronic acid. The ground substance also allows for the transportation of water and nutrients through the tissue.

Gingival Fibers   The free and attached gingivae are attached to the tooth surface through a **connective tissue attachment**. Collagen fibers in the gingiva are arranged in such a way that they maintain the gingiva against the tooth and bone. The collagen fibers are organized in bundles or groups according to their origin and insertion (Schroeder & Listgarten, 1997). The collagen fibers embedded on one end in the cementum are termed Sharpey's fibers (Goldman, 1951). Collectively, the gingival fiber bundles are called the gingival fibers, the supracrestal fiber apparatus (because they are located coronal to the crest of alveolar bone), or the gingival connective tissue attachment. These three terms will be used interchangeably throughout the text. Table 1–1 ■ reviews the primary collagen fiber groups in the gingiva (Figure 1–9 ■), including the circular, dentogingival, dentoperiosteal, alveologingival, and transseptal fibers. Secondary gingival fiber groups include periostogingival, interpapillary, transgingival, intercrevicular, semicircular, and intergingival fibers. Their function is to support and give contour to the free and attached gingivae and firmly connect the attached gingiva to the underlying cementum and alveolar bone. The free gingiva is not actually free nor is it attached to the tooth, but rather it is held in close proximity to the tooth by the gingival fibers, which prevent the free gingiva from being deflected from the tooth during mastication.

Collagen Organization

Collagen fibers are either densely or loosely organized. Dense connective tissue that is found in the lamina propria of the gingiva consists of heavy, tightly packed fibers that function to resist tension. Loose connective tissue, as exemplified by alveolar mucosa, is composed of the collagen fibers that are thin and delicate and do not have a mechanical protective function. Collagen is constantly being synthesized and degraded as part of the normal remodeling or turnover of gingival connective tissue.

Table 1–1	Classification of the Gingival Fibers	
Name of Fiber	*Origin and Distribution*	*Function*
Circular	Encircles the tooth within the free gingiva	Provides support and contour to the free gingiva
Dentogingival	From the cementum at the base of the gingival sulcus, flares coronally into the free gingiva (group A), laterally into the attached gingiva (group B), and apically into the periosteum (group C); found on the facial, lingual, and interproximal surfaces	Contributes to the support of the gingiva
Dentoperiosteal	Extends from the cementum apically over the alveolar crest into the periosteum	Anchors the tooth to the bone
Alveologingival	Extends from the periosteum of the alveolar crestal bone coronally into the connective tissue	Attaches the gingiva to the alveolar bone
Transseptal	Runs from the cementum of one tooth interproximal to the cementum of the adjacent tooth	Keeps teeth in alignment and protects the interproximal bone from the inflammatory infiltrate; resistant to inflammation and will continuously reform when bone and fibers are destroyed

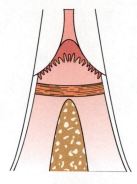

(a) Circular fibers

(b) Dentogingival fibers

(c) Transseptal fibers

■ **FIGURE 1–9**   The major component of the connective tissue of the free and attached gingivae are composed of collagen fibers that are arranged in groups or bundles. The name indicates the origin and insertion of the fibers: circular fibers, dentogingival fibers, dentoperiosteal fibers, and transseptal fibers.

Cellular and Vascular Elements

The cellular part of the lamina propria predominately consists of the following:

- Fibroblasts
- Macrophages
- Mast cells
- Plasma cells, lymphocytes, and neutrophils

Fibroblasts synthesize ground substance, collagen, and collagenase. Collagenase is an enzyme responsible for the breakdown of collagen during remodeling. Thus, fibroblasts play a chief role in the maintenance and remodeling of connective tissue. Other cells in the lamina propria include red blood cells, PMNs, macrophages, lymphocytes, and mast cells, which are involved in the defense of the host against toxins.

A rich vascular complex is found in the lamina propria. Since there is no submucosa, as is found in the alveolar mucosa, the blood supply passes directly to the lamina propria.

Cell-to-Cell Tissue Junction

Epithelial Cell-to-Cell Attachment

Electron microscopy has demonstrated that epithelial cells are held together by intercellular bridges or desmosomes. A desmosome consists of two adjacent attachment plaques, which are continuous with the innermost leaflet of the cell membrane (Figure 1–10 ■). A space exists between adjacent desmosomes, allowing passage of material and fluid through the tissue while holding together epithelial cells. Junctional epithelium has four times fewer desmosomes than oral epithelium, so the intercellular spaces are wider.

Epithelium-Tooth Surface/Connective Tissue Interface

The junctional epithelium adheres to the tooth surface (e.g., enamel) through the epithelial attachment. The basal cells of the junctional epithelium do not contact the enamel or the connective tissue directly. Instead, between the junctional epithelium and the tooth and connective tissue is a basal lamina and hemidesmosomes (Stern, 1965; see also Figure 1–10). The basal lamina and the hemidesmosomes are referred to as the epithelial attachment, and it provides the attachment of the junctional epithelium to the tooth surface as seen under the electron microscope. The epithelial attachment is not synonymous with junctional epithelium, which refers to the entire epithelium. The basal lamina has an outer electron-lucent (lighter) zone called the lamina lucida and an inner electron-dense (darker) zone called the lamina densa. The basal lamina is continuous around the base of the junctional epithelium. These structures lie in a sandwich-like arrangement, one on top of each other.

A hemidesmosome consists of one attachment plaque continuous with the cell membrane and attaches the epithelial (basal) cell to the basal lamina. This in turn attaches to the enamel on one side and the underlying connective tissue on the other side (see Figure 1–10). Connective tissue fibers called anchoring fibrils attach the lamina densa to the underlying connective tissue. This same structural relationship also exists between the oral and sulcular epithelium, where a basal lamina separates the epithelium from the connective tissue.

Dentogingival Unit

The **dentogingival unit** collectively refers to the epithelial attachment and the gingival connective tissue attach-

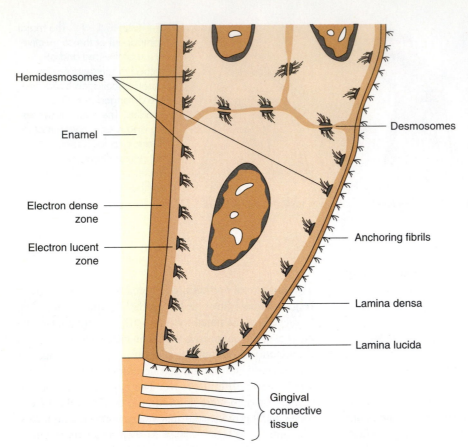

Hemidesmosomes

Enamel

Electron dense zone

Electron lucent zone

Desmosomes

Anchoring fibrils

Lamina densa

Lamina lucida

Gingival connective tissue

■ **FIGURE 1–10** Schematic illustration showing the attachment of the junctional epithelium to the tooth surface and the underlying connective tissue and enamel. The electron-dense zone is a continuation of the lamina densa; the electron-lucent zone is a continuation of the lamina lucida; anchoring fibrils radiate out into the lamina propria. The cell membrane of the epithelial cells harbor hemidesmosomes toward the enamel and the connective tissue. Adjacent epithelial cell membranes also harbor desmosomes, which hold epithelial cells together. (Copyright © 2003 by J. Lindhe and T. Karring. Anatomy of the periodontium, in *Clinical periodontology and implant dentistry,* ed. J. Lindhe, Copenhagen: Munksgaard.)

ment (gingival fibers) to the cementum, both of which are involved in the stabilization of the gingiva to the tooth. Of the two types of attachment, the gingival connective tissue (gingival fibers) forms a firmer one, supporting the epithelium and probably inhibiting movement of the epithelium apically (Bartold & Narayana, 2006)

The combined length of the dentogingival unit has been described in the literature as the **biologic width** (Figure 1–11 ■). A study using human cadaver models determined that the components of the biologic width included the junctional epithelium with a mean length of 0.97 mm and gingival connective tissue attachment with a mean length of 1.07 mm (Gargiulo, Wentz, & Orban, 1961). This soft-tissue dimension is essential to maintain gingival health. Biologic width or the length (coronalapical dimension) of the soft tissue attachments becomes important during periodontal-prosthetic (restorative) treatment. The margin of a restoration should not disturb the biologic width. Thus, the margin of a restoration should not be closer than 2 mm to the alveolar bone crest.

Formation of the Dentogingival Unit

The formation of the dentogingival unit has important clinical implications during the periodontal evaluation and in the healing of the gingiva after periodontal treatment. After completion of the enamel, the ameloblasts produce the primary enamel cuticle as their last function before they degenerate and become part of the reduced enamel epithelium. At the time of tooth eruption, the enamel is still covered with reduced enamel epithelium, which is connected to the enamel by the primary enamel cuticle. As tooth eruption occurs, the reduced enamel ep-

Rapid Dental Hint

Biologic width is important when evaluating a tooth for a crown. There must be an adequate amount of biologic width (soft tissue attachment) for periodontal health. Look at the radiograph to determine the amount of space between the CEJ and the crest of bone.

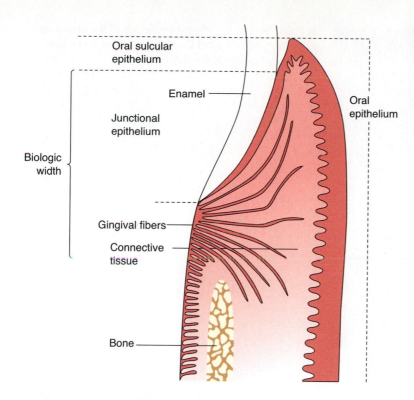

■ FIGURE 1–11 Schematic illustration of the biologic width includes the length of the junctional epithelium (0.97 mm) and the gingival connective tissue attachment (1.07 mm). (Copyright © 2003 by J. Lindhe and T. Karring. Anatomy of the periodontium, in *Clinical periodontology and implant dentistry*, ed. J. Lindhe, Copenhagen: Munksgaard.)

ithelium fuses with the oral epithelium at the base of the sulcus, forming the junctional epithelium. The reduced enamel epithelium forms the lining of the gingival sulcus. The junctional epithelium produces another cuticle between itself and the enamel called the secondary cuticle, which holds the junctional epithelium in close proximity to the tooth. While the tooth erupts into occlusion, the junctional epithelium gradually moves apically down the crown exposing it. Several stages occur during this passive eruption process. Eventually, the junctional epithelium ends at the cementoenamel junction. With gingival

inflammation, the junctional epithelium also migrates onto the cementum, while the *base of the sulcus remains located on the enamel,* at the cementoenamel junction or on the root surface. In other words, the base of the epithelial attachment of the gingiva is at the cementoenamel junction in health and gingivitis. This situation changes in periodontitis, where the junctional epithelium migrates apically along the root surface. This concept of attachment level is important when performing periodontal probing and monitoring periodontal disease progression.

ATTACHMENT APPARATUS

The periodontal ligament, cementum, and alveolar and supporting bone constitute the attachment apparatus (Figure 1–12 ■). The function of these tissues is to support and anchor the teeth within the alveolar process (Hassell, 1993).

Periodontal Ligament

The connective tissue that extends from the cementum covering the root surface to the alveolar bone is termed the periodontal ligament. This connective tissue is continuous with the gingival connective tissue. The periodontal ligament is primarily composed of collagen fibers and islands

RDH **Rapid Dental Hint**

Attachment level refers to the level of attachment of the junctional epithelium to the tooth surface. When probing, this attachment level is what is actually being measured. In periodontal disease, this attachment of the junctional epithelium is "lost" or moves laterally away from the tooth and apically onto the root surface (the term for this is "attachment loss"), thus creating a periodontal pocket where the probing depth will be deeper.

Dentin
Cementicles
Cementum
Periodontal ligament
Alveolar process
Marrow spaces

■ **FIGURE 1–12** Photomicrograph of the attachment apparatus. (Courtesy of Dr. Harvey Wishe, New York University College of Dentistry)

of loose connective tissue, creating interstitial spaces where blood vessels, nerves, lymphatics, and cells are embedded in a ground substance (Beertsen, McCulloch, & Sodek, 1997). The primary cell of the periodontal ligament is the fibroblast, which synthesizes collagen, collagenase, and ground substance. On one side of the periodontal ligament is the alveolar bone, where osteoblasts reside and are involved in bone formation. The other side of the periodontal ligament is the cementum, where cementoblasts reside and are involved in the formation of cementum.

Connective Tissue Attachment: Periodontal Ligament

The primary component of the periodontal ligament is collagen fibers. The fibers are arranged in groups or bundles that blend into one another and are collectively called the principal fibers (see Figure 1–13 ■). This constitutes the second type of connective tissue. The principal fibers are a continuation of the gingival fibers or gingival connective tissue attachment (the other type of connective tissue attachment) in the gingiva and are also named according to their direction of insertion and location. Table 1–2 ■ reviews the principal fiber groups (Hassell, 1993). The ends of the fibers, which are embedded into alveolar bone and cementum, are termed Sharpey's fibers. The first principal fibers formed before the tooth erupts are the alveolar crest fibers. With definitive tooth-to-tooth contact, the oblique fibers mature.

Eventually, with the formation of the apical fibers, the periodontal ligament is established. Since the periodontal ligament contains few elastic fibers, it is the wavy configuration of the principal fibers that permits slight movement of the tooth under function (tooth-to-tooth

Principal Fiber Groups

Apical
Oblique
Horizontal
Interradicular
Alveolar crest

■ **FIGURE 1–13** Schematic diagram showing the location of the periodontal ligament between the alveolar bone proper and the root cementum. The tooth is joined to the bone by bundles of collagen fibers, which can be divided into the following main groups: alveolar crest fibers, horizontal fibers, oblique fibers, interradicular fibers, and apical fibers.

Table 1–2	Classification of the Principal Fiber Groups of the Periodontal Ligament		
Name of Fiber Bundle	*Direction*	*Function*	*Features*
Alveolar crest	Originates from the cementum and runs apically to insert into the alveolar crest	Resists lateral movement of the tooth and keeps tooth in its socket	The first fibers to be formed before tooth eruption has occurred
Horizontal	Originates from cementum and runs at right angles and inserts into bone	Opposes lateral forces	The second fibers to be formed as soon as the first tooth-to-tooth contact has occurred
Oblique	Found in the middle third of the root apical to the horizontal fibers; originates from cementum and runs coronally and diagonally into bone	Absorbs occlusal forces	The most abundant and thus the principal attachment of the tooth
Apical	Originates from cementum of the apex of the root, spreading out apically and laterally into bone	Resists tipping of the tooth	One of the last fibers to form
Interradicular	From the crest of the interradicular septum extending to the cementum in the furcation area	Resists the forces of luxation (pulling out) and tipping	Lost when bone is destroyed in the furcation area in disease

contact). Collagen turnover time is five times faster in the periodontal ligament than in bone or gingiva because of the greater functional demands placed upon it. Besides containing collagen, different types of cells are also present in the periodontal ligament including fibroblasts (make collagen), fibroclasts (resorption collagen), cementoblasts (make cementum), cementoclasts (cementum resorption) osteoblasts (make bone) and osteoclasts (resorb bone).

Periodontal Ligament Space

Although the width of the periodontal ligament varies from tooth to tooth and from different areas on the same tooth, the average width is approximately 0.25 mm. Seen radiographically, a tooth that has heavy occlusal loads placed upon it for long periods of time will have a thicker periodontal ligament space. A tooth that is not in function, such as a tooth without an antagonist, will have a narrower periodontal ligament space.

Functions of the Periodontal Ligament

The periodontal ligament functions include the following:

- Suspensory: Acts like a suspensory mechanism attaching the tooth to the alveolar bone.

- Shock absorption: Acts as a shock absorber transmitting occlusal forces to the alveolar bone. Axial-placed forces, which are parallel to the long axis of the tooth, are more easily absorbed than lateral or rotational forces.
- Remodeling: Serves a remodeling function by providing cells that are involved in the formation and resorption of cementum and bone and itself.
- Formative: Carries a blood supply to the rest of the periodontium for nutrition.
- Sensory: Transmits tactile pressure and pain perception via the trigeminal nerve.
- Proprioceptive: Allows the feeling of localization of pain and pressure to be transmitted through proprioceptive nerve endings (e.g., trigeminal nerve) found in the periodontal ligament. For example, when biting into a hard object, the mouth quickly opens. This quick reflex sensation is a function of the periodontal ligament. The greatest amount of sensory receptors is found in the apical area.

Abnormalities

Histologically, besides collagen fibers, clusters of epithelial cells are found within the periodontal ligament. These clusters are called epithelial rests of Malassez. Epithelial rests of Malassez are considered to be remains of epithelium of Hertwig's epithelial root sheath, which plays an important role in the development of the cementum and the shape of the roots. Their presence and function are controversial, but they may play a role in the formation of dental cysts.

Cementicles are calcified bodies of cementum seen in the periodontal ligament of older adults (see Figure 1–12). Either they are attached to the cementum, embedded within the cementum, or not associated with the root. It is unknown if cementicles present any clinical significance.

Cementum

The cementum is a layer of mineralized tissue covering the root of the tooth and is composed of collagen, ground substance, cells, and calcium and phosphate in the form of hydroxyapatite. The primary function of the cementum is to attach the principal fibers to the root surface.

The cementum is a product of the periodontal ligament and forms in layers or increments. As a layer of uncalcified cementoid forms, adjacent cementoblasts found in the periodontal ligament stop producing. When the layer of cementoid becomes 80 to 90% calcified, more cementoid is laid down. Therefore, the cementum is never fully calcified. Cementoid serves a protective function, resisting resorption. Sharpey's fibers are embedded into cementoid allowing for repositioning of the tooth in response to biting forces.

The surface of the cementum is soft and relatively permeable, allowing bacterial by-products and toxins to easily penetrate the cemental surface. However, it is now

recognized that the toxins are actually not as deeply penetrated into the root surface as was once thought (Nakib, Bissada, Simmelink, & Goldstine, 1982). The cementum is avascular and does not contain lymph vessels or nerves.

Relationship of Cementum and Enamel

The relationship of the cementum to the enamel margin varies (Figure 1–14 ■). In 60 to 65% of the population, the cementum overlaps the enamel. In 30% of the population, the cementum meets exactly with the enamel in an edge-to-edge relationship, and in 5 to 10% of the population, the cementum and enamel do not meet and the dentin is exposed, leaving an area of possible sensitivity.

Types of Cementum

Two kinds of cementum are identified under the light microscope. Acellular cementum, which is formed before tooth eruption, is found on the coronal two-thirds of the root and is approximately 0.1 mm in thickness, with the cementoenamel junction being the thinnest area. Since acellular cementum does not contain cementocytes, it is not involved in the laying down of new cementum. Cellular cementum, which covers the apical third of the root and furcations, has a thickness of about 0.5 mm and is formed much faster than acellular cementum. Cellular cementum can be laid down on top of acellular cementum, or it can comprise the entire thickness of the cementum.

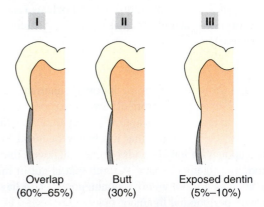

I   II   III

Overlap (60%–65%)   Butt (30%)   Exposed dentin (5%–10%)

■ **FIGURE 1–14**   Schematic illustration of the relationships of the cementum to the enamel at the cementoenamel junction. (Adapted from P. F. Fedi, Jr., and A. R. Vernino, *The Periodontic Syllabus.* Copyright © 2000 by Lippincott Williams & Wilkins.)

Physiologic Features

As teeth wear down (attrition) on either the occlusal surface or incisal edge, there is a compensatory deposition of cellular cementum in the apical area in addition to deposition of bone at the alveolar crest and in the socket. This acts to maintain the vertical dimension of the face and maintain the length of the root. Instead of remodeling (resorption and deposition) like bone, cementum is deposited continuously. Cementum thickens with increasing age, but the production of cementum slows.

Cementum does not resorb as readily as bone due to its avascularity and protective layer of cementoid. This property makes orthodontic movement possible without normally resorbing the roots. However, cementum can be resorbed under certain circumstances such as inappropriate orthodontic movement, cysts, tumors, trauma, replanted teeth, periapical disease, and periodontal disease or for no known reason. Therefore, instead of resorption followed by deposition, a new layer of cementum is formed on the most superficial or oldest layer.

Abnormalities

Hypercementosis is a condition characterized by an atypical thickening of the cementum. It may be localized to one tooth due to factors such as excessive and rapid orthodontic movement, or it may result from excessive occlusal force placed on a tooth.

Alveolar Process

The alveolar process constitutes that part of the maxilla and mandible that forms and supports the sockets or alveoli of the teeth. Periosteum is connective tissue that covers the outer surface of the alveolar process and is well supplied with blood vessels and nerves, some of which enter the bone. Endosteum covers the inner surface of the alveolar process facing the tooth surface.

Parts of the Alveolar Process

There are two parts to the alveolar process: the alveolar bone proper and the supporting bone. It is important to distinguish between the alveolar process and the alveolar bone proper. The alveolar bone proper or cribriform plate is hard compact bone that lines the tooth socket, which is contained within the alveolar process (Figure 1–15 ■). Radiographically, it is referred to as the lamina dura (Figure 1–16 ■). The bone where Sharpey's fibers terminate is called bundle bone and is found at the inner sur-

■ **FIGURE 1–15** A section through the mandible after removal of all teeth. The thin bone lining the tooth socket (cribriform plate or alveolar bone proper) is clearly seen. (Reprinted with permission from A. Schroeder, F. Sutter, D. Buser, and G. Krekeler, *Oral implantology.* Copyright © 1996 by Thieme Medical Publishers, Inc., New York.)

■ **FIGURE 1–16** Radiographic appearance of the lamina dura. The lamina dura is a radiopaque (white) line around the roots of the teeth and the alveolar crest.

face of the tooth socket. The cribriform plate is perforated by numerous openings that carry blood, nerves, and lymphatics from the bone to the periodontal ligament.

The supporting bone is composed of two parts: compact bone and cancellous bone (also called spongy or trabecular bone). Compact bone, which covers the alveolar process, consists of buccal (outer) and lingual (inner) cortical plates that are continuous with the cribriform plate (Figure 1–17a ■). The buccal and lingual cortical plates vary in thickness. Generally, the cortical plate is thicker in the mandible than in the maxilla. In the maxilla, the compact bone is thicker on the palatal than on the buccal surfaces. In the mandible, the bone is thicker in the buccal area of the premolar and molar areas and thinnest in the incisor area.

Cancellous bone fills the area between the buccal and lingual cortical plates and between the alveolar bone proper of adjacent teeth. There may be little or no cancellous bone when there is close root proximity of adjacent teeth. In these cases, the interdental septum is thin and the alveolar bone proper is fused with the cortical plate of bone.

Morphology

The cortical plate of bone covering the roots of the teeth is called radicular bone. Interradicular bone is found between roots of the same teeth (e.g., bi- and trifurcation areas of multirooted teeth). The interdental septum or interproximal bone consists of the cribriform plate of two adjacent teeth and some cancellous bone (Figure 1–17b,c). The alveolar bone crest is the most coronal part of the alveolar bone. It is where the outer cortical plate is continuous with and fuses with the cribriform plate. At this area cancellous bone is absent.

(a)

(b)

Cancellous bone

Interdental bone

Alveolar bone crest

(c)

Alveolar bone crest
Interdental bone

Cancellous bone

■ **FIGURE 1–17**   (a) Dry skull specimen showing the outer cortical plates of bone covering the roots of the teeth. (b) Dry skull of the maxilla. The cortical plates of bone are removed. (c) Dry skull of the mandible. The cortical plates of bone are removed. (Reprinted with permission from A. Schroeder, F. Sutter, D. Buser, and G. Krekeler, *Oral Implantology.* Copyright © 1996 by Thieme Medical Publishers, Inc., New York.)

Alveolar Bone Crest   The shape of the alveolar bone crest is influenced by the width of the interdental space, stage of eruption, position of the teeth in the arch, and shape of the cementoenamel junction. By following the contour of the cementoenamel junction, the alveolar bone crest is relatively flat in the posterior and more convex and pointed in the anterior. In health, the shape of bone takes on a form where the alveolar bone crest is more coronal than the radicular bone. The slope of the alveolar bone crest follows an imaginary parallel line connecting the cementoenamel junction of adjacent teeth (Ritchey & Orban, 1953) and is approximately 2 mm apical to it if the biologic width is taken into consideration (Figure 1–18 ■), but this relationship may vary.

Composition of Bone

The alveolar process is primarily composed of collagen fibers and cells embedded in a ground substance (proteoglycans), which make up the organic component. The inorganic salts of bone are principally calcium and phosphate. The salts allow bone to withstand compression. The combination of fibers and salts makes bone exceptionally strong without being brittle. The cells present in the alveolar and supporting bone are the following:

- Osteoblasts, which synthesize and secrete bone.
- Osteocytes, which are osteoblasts that are embedded within lacunae as bone is being laid down.
- Osteoclasts, which destroy or resorb bone.

Metabolism

Despite its rigid physical characteristic, bone is a vascular tissue and the least stable of all the periodontal tissues. There is a constant remodeling with formation and resorption of bone due to the functional demand placed upon it. This occurs more rapidly in cancellous than compact bone. The normal remodeling of bone occurs by resorption by osteoclasts followed by deposition by osteoblasts. During orthodontic movement, bone is resorbed on the pressure side and laid down on the tension side.

Variations in Anatomy

Roots of teeth are usually contained entirely within the alveolar bony plates. Frequently, the bone may not completely encircle prominent roots of teeth that are rotated, in facioversion, in lingoversion, tipped, or crowded. The resulting defects take the form of windows (fenestrations) where the radicular cortical bone is lost except for the most coronal edge or clefts (dehiscences) where the cortical bone, including the marginal bone (most coronal edge of bone), is lost over the root (Figure 1–19 ■). The etiology of these defects is not definitive. These defects occur more frequently on facial bone than on lingual bone.

Buttressing bone occurs at the margin of bone where it thickens in response to increased functional demands. This is a response to the repair process, with bone resorption and deposition occurring.

PHYSIOLOGY OF THE PERIODONTIUM

The blood to the gingiva is primarily supplied by the vessels of the periosteum (supraperiosteal), periodontal ligament, and alveolar bone (Figure 1–20 ■). The supraperiosteal vessels run along the facial and lingual surfaces of the alveolar bone and give off many little branches as they make their way toward the gingiva. These finally join with blood vessels of the alveolar bone and periodontal ligament to form a gingival plexus located just under the oral epithelium in the laminia propria. Remember that the epithelium contains no blood vessels.

Cementoenamel junction

Alveolar crest

Cementoenamel junction

Alveolar crest

■ **FIGURE 1–18**   The alveolar crest is parallel to a line connecting the cementoenamel junctions of adjacent teeth, even when a tooth is tilted and the cementoenamel junction on one tooth may be lower than the adjacent tooth.

Fenestration

Dehiscence

■ **FIGURE 1–19**   Dry skull specimen of a dehiscence showing loss of radicular cortical bone involving the marginal bone and a fenestration with loss of radicular bone but not involving the marginal bone.

The inferior and superior alveolar arteries supplying the periodontal ligament originate from the apical foramen, the alveolar bone, and the gingiva.

The blood supply to the cortical bone is via branches of the supraperiosteal blood vessels. The vessels that enter the interdental septum, in addition to the vessels that supply the remainder of the alveolar bone, supply blood to the cancellous bone.

Lymphatic drainage from the gingiva starts in the papillae of the connective tissue and drains into the regional lymph nodes, primarily the submandibular nodes. The lymphatic vessels follow the course of the blood vessels.

The nerves supplying the periodontium branch off from the trigeminal nerve (fifth cranial nerve). The nerves follow the course of the blood vessels that supply blood to the periodontium. Gingival branches of the anterior superior alveolar nerve innervate the gingiva overlying the maxillary incisors and canines. The gingival branches of the middle superior alveolar nerve supply the gingiva around the maxillary premolars. The posterior superior alveolar nerve supplies the gingiva around the maxillary molars.

The gingival branches of the inferior alveolar nerve supply the facial gingiva of the mandibular incisors, canines, premolars, and molars. The mental nerve supplies the mandibular facial gingiva of the incisors, canines, and premolars. The gingival branches of the buccal nerve supply the facial gingiva of the mandibular molars. The lingual nerve supplies the mandibular lingual gingiva.

Changes with Aging

With increasing age, certain changes in the hard- and soft-tissue components of the periodontium occur, as well as a thinning of the gingiva with reduced keratinization. The amount of stippling is either reduced or unchanged. Within the lamina propria, there is a decrease in the number of cells and the gingival fibers become less dense. Cementum increases in thickness throughout life, with a greater deposition in the apical area in response to the continuing tooth eruption that compensates for tooth attrition. Cells within the periodontal ligament decrease in number, while the number of elastic fibers increases. The width of the periodontal ligament can be either increased or decreased. Changes in the alveolar bone occur with aging just as in any other bone in the body. There may be a decrease in vascularity and healing. A physiologic tendency with increasing age is for the proximal surface contacts of teeth to wear down (attrition), causing the teeth to migrate in a mesial direction (mesial drifting) while retaining tooth-to-tooth contact. Accordingly, bone

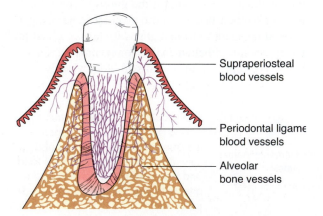

Supraperiosteal blood vessels

Periodontal ligament blood vessels

Alveolar bone vessels

■ **FIGURE 1–20**   The blood supply to the periodontium comes from three sources: (1) supraperiosteal blood vessels, (2) blood vessels from the periodontal ligament, and (3) blood vessels of the alveolar process.

is laid down on the distal surface, which is the tension side, and bone is resorbed on the mesial surface, which is the pressure side.

DENTAL HYGIENE NOTES

This chapter reviewed the structure and functions of the periodontal soft and hard tissues including the gingiva, periodontal ligament, cementum, and supporting and alveolar bone. The periodontium is a dynamic, highly specialized structure that is constantly changing with the demands placed upon it. Knowing the macro- and microstructure of the periodontium in health will help to understand the process that leads to pathological destruction.

KEY POINTS

- The attachment of the soft and hard tissues to the tooth surface contributes to the stability and health of the periodontium.
- The junctional epithelium is a semipermeable structure involved in the movement of fluids, cells, and substances from the lamina propria into the gingival crevice and vice versa.
- The dentogingival unit is involved in the attachment of the gingiva to the tooth.
- The biologic width comprises the length of the junctional epithelium and the gingival fibers.
- The biologic width is important during prosthetic treatment. There must be an adequate amount of bone from the finish line of the crown to the crest of the bone in order not to invade the biologic width. If the biologic width is not adequate, inflammation may occur.

SELF-QUIZ

1. Which of the following structures comprise the attachment apparatus? (p. 15)
   a. gingiva, cementum, alveolar and supporting bone, periodontal ligament
   b. gingiva, cementum, periodontal ligament
   c. cementum, alveolar and supporting bone, periodontal ligament
   d. cementum, alveolar and supporting bone

2. At which one of the following areas is the width of attached gingiva greatest? (p. 5)
   a. mandibular second premolars
   b. mandibular canines
   c. maxillary lateral incisors
   d. maxillary first premolars
   e. maxillary second molars

3. Which one of the following substances is the primary component of the connective tissue of the periodontium? (pp. 11–13)
   a. gingival crevicular fluid
   b. calcium
   c. collagen
   d. proteoglycans

4. Which one of the following structures directly attaches the junctional epithelium to the enamel? (pp. 13–14)
   a. desmosomes
   b. hemidesmosomes
   c. basal lamina
   d. gingival fibers

5. Which one of the following structures is involved in the attachment of the gingiva to the tooth surface? (pp. 13–14)
   a. alveolar mucosa
   b. dentogingival unit
   c. mucogingival junction
   d. desmosomes

6. Which of the following structures comprise the biological width? (p. 14)
   a. gingival sulcus, junctional epithelium, gingival connective tissue attachment
   b. gingival sulcus, sulcular epithelium, gingival connective tissue attachment
   c. junctional epithelium, gingival connective tissue attachment
   d. sulcular epithelium, gingival connective tissue attachment
   e. sulcular epithelium, junctional epithelium, principal fibers

7. Which one of the following types of bone lines the tooth socket? (pp. 19–20)
   a. alveolar
   b. interradicular
   c. interdental
   d. trabecular

8. Which one of the following structures is referred to as a semipermeable structure? (p. 10)
   a. junctional epithelium
   b. oral epithelium
   c. sulcular epithelium
   d. lamina propria
   e. cementum

9. All of the following structures are avascular except one. Which one is the exception? (pp. 11–13)
   a. enamel
   b. cementum
   c. junctional epithelium
   d. lamina propria

10. Arteries that supply blood and lymphatics to the free gingiva originate from all of the following parts of the periodontium except one. Which one is the exception? (pp. 21–22)
    a. supraperiosteal
    b. periodontal ligament
    c. alveolar bone
    d. cementum

REFERENCES

Alfano, M. 1974. The origin of gingival fluid. *J. Theor. Biol.* 47:127–136.

Bartold, P. M. 2006. Periodontal tissues in health and disease. Introduction. *Periodontology 2000* 40(1):7–0.

Bartold, P. M., and A. S. Narayana, 2006. Molecular and cell biology of health and diseased periodontal tissues. *Periodontology 2000* 40(1):29–49.

Beertsen, W., C. A. G. McCulloch, and J. Sodek. 1997. The periodontal ligament: A unique, multifunctional connective tissue. *Periodontology 2000* 13:20–40.

Gargiulo, A., F. Wentz, and B. Orban. 1961. Dimensions and relations of the dento-gingival junction in humans. *J. Periodontol.* 32:261–267.

Goldman, H. M. 1951. The topography and role of the gingival fibers. *J. Dent. Res.* 30:331–336.

Gordon, J. M., C. B. Walker, J. C. Murphy, J. M. Goodson, and S. S. Socransky. 1981. Tetracycline: Levels achievable in gingival crevice fluid and in vitro effect on subgingival organisms. Part 1. Concentrations in crevicular fluid after repeated doses. *J. Periodontol.* 52:609–612.

Hassell, T. M. 1993. Tissues and cells of the periodontium. *Periodontology 2000* 3:9–38.

Kornman, K., R. Page, and M. Tonetti. 1997. The host response to the microbial challenge in periodontitis: Assembling the players. *Periodontology 2000* 14:33–53.

Moss-Salentijn, L., and M. Hendricks-Klyvert. 1990. Oral mucosa-epithelium. In eds. L. Moss-Salentijn & M. Hendricks-Klyvert, *Dental and oral tissues,* 27–44. Philadelphia: Lea & Febiger.

Mukherjee, S. 1985. The significance of crevicular fluid. *Compendium Cont. Educ. Dent.* 6:611–616.

Nakib, N., N. M. Bissada, J. W. Simmelink, and S. N. Goldstine. 1982. Endotoxin penetration into root cementum of periodontally healthy and diseased human teeth. *J. Periodontol.* 53:368–378.

Nanci, A., and D. D. Bosshardt. 2006. Structure of periodontal tissues in health and disease. *Periodontology 2000* 40(1):11–28.

Page, R. C., W. F. Ammons, L. R. Schectman, and L. A. Dillingham. 1974. Collagen fibre bundles of the normal marginal gingiva in the marmoset. *Arch. Oral. Biol.* 19:1039–1043.

Ritchey, B., and B. Orban. 1953. The crests of the interdental alveolar septa. *J. Periodontol.* 24:75–87.

Schroeder, H. E. 1991. Oral mucosa. In *Oral structural biology,* ed. H. E. Schroeder, 350–391. Stuttgart and New York: Georg Thieme Verlag.

Schroeder, H. E., and M. A. Listgarten. 1997. The gingival tissues: The architecture of periodontal protection. *Periodontology 2000* 13:91–120.

Squier, C. A., and M. W. Hill. 1998. Oral mucosa. In ed. A. R. Ten Cate, *Oral histology.* St. Louis, MO: Mosby.

Stern, I. B. 1965. Electron microscopic observations of oral epithelium I. Basal cells and the basement membrane. *Periodontics* 3:224–238.

Tonetti, M. S., M. Imboden, I. L. Gerber, and N. P. Lang. 1995. Compartmentalization of inflammatory cell phenotypes in normal gingiva and peri-implant keratinized mucosa. *J. Clin. Periodontol.* 22:735–742.

Chapter **2**

Epidemiology of Periodontal Diseases

Mary Elizabeth Aichelmann-Reidy

The OUTLINE is a per-chapter table of contents listing.

OUTLINE
Introduction and Definitions
Indices
Accuracy of Methodology
Prevalence of Periodontal Diseases
Incidence and Disease Progression
Epidemiologic Variables
Treatment Needs
Future Trends
Dental Hygiene Notes
Key Points
Self-Quiz
References

EDUCATIONAL OBJECTIVES

Upon completion of this chapter, the reader should be able to:

- Describe epidemiology and its descriptive terms: prevalence, incidence, extent, and severity.
- Explain the significance of epidemiologic data to future treatment.
- Describe the role of indices in private practice and population surveys.
- Describe the prevalence and incidence of periodontal diseases.
- Identify risk factors and risk indicators for periodontal diseases.
- Discuss future periodontal treatment needs and future trends that may have an impact on dental hygiene practice.

GOAL: To provide an understanding of the prevalence, extent, and severity of periodontal diseases in the population.

KEY WORDS

epidemiology 26
extent 26
indices 26
incidence 26
periodontal diseases 26
population surveys 26
prevalence 26
risk factors 26
risk indicators 45
severity 26

INTRODUCTION AND DEFINITIONS

Epidemiology is the study of health and disease in the human population. The rationale for the study of epidemiology is to identify events and **risk factors** in populations that lead to disease so that future health problems can be anticipated, prevented, and controlled. A risk factor is an event or characteristic associated with a given disease. It is important to identify risk factors so that healthcare measures can target people at risk for a particular disease, perhaps altering the future course of the disease (American Academy of Periodontology, 2005). It is important to note that risk is not causative.

Epidemiologic studies focus on populations rather than individuals. Much of what we know about **periodontal diseases** comes from national or **population surveys**. Population surveys evaluate representative samples of individuals within a study population to assess the true risk for disease and quantify how many individuals are or will be affected by disease. This quantification of disease is referred to as disease **prevalence** and **incidence**. Prevalence is the proportion or number of individuals in a population having the disease (old and new cases) at a given time. Incidence is defined as the rate of new cases occurring within a certain period of time. Disease prevalence and incidence can only be understood by looking at a large number of individuals within a population. Population surveys also provide insight into the severity and extent of a particular disease, say, periodontal disease, in populations. **Severity** is defined as the degree or amount of periodontal disease involvement and quantifies the amount of attachment loss, bone loss, or probing depth (Oliver, Brown, & Löe, 1998). The **extent** of periodontal disease refers to the number or percentage of diseased teeth or sites per individual.

Epidemiologic research is used to detect the underlying patterns of a disease and its associated factors to help find the cause of the disease. Trends are detectable when data collected from large numbers of individuals from within a study population are combined. For a survey to be useful, the clinical assessments must be standardized so that population means (averages) can be determined.

Epidemiologic data are collected through the use of a specific methodology that differs from patient evaluations in private practice. Complete, full-mouth periodontal examinations, which are necessary to establish an individual's diagnosis and to determine treatment needs, are too time-consuming for use on a large scale in an epidemiologic survey. The survey methods used to evaluate periodontal diseases in a population usually involve screening tools designed to quantify and simplify the disease assessment. These tools are referred to as **indices** (singular: index). An index is a numerical expression of values, with upper and lower limits, that is used to describe a specific condition. Indices are used in both clinical practice and research as the system of measurement for collecting data. They provide the private practitioner with information for patient treatment planning and the researcher with information about the prevalence and incidence of disease.

INDICES

Significance of Indices

Epidemiology is used to identify disease patterns, and indices are the measurement systems used for collecting the necessary data. For the study of periodontal diseases, assessments of plaque, calculus, gingival inflammation, periodontal attachment level, bleeding, and mobility are necessary to determine individual disease status. An index is a tool for standardized data collection and can measure the presence, absence, or severity of a disease condition on a specific tooth, area, or whole mouth and then can be extrapolated to the population. Unlike subjective clinician assessments of parameters of disease, an index is a numerical expression given to conditions that can then be quantified, tabulated, and used in comparisons to predict disease patterns, progression, and trends in study populations.

If a dental hygienist examines a patient and subjectively describes the condition of oral cleanliness in the mouth as "a fair amount of plaque and calculus on the teeth," this description could be interpreted differently by another clinician and might be interpreted as light or moderate plaque levels. Terms such as fair, light, moderate, and heavy have different meaning for different practitioners and therefore need to be standardized. The use of indices can help to standardize and reproduce findings for the purpose of assessment and monitoring patients' progression in private practice.

Dentists and dental hygienists formulate treatment plans based on full-mouth data collection. Becoming aware of the periodontal problem, assessing its severity, and presenting the findings to the patient require the practitioner to record and chart data in formats that can be compared over time. Periodontal charting forms and indices tabulate the measurements to be interpreted for treatment plans.

Indices measure disease outcomes and so measure past disease. When a dental hygienist supplements a patient's clinical examination with index scores to monitor patient conditions over time, these data, along with information gleaned from population surveys, can help the clinician predict future disease progression and establish a prognosis for the individual patient.

Criteria for Indices

There are many types of indices a practitioner can select from depending on the specific method of data collection and the meaning to be given to the data collected. When selecting an index or set of indices, the following properties should be considered:

- Simplicity or ease of use is critical to provide a fast and reproducible method to collect the data. Reproducibility creates a reliable instrument that can be used by different examiners or the same examiner over time to produce the same results.
- The index should be quick to perform and practical. Whether in the field for research purposes or in a dental practice, the method of data collection must not be time-consuming, costly, or involve many instruments.
- Sensitivity requires the index to detect small changes. Sensitivity determines if the disease is really present and can be seen. A true-positive result would indicate that the disease or condition exists.
- Validity provides the correlation of the disease with the measure employed. If bleeding on probing is to be measured, then the index can be confounded by other variables such as probing pressure, spontaneous bleeding, or instrumentation differences. A valid index must measure what it intended to measure.
- Reliability describes the consistency of a set of measurements. It is the extent to which the indices remain constant over repeated testing of the same subject.

Rapid Dental Hint

Indices are important for patient assessment because indices are intended to be reproducible by other clinicians. Therefore, other clinicians that perform the same index as you will obtain the same results.

6. Risks involved in participation should be acceptable to subjects.
7. Amenable to statistical analysis allows the results of the index to be interpreted through statistics.
8. Clinically significant and meaningful to researchers.

There is no perfect index or one that assesses all categories of inquiry. There are numerous indices, and the practitioner must select the best ones to represent the disease under examination or the health of the patient. There are over forty types of indices in periodontics. They fall into four general categories: oral hygiene indices (plaque and calculus), gingival indices, periodontal (destruction) indices, and treatment needs indices. An overview of historically important and commonly used indices is presented in Table 2–1 ■ and is reviewed briefly below.

Plaque and Debris Indices

Oral cleanliness is quantified by indices that measure plaque and debris and indices that measure calculus. Since bacterial plaque is considered a risk factor of periodontal diseases, methods of measuring plaque (debris) are important epidemiologically and are useful to practitioners treating the disease. Many plaque indices are used today. Some are meant simply as screening tools in clinical practice to assess home-care practices, whereas others are designed to quantify and locate plaque as needed for the evaluation of plaque-control devices or products before and after use.

One of the simplest methods of monitoring patient plaque levels is the use of the O'Leary Plaque Index (O'Leary, Drake, & Naylor, 1972), also called the plaque control record. A visual record of plaque control is made using a disclosing agent. A diagram is made of plaque-covered surfaces that can be shared with patients to visually help them identify problem areas and focus their efforts at home. O'Leary and colleagues (1972) recommended reduction of plaque levels to 10% of the available tooth surfaces as the patient's goal for home-care mastery.

Other common plaque indices are the Plaque Index (PlI) (Silness & Löe, 1964), the Debris Index (DI-S) of the Simplified Oral Hygiene Index (Greene, 1967), and

Did You Know?

Oral biofilm deposits are closely correlated with gingivitis, a relationship long considered one of cause and effect.

Table 2–1   Indices Used for Periodontal Disease Assessments

Index	Type of Measure	Teeth Measured	Method of Measurement	Scale of Measurement	Purpose	Advantages	Disadvantages	Uses
O'Leary (O'Leary, Drake, & Naylor, 1972)	Plaque	All teeth are scored at the cervical third of the tooth. Four surfaces of each tooth (M, B, D, L,) are measured.	A plaque record is made by marking a tooth diagram with the surface location of plaque. Mark each tooth surface with plaque as positive (disclosing agent used).	Calculation: Surfaces with plaque divided by the total number of surfaces. Multiply by 100 to get the percent of surfaces with plaque. Patient goal of 10% or less of plaque is ideal.	Visual record of plaque distribution; shows patients where are insufficient in plaque removal; patient motivation.	Complete assessment of all tooth surfaces to determine areas of cleaning deficiency.	Will not pick up changes in plaque quantity at each tooth surface; time-consuming.	Private practice.
Plaque Index (PII) (Silness & Löe, 1964)	Plaque	All teeth (distal, facial, mesial, lingual) or selected teeth.	Sweep a probe along the tooth surface at the gingival margin. (No disclosing agent is used.) The score (0, 1, 2, or 3) per tooth is obtained by summing the four different surface scores and dividing by four. Adding each tooth score and dividing by the number of teeth evaluated	0 No plaque. 1 A thinly adherent layer of plaque visible only when a probe is run across the tooth. 2 A visible layer of plaque, which is thin to moderately thick. 3 Heavy plaque accumulation in the crevice and the gingival margin.	Measures the thickness or amount of plaque along the gingival margin.	Good for research purposes because qualitative changes can be measured; not as time-consuming if selected teeth are used.	Somewhat subjective; limited to the cervical portion of the tooth, not for patient motivation.	Clinical studies, epidemiologic surveys.

Table 2–1 Indices Used for Periodontal Disease Assessments (continued)

Index	Type of Measure	Teeth Measured	Method of Measurement	Scale of Measurement	Purpose	Advantages	Disadvantages	Uses
			generates a patient score. Excellent: 0 Poor: 2.0–3.0					Epidemiologic and research projects.
Simplified Debris Index (DI-S) of the Simplified Oral Hygiene Index (OHI-S) (Greene & Vermillion, 1964)	Soft debris	Six tooth surfaces per mouth are scored: facial surfaces of teeth nos. 3, 8, 14, 24, and lingual surfaces of teeth nos. 19, 30. If the first molars are missing, choose the first fully erupted tooth distal to the second premolar.	Each tooth is divided into gingival, middle, and incisal thirds. Scoring is done by moving a no. 23 explorer from the incisal third toward the gingival third of the tooth. No disclosing agent is used. Score as 0, 1, 2, 3. Calculation: Total of surface scores divided by the number of surfaces scored Good score: 0.0–0.6 Poor score: 1.9–3.0	0 No stain or debris. 1 Soft deposit covering ≤ 1/3 of the surface or the presence of extrinsic stain. 2 Soft deposit covering more than 1/3 but less than 2/3 of the tooth surface. 3 Soft deposit covering > 2/3 of the tooth surface.	Measures plaque surface area.	Measures the quantity of debris rather than the presence or absence; not as time-consuming.	Somewhat subjective.	

(continues)

Table 2-1   Indices Used for Periodontal Disease Assessments (continued)

Index	Type of Measure	Teeth Measured	Method of Measurement	Scale of Measurement	Purpose	Advantages	Disadvantages	Uses
Turesky Modification of the Quigley-Hein Index (Turesky, Gilmore, & Glickman, 1970)	Plaque	Facial and lingual surfaces of all teeth excluding the third molars.	Score as 0, 1, 2, 3, 4, 5. Disclosing agent is used. Calculation: Total of all scores divided by the number of surfaces examined.	0 No plaque. 1 Flecks of plaque at the cervical margin. 2 Thin, continuous band of plaque (≤1 mm) at the cervical margin. 3 Band of plaque wider than 1 mm but covering less than 1/3 of crown. 4 Plaque covering at least 1/3 but less than 2/3 of the crown. 5 Plaque covering more than 2/3 of the crown.	Measures surface area of plaque.	The additional scoring categories allow the researcher to quantify improvement or change in plaque levels after the use of a plaque-control device or topical antimicrobial.	Somewhat subjective; time-consuming.	Index of choice in clinical trials.
Simplified Calculus Index (CI-S); part of the OHI-S (Greene, 1967)	Calculus	Six tooth surfaces per mouth are scored: facial surfaces of teeth nos. 3, 8, 14, 24, and lingual surfaces of teeth nos. 19, 30. If the first molars	Score as 0, 1, 2, 3. Calculation: Total calculus scores divided by the number of surfaces scored. To tabulate the total OHI-S,	0 No calculus present. 1 Supragingival calculus covering ≤ 1/3 of the exposed tooth. 2 Supragingival calculus covering more than 1/3 but	Quantifies calculus.	Well-defined criteria, allows for interexaminer reproducibility.	Combines location and quantity.	Epidemiologic and longitudinal studies.

Table 2-1 Indices Used for Periodontal Disease Assessments (continued)

Index	Type of Measure	Teeth Measured	Method of Measurement	Scale of Measurement	Purpose	Advantages	Disadvantages	Uses
		are missing, choose the first fully erupted tooth distal to the second premolar.	add the DI-S + CI-S. Combined OHI-S: Good: 0.0–1.2 Poor: 3.1–6.0	2/3 or less of exposed tooth or separate flecks of subgingival calculus in the cervical region. 3 Supragingival calculus covering more than 2/3 of exposed tooth or a continuous heavy band of subgingival calculus.				
Volpe Manhold Calculus Assessment (Volpe, Manhold, & Hazen, 1965)	Calculus	Mandibular incisors and cuspids (lingual surfaces).	With a probe, the coronal extension of supragingival calculus is measured in millimeters. Three readings are made bisecting the dimension of calculus at the direct lingual and mesial and distal line angles. These readings are averaged to generate a	Readings are scored in millimeter markings from the probe.	Measures the height or dimension of calculus.	Ability to measure the rate of calculus formation.	Difficult to master.	Clinical studies and epidemiologic studies.

(continues)

Table 2-1 Indices Used for Periodontal Disease Assessments (continued)

Index	Type of Measure	Teeth Measured	Method of Measurement	Scale of Measurement	Purpose	Advantages	Disadvantages	Uses
			tooth score, and the individual tooth scores are averaged to provide the total patient score.					
Calculus Index of the National Institute of Dental Research (Miller et al., 1987)	Calculus	Mesiobuccal and midbuccal surfaces of all fully erupted permanent teeth present in two randomly selected quadrants (one mandibular and the other maxillary).	Detected by explorer or probe.	0 No calculus. 1 Supragingival calculus only (calculus on the crown and root not extending more than 1 mm below the gingival margin). 2 Subgingival calculus is detected with or without supragingival calculus.	Presence or absence and location supra- or subgingival.	Simple.	Unable to quantify amount of calculus.	Used in the National Health and Nutrition and Examination Survey (NHANES III).
Gingival Index (GI) (Löe, 1967)	Gingival inflammation	Four gingival areas (buccal, mesial, distal, and lingual) for all teeth or select teeth.	Probe is inserted into the gingival crevice and moved with a sweeping along the pocket wall. Probe is also pressed lightly against the gingiva to	0 Normal gingiva. 1 Mild inflammation with slight changes in color and edema (swelling); no bleeding on probing. 2 Moderate inflammation	Measures severity of gingivitis.	Can detect change in degree of inflammation.	Somewhat subjective, time-consuming.	Epidemiologic and clinical studies.

Table 2–1 Indices Used for Periodontal Disease Assessments (continued)

Index	Type of Measure	Teeth Measured	Method of Measurement	Scale of Measurement	Purpose	Advantages	Disadvantages	Uses
			determine its firmness. Calculation: Each of the four gingival areas per tooth is given a GI score of 0 to 3. Total the scores for each area and divide by the number of teeth scored. Good: 0.0–1.0 Fair: 1.1–2.0 Poor: 2.1–3.0	with redness, edema, and glazing; bleeding on probing. 3 Severe inflammation with marked redness and edema; tendency to spontaneously bleed.				
Sulcus Bleeding Index (Mühlemann & Son, 1971)	Gingival inflammation	Three gingival areas (facial and lingual marginal gingival and mesial and distal interdental papillae) for all teeth.	Insert probe in the sulcus and withdraw it. Wait 30 seconds to score the area. Calculation: Total the scores for each tooth, and divide by the number of teeth.	0 Healthy appearance with no bleeding on probing. 1 Healthy but with bleeding on probing. 2 Bleeding on probing and color change but no swelling. 3 Bleeding on probing, color change, and slight edema. 4 Bleeding on probing and	Presence or absence and severity of gingival inflammation.	Less subjective, more gradations of severe inflammation.	Criticized for scores beyond clinical gingivitis.	Clinical and epidemiologic studies.

(continues)

Table 2–1 Indices Used for Periodontal Disease Assessments (continued)

Index	Type of Measure	Teeth Measured	Method of Measurement	Scale of Measurement	Purpose	Advantages	Disadvantages	Uses
				obvious swelling with or without color change. 5 Bleeding on probing and spontaneous bleeding and color change, marked swelling with or without ulceration.				
Periodontal Index (PI) (Russell, 1967)	Inflammation, pocket depth, tooth mobility (visual assessment, without periodontal probing)	All teeth.	Each tooth is given a score from 0 (no disease) to 8 (severe disease) Calculation: Add up the scores for all teeth, and divide by the number of teeth scored. 0.0–0.2: Normal periodontal condition. 0.3–0.9: Simple gingivitis. 0.–1.9: Early destructive periodontitis.	0 Tooth with healthy periodontium. 1 Mild gingivitis, localized and does not involve the entire tooth. 2 Gingivitis encircling the entire tooth. 6 Gingivitis with pocket formation with no loss of function or mobility. 8 Advanced destruction with tooth mobility.	Measures the severity of the periodontal condition.	Objective measures.	Visual assessment that often underestimates disease; evaluates both gingivitis and periodontitis in the same index.	National epidemiologic surveys including the National Health and Nutrition Examination Survey (1971–1974).

Table 2–1 Indices Used for Periodontal Disease Assessments (continued)

Index	Type of Measure	Teeth Measured	Method of Measurement	Scale of Measurement	Purpose	Advantages	Disadvantages	Uses
			1.6–5.0: Established periodontitis. 3.8–8.0: Terminal disease.					
Community Periodontal Index of Treatment Needs (Ainamo et al., 1982)	Periodontal pockets, calculus, gingival bleeding	Ten teeth: 2, 3, 8, 14, 15, 18, 19, 24, 30, 31	A 0.5 mm ball-tip probe with demarcations for shallow (3.5 mm) and deep (5.5 mm) pockets (CPITN probe) is used to detect and record the presence of bleeding, calculus, and periodontal pockets. The individual is scored by sextant assigning the worst tooth score per sextant as the overall sextant score. Treatment needs are assigned based on the highest code received	Code 0: No pocketing or inflammation. Code 1: Bleeding on probing. Code 2: Calculus present. Code 3: Pocketing extending in to the black area of the probe (4–5 mm). Code 4: Pocketing extending beyond the black area of the probe ($\leq$ 6 mm).	Measures severity of the periodontal condition and treatment needs.	Simple.	Only selective teeth are measured, which may underestimate the disease.	Epidemiologic surveys (specifically designed by the WHO to compare population surveys internationally).

(continues)

Table 2–1 Indices Used for Periodontal Disease Assessments (continued)

Index	Type of Measure	Teeth Measured	Method of Measurement	Scale of Measurement	Purpose	Advantages	Disadvantages	Uses
			by each sextant. 0 No further therapy needed. 1 Patient only requires oral home-care instruction. 2 Patient requires oral hygiene improvement and professional debridement. 3 Patient requires oral hygiene improvement and professional debridement. 4 Patient requires complex treatment (scaling and root planing with dental anesthesia and may require periodontal surgery).					

Table 2–1   Indices Used for Periodontal Disease Assessments (continued)

Index	Type of Measure	Teeth Measured	Method of Measurement	Scale of Measurement	Purpose	Advantages	Disadvantages	Uses
Periodontal Screening and Recording (PSR)	Periodontal pockets, calculus, bleeding, and defective restorations	Mouth is divided into sextants. All teeth are measured.	Each tooth in the sextant is probed, and the tooth with the worst score determines the sextant score. The highest-scoring sextant determines the individual's overall management. If two or more sextants have a score of 3 or any one sextant has a score of 4, then a complete periodontal charting is advised. Scores of 0 or 1 require preventive measures inclusive of home-care instructions.	Code 0: No calculus, defective margins, or bleeding, and the black band of the probe is completely visible (probing depth less than 3.5 mm). Code 1: No calculus or defective margins, but there is bleeding, and the black band of the probe is completely visible. Code 2: Supragingival or subgingival calculus or defective markings are present, but the black band is still visible. Code 3: Calculus, defective restorations,	Screening of periodontal disease in private practice.	Simplifies the charting of an individual's periodontal condition when extensive treatment is not required.	Cannot be substituted for a complete periodontal charting necessary for the treatment of periodontitis patients.	Private practice.

(continues)

Table 2–1 Indices Used for Periodontal Disease Assessments (continued)

Index	Type of Measure	Teeth Measured	Method of Measurement	Scale of Measurement	Purpose	Advantages	Disadvantages	Uses
			Scores of 2 or greater require the patient to have additional professional cleaning and correction of defective restorations.	and bleeding may or may not be present, and the black band is partly visible (probing depth more than 3.5 mm but less than 5.5 mm). Code 4: The black band of the probe is not visible (probing depth more than 5.5 mm). An asterisk (*) is added if any additional pathology is present, such as furcations.				
Miller Index of Tooth Mobility (Miller, 1950)	Pathologic tooth mobility	All teeth in dentition.	Take blunt end of two instruments (e.g., probe and mirror). Using finger rests apply ends of instruments to the labial and lingual surfaces of teeth. Move tooth in facial-lingual direction.	0 = No pathologic movement. I = First distinguishable sign of tooth movement in a facial/lingual direction. II = Movement of the crown in a facial/lingual direction up to 1 mm.	Determine the amount of movement of a tooth.	Results are reproducible.	This index is actually the only referenced index for tooth mobility. There are no disadvantages	Private practice.

Table 2-1 Indices Used for Periodontal Disease Assessments (continued)

Index	Type of Measure	Teeth Measured	Method of Measurement	Scale of Measurement	Purpose	Advantages	Disadvantages	Uses
				III = Movement of the crown in a facial/lingual direction more than 1 mm and/or depressed in a vertical direction.				

the modified Quigley-Hein Plaque Index (Turesky, Gilmore, & Glickman, 1970). These plaque indices provide subjective numerical values that quantify the amount of plaque present, unlike the O'Leary Index, which merely indicates the presence or absence of plaque and is most suited for patient education and motivation in private practice rather than epidemiologic surveys.

The Plaque Index (PlI) (Silness & Löe, 1964) scores the plaque thickness along the gingival margin of the tooth, whereas the Debris Index (DI-S) measures plaque surface area. The Debris Index is a component of the Simplified Oral Hygiene Index (OHI-S) developed by Greene and Vermillion (1964). The other component of the OHI-S is a Calculus Index (CI-S). The OHI-S is used primarily for epidemiologic and longitudinal dental studies.

Another plaque index used more specifically for clinical trials is the Turesky Modification of the Quigley-Hein Index (Turesky et al., 1970). Plaque is assessed on all facial and lingual tooth surfaces (excluding third molars) after a disclosing agent is applied. The additional scoring categories of this index allow researchers to quantify improvement or change in plaque levels after the use of a plaque-control device or topical antimicrobial. Both the modified Quigley-Hein Index and the Plaque Index (PlI) are suitable for the evaluation of topical antimicrobials and plaque-removal devices (Fischman, 1986).

In summary, a number of plaque indices are used today. Four plaque indices were presented, and each serves different purposes. The plaque control record (O'Leary et al., 1972) is used most commonly in periodontal practice, whereas the others are used more frequently in clinical trials and population surveys.

Calculus Indices

In clinical practice, calculus is not monitored by a numeric index, but it is in epidemiologic surveys. Numerous methods have been devised to quantify this deposit, and three commonly used calculus indices will be presented here (see Table 2–1).

The simplified Calculus Index (CS-1), which is part of the OHI-S mentioned previously (Greene, 1967), is valuable for epidemiologic surveys and longitudinal studies. It quantifies calculus by location and surface area. Another common calculus evaluation is the Volpe Manhold Calculus Assessment (Volpe, Kupczak, & King, 1967; Volpe, Manhold, & Hazen, 1965), which measures the height and dimension of the calculus present. It was designed originally for use on the lingual sur-

faces of the mandibular incisors but can be used throughout the mouth.

National epidemiologic studies, conducted through the National Institute of Dental Research (NIDR), have developed and used their own calculus index (Miller, Brunelle, Carlos, Brown, & Löe, 1987). The NIDR Index merely indicates the presence or absence of calculus supragingivally or subgingivally. This index was used for the third National Health and Nutrition Examination Survey (NHANES III), conducted by the National Center for the Health Statistics in collaboration with the National Institute for Dental Research from 1988 to 1991.

Gingival Indices

The epidemiologic tool used to quickly assess gingival inflammation is the gingival index. A gingival index is designed to measure the degree of visible inflammation of the gingival tissues. Visible signs of gingival inflammation are bleeding, redness, and swelling. These are accepted clinical signs of inflammation and also have been incorporated into indices for evaluation of the periodontal status of individuals and populations.

The Gingival Index (GI) of Löe and Silness (Löe, 1967) is based on the subjective assessment of the visual indicators of gingival inflammation. The degree of inflammation is subdivided into three categories, with moderate inflammation determined by the presence of bleeding and severe inflammation determined by spontaneous bleeding. The GI historically has been used for epidemiologic studies. Lobene, Weatherford, Ross, Lam, and Menaker (1986) modified this index for use in clinical trials evaluating plaque-control products. The Modified Gingival Index (Lobene et al., 1986) assesses gingival health by looking only at qualitative changes in the gingiva. Unlike the GI, which uses bleeding as an indicator of increasing severity of gingival inflammation, this index does not use bleeding on probing and has more gradations. The Modified Gingival Index is scored to pick up subtle changes earlier with four different scores for gingival inflammation.

> **Did You Know?**
>
> In a national survey of employed adults conducted in 1985–1986, 47% of males and 39% of females aged 18 to 64 exhibited at least one site that bled on probing.

Other gingival indices based primarily on bleeding include the Sulcus Bleeding Index (Mühlemann & Son, 1971) and the Eastman Interdental Bleeding Index (Caton & Polson, 1985). Gingival bleeding as a measure of gingival inflammation is considered a more objective measure, whereas gingival color and consistency are more subjective. For this index, gingival bleeding is determined by gently inserting a probe in the sulcus and withdrawing it. Mühlemann and Son (1971) based the Sulcus Bleeding Index on bleeding being the earliest symptom of gingivitis, but it has been criticized because distinctions are not made beyond the clinical point of gingivitis.

A novel approach to determining bleeding is the use of a triangular toothpick (e.g., Stimudent) rather than a periodontal probe. The Interdental Bleeding Index (Caton & Polson, 1985) uses interdental cleaners to evaluate bleeding in the midproximal gingival tissues where periodontal changes are most likely to be found. The interdental cleaner is inserted between teeth and removed, depressing the interdental papilla 1 to 2 mm. Fifteen seconds after insertion and removal, bleeding is recorded.

In an attempt to achieve a more objective measure, gingival bleeding is being used increasingly for the determination of gingival changes in epidemiologic studies. The presence or absence of bleeding has been used in current demographic studies, in the NIDR Adult Survey (1985–1986) (Brown, Oliver, & Löe, 1989), and in NHANES III (1988–1991) (Brown, Brunelle, & Kingman, 1996). Gingival bleeding also has been used to monitor patient home oral hygiene practices. The percentage of bleeding sites is considered a more accurate representation of the patient's true level of daily home care. Bleeding and gingival indices also have been monitored along with individual attachment levels and pocket bacteria to find markers or predictors of disease activity.

Indices of Periodontal Destruction

Another essential measure employed in epidemiologic studies is evaluation of periodontal destruction. Indices of periodontal destruction are designed to measure disease severity and extent by observing the outcomes of periodontal destruction. This is done by measuring clinical attachment loss and probing depth and recording bone loss and loss of function. Current national studies use direct measures of these disease outcomes. These measures are taken at the midbuccal and mesiobuccal levels of all fully erupted teeth (Brown et al., 1996). Even though current national surveys do not employ periodon-

tal indices or directly measure the outcome of destruction, much of the historical data pertinent to periodontal diseases in the United States have been compiled using periodontal indices.

The Periodontal Index (PI) (Russell, 1967) has been a standard measure for the large national surveys that are responsible for early views of periodontal disease prevalence and incidence in the United States. The PI is a visual index and does not use a periodontal probe. The presence of inflammation, pocket formation, and loss of function is assessed visually as criteria for numeric scoring of teeth.

Two additional indices of epidemiologic importance evaluate periodontal destruction and designate treatment needs. The Community Periodontal Index of Treatment Needs (CPITN; Ainamo, Barmes, Beargie, Cutress, & Martin, 1982) was developed by an initiative of the World Health Organization (WHO) expressly for population studies. Its primary focus is to assess treatment needs.

The CPITN was modified to the Periodontal Screening and Recording (PSR) system for general-practice use. The PSR system was developed to evaluate individual treatment needs and to be used as a quick screening tool to document new patient periodontal findings in lieu of a complete periodontal charting. It has been endorsed by the American Academy of Periodontology and the American Dental Association as a quick and easy method to record the periodontal status of a patient in the private-practice setting. This screening tool reduces the number of patients who need a complete periodontal charting simply by identifying those with periodontal treatment needs and therefore the need for a complete periodontal charting.

The CPITN probe is used in the PSR system, and the same parameters employed by the CPITN are evaluated—bleeding, calculus, and probing depth. The CPITN probe has a ball tip to aid in calculus detection and a black band that demarcates probing depth from 3.5 to 5.5 mm. It was developed to increase the recognition and treatment of periodontal disease in the general dental practice. Generation of the PSR score is the responsibility of the dental hygienist, especially for recall visits.

ACCURACY OF METHODOLOGY

Thus far the tools used for assessing the periodontal condition in epidemiologic studies have been described. These tools define or identify individuals within a population with periodontal disease. The sampling methodology for population studies differs from that used in clinical peri-odontics and can influence the accuracy of the data obtained. Epidemiologic data-collection tools do not measure all the periodontal findings a clinician might use to establish a diagnosis and prognosis, such as furcation involvement or tooth mobility. Population studies, because of their large sample sizes, use indices as assessment tools, unlike diagnostic evaluations in clinical practice, and thus only score a portion of the mouth. To streamline the examination process, partial mouth scores are incorporated into indices. Partial mouth observations improve study efficiency but reduce the accuracy of overall reporting of periodontal disease prevalence and incidence.

For example, the CPITN measures only ten teeth in the mouth. Baelum, Manji, Fejerskov, and Wanzala (1993) found that the prevalence of teeth with moderate to deep pockets was underreported in the partial mouth scores of the CPITN. This was especially true for severe periodontal conditions. In another report, Baelum, Manji, Wanzala, and Fejerskov (1995) concluded that the CPITN scores tend to underestimate prevalence and severity in younger age groups and overestimate the same in the elderly. The methodology employed by the NIDR for the most recent survey, NHANES (1999–2000) (Borrell, Burt, & Taylor, 2005), also involves a partial mouth evaluation. As described earlier, periodontal probing is performed in half the mouth. When half-mouth and full-mouth scores were compared (Hunt & Fann, 1991), the results were similar. Half-mouth examination was considered accurate in estimating the prevalence of periodontal disease but still underestimated the percentage of the population with more advanced disease (periodontal attachment loss). A review by Papapanou (1996) concluded that the current NIDR methodology is inadequate because it is a combination of partial scores (e.g., only two sites per tooth are measured in only one-half of the mouth). Papapanou contended that the location of the pocket and the number of probing measures could have a profound influence on the outcome of the study. Partly because previous studies comparing half-mouth scores with full-mouth scores had used partial scores for their comparison, not all probing sites encircling a tooth were measured. When combining partial mouth scores with measures at only the midbuccal and mesiobuccal sites, current methodology actually could produce a mean percentage underestimation of deep pockets of 40% and an underestimation of the prevalence of these deep pockets of 58%.

The validity of an index in describing a population also can be affected by tooth loss. Missing teeth may have been the ones most severely affected by periodontitis. Since they are no longer present to be measured, there is a built-in selection bias for the healthier teeth still present, potentially underestimating both severity and prevalence of the disease (periodontitis). Thus the overall reliability of an index is affected by the method of data collection. It is difficult to have one tool that will be representative, accurate, and efficient at the same time for all periodontal measures. Historical and modern data are based on methodologies that have been criticized, but some researchers contend that they still render an adequate estimation of disease.

PREVALENCE OF PERIODONTAL DISEASES

National surveys have helped build our knowledge of the prevalence, severity, and extent of periodontal diseases in the United States. Based on the results of these surveys, the commonly accepted model for periodontal diseases has changed and evolved. Historically, periodontal disease was considered inevitable, and all individuals were susceptible to advanced periodontal disease, gingivitis being its precursor. In essence, periodontal disease was considered universal, and the susceptibility to periodontitis increased with age (Waerhaug, 1966).

Information gathered from more recent national surveys, however, suggests otherwise. More severe disease (advanced periodontitis) was found in only 5 to 20% of adults (U.S. Public Health Service, 1987), and moderate disease (periodontitis) was found in the majority of adults (U.S. Public Health Service, 1987). Thus only a few individuals will be susceptible to advanced disease. Today, periodontitis is not considered part of the aging process but occurs because of the interaction of bacteria and the immune response of the individual.

Prevalence of Gingivitis

Gingivitis is the most common form of periodontal disease found in individuals of all ages; it can even occur in early childhood (Ayers, Abrama, & Lausten, 1979). In the U.S. Health and Resources and Service Administration (HRSA) study of 1981 (Brown, Oliver, & Löe, 1989), 54% of adults over age 18 were affected with gingivitis involving at least six or more teeth. Another national study of employed adults between the ages of 18 and 64, the NIDR Adult Survey (1985–1986), reported less gingivitis, finding that 44% of the sample had gingivitis (defined by gingival bleeding) (Miller et al., 1987). The average involvement was 2.7 sites per person, and the extent of gingivitis increased with age. In NHANES III study (Brown et al., 1996), gingival bleeding was present in 63% of those examined, and 12% of all sites examined bled on probing. Gingivitis was slightly more prevalent in teenagers (13 to 17 years). The extent was similar among all age groups, ranging from 10 to 15% of the sites examined. Plaque and calculus deposits correlated with the prevalence of gingivitis and subgingival calculus were found in 67% of the population and at 22% of the sites evaluated. Compared with the more recent NHANES (Borrell, Burt, & Taylor, 2005) there has been a decrease in bleeding compared to the NHANES III.

When compared with earlier national surveys, gingivitis has declined in the United States most likely due to the current focus on oral hygiene as part of a daily personal hygiene routine (Burt, 1996). In the early 1960s, visual assessments revealed that 85% of men and 79% of women had gingivitis. Current surveys report that 63% of the population has gingival bleeding and that gingivitis is found in 44 to 54% of the population. This differs considerably from reports from third-world countries, where gingivitis in the presence of extensive plaque and calculus is considered normal among adults (Löe, Anerud, Boysen, & Smith, 1978).

Prevalence of Periodontitis

Chronic periodontitis, a more severe form of periodontal disease, is not commonly found among young individuals and is more prevalent with age. The NHANES III study (1988–1994) (Brown et al., 1996) (*n* = 7,447 surveyed) found that over 90% of individuals over age 13 had some attachment loss, with only 15% of the population having advanced disease (defined as 5 mm or more of attachment loss). If the definition of attachment loss were limited to 3 mm or more, the prevalence was 40%. One-quarter of the individuals surveyed showed moderate attachment loss (3–4 mm). With increasing age, the prevalence of moderate and severe attachment loss increased, but the prevalence of pockets 4 mm or greater and 6 mm or greater in size remained the same. Since the extent and prevalence of attachment loss were found to increase with age and the prevalence of 4 mm or greater pocket depths did not, increased gingival reces-

sion was deemed responsible for the increased attachment loss experienced with age (Oliver et al., 1998).

A recent study (Borrell et al., 2005) examined change in the prevalence of periodontitis between the NHANES III and the NHANES 1999–2000, and differences in the prevalence of periodontitis among racial/ethnic groups in the United States. Results showed that the prevalence of periodontitis has *decreased* between the NHANES III and the NHANES 1999–2000 for all racial/ethnic groups in the United States. This may be attributed to awareness and changes in health risk behaviors such as smoking. The overall prevalence of periodontitis for the NHANES III was 7.3%, while for the NHANES 1999–2000 it was 4.2%.

In the HRSA survey (Brown et al., 1989), periodontitis (at least one tooth with a pocket 4 mm or deeper) was found in 36% of the 7,078 individuals examined. The prevalence of the disease increased with age. Twenty-nine percent of individuals in the 19- to 44-year-old age group were affected, whereas almost 50% of individuals 45 years of age or older were affected. The percentage of elderly individuals (age 65 and older) with pockets was similar to that of the 45- to 64-year-old age group, although the number of teeth present decreased. Periodontitis, when present, usually involved only a few teeth, and advanced periodontitis was relatively rare.

In the NIDR study of employed adults between the ages of 18 and 64 (Brown et al., 1990), almost all had some attachment loss, with 44% experiencing attachment loss of 3 mm or more. Moderate pocket depths (4 to 6 mm) were present in only 13.4% of those examined, generally affecting only one to two sites. More advanced disease again was considered rare and was found in only 0.6% of the study population. Males experienced more disease than females, and blacks were more affected than whites.

In the NHANES III study (Brown et al., 1996), racial and gender differences were reported as well. Females overall were in better periodontal health than their male counterparts, and non-Hispanic whites had less periodontal disease than non-Hispanic blacks or Mexican

 Rapid Dental Hint

Attachment loss is defined as the loss of collagen fiber attachment to the tooth with subsequent apical migration of the junctional epithelium.

> **Did You Know?**
>
> For many years, periodontitis was primarily viewed as the outcome from infection. It is now seen as resulting from a complex interplay between bacterial infection and host response, often modified by behavioral factors.

> **Did You Know?**
>
> Cats and dogs can also develop periodontal disease!

Americans. Overall, the United States has a relatively low prevalence and severity of periodontal disease compared with the rest of the world, and the severity and extent of disease have declined in the past thirty years (Oliver et al., 1998).

Prevalence of Aggressive Periodontitis

The prevalence of aggressive periodontitis (replaces the older term "early-onset periodontitis"), has been estimated to be less than 1% of the general population (Papapanou, 1996). It is considered a rare form of periodontal disease. A review of national population studies indicates that approximately 3.6% of individuals between the ages of 18 and 34 (NIDR Adult Survey, 1985–1986; Oliver et al., 1998) have moderate periodontal disease. Among 14- to 17-year-olds (Löe & Brown, 1991), the prevalence of all forms of aggressive periodontitis was 2.27%, 0.53% were affected by localized aggressive periodontitis, and 0.13% were estimated to be affected by generalized aggressive periodontitis.

Racial differences also have been reported. Blacks were affected more often than whites by all forms of aggressive periodontitis. Ironically, racial and gender prevalences reported by recent national surveys do not match diagnostic criteria used to define and distinguish forms of aggressive periodontitis from chronic periodontitis. In a national (NIDR) study of over 11,000 adolescents between the ages of 14 and 17, gender differences existed and were influenced by race. For example, black males

Rapid Dental Hint

Gingivitis is defined as inflammation of the gingival tissue without loss of connective tissue attachment.

Periodontitis is defined as inflammation and loss of the connective tissue of the supporting or surrounding structure of teeth with loss of attachment.

were 2.9 times more likely to have localized aggressive periodontitis than black females, and white females were more frequently affected by localized aggressive periodontitis than white males by the same amount. Males, in general, were 4.3 times more likely to have generalized aggressive periodontitis than females. When these results were extrapolated to the racial mix of the U.S. population in general, about 87,000 cases of localized and generalized aggressive periodontitis were estimated among 13 million 14- to 17-year-olds (Oliver et al., 1998).

Traditionally, black females have been reported to be two to three times more likely to have aggressive periodontitis than white females. It has been suggested that clinical trials and case reports used to establish this racial and gender predilection may have been skewed by ascertainment bias because more females will seek dental treatment and participate in clinical trials than males (Oliver et al., 1998). Thus, a national survey that does not start out with this selection bias may more accurately reflect the national population prevalence.

In summary, the national status of periodontal disease has been gleaned by three recent national surveys: the NIDR, NHANES, and HRSA surveys. About 50% of all U.S. adults have gingivitis involving three to four teeth. Periodontitis is experienced in over 90% of the population over 13 years of age, but only 15% have severe disease. There is a specific small subset of the population that has more advanced disease. Aggressive periodontitis is considered a rare disease in the United States and affects only 0.53 to 3.6% of individuals under age 35. Overall, the national prevalence of gingivitis has declined over the past thirty years. However, the prevalence of periodontitis has remained the same, but the severity of disease has decreased (Capilouto & Douglass, 1988).

INCIDENCE AND DISEASE PROGRESSION

National surveys used to estimate disease prevalence are cross-sectional, which means that the study population is evaluated at only one point in time. To determine the natural progression of periodontal diseases, longitudinal studies are necessary, where individuals are examined at multiple intervals. Few longitudinal studies are available because of the difficulty of conducting them. In a fifteen-year longitudinal study by Löe and colleagues (1986), 480 Sri Lankan tea workers with untreated disease were evaluated. About 8% had rapid progression of their periodontitis, and most had a moderate rate of disease progression. A small portion of this population (11%) showed no progression beyond gingivitis despite the presence of heavy plaque and calculus.

A parallel study run in Norway (Löe et al., 1978) showed a different rate of disease progression. No cases of aggressive periodontitis were found, unlike the Sri Lankan study. The mean annual rate of attachment loss was 0.08 mm for interproximal and 0.1 mm for buccal surfaces as individuals approached 40 years of age. In patients with moderate periodontitis, progression occurred slowly at any given site. The rate of periodontal destruction did not increase with age, and therefore, the progression of periodontitis (extent and severity) appeared to be slow and continuous in this population.

In a report by Beck, Koch, and Offenbacher (1994) detailing a longitudinal study of adults between the ages of 65 and 80 in North Carolina identified with extensive attachment loss, additional evidence of slow disease progression also can be found. Only 12% of this population experienced 3 mm or more of attachment loss on one or more teeth during the three-year study period. Again, it appears that subjects with a past history of periodontitis can be quite resistant to future disease (breakdown). Future attachment loss was associated with greater baseline probing depths, but the vast majority of sites that lost attachment had probing depths of 3 mm or less at baseline. Individuals who experienced attachment loss in the first eighteen months of the study were more likely to experience attachment loss in the subsequent eighteen-month period.

Racial differences also were detected. Blacks tended to experience more attachment loss during both eighteen-month periods of the study. Only 45% of blacks had no attachment loss during the three-year period, whereas 63% of whites were free of attachment loss. Despite having advanced attachment loss at the outset of the study, both blacks and whites had a high frequency of no further disease progression. Similarly, adult subjects with gingivitis monitored over a three-year period had no detectable increase in probing depth (Listgarten, Schifter, & Laster, 1985). In a review by Stamm (1986),

the incidence of gingivitis was greatest at puberty, declined through age 17, and then remained steady.

These studies imply that only select individuals or a small portion of the population will have new disease or disease progression. In another U.S. study by Löe and Brown (1991), only a small portion of the study population had the highest rate of disease progression, as noted by attachment loss; this subset of the population was identified with aggressive periodontitis. In the Beck and colleagues (1994) study of elderly adults, disease progression was more likely when extensive bone loss and tooth loss were experienced at a young age, again alluding to a specific subset of the population with a higher incidence of disease. In sum, only a small portion of the population will experience incidence and progression of severe attachment loss. This attachment loss will not progress at the same rate but may be episodic. The progression of periodontal disease appears to be influenced by education level, socioeconomic factors, gender, and race. These variables will be discussed in the next section of this chapter.

EPIDEMIOLOGIC VARIABLES

Risk Indicators

Risk indicators are demographic, behavioral, and socioeconomic characteristics that are associated with disease but not considered causal for the disease. Aging is considered a risk indicator for periodontal disease, but does not cause periodontal disease. With increasing age, the prevalence of periodontal disease increases, but the aging process is not responsible for the disease. It is believed that there is more disease with age because there is more exposure to plaque-induced inflammation over time. Other characteristics associated with an increased frequency of disease are the level of education, gender, and race. Females have less periodontal disease than males (Sheiham & Striffler, 1970). It is hypothesized that these differences are due to the availability and use of dental services, oral home care, and preventive practices. For example, the higher levels of periodontal disease reported in males versus females are attributed to higher levels of plaque and less use of dental services. More education, higher income, and dental insurance reduce the risk of oral disease. Where extensive plaque, calculus, and gingival inflammation are considered normal among adults in third-world countries, an association is found with less education and low income, and generally, there is more attachment loss than in industrial nations of the Western world.

Risk Factors

Risk factors are characteristics that have been shown to possibly put an individual more at risk for developing periodontal disease. Risk factors are used to predict the occurrence of disease. The presence of even a strong risk factor does not necessarily mean that an individual is very likely to get the disease. Also, just because risk factors predict disease, it does not necessarily follow that they will cause disease (Fletcher & Fletcher, 2005). Risk factors may or may not be causal (Fletcher & Fletcher, 2005). A risk factor that does not cause a disease is called a *marker of disease* because it marks the increased probability of disease (Fletcher & Fletcher, 2005). Even though a risk factor may not cause the disease, it is important to identify potential causal relationships so that oral disease can be prevented if a risk factor is modifiable. *Note that when the term risk factor is used throughout this textbook it is referring to factors that predispose an individual to periodontal disease.* For example, it is accepted that bacteria in bacterial biofilms causes gingivitis, and thus biofilms are considered a risk factor for gingivitis. Poor oral hygiene has been correlated strongly with periodontal disease. The NHANES I data showed an inverse relationship between tooth loss and good oral hygiene. The periodontal index (PI) and oral hygiene (OHI-S) index scores were significantly better in individuals with the least tooth loss (Burt, Ismail, & Eklund, 1985). However, the causal relationship is not clear-cut with periodontitis. Supragingival plaque and supragingival calculus are not as strongly correlated with periodontitis as with gingivitis (Bakdash, 1994; Löe et al., 1978). In a recent appraisal by Oliver and colleagues (1998), the presence of subgingival calculus appeared to be a better predictor of periodontitis but was not considered causal because there was an inconsistent relationship among the epidemiologic data regarding oral hygiene, plaque and calculus, and periodontitis. In the NHANES III survey (Brown et al., 1996), no bleeding was found 88% of the time when subgingival calculus was present. Additionally, gingivitis does not always progress to periodontitis, which means that periodontitis will not always occur in the presence of plaque and calculus. One could infer from this inconsistency that poor oral hygiene is an important risk factor in individuals who are more susceptible based on their immune response to bacterial plaque. The NHANES study reported a decrease in bleeding for all ethnic/racial groups compared to the NHANES III (Borrell et al., 2005)

Other risk factors for periodontitis are diabetes and tobacco use. The prevalence and extent of periodontal pockets are greater in diabetics than in nondiabetics. This is especially true for poorly controlled diabetics, who experience more attachment and bone loss than well-controlled diabetics with similar plaque levels (Seppälä, Seppälä, & Ainamo, 1993). Oliver and Tervonen (1994) outlined diabetes as a risk factor for extensive, severe periodontitis when the individual's diabetes is poorly controlled and the individual has extensive subgingival calculus from poor home care and lack of professional cleanings. In a recent report (Taylor et al., 1998), subjects with type 2 diabetes had more severe alveolar bone loss progression over a two-year period than those without diabetes.

Smoking has been well documented as a risk factor for periodontitis. An early National Health and Nutrition Survey (NHANES I) in 1971–1974 first demonstrated the relationship between smoking and periodontitis (Ismail, Burt, & Eklund, 1983) in the United States. More recent longitudinal studies confirm this relationship. One longitudinal study showed that smokers lost proximal bone twice as fast as nonsmokers (Bolin, Eklund, Frithiof, & Lavstedt, 1993). Even when plaque accumulation is minimal, smokers have more teeth with deeper pockets and alveolar bone loss than nonsmokers (Bergström & Eliasson, 1987; Bergström & Floderus-Myrhed, 1983). In a three-year study conducted by Beck, Koch, and Offenbacher (1995), disease was more likely to progress if the subject was a cigarette smoker, had the presence of gram-negative anaerobes in his or her subgingival microbiota (especially *Porphyromonas gingivalis*), or had financial stress. All led to an increased risk for disease progression. Thus it is apparent that microbiota and stress could be considered risk factors for periodontitis.

Another longitudinal study running from 1959 to 1985 in Tecumseh, Michigan (Ismail, Morrison, Burt, Cafesse, & Kavanaugh, 1990), reported age, smoking, and the presence of tooth mobility as risk markers for future attachment loss (2 mm or more). It has been hypothesized (Papapanou, 1996) that periodontitis actually may have different factors associated with its initiation than those involved in its progression. Multiple factors may play a role in the induction and progression of periodontal disease. The commonly accepted risk factors are lack of oral cleanliness, smoking, and systemic disease (diabetes). Specific subgingival bacteria and socioeconomic stress also have been linked causally to periodontal disease through epidemiologic studies, but further evaluation is ongoing. Gender, race, and age may play a role in disease expression but are not causally linked to periodontal disease.

 Rapid Dental Hint

A *risk factor* is an environmental exposure, aspect of behavior, or an inherent characteristic that is associated with a disease. Risk factors predispose an individual to a disease; they don't necessarily cause the disease.

A *risk indicator* describes plausible correlates of disease identified in cross-sectional studies.

Did You Know?

A recent review reports that the risk of destructive periodontal disease is five- to twenty-fold higher for a smoker compared with a never-smoker.

TREATMENT NEEDS

Information provided by epidemiologic surveys regarding gingival bleeding (gingival inflammation), subgingival calculus, and probing depths of 4 mm or greater is of great importance to the dental hygienist. These data represent clinical parameters used to decide when treatment of periodontal disease is necessary. Most individuals will need periodontal preventive care (Oliver et al., 1998), which is provided by the hygienist. Over 90% of people surveyed (NHANES III) have attachment loss, and only 15% of the population has advanced disease, suggesting that much of the treatment needs of the United States can be fulfilled by hygienists. More extensive, severe disease is found among minorities and those with less income and education. However, these are the same individuals who are less likely to seek or perceive the need for dental services. Tooth loss due to periodontal disease remains high in the United States (Brown et al., 1989). This suggests that public awareness and education about the preventive services of dental hygienists are paramount if those individuals who are most affected are to be treated before tooth loss due to periodontitis occurs.

FUTURE TRENDS

The hygienist in the general dentist's office plays an important role in the treatment of periodontal patients. Prevention and education are important responsibilities of the dental clinician. As epidemiologic studies elaborate and refine the interrelationship between periodontal infections and the systemic health of the patient, hygienists will need to include this information in patient education sessions. It has been documented that systemic conditions can contribute to the expression of periodontal disease. In recent years there is increasing evidence that supports the concepts that the relationship between systemic and oral health is bidirectional (Williams & Offenbacher, 2000). As patient awareness of periodontal disease and its systemic implications increases, more individuals will specifically seek the preventive and periodontal debridement services of the dental hygienist.

Recent technological advances have revolutionized the ability to understand and apply genetic principles to the study of human diseases. These developments may soon alter the management of periodontal diseases (American Academy of Periodontology, 2005).

Did You Know?

Periodontal diseases are possible risk factors for cardiovascular disease, diabetes, lung disease, and preterm low-birth weight babies.

DENTAL HYGIENE NOTES

Epidemiology of the periodontal diseases is an important concept for the dental hygienist to know because it gives an overall assessment of the prevalence and incidence of periodontal disease in the general population. It is important to have healthcare programs for young adults for the early detection of periodontal diseases (Costa et al., 2007).

KEY POINTS

- Epidemiologic measurements used to assess periodontal diseases include plaque, calculus, gingival, and periodontal indices.
- Indices measure past disease activity rather than current disease activity or future periodontal breakdown.
- Gingivitis is the most common form of periodontal disease.
- Aggressive periodontitis is not common in the general population.
- Chronic periodontitis is prevalent in the general population.
- Risk factors are used to predict occurrence of disease; risk factors are not causal.
- Even though risk factors are not causal, they predict the probability of disease.

SELF-QUIZ

1. Which one of the following modalities would best determine disease prevalence? (p. 26)
   a. Comprehensive periodontal charting
   b. Epidemiologic population surveys
   c. Patient questionnaires
   d. National dental hygiene expenditures
2. Which one of the following terms describes the rate of new cases of periodontal disease occurring in a given time period? (p. 26)
   a. Prevalence
   b. Incidence
   c. Severity
   d. Extent
   e. Index
3. An individual has been identified with advanced attachment loss at one point in time. Is it highly unlikely (infrequent) that this individual will again experience rapid attachment loss (>3 mm) within the next three years? (p. 45)
   a. The first statement is true, and the second statement is false.
   b. The first statement is false, and the second statement is true.
   c. Both statements are true.
   d. Both statements are false.
4. Which one of the following indices is best used to monitor a patient's plaque control in private dental practice? (pp. 27–30, Table 2–1)
   a. Quigley-Hein Plaque Index
   b. Plaque Record (O'Leary)

   c. Periodontal Screening and Recording (PSR) system
   d. Sulcus Bleeding Index
5. Which one of the following best measures the severity of periodontal disease in a population? (pp. 26–27)
   a. Radiographs
   b. Intraoral cameras
   c. Indices
   d. Surgical costs
6. All of the following are potential risk factors for periodontal disease except one. Which one is the exception? (pp. 45–47)
   a. Age
   b. Smoking
   c. Diabetes
   d. Oral cleanliness
7. A risk indicator differs from a risk factor in that there is no causal relationship of the associated characteristic with the disease. Low income and less education are risk indicators for periodontal disease. (p. 45)
   a. The first statement is true, and the second statement is false.
   b. The first statement is false, and the second statement is true.
   c. Both statements are true.
   d. Both statements are false.
8. According to recent surveys, which of the following percentages of the U.S. adult population has severe periodontal disease (advanced periodontitis)? (pp. 42–44)
   a. 5–20
   b. 40–50
   c. 70–80
   d. 90–100
9. Which one of the following describes how has the prevalence of gingivitis changed over the past thirty years? (pp. 42–43)
   a. Increased
   b. Decreased
   c. Remained the same
   d. Increased in the first ten years and then decreased
10. Which one of the following describes the prevalence of aggressive periodontitis in the general population? (p. 44)
    a. Rare
    b. Frequent
    c. Universal
    d. Nonexistent

REFERENCES

Ainamo, J., D. Barmes, G. Beargie, T. Cutress, and J. Martin. 1982. Development of the World Health Organization (WHO) Community Periodontal Index of Treatment Needs (CPITN). *Int. Dent. J.* 32:281–291.

American Academy of Periodontology. 2005. Epidemiology of periodontal diseases. Position Paper.

American Academy of Periodontology. 2005. Implications of genetic technology for the management of periodontal diseases. *J. Periodontol.* 76:850–857.

Ayers, C., A. Abrama, and L. Lausten. 1979. Oral health assessment of inner city preschoolers. *Dent. Hygiene* 53:465–468.

Baelum, V., F. Manji, O. Fejerskov, and P. Wanzala. 1993. Validity of CPITN's assumptions of hierarchical occurrence of periodontal conditions in a Kenyan population aged 15–65 years. *Commun. Dent. Oral Epidemiol.* 21:347–353.

Baelum, V., F. Manji, P. Wanzala, and O. Fejerskov. 1995. Relationship between CPITN and periodontal attachment loss findings in an adult population. *J. Clin. Periodontol.* 22:146–152.

Bakdash, B. 1994. Oral hygiene and compliance as risk factors in periodontitis. *J. Periodontol.* 65:539–544.

Beck, J., G. Koch, and S. Offenbacher. 1994. Attachment loss trend over 3 years in community-dwelling older adults. *J. Periodontol.* 65:737–743.

Beck, J., G. Koch, and S. Offenbacher. 1995. Incidence of attachment loss over 3 years in older adults: New and progressing lesions. *Commun. Dent. Oral Epidemiol.* 23:291–296.

Bergström, J., and S. Eliasson. 1987. Cigarette smoking and alveolar bone height in subjects with high standard oral hygiene. *J. Clin. Periodontol.* 14:466–469.

Bergström, J., and B. Floderus-Myrhed. 1983. Co-twin study of the relationship between smoking and some periodontal disease factors. *Commun. Dent. Oral Epidemiol.* 11:113–116.

Bolin, A., G. Eklund, L. Frithiof, and S. Lavstedt. 1993. The effect of changed smoking habits on marginal alveolar bone loss: A longitudinal study. *Swed. Dent. J.* 17:211–216.

Borrell, L. N., B. A. Burt, and G. W. Taylor. 2005. Prevalence and trends in periodontitis in the USA: From the NHANES III to the NHANES. *J. Dent. Res.* 84(10):924–930.

Brown, L., J. Brunelle, and A. Kingman. 1996. Periodontal status in the United States, 1988–91: Prevalence, extent, and demographic variation. *J. Dent. Res.* 75 (spec issue): 672–683.

Brown, L., R. Oliver, and H. Löe. 1989. Periodontal diseases in the U.S. in 1981: Prevalence, severity, extent and role in tooth mortality. *J. Periodontol.* 60:363–371.

Brown, L., R. Oliver, and H. Löe. 1990. Evaluating periodontal status of U.S. employed adults. *J. Am. Dent. Assoc.* 121: 226–232.

Burt, B. 1996. Epidemiology of periodontal diseases. *J. Periodontol.* 67:935–945.

Burt, B., A. Ismail, and S. Eklund. 1985. Periodontal disease, tooth loss and oral hygiene among older Americans. *Commun. Dent. Oral Epidemiol.* 13(2):93–96.

Capilouto, M., and C. Douglass. 1988. Trends in the prevalence and severity of periodontal disease in the U.S.: A public health problem? *J. Public Health Dent.* 48:245–251.

Caton, J., and A. Polson. 1985. The Interdental Bleeding Index: A simplified procedure for monitoring gingival health. *Comp. Cont. Educ. Dent.* 6:88–92.

Costa, F. O., L. O. M., Costa, J. E. Costa, and I. A. Pordeus. 2007. Periodontal disease progression among young subjects with no preventive dental care: A 52-month follow-up study. *J. Periodontol.* 78:198–203.

Fischman, S. 1986. Current status of indices of plaque. *J. Clin. Periodontol.* 13:371–374.

Fletcher, R. W., and S. W. Fletcher. 2005. Risk: Looking forward. In: eds. R. W. Fletcher and S. W. Fletcher, *Clinical epidemiology. The essentials,* 4th ed., 75–90. Hagerstown, Maryland: Lippincott, Williams and Wilkins.

Greene, J. 1967. The Oral Hygiene Index. Development and uses. *J. Periodontol.* 38:625–637.

Greene, J., and J. Vermillion. 1964. The Simplified Oral Hygiene Index. *J. Am. Dent. Assoc.* 68:7–13.

Hunt, R., and S. Fann. 1991. Effect of examining half the teeth in a partial periodontal recording of older adults. *J. Dent. Res.* 70:1380–1385.

Ismail, A., B. Burt, and S. Eklund. 1983. Epidemiologic patterns of smoking and periodontal disease in the United States. *J. Am. Dent. Assoc.* 106:617–621.

Ismail, A., E. Morrison, B. Burt, R. Cafesse, and M. Kavanaugh. 1990. Natural history of periodontal disease in adults: Findings from the Tecumseh Periodontal Disease Study, 1959–1987. *J. Dent. Res.* 69(2):430–435.

Listgarten, M., C. Schifter, and L. Laster. 1985. Three-year longitudinal study of the periodontal status of an adult population with gingivitis. *J. Clin. Periodontol.* 12:225–238.

Lobene, R., T. Weatherford, N. Ross, R. Lam, and L. Menaker. 1986. A modified gingival index for use in clinical trials. *Clin. Prev. Dent.* 8(1):3–6.

Löe, H. 1967. The gingival index, the plaque index, and the retention index. Systems (Part II). *J. Periodontol.* 38: 610–616.

Löe, H., A. Anerud, H. Boysen, and E. Morrison. 1986. Natural history of periodontal disease in man: Rapid, moderate and no loss of attachment in Sri Lankan laborers 14–46 years of age. *J. Clin. Periodontol.* 13:431–446.

Löe, H., A. Anerud, H. Boysen, and M. Smith. 1978. The natural history of periodontal disease in man: The rate of periodontal destruction before 40 years of age. *J. Periodontol.* 49(12):607–620.

Löe, H., and L. Brown. 1991. Early-onset periodontitis in the United States of America. *J. Periodontol.* 62: 608–616.

Miller S. C. 1950. *Textbook of periodontia,* 3rd ed., 125. Philadelphia: Blakiston.

Miller, A., J. Brunelle, J. Carlos, L. J. Brown, and H. Löe. 1987. *Oral health of United States adults. National findings*

1985–1986. Bethesda, MD: U.S. Public Health Service, U.S. Dept. of Health and Human Services.

Mühlemann, H. R., and S. Son. 1971. Gingival sulcus bleeding: A leading symptom in initial gingivitis. *Helv. Odont. Acta* 15:107–113.

O'Leary, T. J., R. Drake, and J. Naylor. 1972. The Plaque Control Record. *J. Periodontol.* 43(1):38.

Oliver, R., L. Brown, and H. Löe. 1998. Periodontal disease in the United States population. *J. Periodontol.* 69:269–278.

Oliver, R., and T. Tervonen. 1994. Diabetes: A risk factor for periodontitis in adults. *J. Periodontol.* 65:530–538.

Papapanou, P. 1996. *Annals of periodontology, section 1A: Periodontal diseases: Epidemiology.* 1996 World Workshop in Periodontics, Lansdowne, VA.

Russell, A. L. 1967. The Periodontal Index. *J. Periodontol.* 38:585–591.

Seppälä, B., M. Seppälä, and J. Ainamo. 1993. A longitudinal study on insulin-dependent diabetes mellitus and periodontal disease. *J. Clin. Periodontol.* 20:161–165.

Sheiham, A., and D. Striffler. 1970. A comparison of four epidemiological methods of assessing periodontal disease: I. Population findings. *J. Periodont. Res.* 5:148–154.

Silness, J., and H. Löe. 1964. Periodontal disease in pregnancy: II. Correlation between oral hygiene and periodontal condition. *Acta Odontol. Scand.* 22:121–135.

Stamm, J. 1986. Epidemiology of gingivitis. *J. Clin. Periodontol.* 13:360–366.

Taylor, G. W., B. A. Burt, M. P. Becker, R. J. Genco, M. Schlossman, et al. 1998. Non-insulin-dependent diabetes and the progression of bone loss over a two-year period. *J. Periodontol.* 68:76–83.

Turesky, S., N. Gilmore, and I. Glickman. 1970. Reduced plaque formation by the chloromethyl analogue of vitamine C. *J. Periodontol.* 41:41–43.

U.S. Public Health Service, NIDR. 1987. *Oral health in United States adults: National findings* (NIH Publication No. 87-2868), pp. 1–168. Bethesda, MD: National Institute of Health, NIDR.

Volpe, A., L. Kupczak, and W. King. 1967. In vivo calculus assessment: III. Scoring techniques, rate of calculus formation, partial mouth exams versus full mouth exams, and intra-examiner reproducibility. *Periodontics* 5:184–193.

Volpe, A., J. H. Manhold, and S. P. Hazen. 1965. In vivo calculus assessment: I. A method and its examiner reproducibility. *J. Periodontol.* 36:292–298.

Waerhaug, J. 1966. Epidemiology of periodontal disease: A review of literature. In *World workshop in periodontics,* 179–212. Ann Arbor: University of Michigan.

Williams, R.C., and S. Offenbacher. 2000. Periodontal medicine: The emergence of a new branch of periodontology. *Periodontol 2000* 23(1): 9–12.

Chapter 3

Dental Biofilms: Microbiology of Periodontal Diseases

Raymond A. Yukna

John D. Mason

OUTLINE
Primary Etiology: Bacteria and Their Products
Periodontal Diseases: The Future
Dental Hygiene Notes
Key Points
Self-Quiz
References

GOAL: To introduce the concept of dental biofilms as one of the primary risk factors for periodontal diseases.

EDUCATIONAL OBJECTIVES

Upon completion of this chapter, the reader should be able to:

- Describe dental plaque (biofilm) formation as well as its composition in the supra- and subgingival environment.
- Describe the features of subgingival biofilms.
- Describe the bacteria associated with the periodontal diseases.
- Describe the relationship between the mechanisms of bacterial action and host responses in the initiation and progression of periodontal diseases.

KEY WORDS

acquired pellile 55	dental plaque 52
asaccharolytic 53	lipooligosaccharide 61
adhesins 56	microorganisms 52
biofilm 52	saccharolytic 53
cytotoxic agents 61	

INTRODUCTION

Inflammatory periodontal diseases are not a single entity and are not caused by a single causative factor. As mentioned in Chapter 2, risk factors may not be causal, but they are used to predict the occurrence or predisposition of a disease. So, the term "risk factors" mentioned throughout this textbook are actually referring to factors that may predispose an individual to periodontal disease but are not an actual cause of the disease. In this context the term "marker" may be a better term than risk factor. Risk factors or markers are important to identify so that oral disease can be prevented if the risk factor is modifiable. For example, it is accepted that dental biofilms cause gingivitis and so are considered a marker for gingivitis. A major triad of etiologic and risk factors (or markers) exists in affecting periodontal health (Box 3–1) (Page, Offenbacher, Schroeder, Seymour, & Kornman, 1997): (1) local factors—environmental forces that predispose to inflammatory periodontal diseases; (2) systemic factors—those medical conditions that predispose to inflammatory periodontal diseases; and (3) host factors—the influences of one's own body (e.g., individual susceptibility to disease).

PRIMARY ETIOLOGY: BACTERIA AND THEIR PRODUCTS

Inflammatory periodontal diseases are initiated and progress as the result of the accumulation of **dental plaque (biofilm)** in the area of the gingival sulcus (Figure 3–1 ■). Dental plaque is defined as a dense, nonmineral-ized, complex mass of bacterial colonies living in a gel-like intermicrobial matrix. **Microorganisms,** in addition to bacteria, can live in this mass, including yeasts and viruses. Other constituents of dental biofilms include cells of various types.

The degree of tissue damage is dependent on the interaction between plaque bacteria and host defense mechanisms. Local contributing factors (e.g., calculus) may encourage the accumulation of dental biofilms, and systemic and local modifying factors may alter the host response to the bacterial challenge. However, if dental plaque is regularly removed and not allowed to accumulate, then gingival health can be maintained, in spite of other factors.

Bacterial Factors

Dental biofilm is the major etiologic or risk factor in the initiation and progression of inflammatory periodontal diseases. Löe, Theilade, and Jensen (1965) provided the first direct scientific evidence of the causal relationship between plaque and gingival inflammation. In this classic "experimental gingivitis model" study, when subjects with excellent gingival health and little plaque did not perform oral hygiene procedures for 21 days, plaque accummulation increased and gingivitis developed. Resuming good oral hygiene eliminated dental plaque, resolved gingival inflammation, and restored gingival health. Many other studies have since demonstrated a similar strong positive association between plaque accumulation and the presence of gingivitis.

(a)

(b)

■ **FIGURE 3–1** Clinical cases of healthy gingiva and inflamed gingiva: (a) healthy gingiva with good color, contour, and texture; (b) inflamed gingiva with bluish red color, puffiness, and altered contour due to dental plaque accumulation.

Box 3–1 **Risk Factors (Markers) and Indicators for Periodontal Diseases**

- Poor oral hygiene
- Tobacco smoking
- Genetics/heredity
- Advancing age
- Stress
- Past history of periodontitis
- Systemic diseases
- Male gender
- Compromised host defense
- Race, ethnicity
- Regularity of dental care
- Interleukin-1 production

Dental Biofilms

Dental plaque has all of the characteristics of a biofilm. Dental biofilms are defined as matrix-enclosed bacterial populations adherent to each other and/or to surfaces or interfaces (Costerton et al., 1994). Microorganisms in biofilms are not evenly distributed and are arranged in microcolonies surrounded by an intermicrobial matrix, which serves as a protective barrier to protect the bacteria in the biofilm from systemically and locally applied antimicrobials. Currently, the only way to remove dental biofilms is mechanically with tooth brushing or scaling/root planing; however, once it is removed, it quickly reforms. Bacteria in the film communicate with one another, build intricate intertwined structures, and even have a primitive circulatory system. Biofilms contain multiple microenvironments that vary greatly in pH, oxygen tension, and availability of specific nutrients. Subgingival dental biofilms have some loosely attached and unattached bacteria on their surface that contact the adjacent epithelium of the pockets. Microorganisms in biofilms are resistant to antibiotics and antimicrobials unless the biofilms are mechanically disrupted.

Did You Know?

A biofilm is a complex aggregation of microorganisms marked by the excretion of a protective and adhesive matrix. Biofilms are found everywhere, not only in the mouth. Biofilms are also found on solid material submerged in or exposed to an aqueous solution. For example, biofilms grow in hot, acidic pools in Yellowstone National Park and on glaciers in Antartica.

Morphology/Types

Over 700 kinds of bacteria present in biofilms normally inhabit the oral cavity, but only about twenty species (< 10%) are considered to be pathogenic for periodontal diseases (Fine, 1995; Moore & Moore, 1994; see Table 3–1 ■). The rest constitute normal oral biota. The mere presence of one or more pathogenic species is not necessarily associated with progressing disease. Both protective host factors and interactions among the components of the dental plaque limit their pathogenicity. For individual species or groups of bacteria to be considered important in the etiology of periodontal diseases, the following criteria are considered important:

- They are found in high numbers in advancing lesions or sites, and in relatively low numbers at healthy or nonprogressing sites.
- Clinical healing occurs with elimination of the pathogen.
- They are present prior to clinical changes becoming evident.
- They create a tissue reaction.
- They can be shown to produce disease in experimental animal or human studies.

Bacteria present in the oral cavity come in a wide variety of shapes from round coccoid forms to simple, short rods to complicated corkscrew shapes. Both Gram-positive (cell wall intact) and Gram-negative (permeable cell wall) forms are present. Some are oxygen using (aerobic), and some cannot tolerate any oxygen (anaerobic), with many forms being somewhat in between (facultative aerobic, microaerophilic, or facultative anaerobic). Within each category are both motile and nonmotile forms. Some bacteria utilize carbohydrates as food (**saccharolytic**), while others prefer proteins obtained in part from the tissue destruction they cause as a substrate (**asaccharolytic**). Some bacteria, such as spirochetes, do not readily fit any of these categories. In general terms, health-associated bacteria are Gram-positive, aerobic, saccharolytic, and nonmotile, while disease-associated bacteria tend to be Gram-negative, anaerobic, asaccharolytic, and motile (Table 3–2 ■).

The right combination of bacteria must be present in sufficient numbers to produce periodontal diseases. The presence of beneficial or good bacteria may modify the effects of known pathogens, thereby reducing the likelihood of disease progression. The presence of a single pathogen does not indicate active disease.

Table 3–1	Specific Bacteria Associated with Periodontal Diseases
Strong Evidence for Etiology	**Primary Association**
Actinobacillus actinomycetemcomitans	Aggressive periodontitis (also in chronic periodontitis and refractory periodontitis)
Porphyromonas gingivalis	Chronic periodontitis
Tannerella forsythensis	Chronic periodontitis
Moderate Evidence for Etiology	
Campylobacter rectus	Aggressive periodontitis, refractory periodontitis
Eikenella corrodens	Chronic periodontitis
Eubacterium nodatum	Chronic periodontitis
Fusobacterium nucleatum	Chronic periodontitis
Prevotella intermedia	Pregnancy gingivitis, puberty gingivitis, necrotizing ulcerative periodontal diseases
Peptostreptococcus micros	Refractory periodontitis
Capnocytophaga species	Aggressive, localized periodontitis
Treponema denticola	Chronic periodontitis, necrotizing ulcerative periodontal diseases
Streptococcus intermedius-complex	Gingivitis
Actinomyces species	Gingivitis
Fusobacterium species	Gingivitis

In health, the primary bacteria that live in the oral cavity are *Streptococcus sanguis, Streptococcus mitis, Veillonella* sp., *Actinomyces naeslundii,* and *Actinomyces viscosus.* In gingivitis there are increased numbers of all of the bacteria seen in health, especially *Prevotella intermedia* and spirochetes. Table 3–1 lists specific bacteria associated with various forms of periodontal diseases. In periodontitis other bacteria proliferate, including

Table 3–2	Health and Disease Associated Bacterial Characteristics	
Health	**Disease**
Gram-positive	Gram-negative
Aerobic	Anaerobic
Nonmotile	Motile
Saccharolytic	Assaccharolytic

Actinobacillus actinomycetemcomitans, Tannerella forsythensis (Honma et al. 2007), *Porphyromonas gingivalis, Capnocytophaga ochraceus,* and *Eikenella corrodens* (Table 3–3 ■). *Porphyromonas gingivalis, Tannerella forsythensis,* and *Treponema denticola* are found primarily at the later stages of plaque development. *Tannerella forsythensis* used to be called *Bacteroides forsythsus.* Name changes occur throughout the field of microbiology because of reclassification based upon molecular methods that are based on identification and characterization of certain molecules and gene sequences of a pathogen's genetic makeup.

There is an association between subgingival bacterial species. There is a specific subgingival microbial complex that is associated with early colonizers and late colonizers. Figure 3–2 ■ is a diagram showing the association among subgingival species. The left side (blue, yellow, and green circles) is early bacterial colonizers on the tooth surface, while the red circles (to the right) are more dominant at late stages in plaque development. The

Table 3–3	Nomenclature of Common Periodontal Microorganisms	

Gram-Positive Bacteria	*Gram-Negative Bacteria*
Gram-positive facultative cocci	**Gram-negative facultative rods**
Streptococcus sanguis, mitis, and *salivarius*	*Eikenella corrodens*
Gram-positive anaerobic cocci	*Capnocytophaga ochracea*
Peptostreptococcus micros	*Actinobacillus actinomycetemcomitans¶*
Gram-positive facultative rods	**Gram-negative obligate anaerobic rods**
Actinomyces viscosus, israelii, and *naeslundii*	*Porphyromonas gingivalis*
Corynebacterium matruchotii	*Prevotella intermedia*
Gram-positive obligate anaerobic rods	*Tannerella forsythensis**
Eubacterium lentum	*Fusobacterium nucleatum*
Yeasts	**Gram-negative obligate anaerobic cocci**
Candida albicans	*Veillonella alcalescens*
	Gram-negative anaerobic spirochetes
	Treponema denticola

¶ Proposed name change for *Actinobacillus actinomycetemcomitans* is *Aggregatibacter actinomycetemcomitans.* Not yet changed. See Norskov-Lauritsen & Kilian, 2006.

*In 2002 Sakamoto et al. (Sakamoto et al. 2002) proposed a new genus for *Bacteroides forsythus.* This new genus is *Tannerella* and the species is *Tannerella forsythensis (*Tanner & Izard, 2006).

orange complex (middle) becomes more dominant and bridges the early and later colonizers.

Actinobacillus actinomycetemcomitans, a Gram-negative bacteria, has been linked to the initiation, progression, and recurrence of disease in localized aggressive periodontitis and chronic periodontitis, as well as being isolated from patients with endocarditis (Fine et al., 2006).

Did You Know?

Bacteria are used to make cheese, milk, sourdough bread, and yogurt.

Microorganisms of Dental Biofilms

The types of microorganisms found in dental biofilms vary among individuals and sites within the mouth. Based upon the surface of the tooth in relationship to the gingival margin, dental biofilms can be identified as supragingival or subgingival.

Supragingival Plaque

The sequence of events involved in the formation of deposits on teeth starts with the deposition of a pellicle, also called salivary or **acquired pellicle.** When the tooth erupts, it has the organic coating of the enamel cuticle. This is lost early due to abrasion or digestion from bacteria. Within seconds after the saliva contacts the natural tooth, a coating of salivary glycoproteins forms on the tooth as an amorphous, tenacious membrane. The pellicle is thought to be acellular in that bacteria are not needed for its formation. The pellicle allows and encour-

 Rapid Dental Hint

Some bacteria, such as *Actinobacillus actinomycetemcomitans* and *Porphyromonas gingivalis,* don't just stay in the pocket area but invade into underlying gingival connective tissue. Thus, systemic antibiotics are necessary to eliminate them. This problem is seen in patients with aggressive periodontitis.

SUBGINGIVAL MICROBIAL COMPLEXES

Actinomyces species

V. parvula
A. odontolyticus

S. mitis
S. oralis
S. sanguis

Streptococcus sp.
S. gordonii
S. intermedius

C. gracilis

C. rectus

S. constellatus

P. intermedia
P. nigrescens
P. micros
F. nuc. vincentii
F. nuc. nucleatum
F. nuc. polymorphum
F. periodonticum

E. nodatum

P. gingivalis
B. forsythus
T. denticola

C. showae

E. corrodens
C. gingivalis
C. sputigena
C. ochracea
C. concisus
A. actino. a

A. actino. b

S. noxia

N subjects = 185
N samples = 13,261
Cluster analyses
Community ordination

■ **FIGURE 3–2**   Diagram of the association among subgingival species. The complexes to the left are comprised of species thought to colonize the tooth surface and proliferate at an early stage. The orange complex becomes numerically more dominant later and is thought to bridge the early colonizers and the red complex species, which become numerically more dominant at late stages in plaque development. (From Lindheard Karing. *Microbiology of Periodontal Disease.* Copenhagen: Munksgaard.)

ages the colonization of bacteria on the tooth surface, and therefore it participates in plaque formation. Adsorption of bacteria to the pellicle is important since the pellicle is formed from glycoproteins that bind selectively to the tooth, and not all of the bacteria available in the saliva can attach to the pellicle. The pellicle can form on the surface of the tooth as a surface pellicle, or it can adhere in fingerlike projections to the millions of imperfections of the enamel or areas of demineralization. This pellicle

is called subsurface pellicle. Subsurface pellicle is significant because it connects the protein of the pellicle with the protein of the component of the enamel. The pellicle can be removed during prophylaxis but begins to reform within minutes. The formation is complete in 2 hours.

Bacteria adhere to the tooth surface via molecules called **adhesins** located on the bacterial cell surface. Adhesins that are proteins and those that recognize carbohydrate structures are called **lectins.** These adhesins, or lectins, recognize and then link to specific carbohydrate structures in the glycoproteins of the pellicle.

Dental Biofilm Formation   Dental biofilm formation begins as the bacteria adhere to the pellicle and

---

Did You Know?

Name change of *Bacteriodes forsythus* to *Tanneralla forsythensis:* Change of name is in accordance with the first Principle of the *International Code of Nomenclature of Bacteria,* which aims at the stability of names to reduce the possibility of errors or confusion.

Did You Know?

Scientists estimate that bacteria produce nearly half the oxygen found in the atmosphere.

Rapid Dental Hint

Actinobacillus actinomycetemcomitans is an oral bacterium that causes localized aggressive periodontitis.

begin to colonize. The pellicle serves as a nutrient source for the bacteria. As the salivary proteins are metabolized, they release peptides and amino acids.

The general pattern of bacterial succession in supragingival plaque is coccoid forms followed by short rods followed by larger rods and then motile forms including spirochetes. The majority of these bacteria are Gram-positive and aerobic (living entirely in an oxygen environment); however, most aerobic bacteria do not survive on total oxygen but rather are considered facultative, living with or without oxygen. Then a shift toward increased numbers of Gram-negative microorganisms and more motile forms occurs. Supragingival plaque is usually detected by visual inspection of the teeth, with or without disclosing solution (Figure 3–3 ■).

When a tooth begins to erupt, it is exposed to saliva, which contains all the acquired bacteria. At this point, the formation of dental plaque begins (Newman & Listgarten, 1999). The initial plaque formation is characterized by the numbers and kinds of bacteria that colonize the pellicle. Phase I, or initiation, begins in one to two days of plaque accumulation with no removal techniques. The microorganisms form as individual clones that extend both laterally and perpendicularly from the tooth surface to form parallel, palisading layers of bacteria (Fine, 1995; Figure 3–4 ■). The first colonies of bacteria are Gram-positive cocci and short rods, including *Streptococcus mutans* and *Streptococcus sanguis*.

In the oral cavity, streptococci and *Actinomyces* form a essential component of the indigenous microbiota, being among initial colonizers in polymicrobial biofilms. The significance of *Actinomyces* is based on the ability to adhere to surfaces such as on teeth and to co-aggregate with other bacteria.

Rapid Dental Hint

Remember that the names of two bacteria have been changed. *Actinobacillus actinomycetemcomitans* and *Bacteriodes forsythus* are now *Tannerella forsythensis*.

■ **FIGURE 3–3**   Clinical picture of supragingival plaque on teeth made more evident with disclosant.

Phase II begins in two to four days after abstaining from daily toothbrushing or leaving individual areas undisturbed. The early plaque masses provide the base for the next phase of colonies to infiltrate. The next bacteria to form are Gram-positive rods and Gram-negative cocci. The space between the layers of the first plaque provides an anaerobic environment for the arrival of anaerobic and facultative anaerobic (living with or without oxygen) bacteria. The cocci still dominate the plaque; however, filamentous forms and slender rods compete for the space (Fine, 1995; see Figure 3–4).

The matrix begins to form around the bacterial colonies derived mainly from salivary material, exudates (e.g., gingival crevicular fluid), and intermicrobial substances. Bacteria can form extracellular polysaccharides (carbohydrates) from sucrose. These glucans, levans, and fructans are significant to the adhesion process, and their insolubility increases the plaque resistance to removal. The levans and soluble glucans are an energy source for bacteria.

Days 4 to 7 mark Phase III of plaque formation with an increase in the filamentous bacteria. The rods, filaments, and fusobacteria commingle and interact with each other as nonmotile bacteria move with motile bacteria around the gingival margins. As the plaque matures, vibrios and spirochetes can colonize. New plaque may lie on the surface of mature plaque or spread coronally at the margin. This new plaque is characterized by cocci as before. The filaments at the edge of the plaque serve as binding sites for these cocci, and a corncob formation appears (Listgarten, Mayo, & Tremblay, 1975; Figure 3–5 ■). Gram-positive facultative filaments such as

Plaque Formation: Phase I

Clinical Thin continuous band at gingival margin with a clear zone

Histological Palisading layers of Gram + bacteria; clonal expansion lateral, perpendicular to tooth

Plaque Formation: Phase II

Clinical Zone obliterated; marginal band thicker

Histological Gram + rods and Gram − species; anaerobes begin to occupy interstices

Plaque Formation: Phase III

4 to 7 days

Clinical Plaque extends coronally, thickens; PMNs increase in crevice

Histological Gram + rods and palisades obliterated; difficult to distinguish rows

7 to 11 days

Clinical Inflammation at subclinical level; PMNs, enlargement of gingiva

Histological Bacteria migrate subgingival; move toward chemoattractants; others piggyback apically by coaggregation

■ **FIGURE 3–4** Illustration of different phases of plaque formation.

Enamel —

■ **FIGURE 3–5** Electron micrograph of three-week-old supragingival plaque. The central filament is attached to the enamel surface. The filaments are usually composed of *Actinomyces* sp. or *Fusobacterium nucleatum*. Corncob formations extend from the enamel surface and are usually cocci such as *Streptococcus sanguis*. (From M. Listgarten, *J. Periodontol.* 51:1–18 [1976]. Copyright 1976 by the American Academy of Periodontology. Reprinted by permission.)

Actinomyces species bind with cocci such as *Streptococcus sanguis*.

Phase III continues as the plaque continues to mature over days 7 to 11. Due to a change in the environment at the tooth surface, spirochetes continue to multiply and new species such as vibrios appear (see Figure 3–4). The host response to the plaque masses begins with early signs of inflammation observable in the gingiva. This inflammatory response is easily reversed by plaque removal.

Subgingival Biofilms

Bacteria living without oxygen are considered strict or obligate anaerobes. Anaerobic microbes thrive in the depths of subgingival biofilms. As the days progress from 14 to 21, the vibrios and spirochetes remain prevalent in the depths of the mass. The growth, accumulation, and pathogenicity of subgingival dental plaque are strongly influenced by the presence of supragingival dental plaque. Inflammation of the gingiva caused by supragingival plaque changes the relationship between the gingival margin and the tooth. In addition, swelling (edema)

┌─ **Did You Know?** ─────────────────
│ There are more microbes on your body than there are humans on the entire planet.
└──────────────────────────────────────

causes gingival enlargement, which alters the anatomic relationship between the tooth surface and the gingival margin and allows bacteria to invade the subgingival space and to form subgingival dental plaque on the root surface or adjacent to the epithelial tissue in the sulcus (Figure 3–6 ■). This newly created subgingival space, which is protected from physiologic and mechanical oral cleansing mechanisms, facilitates further bacterial multiplication. The microbiota of subgingival plaque is generally more anaerobic, more Gram-negative, more motile, and more asaccharolytic. There are also many motile organisms that are completely unattached to the plaque matrix. These microbes produce toxins, enzymes, and metabolic products that cause direct injury to the periodontium. More importantly, they act as antigens, and as the host responds to the irritant present, some destruction of the periodontal tissues occurs. Thus, elimination of subgingival plaque is critical to the prevention of periodontal diseases.

Types of Subgingival Plaque   Subgingival plaque can be separated into three types based on location: (1) tooth associated (attached), (2) tissue associated, and (3) unattached subgingival plaques. They have been identified with varying characteristics (Box 3–2; Figure 3–7 ■). *Unattached Gram-negative anaerobic microorganisms are in close proximity to the epithelium*

■ **FIGURE 3–6**   Histology of shallow pocket with plaque present.

The growth, accumulation, and pathogenicity of subgingival dental plaque are strongly influenced by the presence of supragingival dental plaque.

and appear to play an important role in the initiation and progression of periodontitis. Filaments surrounded by rods can occur, creating a test-tube or bristle-brush effect on the surface plaque (Figure 3–8 ■).

Nutrients

Nutrients from the crevicular fluid in the pocket are readily available, so bacteria that use proteins as energy sources are favored over those that require carbohydrates. For example, hemin-containing compounds found in crevicular fluid enhance the growth of *Porphyromonas* and *Prevotella* species; *Prevotella intermedia* use menadione, a by-product of estrogen metabolism. Thus, the final proportions of various bacteria found in the subgingival area are the sum of a large variety of intertwining processes.

Tissue Invasion

Several studies have shown that plaque bacteria such as *Actinobacillus actinomycetemcomitans, Porphyromonas gingivalis,* and spirochetes can be found within the tissues, including the epithelium, gingival connective tissues, and the alveolar bone (Renvert, Wikström, Dahlen, Slots, & Egelberg, 1990; Saglie, Carranza, Newman, Cheng, & Lewin, 1982). Although the bacteria seem to be present in these tissues, they have shown no evidence of local activity or multiplication, so they may be inactive in those locations. In addition, the severity of the periodontal disease and associated tooth mobility, as well as the trauma associated with tooth extraction, suggest that the bacteria may actually be pushed into the tissues,

Rapid Dental Hint

Remember, when you are probing that there are many good (beneficial) and bad (pathogenic) bacteria down in the pocket. Many of these pathogens may contribute to an individual's risk of heart disease and diabetes mellitus.

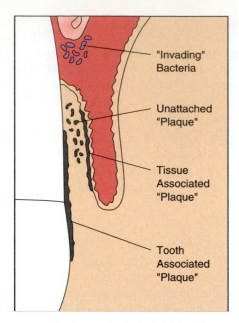

■ **FIGURE 3–7** Schematic of the three types of subgingival plaque plus the depiction of "invading" microorganisms.

■ **FIGURE 3–8** Electron micrograph of subgingival plaque. Subgingival bacteria gather to form a test-tube or bristle-brush configuration composed of Gram-negative rods (bristles) attaching to filamentous bacteria such as *Actinomyces* sp. (From M. Listgarten, *J. Periodontol.* 51:1–18 [1976]. Copyright by the Academy of Periodontology. Reprinted with permission.)

rather than invading. However, invasion of the deeper periodontal tissues by bacteria may be important to the pathogenesis of certain periodontal diseases.

Microorganisms of Dental Implants

Clinical studies have demonstrated that the microbiota of healthy, stable dental implants are similar to that of healthy teeth (Gram-positive, nonmotile, aerobic/facultative anaerobic, cocci), while implants that are unstable and failing have bacteria similar to natural teeth with periodontitis (Gram-negative , motile, anaerobic rods, spirochetes) (Nowzari et al., 2008; Rams & Link, 1983). Dental plaque must be removed around implants just as for natural teeth, but using special dental implant instruments (i.e., plastic) that will not scratch the implant.

Gram-negative anaerobes may play a role in periimplant infections, and that their elimination leads to improvement of the clinical condition (Mombelli, 1993). Gram-negative anaerobic bacteria, particularly fusobacteria, spirochetes, and black-pigmenting organisms such as *Prevotella intermedia* were often present in high proportions (Mombelli, 1993) (Table 3–4).

Other Components of Plaque

Cells

Although bacteria are the primary constituents of plaque, several types of cells are also present. Epithelial cells are found almost universally in samples of plaque in a variety of anatomic forms ranging from cells recently shed from the surface with discrete nuclei and clearly defined cell walls to what may be described as empty "ghosts" of cells filled with bacteria. White blood cells, particularly polymorphonuclear neutrophils (PMNs), are often also found in plaque. Red blood cells are commonly seen in samples taken from tooth surfaces adjacent to pockets with bleeding on probing, indicating a break in the pocket epithelial lining.

Did You Know?

There over 700 types of bacteria in the mouth!

Rapid Dental Hint

Since periodontal bacteria dislike oxygen, they move toward the inner part of the periodontal tissue, where oxygen partial pressure is low.

Other Tooth-Accumulated Materials

Several other tooth-accumulated materials (TAMs) besides dental biofilm and pellicle are found in the region of the gingival sulcus. Food debris is the most commonly found TAM. Materia alba is also a bacterial aggregation with food debris, but it differs from plaque in that it is not strongly adherent to the tooth. There is no definite architecture as with dental plaque, and it is minimally implicated in periodontal diseases. While these tooth-accumulated materials may stain with disclosant and be visible on the tooth surface, they are readily dislodged by rinsing or a water spray, unlike pellicle or dental biofilm.

Box 3–2   Types of Subgingival Dental Biofilm

Tooth Associated
- Densely packed strongly adherent to tooth surface (biofilm)
- Gram-positive rods, cocci, and filamentous bacteria
- Facultative aerobic or facultative anaerobes
- Removed by scaling and root planing
- Less virulent (limited ability to cause disease)

Tissue Associated
- Loosely packed, loosely adherent to soft tissue wall
- Gram-negative, motile, anaerobic
- Spirochetes, "bottle-brush" types
- More virulent (able to cause disease)
- Cannot be removed by scaling and root planing; needs to be surgically removed

Unattached
- Free swimming in pocket (not a biofilm)
- Gram-negative, motile, anaerobic
- Spirochetes and others
- More virulent (able to cause disease)
- Removed by flushing

Mechanisms of Bacterial Action

In order for a periodontal pathogen to cause disease, the following are essential for the bacteria to be able to colonize and multiply in the subgingival area and produce factors that either directly damage the host tissue or lead to the host tissue damaging itself (Li et al, 2004). Different combinations of indigenous (living-in-the-mouth) bacteria, rather than just a single species, produce the pathogenic potential necessary to cause progression from gingivitis to destructive periodontitis.

Once pathogenic microbiotas are established, the microorganisms appear to incite destruction of the supporting structures by both direct toxic effects on adjacent tissues and by the indirect activation of host immune and inflammatory cells.

Direct Effect

Cytotoxic Agents   The subgingival unattached dental biofilm has **cytotoxic agents** such as endotoxins, which are called **lipooligosaccharide** (LOS). Lipooligosaccharides, which are found in the cell wall of Gram-negative bacteria, can initiate inflammation, cause soft-tissue destruction, and stimulate bone resorption. Endotoxins are released from the cell wall upon death of Gram-negative bacteria. LOS is found in the cementum of untreated periodontally involved root surfaces.

Exotoxin is a toxin released by some bacteria such as *Actinobacillus actinomycetemcomitans* that can cause damage to the host by killing polymorphonuclear neutrophils.

Enzymes   Many of the bacteria present in the various dental biofilm environments of the sulcus/pocket produce a variety of enzymes, which can adversely affect the gingival and periodontal tissues. These enzymes accumulate in the sulcus and can penetrate through intact epithelium into the deeper tissues. Enyzmes function to destroy the connective tissue by breaking down collagen and ground substance. Some of the enzymes that have been identified as important products of plaque bacteria are shown in Box 3–3.

Host-Derived Enzymes   New information regarding *host-mediated* degradation (breakdown) of connective tissues has focused on the matrix metalloproteinases (MMPs) (Birkedal-Hansen, 1993). This group of structurally similar enzymes is produced by stimulated host cells and includes the collagenases, gelatinases, and stromelysins. These enzymes are responsible for cleaving the collagen molecule (the major component of connective tissue), degrading proteoglycans (part of the

> **Box 3–3 Common Enzymes That Break Down Periodontal Tissues**
>
> **Collagenase:** This degrades collagen fibers, the major-formed elements in the gingiva and periodontal ligament. It is produced by both bacteria and the host cells in the body (e.g., PMNs and fibroblasts) and is included in the family of enzymes called matrix metalloproteinases (MMPs).
>
> **Hyaluronidase:** This breaks down hyaluronic acid, an important polysaccharide (carbohydrate) that helps hold tissue and cells together. It can act as a "spreading" factor to increase tissue permeability. This enzyme is also produced both by bacteria and by the host.
>
> **Chondroitin sulfatase:** This breaks apart chondroitin sulfate, another cell- and tissue-cementing polysaccharide (carbohydrate).
>
> **Proteases:** These are a large group of enzymes that contribute to the breakdown of noncollagenous proteins (proteins in the connective tissue other than collagen) and increase capillary permeability.
>
> **Elastases:** This affects the elastin (elastic) fibers of the mucosa and blood vessels, thereby reducing tissue integrity.

ground substance) and other proteins making up the connective tissues, and causing osteoclastic bone resorption.

Indirect Effect

Immunopathologic Mechanisms Several bacterial antigens induce inflammation in the periodontal tissues by stimulating the immune response. Both the humoral (antibody-based) and the cell-mediated (lymphocyte-based) types of immune responses have been observed in patients with periodontitis. The role of the immunologic response in periodontal disease is not completely understood; however, the potential to cause tissue destruction, as well as to be protective, is apparent. Rather than always being protective, the host immune response may contribute to the tissue destruction.

Combined Mechanisms

While not truly contagious, transmission of pathogenic bacteria has been shown to occur between individuals.

Actinobacillus actinomycetemcomitans can be transmitted from parent to child and from dogs to humans (Asikainen, Chen, Alaluusua, & Slots, 1997). There is some evidence that *Porphyromonas gingivalis* is transmitted among individuals in a household, including spouses (Asikainen et al., 1997). The most common route of transmission is via saliva. It is probable that more than one mechanism is involved in the initiation and progression of gingivitis and periodontitis. It is possible that bacterial enzymes and/or cytotoxic substances exert a direct effect on the sulcular and subsulcular tissue, and at the same time initiate an indirect immune response. Therefore, there are multiple mechanisms of action of dental plaque.

PERIODONTAL DISEASES: THE FUTURE

The scenario following the accumulation of oral biofilms on tooth surfaces will continue unless treatment is started. Without treatment, the supporting structures may be destroyed. Thus, current periodontal disease is a local contributing factor for further and future periodontal disease.

Population genetic analysis of oral bacteria can reveal new insight into the molecular mechanisms of the genetic diversity that exists in the oral microflora, which may provide a better understanding of the etiology of oral diseases (Kilian et al. 2006).

DENTAL HYGIENE NOTES

Periodontal diseases have multiple risk factors. Therefore, it should not be expected that one risk factor will consistently be associated with the development of this kind of disease, and it should not be expected that control of one risk factor will completely eliminate the risk of developing the disease.

Dental biofilm is the primary etiologic factor in periodontal diseases. However, other local and systemic factors play an important role. By taking a thorough health and social history, and correlating known local and systemic risk factors with periodontal clinical findings, clinicians can make patients who are at increased risk aware of the impact of these factors and the influence the factors have on their periodontal condition. Especially when treatment is unsuccessful, reevaluation of primary and secondary risk factors might improve future treatment results.

Metabolic interactions among different bacterial cell types probably play a dominant role in the changes in community composition during plaque maturation. Communication among different bacterial communities may help with nutrient availability and oxygen removal, favoring the proliferation of specific bacterial species (Kolenbrander et al., 2006)

The *Parameters of Care* published by the American Academy of Periodontology (2000) suggest that the initial therapy for patients with periodontal inflammation should include the elimination, alteration, or control of risk factors that may contribute to chronic periodontitis. This represents significant progress since it is clear that periodontal diseases are infections initiated by bacteria and may have several associated risk factors. Management of these risk factors is likely to be the most successful approach to preventing periodontitis in the future. Physical removal of subgingival biofilms results in only a brief reduction in the numbers of colonizing bacteria. Within two to seven days the bacterial mass of dental biofilms starts to be recolonized. Some bacteria such as *Streptococcus* recolonize very rapidly, while *T. forsythensis, P. gingivalis,* and *T. denticola* return slowly after mechanical debridement (Haffejee, Teles, & Socransky, 2006).

Also, since the presence of periodontitis is recognized as a risk factor for future and more severe periodontal disease (past attachment loss is a risk factor for future attachment loss), proper diagnosis and therapy of an existing condition is very important in helping prevent future occurrences.

KEY POINTS

- Dental plaque is a biofilm.
- Currently, evidence-based dentistry supports the use of risk assessment techniques to guide clinical decisions in the treatment of periodontal diseases.
- Important risk factors for periodontal diseases include certain periodontal bacteria (plaque biofilm).
- Formation of dental biofilm begins with tooth eruption.
- Inflammatory periodontal diseases are infections caused by bacteria.
- Attempts to manage risk factors are important in the prevention and treatment of periodontal diseases.

SELF-QUIZ

1. All of the following are harmful products produced by bacteria that affect the periodontal tissues except one. Which one is the exception? (pp. 61–62)
    a. Enzymes
    b. Lipooligosaccharides
    c. Waste products
    d. Crevicular fluid
2. Which one of the following types of bacteria found in subgingival plaque is considered pathogenic for periodontitis? (pp. 54–56)
    a. *Porphyromonas gingivalis*
    b. *Actinomyces viscosis*
    c. *Streptococcus sanguis*
    d. *Corynebacterium matruchotii*
3. Which one of the following is the primary risk factor for periodontal diseases? (p. 53)
    a. Dental calculus
    b. Dental biofilms
    c. HIV/AIDS infection
    e. Systemic drugs
4. Which one of the following features makes bacteria an important risk factor for periodontal diseases? (pp. 53, 58–59)
    a. Colonize and multiply in subgingival area
    b. Irritate the epithelial lining of the pocket
    c. Break down in the epithelial cells in the gingiva
    d. Cause tissue erosion
5. Which of the following bacteria is primarily found in pregnancy gingivitis? (p. 55)
    a. *Porphyromonas gingivalis*
    b. *Streptococcus sanguis*
    c. *Prevotella intermedia*
    d. *Actinomyces viscosis*
6. Löe and coworkers proved that there is a direct relationship between dental plaque and periodontal diseases because the removal of dental plaque improves gingival health. (p. 52)
    a. Both the statement and reason are correct and related.
    b. Both the statement and reason are correct but not related.
    c. The statement is correct, but the reason is not.
    d. The statement is not correct, but the reason is correct.
    e. Neither the statement nor reason is correct.
7. From which of the following sources do subgingival bacteria receive nutrition? (pp. 58, 59)
    a. Saliva
    b. Dental calculus
    c. Crevicular fluid
    d. By-products of bacterial metabolism
    e. Endotoxins from supragingival plaque

8. Which of the following types of subgingival plaque cannot be removed with periodontal debridement? (pp. 58–60)
   a. Tooth-associated
   b. Tissue-associated
   c. Unattached
   d. Invading
9. In which of the following phases of plaque formation does supragingival bacteria migrate subgingivally? (pp. 57, 58)
   a. Phase I
   b. Phase II
   c. Phase III/4 to 7 days
   d. Phase III/7 to 11 days
10. All of the following bacteria are strongly associated with invading epithelium and gingival connective tissue except one. Which one is the exception? (p. 59)
    a. Spirochetes
    b. *Actinobacillus actinomycetemomitans*
    c. *Prevotella intermedia*
    d. *Porphyromonas gingivalis*

REFERENCES

American Academy of Periodontology. 2000. Parameters of Care. *J. Periodontol.* 71(5):847–883.

Asikainen, S., C. Chen, S. Alaluusua, and J. Slots. 1997. Can one acquire periodontal bacteria and periodontitis from a family member? *J. Am. Dent. Assoc.* 128:1263–1271.

Birkedal-Hansen, H. 1993. Role of matrix metalloproteinases in human periodontal diseases. *J. Periodontol.* 64:474–484.

Costerton, J. W., Z. Lewandowski, D. DeBeer, D. Caldwell, D. Korber, and G. James. 1994. Biofilms, the customized microniche. *J. Bacteriol.* 176:2137–2142.

Fine, D. 1995. Chemical agents to prevent and regulate plaque development. *Periodontology* 8:87–107.

Fine, D., J. B. Kaplan, S. C. Kachlany, and H. C. Schreiner. 2006. How we got attached to *Actinobacillus actinomycetemcomitans:* A model for infection diseases. *Periodontology 2000* 42(1):114–157.

Haffejee, A. D., R. P. Teles, and S. S. Socransky. 2006. The effect of periodontal therapy on the composition of the subgingival microbiota. *Periodontology 2000* 42(1):219–258.

Honma, K., S. Inagaki, K. Okuda, et al. 2007. Role of a *Tannerella forsythensis* exopolysaccharide synthesis operon in biofilm development. *Microbial Pathogenesis* 42(4):156–166.

Kilian, M., E. V. G. Frandsen, D. Haubek, and K. Poulsen. 2006. The etiology of periodontal disease revisited by population genetic analysis. *Periodontology 2000* 42(1):158–179.

Kolenbrander, P. E., R. J. Palmer., A. H. Rickard., N. S. Jakubovics, et al. 2006. Bacterial interactions and successions during plaque development. *Periodontology 2000* 42(1):47–79.

Li J., E. J. Helmerhorst, C. W. Leone, et al. 2004. Identification of early microbial colonizers in human dental biofilm. *J. of applied microbiology* 97:1311–1318.

Listgarten, M. A., H. E. Mayo, and R. Tremblay. 1975. Development of dental plaque on epoxy resin crowns in man. A light and electron microscopic study. *J. Periodontol.* 46:10–26.

Löe, H., E. Theilade, and S. Jensen. 1965. Experimental gingivitis in man. *J. Periodontol.* 49:117–187.

Mombelli, A. 1993. Microbiology of the dental implants. *Adv. Dental Res.* 7:202–206.

Moore, W. E. C., and L. V. H. Moore. 1994. The bacteria of periodontal diseases. *Periodontology 2000* 5:66–77.

Newman, H. N., and M. A. Listgarten. 1999. The development of dental plaque: From preeruptive primary cuticle to acquired pellicle to dental plaque to calculus formation. In eds. N. O. Harris and F. Garcia-Godoy, *Primary preventive dentistry,* 5th ed., 21–39. Stamford, CT: Appleton and Lange.

Norskov-Lauritsen N., and M. Kilian. 2006. Reclassification of *Actinobacillus actinomycetemcomitans, Haemophilus aphrophilus, Haemophilus paraphrophilus* and *H. segnis* as *Aggregatitbacter actinomycetemcomitansgen.* Nov., comb. Nov., *Actinobacillus aphrophilus comb.nov.* and *Actinobacillus sengis comb.nov.,* and emended description of *Actinobacillus aphrophilus to include V factor-dependent and V factor-independent isolate. Int. J. Syst. Evol. Microbiol.* 56:2135–2146.

Nowzari, H., J. E. Botero, M. Degiacomo, M. C. Villacres, and S. K. Rich. January 24, 2008. Microbiology and cytokine levels around healthy dental implants and teeth. *Clin. Implant. Dent. Relat. Res.* Online.

Page, R. C., W. Offenbacher, H. E. Schroeder, G. J. Seymour, and K. S. Kornman. 1997. Advances in the pathogenesis of periodontitis: Summary of developments, clinical implications and future directions. *Periodontology 2000* 14:216–248.

Rams, T. E., and C. C. Link, Jr. 1983. Microbiology of failing dental implants in humans: Electron microscopic observations. *J. Oral Implantol.* 11:93–100.

Renvert, S., M. Wikström, G. Dahlen, J. Slots, and J. Egelberg. 1990. On the inability of root debridement and periodontal surgery to eliminate *Actinobacillus actinomycetemcomitans* from periodontal pockets. *J. Clin. Periodontol.* 17:351–355.

Saglie, R. F., F. A. Carranza, Jr., M. G. Newman, L. Cheng, and K. J. Lewin. 1982. Identification of tissue-invading bacteria in human periodontal disease. *J. Periodontol. Res.* 17:452–455.

Sakamoto, M., M. Suzuki, M. Umeda, L. Ishikawa, and Y. Benno. 2002. Reclassification of *Bacteroides forsythus* as *Tannerella forsythensis corrig., gen. nov., comb. nov. Int. J. Syst. Evol. Microbiol.* 52(Pt 3):841–849.

Tanner A., and J. Izard. 2006. *Tannerella forsythensis,* a periodontal pathogen entering the genomic era. *Periodontolgy 2000* 42(1):88–113.

Chapter 4

Bacteria–Host Response: Inflammatory and Immunology Fundamentals

Mea A. Weinberg

GOAL: To provide an understanding of host response to the bacteria present in dental biofilms (plaque).

OUTLINE

Introduction
Periodontal Disease Activity
The Bacteria–Host Challenge
Oral Defense Mechanisms
The Inflammatory Response and the Immune Response: Host Response to the Periodontal Diseases
Dental Hygiene Notes
Key Points
Self-Quiz
References

EDUCATIONAL OBJECTIVES

Upon completion of this chapter, the reader should be able to:

- List three theories of periodontal disease activity.
- Describe the progression of gingivitis into periodontitis.
- Discuss bacterial components that stimulate the initiation of the inflammatory and immune systems.
- Describe the different levels of oral defense mechanisms.
- Describe the inflammatory/immune host responses to plaque-induced periodontal diseases.
- Describe the process of phagocytosis.
- Compare and contrast humoral immunity and cellular immunity.

KEY WORDS

antibodies 76
antigens 68
cellular immunity 75
chemotaxis 73
connective tissue attachment loss 66
complement system 74
cytokines 74
gingivitis 66
host response 67
humoral immunity 75
immunoglobulins 76
inflammatory process 69
opsonins 74
periodontitis 66
periodontal disease activity 66
phagocytosis 73
prostaglandins 71

INTRODUCTION

Gingivitis is defined as inflammation confined to the gingiva without clinical connective tissue attachment loss and bone loss. Gingivitis is a direct response of the host (body) to the accumulation of supragingival dental biofilms at the gingival margin. **Periodontitis** is defined as the loss of clinical connective tissue attachment (also referred to as clinical attachment loss) and alveolar bone loss with the formation of a periodontal pocket. **Connective tissue attachment loss** refers to the pathological detachment of collagen fibers from the cemental surfaces with the concomitant apical migration of the apical part of the junctional epithelium onto the root surface (Armitage, 1995). The events leading to clinical connective tissue attachment loss also result in the destruction of alveolar and supporting bone. The *inflammatory process* involved in the development of **gingivitis** and periodontitis is influenced by the *immune response* of the individual.

PERIODONTAL DISEASE ACTIVITY

The development of chronic inflammatory periodontal diseases involves a series of host responses or reactions of the body to bacteria present in the dental biofilm, which is considered the invader or irritant. Host cells or cells normally found in the body are needed to fight this infection. Examples of host cells include blood cells present in the body, such as macrophages, lymphocytes, and polymorphonuclear leukocytes (PMNs) or, as they are sometimes called, neutrophils. PMNs are a type of white blood cell involved in the host defense system. The host defense is constantly being called upon to ward off attacks of the microorganisms that are colonizing the oral cavity at any given time. This balance of host defense mechanisms against the microbial attack is kept in check until the microorganisms overtake the defense system, at which time infection and tissue damage develop. It is assumed that host cells mediate the destruction of soft and hard connective tissue because of the reaction to bacteria in the plaque.

    Periodontal disease activity (PDA) is defined as the *ongoing* loss of clinical connective tissue attachment and alveolar and supporting bone (Greenstein & Caton, 1990) at a certain point in time (e.g., at the clinical examination appointment). Detection of areas in the mouth that are in the active stage of destruction may be important in the implementation of treatment. However, it is

Rapid Dental Hint

It is very difficult to determine or predict that a specific periodontal site in the mouth is "breaking down" and losing attachment and bone. It has been suggested that a 2 to 3 mm change in attachment level (level of the junctinal epithelium, which is your probing depths measured from the CEJ) is required for a site to be disease active.

extremely difficult to determine at a given time if a site is actively breaking down or will break down in the future.

Rapid Dental Hint

Loss of connective tissue attachment (or loss of attachment, as it is sometimes referred to) is defined as the destruction of gingival connective tissue attachment (e.g., gingival fibers) due to disease, followed by apical migration of the junctional epithelium along the root surface.

Models of Disease Activity

Currently, three theories of periodontal disease activity have been described:

1. The continuous model theory
2. The random burst theory
3. The asynchronous multiple burst theory

    The continuous model theory is based on the concept that periodontal destruction is slow and constant until tooth loss and the severity of the disease increase with age (Löe, Anerud, Boysen, & Morrison, 1986). However, epidemiologic studies have not demonstrated whether destruction is continuous or new diseased sites actually develop (Greenstein & Caton, 1990).

    The next theory is the random burst theory (Socransky, Haffajee, Goodson, & Lindhe, 1984). This theory states that periodontal diseases progress in short bursts of exacerbation (actively losing attachment), followed by a period of remission or quiescence where there is no progressive attachment loss (Goodson, 1992; Socransky et al. 1984). Another proposed name for this theory is the episodic burst theory, which reflects the fact that periodontal diseases are site specific, and not all sites in the mouth are equally susceptible (Zimmerman, 1986).

The third concept, the asynchronous multiple burst hypothesis, states that periodontal disease activity occurs during a limited time period (e.g., acne during childhood may resolve during adulthood) followed by remission (Greenstein & Caton, 1990; Socransky et al., 1984).

In reality, all of the above theories may be interacting to explain periodontal disease progression. No one theory alone can explain the disease progression. It cannot be assumed that all sites will continuously get worse. Also, treatment should not wait until a burst of bone destruction has occurred. Periodontal destruction is cumulative over time. Since it is difficult to actually determine if a site is disease active, it is prudent to treat all inflamed sites (Greenstein & Caton, 1990).

Progression of Gingivitis into Periodontitis

Gingivitis must precede periodontitis. That is, periodontitis does not develop unless gingivitis existed previously. However, gingivitis may, but does not always, progress to periodontitis.

Why does periodontitis develop in some individuals while in others gingivitis does not progress into periodontitis? Currently, the *exact* cause for the progression of gingivitis into periodontitis is relatively unclear. Approximately 80% of the population is susceptible to periodontal diseases (Brown & Löe, 1993). Susceptibility to periodontal diseases involves changes in bacteria–host equilibrium. A failure of this equilibrium results in the

Rapid Dental Hint

Periodontitis does not develop unless gingivitis existed previously. Gingivitis may, but does not always, progress to periodontitis.

initiation of periodontal disease. However, although bacteria are essential to this process, their presence alone is not enough to cause destructive periodontal disease. There must be a decrease in the number of beneficial (good) bacteria such as *Streptococcus* sp., a critical mass of pathogenic (disease-producing) bacteria, a conducive or favorable environment to cause disease, and a susceptible host that reacts to the pathogen. Gingivitis may progress into periodontitis if the host resistance decreases and if bacteria overwhelm the defense system and penetrate soft tissue. Some reasons for a decrease in host resistance include stress, chemotherapy, local tissue trauma, uncontrolled diabetes, leukemia, steroids, and fully developed acquired immunodeficiency syndrome (AIDS).

The **host response** is in nature a defense mechanism (Kinane & Bartold 2007; Shikawa, 2007). It is a natural response of the body to protect and defend the individual after the person's body has been challenged by an injurious agent such as a bacterium or virus. This same host response that provides protection to host tissues frequently also causes host tissue destruction (Figure 4–1 ■). When the repair of tissue is greater than its destruction, the tissue starts healing. Fortunately, host tissue destruction usually is not permanent since tissues have a great capacity for healing.

Poor oral hygiene with/without contributing environmental systemic and acquired factors (a susceptible host)

↓

Accumulation of dental biofilms and other antigens at the gingival margin and in the gingival crevice; bacteria release antigenic substances through the crevice into the connective tissue

↓

Host's inflammatory and immune systems activated

↙ ↘

Protective
PMN and macrophage phagocytosis; plasma cell production of antibodies

Destructive
Prostaglandin E_2, cytokines, collagenases (matrix metalloproteinases (MMPs)) and lysosomal enzymes cause connective tissue destruction including bone destruction

■ **FIGURE 4–1** Pathway of pathogenesis showing the sequence of events leading to periodontal destruction.

THE BACTERIA–HOST CHALLENGE

Microbiology

Bacteria that colonize early on the tooth surface at the gingival margin are predominately supragingival Gram-positive facultative (i.e., can live with or without oxygen) *Streptococci* and *Actinomyces* species. If plaque is not disrupted by toothbrushing and flossing, a more established and varied microbial colony develops. With increasing time and poor plaque control, periodontitis-associated microbiota populate the subgingival pocket area, including Gram-negative anaerobes (oxygen intolerant) such as *Fusobacterium nucleatum, Porphyromonas gingivalis, Eikenella corrodens, Actinobacillus actinomycetemcomitans,* and *Prevotella intermedia* (Listgarten, 1994) (Figure 4–2 ■, 4–3 ■). In addition to the subgingival anaerobic bacteria found in the deeper subgingival plaque, the bacteria found in direct contact with the junctional epithelium may be or has the potential to become pathogenic and cause disease. Anaerobic bacteria become established as the bacteria multiply and become thicker with less oxygen available to the bacteria. The rate of subgingival plaque recolonization may depend upon supragingival plaque accumulation.

　　Bacteria, their metabolic wastes or by-products, and toxins they synthesize and release into the subgingival environment are foreign to the body and are termed **antigens.** Long-standing, chronic bacterial accumulation causes an excessive and persistent antigenic stimulus to the host response mechanisms. Thus, while bacteria initiate the disease process, it is enzymes and by-products

■ FIGURE 4–3　Dental biofilms initiate inflammation and host immunity determines the response. (Courtesy of Procter & Gamble)

produced by the host that are actually responsible for most of the breakdown of periodontal tissues. As a side effect, the reactions activated by the host response result in tissue inflammation in which surrounding cells, connective tissue, and bone are destroyed. Thus, host responses are basically protective by destroying antigens, but if the body is overwhelmed then the host responses are destructive, causing soft- and hard-tissue destruction.

Bacterial Components

Bacteria release metabolic substances proven to be toxic to cells and tissues. These stimulate the initiation of the inflammatory and immune systems. The following substances are released from bacteria that affect the host:

- Endotoxin, a lipopolysaccharide (also termed lipooligosaccaride), is part of the outer membrane of all Gram-negative bacteria. Endotoxins, which are released when the bacteria die and lyse (break apart), stimulate biologic activities that cause tissue damage and bone destruction (Figure 4–4 ■).
- Leukotoxin, an exotoxin produced by *Actinobacillus actinomycetemcomitans,* can kill PMNs.
- Bacteria synthesize and release various waste products (by-products) such as ammonia, which is toxic to many host cells, and hydrogen sulfide, which increases the permeability of the epithelium so that antigenic substances can more easily enter the lamina propria.
- Bacteria synthesize and secrete enzymes, which can break down tissue. Hyaluronidase, an enzyme found in periodontal pockets, may break down or

■ FIGURE 4–2　Gram-negative microorganisms live in the subgingival pocket environment and are no longer subjected to normal oral hygiene procedures.

■ **FIGURE 4–4**   Endotoxins amplify the inflammatory process. (Courtesy of Procter & Gamble)

degrade the "cementing substance" between epithelial cells, causing widening of the intercellular spaces and increased permeability.

Matrix metalloproteinases (MMPs) are a family of enzymes that cleave or break down the components of the extracellular matrix. This family of enzymes includes more than twenty-five members that are divided into collagenases (MMP 1,8,13), gelatinases (MMP 2,9), stromelysins (MMP 3, 10), matrilysins (MMP 7, 26), and membrane-type MMPs (MMP 14-17, 24) (Birkedal-Hansen, 1993). Collagenase may break down collagen, and proteases degrade the connective tissue ground substance. Host cells such as PMNs and fibroblasts also secrete collagenase. Thus, these enzymes that bacteria and host cells synthesize and release prepare the tissues for absorption of toxic and otherwise harmful bacterial products.

ORAL DEFENSE MECHANISMS

The host interacts with microorganisms at three different areas in the periodontium:

1. The supragingival environment
2. The gingival crevice
3. The gingival connective tissue

Rapid Dental Hint

Host responses are basically protective by destroying antigens. If the body is overwhelmed then the host responses are destructive, causing soft- and hard-tissue destruction.

The first attempt at self-protection comes from the supragingival environment and involves nonspecific defenses. These responses are important in the prevention of the extension of supragingival plaque into the subgingival area (the gingival crevice). Defense mechanisms include the following:

- Saliva, which contains numerous defensive substances such as antibacterial factors (lysozyme, lactoferrin, lactoperoxidase, myeloperoxidase) and antibodies (secretory immunoglobulin A [sIgA]). Antibodies called immunoglobulins are proteins present in the blood serum and mucosal secretions (e.g., saliva, tears, sweat, nasal fluids) produced following interaction with an antigen.
- Gingival crevicular fluid (GCF) functions as an outward flow cleansing the sulcus. The increased volume of GCF produced during the **inflammatory process** also serves to deliver more antimicrobial products from the deeper tissue toward the main site of supragingival bacterial colonization (e.g., tooth surface). These are the first substances to interact with the antigenic challenge (bacteria) to try to neutralize, isolate, or kill it.
- Oral epithelium also serves to prevent bacteria and their by-products from entering the underlying tissues. This is attained by the surface keratin and the close attachment of the epithelial cells.
- Shedding of epithelial cells from the oral mucosa into the oral cavity.

Did You Know?

A person cannot taste food unless it is mixed with saliva.

THE INFLAMMATORY RESPONSE AND THE IMMUNE RESPONSE: HOST RESPONSE TO THE PERIODONTAL DISEASES

If the body is unsuccessful in eliminating the pathogenic bacteria at the supragingival level, the inflammatory/immune response, working together, is further stimulated to eliminate the irritant and prevent the spread of infection. This system is activated when antigens (e.g., endotoxins, bacterial enzymes, and by-products) present in the plaque mass in the gingival crevice pass through the

Rapid Dental Hint

Many substances or markers for periodontal disease are found in GCF, including collagenase, β-glucuronidase, and prostaglandinE₂.

protective wall of PMNs (leukocyte wall) interposed between the plaque mass and the lining of the gingival crevice and junctional epithelium. After the antigens cross the junctional epithelial barrier, the deeper tissues are penetrated (Miyasaki, 1991; see Figure 4–5 ■). Only a few bacteria themselves actually enter the connective tissue. Usually, it is the products from the bacteria that enter the tissues while the bacteria remain in the crevice. However, it has been demonstrated that *Actinobacillus actinomycetemcomitans, Porphyromonas* gingivalis, and spirochetes invade connective tissue (de Graaf, van Winkelhoff, & Goené, 1989; Renvert, Winström, Dahlén, Slots, & Egelberg, 1990; Saglie, Carranza, Newman, Cheng, & Lewin, 1982). Activation of the inflammatory/immune system results in the following: (1) elimination or retardation of the invader (bacteria); (2) the limiting of further tissue destruction; and (3) the beginning of healing.

The Inflammatory Response

The inflammatory response to a bacterial challenge is a nonspecific reaction intended to prevent the spread of invading bacteria and, if possible, to destroy the damaging agent. This is accomplished through the process of inflammation.

   When bacteria cause irritation to the gingival or periodontal tissues, a series of responses mediated by host defense cells is initiated. First, an acute inflammatory response occurs. Box 4–1 lists the cells involved in the inflammatory response (Van Dyke, 2007). If this is ineffective—the stimulus is not removed and healing does not occur—inflammation becomes chronic and additional defense cells from the immune system become involved. After the events in the periodontal areas subside, the tissues are cleansed, repaired, and rebuilt. Unfortunately, sometimes the damage to some of these tissues is permanent and is present even after the infection is eliminated.

Elements of the Inflammatory System

A clinically healthy gingiva that is relatively plaque-free is characterized by a salmon pink color, firm consistency,

■ FIGURE 4–5   As the protective wall of neutrophils between the plaque mass and the gingival crevice and junctional epithelium becomes compromised, the inflammatory response becomes magnified by the immune system. Once the antigens in the pocket pass through the wall of white blood cells and touch or penetrate the gingival connective tissue, a burst of immunological response results in gingival tissue damage and alveolar and supporting bone destruction.

Box 4–1   **Key Elements in the Inflammatory Response**

- Polymorphonuclear leukocytes (PMNs) or neutrophils (a white blood cell involved in phagocytosis or engulfing bacteria)
- Macrophages (phagocyte in connective tissue)
- Mast cells (cell found in connective tissue that contains granules and releases substances such as heparin and histamine)
- Serum complement (serum proteins that work with [*complement*] antibody activity to eliminate pathogens; stimulate inflammation)
- Gingival crevicular fluid (fluid found in small amounts in gingival crevice; important in cleansing substances from crevice and has antimicrobial properties)

no bleeding from the gingival crevice, and shallow sulci. In the healthy gingiva the junctional epithelium does not have long epithelial ridges and overlies the highly oriented collagen fiber bundles. Although clinically there may appear to be no inflammation, at a microscopic level there may be a mild inflammatory reaction. Thus, in the junctional epithelium of clinically healthy gingiva there are always inflammatory cells, primarily PMNs, which form a protective wall between the epithelium and the bacteria. PMNs constantly migrate from the junctional epithelium into the gingival crevice where the older cells are shed into the oral cavity. With severe inflammation, a greater number of these cells are present.

The Inflammatory Process

Table 4–1 ■ describes three phases of the inflammatory process. If dental plaque is allowed to accumulate at the gingival margin and is not disrupted, inflammation or gingivitis results. Plaque removal every 48 hours can prevent gingivitis, but if allowed to accumulate for 72 hours, gingivitis will develop (Van Dyke, Offenbacher, Pihstrom, Putt, & Trummel, 1999). The gingiva reacts to the bacteria and its products by the first three days of plaque accumulation at the gingival margin with signs of acute inflammation. The first inflammatory response to injury is vascular changes in the gingival connective tissue; the epithelium is avascular. Vasodilation of the blood vessels in the connective tissue results in the outflow of blood, fluids, proteins, and cells (PMNs) into the connective tissue (Figure 4–6 ■). The primary substance responsible for the vasodilation and increased permeability of the blood vessel wall is histamine, which is released from mast cells found in the connective tissue. Another substance that is involved in the vasodilation is prostaglandin. **Prostaglandins** are fatty acids found in most cell membranes, are synthesized in large amounts during gingivitis and periodontitis, and may be responsible for the pain and bone loss seen in

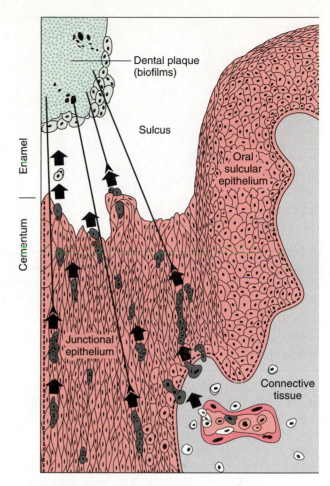

■ **FIGURE 4–6** Schematic drawing of the relationship of the gingival sulcus to the epithelium and connective tissue in health. Note the dental plaque on the tooth surface at the entrance to the gingival sulcus. Neutrophils are leaving blood vessels in the connective tissue and moving chemotactically through the semipermeable junctional epithelium but not through the oral sulcular epithelium of the lateral wall of the sulcus.

Table 4–1	**Phases of the Inflammatory Process**
Phase	*Features*
Acute transient phase	Local vasodilation and increased capillary permeability
Delayed subacute phase	Migration of PMNs and other phagocytic cells into the tissue
Chronic phase	Tissue destruction

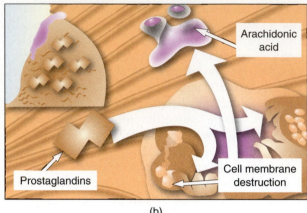

(a)   (b)

■ **FIGURE 4–7** (a) Prostaglandins (PGs) are fatty acids produced in the body by the initiation of an inflammatory response involving the release of substances from the injured cell membrane of the tissue followed by production of PGs via arachadonic acid. (b) Prostaglandins are involved in the entire body process. Specifically, PGE_2 is involved in inflammatory periodontal disease, including destruction of alveolar bone.

periodontal diseases (Offenbacher, Heasman, & Collins, 1993) (Figure 4–7a, b ■). Vasodilation clinically shows as gingival edema and erythema (redness). Thus, tissue edema or swelling is due to the increase of permeability of blood vessels, which causes the migration and accumulation of cells and fluid from the vessels to surrounding tissue. With the initiation of inflammation, the flow of gingival crevicular fluid increases from the connective tissue out through the junctional epithelium into the gingival crevice. Migration of PMNs through the junctional epithe-

lium into the gingival sulcus and crevicular fluid flow both peak six to twelve days after the onset of clinically detectable gingivitis (Kowashi, Jaccard, & Cimasoni, 1980; Zappa, 1995). Table 4–2 ■ describes the differences between the acute and chronic inflammatory responses.

Gingival bleeding at the gingival crevice is an early and important sign of gingival inflammation. When the crevice is probed or stroked, it may bleed immediately because the sulcular epithelium (epithelium lining the sulcus) becomes ulcerated with tears in the epithelial lin-

Table 4–2	Acute versus Chronic Inflammatory Responses	
	Acute Inflammation	*Chronic Inflammation*
What causes it?	Antigen such as bacteria in dental plaque	Unresolved acute inflammation; continued presence of antigens
What cells are involved in the bodies response to the causative agent?	PMNs, mononuclear cells (e.g., macrophages)	Monocytes, macrophages, lymphocytes, plasma cells
What substances (or mediators) are released from the cells that causes the signs and symptoms of inflammation?	Vasoactive amines (e.g., histamine, bradykinin)	Cytokines, growth factors, reactive oxygen species, hydrolytic enzymes
When does this inflammatory response first appear?	Immediate onset	Delayed onset
How long does this response last?	Several days	Long time (months to years)
After the response over, what happens to the tissues?	Healing occurs if the inflammation is resolved	Tissue destruction

ing. The bleeding on probing comes from the underlying vascular gingival connective tissue (lamina propria), which is engorged with blood because of the disease process (Rizzo, 1970).

The Neutrophil: The Phagocytic Cell   The neutrophil has been referred to as a "first line of defense" and the "hallmark of acute inflammation," meaning that it is one of the first defensive cells to be recruited to a site of inflammation (Figure 4–8 ■). PMNs are the first cells to migrate from inside the blood vessels into the surrounding connective tissue and enter the gingival crevice and junctional epithelium in response to chemotactic substances such as toxins released by the bacteria and complement, which are proteins found in the serum (Miyasaki, 1991). **Chemotaxis** is the movement of cells in the direction of a chemical attractant. The PMNs create a wall between swimming, unattached bacteria and the junctional and sulcular epithelium. Once in the tissue, the neutrophil is ready to kill the foreign invader. Once the PMN comes in contact with the bacteria, **phagocytosis** occurs. The PMN is the major phagocytic cell, whose fast arrival from the blood vessels in the connective tissue into the junctional epithelium and crevice plays an important part in removing bacteria and other foreign substances. Neutrophils

live a very short time. They come out of the bone marrow programmed to die in an average of about five days. Once at the site of injury, phagocytosis occurs where PMNs recognize the foreign material (bacteria, toxins, and by-products) and "eat and digest" it. Once inside the PMN, the bacteria are degraded by enzymes called lysosomes. As the bacteria are engulfed, lysosomal enzymes "leak" out of the cell into the surrounding tissue causing destruction of host tissue. Examples of lysosomal enzymes include collagenase, beta-glucuronidase, and alkaline phosphatase. High levels of these enzymes can be detected in the GCF during periodontitis.

Genetically, impaired PMN function is seen in patients with certain medical conditions. A depressed PMN chemotaxis and depressed phagocytic ability is seen in localized aggressive periodontitis and diabetes type 1. A depressed PMN chemotaxis is seen in Chediak-Higashi syndrome and Papillon-Lefévre syndrome. A decreased number of circulating PMNs are seen in drug-induced agranulocytosis, cyclic neutropenia, and leukemia (Genco & Slots, 1984).

The Macrophage: The Other Phagocytic Cell The other important phagocytic cell is the macrophage (Figure 4–9 ■). Monocytes (a type of white blood cell)

■ **FIGURE 4–8**   PMNs are the first cells to migrate to the infection site. They comprise more than 90% of the circulating granulocytes, and they move by chemotaxis.

Macrophage ingests foreign protein...

...Gives antigen to lymphocyte

Lymph Node

Soft tissue and bone destruction: Interaction of macrophages and lymphocytes

■ **FIGURE 4–9**   A macrophage is a phagocyte that ingests foreign material such as periodontal bacteria.

in the blood differentiate or change into macrophages and migrate from the blood vessel into the inflamed connective tissues by chemotaxis and a few continue into the gingival crevice. Similar to PMNs, macrophages kill bacteria by phagocytosis. Although neutrophils and macrophages arrive at the same time at the site of inflammation, neutrophils predominate initially because of their higher concentration in the circulation. The majority of macrophages remain in the inflamed connective tissue for months, where they function to clean up the body's damaged tissue and secrete prostaglandins and cytokines. **Cytokines** are proteins that are involved in regulating the activity of the cells that release them, as well as other cells (Kjeldsen, Holmstrup, & Bendtzen, 1993). The major cytokines released by macrophages as a result of phagocytosis are interleukin (IL-1) and tumor necrosis factor (TNF).

IL-1 worsens inflammation by stimulating mast cells to release histamine and attracts more PMNs and macrophages into the tissues (Offenbacher, 1996). As with PMNs, macrophages can also damage host tissue most likely a result of cytokines. IL-1 can increase the number of osteoclasts, which stimulate bone resorption seen in periodontitis (Ishikawa et al., 1997; Tatakis, 1993), and stimulates other cells to secrete prostaglandins, which are also involved in bone resorption. TNF is a less potent stimulator of bone resorption (Stashenko, Dewhirst, Peros, Kent, & Apo, 1987).

Phagocytosis: Opsonization The process of phagocytosis is more effective if **opsonins** are present. Opsonins are antibodies or complement that bind to the surface of the bacteria, coating the bacteria so they are easier to be identified by PMNs and to be "swallowed."

The Complement System: A Group of Proteins Besides blood cells (e.g., PMNs) and fluids migrating from the blood vessels into the gingival tissues and crevicular area during inflammation, there is also a series of about twenty to thirty different plasma proteins called the **complement system.** The complement system works together with the rest of the immune system to destroy invaders and to signal to other immune system cells that the attack is occurring. The complement system plays an important role in the inflammatory and immune response by generating chemotactic factors, which attract PMNs,

macrophages, and other leukocytes to the inflamed area. Also, it directly kills and lyses (breaks apart) bacteria.

As with everything else in the immune system, the complement system must be activated before it can function. One way it is activated is when antibodies (proteins produced by plasma cells during the immune response) bind to the surface of bacteria (the antigen). This is called the "classical" pathway. The second way is called the "alternative" pathway, whereby endotoxins (lipooligosaccarides) activate the system. A third pathway involves the binding of specific proteins to proteins or carbohydrates on bacteria (Dennison & Van Dyke, 1997).

The Immune Response

If, for any reason, inflammation does not subside within about seven days, it will become a chronic reaction. Usually gingival inflammation progresses quickly into a chronic condition (Figure 4–10 ■). When the PMNs and macrophages are not strong enough to destroy the invaders, the immune system is further activated, although the inflammatory cells remain in the area.

Activation of the "specific host response" or adaptive immune system is the next line of defense, with the purpose of the host developing immunity or resistance to specific antigens (e.g., bacteria and toxins) (Figure 4–11 ■) (American Academy of Periodontology, 2002; Ishikawa, 2006; Nagasawa et al., 2006). The objective of the immune response is to recognize the antigen and communicate with other defense cells to destroy or suppress the antigen. There is an interrelationship between the inflammatory and immune reactions. The same reactions and cells seen in the inflammatory level are also seen in the chronic state (e.g., PMNs and macrophages

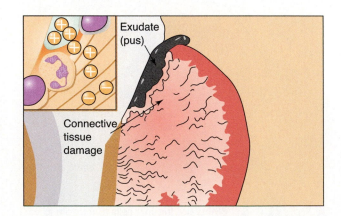

■ **FIGURE 4–10** The inflammatory response triggers an immunologic response resulting in periodontal destruction.

> ### Did You Know?
> Phagocyte means, "eating cell," or "cell eater."

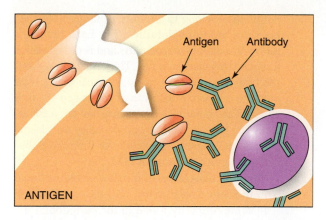

■ FIGURE 4–11   An antigen is any foreign material in-cluding bacteria. Antigens will eventually bind to antibod-ies with the intention of being eliminated from the body.

Box 4–2   **Key Elements in the Immune Response**

- B-lymphocytes
- Antibodies
- Macrophages
- Cytokines
- T-lymphocytes
    T-killer—directly involved
    T-helper—"help" plasma cells

also belong to the immune system), but more cells are involved. There are two parts to the immune reaction: **humoral immunity** and **cellular immunity.**

Immune System: Cells

The major cells in the immune system are white blood cells called lymphocytes (Box 4–2). The role of the im-mune system is to "patrol" the body, identifying foreign pathogens such as bacteria and viruses, cancer cells, or damaged tissue and eliminating them. There are two kinds of lymphocytes that originate in the bone marrow and travel to other areas of the body (Figure 4–12a ■). In fact, all cells in the inflammatory and immune systems,

including blood cells, are made in the bone marrow from a stem cell. A stem cell is a cell from which all blood cells "stem" or originate. Lymphocytes predominate in the gingival connective tissue (Page & Schroeder, 1976). T-lymphocytes, also referred to as *T-cells,* are the medi-ators of cellular immunity. B-lymphocytes, or *B-cells,* are the mediators of humoral immunity (Figure 4–12b).

Humoral Immunity

Humoral immune mechanisms are most effective against bacteria such as those found in periodontitis. Although both the humoral and cellular immunity reactions occur almost at the same time, one or the other cells may pre-dominate during a particular stage of periodontal diseases.

B-lymphocytes or B-cells are so named because much of the early research was done on chickens, in which the bursa (hence "B") of Fabricius is a center of B-cell activation; there is no direct equivalent of this bursa

(a)

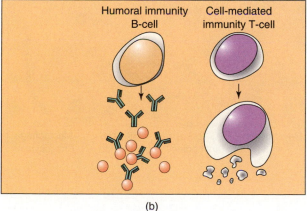

(b)

■ FIGURE 4–12   The antigen–antibody reaction involves the B-lymphocytes and T-lymphocytes.

in human beings. B-cells originate and mature in the bone marrow and then migrate and deposit in the blood and various lymphatic tissues (e.g., lymph nodes) (Berglundh, Donati, & Zitzmann, 2007)

Humoral Immunity and Periodontal Disease
The following events depict the humoral response to plaque accumulated at the gingival margin (Figure 4–13 ■):

1. In periodontal diseases, bacteria and their products, such as toxins and enzymes, accumulate in the gingival crevice. Then they penetrate through the protective wall of neutrophils and through the junctional epithelium, entering the lamina propria. Once this happens an inflammatory/immune response is set off. As previously stated, if the inflammatory reaction cannot eliminate the antigens effectively, the immune response comes into play.

2. From the tissues, these antigenic substances are carried to the local lymph nodes, probably by macrophages.

3. In the lymph nodes, the macrophages either present the antigens to B-cells or the B-cells by themselves recognize the antigens. The B-cells then transform into plasma cells and memory cells.

4. Plasma cells make **antibodies** in the lymph nodes with the assistance from T_H-cells. They also circulate in the blood to seek out and destroy the antigens.

5. The memory B-cells remain inactivated, ready to respond should the same antigens appear again.

6. The plasma cells remain in the lymph nodes and secrete antibodies into the bloodstream. A local antibody response is also seen in the gingival tissues.

7. Antibodies belong to a family of large molecules known as **immunoglobulins** (Ig). Each immunoglobin has about a dozen parts and is designed for a specific invader (antigen). They float throughout the body and wait for invaders. Antibodies lock onto the antigen of the invader like a key fits into a lock. They neutralize the enemy and tag it for attack. The primary antibody produced by the plasma cells is IgG (Note: "Ig" stands for immunoglobulin) with lesser amounts of IgM.

   • There are five classes of immunoglobulins found in the serum, secretions, and tissues. IgG and IgM are primarily found in the periodontal tissues and SIgA ("S" stands for secretory) is found in the saliva. IgE is found on mast cells and is responsible for the release of histamine causing vasodilation and allergy. Additionally, there is IgD.

   • Antibodies (e.g., IgG) are proteins that directly bind to and neutralize bacterial toxins (foreign antigens) forming an immune complex. This immune complex may activate the complement system or be phagocytosed by PMNs or macrophages for elimination.

8. Once the antigens and the surrounding tissue are destroyed, the tissue macrophages phagocytize and digest the debris and stimulate repair.

9. After the antigens have been eliminated, the short-lived plasma cells disappear into the gingival crevicular fluid and out through the gingival crevice, but the long-lived memory cells remain in circulation

(a)

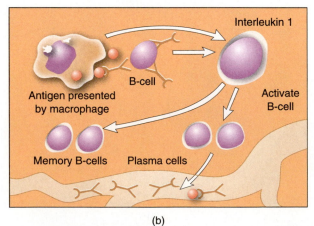

(b)

■ **FIGURE 4–13**   B-lymphocytes function in periodontal disease (a) T-cell and (b) B-cell and are capable of maturing very rapidly into plasma cells if the antigens are encountered again.

Antibodies to various periodontal pathogens have been found in both serum and gingival crevicular fluids of patients with periodontal diseases (Ebersole & Taubman, 1994; Genco & Slots, 1984). Immune complex and complement will cause the release of prostaglandins from cell membranes of macrophages and PMNs. Prostaglandins of the E series (PGE_2) are potent stimulators of osteoclast activity responsible for bone resorption. B lymphocytes also release cytokines such as IL-1. Thus, it has been suggested that B-cells may play a role in alveolar bone loss (Han, Kawai, Eastcott, & Taubman, 2006). Humoral immunity is activated in severe gingivitis and periodontitis. Thus, the proportion of B-cells in connective tissue at sites with periodontitis can be as high as 90%.

Cellular Immunity

T-cells undergo further maturation in the thymus gland located in the chest cavity. From the thymus gland, the T-cells migrate into the bloodstream and lymph nodes. From the bloodstream, T-cells enter the gingival tissues where they "watch" the tissues (Figure 4–14 ■).

There are two major types of T-cell: helper T-cells (T_H) and cytotoxic T-cells. Both T-cells have protein receptors on the surface of their plasma membranes (Gemmell, Yamazaki, & Seymour, 2006). The helper T-cells have a CD4 receptor and the cytotoxic T-cells have a CD8 receptor. There is a reduction in CD4 T_H-cells in AIDS patients. Once the helper T-cells are stimulated, they secrete cytokines (referred to as lymphokines when produced by

> ### Did You Know?
>
> B-cells may play an active role in alveolar bone resorption, more research is needed.

lymphocytes) that activate phagocytic cells to destroy target antigens (Box 4–3). T-cells can directly cause alveolar bone loss through stimulation the synthesis of osteoclasts or indirectly through production of IL-1. They also activate other immune cells such as B-cells. Cytotoxic T-cells are sometimes called killer T-cells, and they can directly kill virus-infected cells, cancer cells, parasites, and certain bacteria by making holes in them. Thus, cellular immunity is most effective against fungi, viruses, cancer, and foreign tissue such as transplanted organs and does not play an important role in periodontal diseases.

Cellular Immunity: Process   When a macrophage presents a foreign antigen to a T-cell, it is stimulated to produce more T-cells and cytokines. T-cells are the target of the human immunodeficiency virus (HIV). AIDS is a manifestation of what happens when T-cells are destroyed, showing the importance of T-cells for a properly functioning body. This type of response is responsible for organ or tissue rejection in a transplant case. Few lymphocytes within the gingival connective tissue are seen in healthy gingiva, with T-lymphocytes mostly seen in gingivitis. The T-cells actually kill other cells on contact when the latter are recognized as foreign or have antigens attached. Unfortunately, T-cells also have the capacity to contribute to permanent tissue damage by the production of cytokines, which activate macrophages.

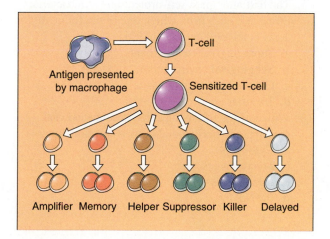

■ **FIGURE 4–14**   Cellular immunity involving T-lymphocytes.

Box 4–3   **Lymphokines Implicated in Periodontal Pathology**

- IL-1 interleukin-1
- TNF tumor necrosis factor
- MAF macrophage activating factor
- MIF macrophage migration inhibitory factor
- CTX leukocyte-derived chemotatic factor

RDH   **Rapid Dental Hint**

B-cells mature in the bone and T-cells mature in the thymus.

DENTAL HYGIENE NOTES

The pathway of destruction of inflammatory periodontal diseases is complicated, involving the host inflammatory and immune cells. Ideally, the overall outcome of these reactions is to eliminate harmful pathogens and prevent the spread of infection, while protecting the host tissues.

The basic concepts of plaque control via periodontal debridement and patient oral home care both involve the inflammatory/immune pathways.

KEY POINTS

• Overall, the host defenses are extremely successful in preventing infection around the teeth and in preventing destructive inflammatory periodontal diseases.

• There are two separate functions that lead to the damage seen in periodontal diseases: (1) direct effects of bacteria (e.g., enzymes, endotoxins) and (2) indirect effects of the body's own immune response.

• The host immune defense and inflammatory reactions are a double-edged sword; while being protective, they can also cause the host to suffer tissue damage.

• Bacterial products can enter the connective tissue and cause direct damage, but their effects are limited by the effectiveness of the host response.

• Weakened host defenses (e.g., because of a systemic disease) will not allow the host to ward off infection; the host will then develop signs and symptoms of destructive periodontal diseases.

• Neutrophils and macrophages are considered capable and efficient agents of phagocytosis.

• Clinical signs of gingival inflammation are first evident in the early lesion of gingivitis.

• B-cells/plasma cells predominate in the body's response to periodontitis.

• Within the last decade, B-cells have been found to also be involved in bone resorption.

• Elevated serum antibodies are seen in periodontitis.

SELF-QUIZ

1. Which one of the following types of cells is primarily recruited in high numbers to the site of acute inflammation? (p. 73)
   a. Mast
   b. Macrophage
   c. Neutrophil
   d. Lymphocyte

2. Which one of the following cells is phagocytic? (pp. 73–74)
   a. Mast
   b. Lymphocyte
   c. Macrophage
   d. Melanocyte

3. Which one of the following cells is mainly involved in the body's immune response to invading bacteria? (pp. 69–70)
   a. Lymphocytes
   b. Mast
   c. Macrophages
   d. Neutrophils

4. Periodontal diseases are considered a group of infections characterized by destruction of the periodontium. The direct effects of the bacteria and indirect effects by the body's own immune response are primarily responsible for the destruction. (pp. 66–70, 73)
   a. Both statements are true.
   b. Both statements are false.
   c. The first statement is true, the second is false.
   d. The first statement is false, the second is true.

5. The first attempt at self-protection from bacterial invasion comes from which one of the following areas in the oral cavity? (p. 69)
   a. Supragingival environment
   b. Subgingival environment
   c. Gingival connective tissue
   d. Tonsillar area

6. Which of the following cells (substances) can contribute to periodontal bone resorption? (p. 74)
   a. Cytokines
   b. Macrophages
   c. Neutrophils
   d. PMNs

7. Which of the following cells is responsible for "patrolling" the body? (p. 75)
   a. PMNs
   b. Macrophages
   c. Lymphocytes
   d. Neutrophils

8. Which of the following cells/substances is involved in regulating the activity of other cells? (p. 74)
   a. Macrophages
   b. Cytokines
   c. Lymphocytes
   d. Neutrophils

9. Which of the following substances are released from all Gram-negative bacteria and cause damage to the periodontium? (p. 68)
   a. Hyaluronidase
   b. Collagenase
   c. Leukotoxin
   d. Endotoxin

10. Which of the following are theories of periodontal disease activity? (p. 66)
    a. Continuous model
    b. Random burst
    c. Asynchronous, multiple burst
    d. All of the above

REFERENCES

American Academy of Periodontology. 2002. Modulation of the host response in periodontal therapy. *J. Periodontol.* 7:460–470.

Armitage, G. C. 1995. Clinical evaluation of periodontal diseases. *Periodontology 2000* 7:39–53.

Berglundh, T., M. Donati, and N. Zitzmann. 2007. B cells in periodontitis–friends or enemies? *Periodontology 2000* 45(1):51–66.

Birkedal-Hansen, H., W. G. Moore, M. K. Bodden, et al. 1993. Matrix Metallo proteinase: A review. *Crit. Rev. Oral Biol. Med.* 4:197–250.

Brown, L. J., and H. Löe. 1993. Prevalence, extent, severity and progression of periodontal disease. *Periodontology 2000* 2:57–71.

de Graaf, J., A. J. van Winkelhoff, and R. J. Goené. 1989. The role of *Actinobacillus actinomycetemcomitans* in periodontal disease. *Infection* 17:269–271.

Dennison, D. K., and T. E. Van Dyke. 1997. The acute inflammatory response and the role of phagocytic cells in periodontal health and disease. *Periodontology 2000* 14:54–78.

Ebersole, J. L., and M. A. Taubman. 1994. The protective nature of host responses in periodontal diseases. *Periodontology 2000* 5:112–141.

Gemmell, E., K. Yamazaki, and G. J. Seymour. 2006. The role of T cells in periodontal disease: homeostasis and autoimmunity. *Periodontology 2000* 43:14-40.

Genco, R. J., and J. Slots. 1984. Host response in periodontal diseases. *J. Dental Res.* 63:441–451.

Goodson, J. M. 1992. Diagnosis of periodontitis by physical measurement: Interpretation from episodic disease hypothesis. *J. Periodontol.* 63:373–382.

Greenstein, G., and J. Caton. 1990. Periodontal disease activity: A critical assessment. *J. Periodontol.* 61:543–552.

Han, X., T. Kawai, J. W. Eastcott, and M. A. Taubman. 2006. Bacterial-responsive B lymphocytes induce periodontal bone resorption. *The Journal of Immunology* 176:625–631.

Ishikawa, I. K. 2006. Host responses in periodontal diseases: A preview. *Periodontology 2000* 43:9–13.

Ishikawa, I., K. Nakashima, T. Koseki, T. Nagasawa, H. Watanabe, et al. 1997. Induction of the immune response to periodontopathic bacteria and its role in the pathogenesis of periodontitis. *Periodontology 2000* 14:79–111.

Kinane, F., and P. M. Bartold. 2007. Clinical relevance of the host responses of periodontitis. *Periodontology 2000* 44(1):278–293.

Kjeldsen, M., P. Holmstrup, and K. Bendtzen. 1993. Marginal periodontitis and cytokines: A review of the literature. *J. Periodontol.* 64:1013–1022.

Kowashi, Y., F. Jaccard, and G. Cimasoni. 1980. Sulcular polymorphonuclear leukocytes and gingival exudate during experimental gingivitis in man. *J. Periodontol. Res.* 15:151–158.

Listgarten, M. A. 1994. The structure of dental plaque. *Periodontology 2000* 5:52–65.

Löe, H., A. Anerud, H. Boysen, and E. Morrison. 1986. Natural history of periodontal disease in man. Rapid, moderate and no loss of attachment in Sri Lankan laborers 14 to 46 years of age. *J. Clin. Periodontol.* 13:431–440.

Miyasaki, K. T. 1991. The neutrophil: Mechanisms of controlling periodontal bacteria. *J. Periodontol.* 62:761–774.

Nagasawa, T, M. Kiji, R. Yashiro, et al. 2006. Roles of receptor activator of nuclear factor-κB ligand (RANKL) and osteoprotegerin in periodontal health and disease. *Periodontology 2000* 43:65–84.

Offenbacher, S. 1996. Periodontal diseases: Pathogenesis. *Ann. Periodontol.* 1:821–878.

Offenbacher, S., P. A. Heasman, and J. G. Collins. 1993. Modulation of host PGE_2 secretion as a determinant of periodontal disease expression. *J. Periodontol.* 64:432–444.

Page, R. C., and H. E. Schroeder. 1976. Pathogenesis of inflammatory periodontal disease. A summary of current work. *Lab Investigations* 33:235–249.

Renvert, S., M. Wikström, M. Dahlén, G. Slots, and J. Egelberg. 1990. On the inability of root debridement and periodontal surgery to eliminate *Actinobacillus actinomycetemcomitans* from periodontal pockets. *J. Clin. Periodontol.* 17:351–355.

Rizzo, A. 1970. Histologic and immunologic evaluation of antigen penetration into oral tissues after topical application. *J. Periodontol.* 41:210–213.

Saglie, F. R., F. A. Carranza, Jr., M. G. Newman, L. Cheng, and K. J. Lewin. 1982. Identification of tissue-invading bacteria in human periodontal disease. *J. Periodontol. Res.* 17:452–455.

Shikawa, I. 2007. Host responses in periodontal disease: A preview. *Periodontology 2000* 44(1):9–13.

Socransky, S. S., A. D. Haffajee, J. M. Goodson, and J. Lindhe. 1984. New concepts of destructive periodontal diseases. *J. Clin. Periodontol.* 11:21–32.

Stashenko, P., F. E. Dewhirst, W. J. Peros, R. L. Kent, and J. Apo. 1987. Synergistic interactions between interleukin-1, tumor necrosis factor and lymphotoxin in bone resorption. *J. Immunol.* 138:1484–1468.

Tatakis, D. N. 1993. Interleukin-1 and bone metabolism: A review. *J. Periodontol.* 64:416–431.

Van Dyke, T. 2007. Control of inflammation and periodontitis. *Periodontology 2000* 45(1):158–166.

Van Dyke, T., S. Offenbacher, B. Pihstrom, M. Putt, and C. Trummel. 1999. What is gingivitis? Current understanding of prevention, treatment, measurement, pathogenesis and relation to periodontitis. *J. International Acad. of Periodontol.* 1:3–10.

Zappa, U. 1995. Histology of the periodontal lesion: Implications for diagnosis. *Periodontology 2000* 7:22–38.

Zimmerman, S. O. 1986. Discussion: Attachment level changes in destructive periodontal diseases. *J. Clin. Periodontol.* 13:473–475.

Chapter 5

Local Contributory Factors for Periodontal Diseases

Raymond A. Yukna

John D. Mason

OUTLINE
Introduction
Dental Calculus
Anatomic Factors
Iatrogenic Factors
Traumatic Factors
Dental Hygiene Notes
Key Points
Self-Quiz
References

EDUCATIONAL OBJECTIVES

Upon completion of this chapter, the reader should be able to:

- List and explain contributing local factors.
- Describe the clinical significance of dental calculus.
- Discuss the specific role of dental calculus as a contributory factor for the periodontal diseases.

GOAL: To introduce the role of local contributory factors for the periodontal diseases.

KEY WORDS

anatomic factors 85
contributory 82
dental calculus 82

iatrogenic factors 87
palatogingival
   grooves 85

INTRODUCTION

Many local factors can increase plaque deposition and retention, inhibit plaque control, and contribute to the development of gingivitis and periodontitis. These factors are termed **contributory** because they do not by themselves initiate gingival inflammation, but foster increased or long-standing plaque accumulation and make plaque removal more difficult. Awareness of these local factors can help the dental hygienist to design more specific plaque-control activities, encourage patients to seek further corrective dental treatment, and contribute to the comprehensive care of periodontal patients.

Perhaps the most significant dentally related local factor strongly associated with an increased probability of developing periodontal diseases, but not directly involved in causing the disease, is the presence of established periodontal disease. Sites already or previously affected by periodontitis are at the greatest risk for future episodes (Douglass, 1998). More frequent professional care has been shown to reduce the risk.

DENTAL CALCULUS

Dental calculus is considered the most important *local* contributing factor. Calculus is not the cause of disease but rather the bacterial challenge. Calculus is essentially calcified dental plaque, but may form even in the absence of bacteria. Mineralization within plaque initially occurs supragingivally, but the rate of formation varies between individuals. Subgingival calculus forms more slowly in a thinner layer and, being firmly attached to the root, is usually more difficult to remove. Calculus is always covered by plaque and retains toxic bacterial products (Figure 5–1 ■).

Subgingival calculus is commonly deposited in rings or ledges on root surfaces, but may also appear in a veneer form and is associated with progressive periodontal disease (Figure 5–2 ■). It is porous and can provide a reservoir of bacteria and endotoxin. Long-term studies of periodontal patients support calculus removal to promote healing and prevent further loss of attachment (Pihlstrom, McHugh, Oliphant, & Ortiz-Campos, 1983).

"Tartar" is the common layman's term for dental calculus and is often used by patients when referring to calculus. Tartar is used to describe the sediment or crust on the side of a wine cask. The term was coined by a Swiss-German physician who identified all stony accretions in humans as tartars because they were similar in

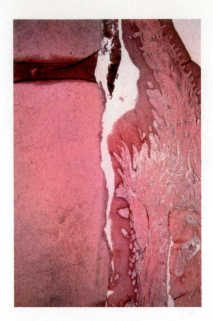

■ **FIGURE 5–1** Histology of calculus with a plaque coating in a deep periodontal pocket.

composition to the potassium bitartrate deposits on wine casks (Mandel, 1990). The term *calculus* is a Latin-rooted word meaning *pebble* or *stone*. Needless to say, the population has become more aware of the word *tartar* because of the advertising of "tartar-control" toothpaste and rinses, which reinforces the use of the common name.

Radiographic evaluation of calculus is not an effective diagnostic method. Only about 45% of surfaces with clinically visible calculus are detected radiographically (Figure 5–3 ■).

Rapid Dental Hint

Calculus is calcified plaque consisting of organic secretions and food particles deposited in various salts, such as calcium carbonate between and within remnants of formerly live microorganisms.

Clinical Significance of Calculus

The population is more aware of supragingival plaque and calculus and their relationship to gingivitis than it is of subgingival plaque and calculus and their relationship

(a)

(b)

■ **FIGURE 5–2**   Clinical photographs of nodular calculus vs. veneer-type calculus. (a) Nodular calculus is evident more coronally while (b) veneer-type calculus is often found more apically.

to periodontitis. Awareness is still lacking in the need to remove plaque to prevent periodontal disease and how to remove supragingival and subgingival plaque. The situation becomes increasingly confusing when descriptions are added of mineralized plaque becoming calculus or of loosely adherent plaque residing on top of mineralized

calculus. Because calculus that forms above the gingival margin is both hard and visible, it has become the focus of consumers for removal based on aesthetic reasons. Rather than being a mechanical irritant, as was once thought (Carranza, 1996), calculus contributes to the accumulation of plaque by having a porous surface. It is

(a)

(b)

■ **FIGURE 5–3**   Radiographs of teeth in the same patient (a) with and (b) without calculus evident. Absence of calculus on radiographs does not mean that it is not present clinically (radiographs produce many false negatives).

> **Did You Know?**
>
> Cats and dogs also develop calculus buildup.

unknown if calculus covered with bacterial plaque is more damaging to tissues than plaque alone (Mandel, 1995).

Dental calculus can be defined as mineralized (calcified) plaque, although calculus has been shown to develop in germ-free animals. As with plaque, described according to its location in relationship to the gingival margin, calculus is also described as supragingival and subgingival. The mineralization process occurs separately for supragingival and subgingival plaque, and because of this, varying amounts of calculus can be found in the supragingival and subgingival areas.

Supragingival calculus can occur on any clinical crown, exposed root surface, prosthesis, or restoration. It is associated most frequently with sites that are adjacent to a salivary source, such as the parotid gland (maxillary molar area; Figure 5–4a ■) or floor of the mouth

Rapid Dental Hint

Calculus is a LOCAL contributing factor for periodontal disease—it is NOT the cause of the disease. Plaque adheres to the surface of calculus.

and salivary caruncle (lingual surfaces of mandibular anterior teeth; Figure 5–4b). Any retention site, such as a maligned tooth, a missed area of plaque removal, or an area where mastication does not remove all debris, is a primary site for supragingival calculus formation. The mineral components of supragingival calculus are derived from saliva.

The formation of supragingival calculus occurs in layers beginning closest to the tooth. The minerals are deposited within 24 to 72 hours of plaque formation. Minerals from the saliva are deposited in the plaque matrix and around the filamentous bacteria. The process can take approximately twelve days or less for rapid formers. The actual mineralization process can occur in as few as 24 to 48 hours. Formation time varies according to the individual, the contents of the saliva, and the ability to remove plaque on all surfaces or various retention sites.

Subgingival calculus is derived from gingival crevicular fluid and any inflammatory exudates. More minerals become available as the inflammatory process continues, and the calculus contains more calcium, magnesium, and fluoride than supragingival calculus (Mandel, 1990). It most often forms in rings around the roots of the tooth or in ledges.

The mineralization process continues as crystals of hydroxyapatite, brushite, and whitlockite form. These crystals have different proportions of calcium and phosphate in combination with other ions, such as magnesium, zinc, fluoride, and other carbonates (Ellwood,

(a)

(b)

■ **FIGURE 5–4**   (a) Supragingival calculus on the maxillary first molar opposite Stensen's duct. (b) Supragingival calculus on the lingual surface of the mandibular anteriors in relation to the opening or orifice of the submandibular and sublingual salivary glands.

Melling, & Rutter, 1979). The crystals form in the matrix and then on the surface of the bacteria; finally, they calcify the bacteria.

Other differences in subgingival calculus and supragingival calculus are the hardness of the calculus and the difficulty in removing it. Supragingival calculus is 30% mineralized, whereas subgingival calculus is 60% mineralized. Subgingival calculus is more difficult to remove because of this hardness. The color of the two calculus types varies from yellow-white for supragingival calculus to gray or black for subgingival calculus. Unless the subgingival calculus is minutely visible at the gingival margin, this coloration adds little to its removal. The gray or black color derives from the bacterial and blood pigments from the crevicular fluid.

The structure of calculus was described as layers in supragingival calculus. These layers build into incremental lines on the surfaces of a tooth. The surface of the calculus is irregular and rough. Plaque accumulates on the surface of the calculus. It can lodge in the pits and valleys of the calculus surface. In the subgingival calculus the outer surface may be less calcified. Again, subgingival plaque can accumulate. In either case, the plaque on the surface of the calculus contains living bacteria and is detrimental to the tissue. In this sense, calculus is a contributing factor for periodontal diseases. The calculus acts as an irritant to the gingival margin or the sulcular tissue. The overlying bacterial plaque continues to be the etiologic factor in periodontal disease.

There are many types of attachment of calculus to root surfaces. Calculus attaches to both tooth and implant surfaces. A classic article recognizes four modes of attachment of subgingival calculus to root surfaces (Zander, 1953):

1. Attachment by means of mechanical locking into irregularities in the cementum.
2. Attachment into areas of cementum resorption.
3. Attachment by means of an organic pellicle.
4. Attachment by penetration into bacteria (not accepted by all researchers).

Both the bacterial plaque and the pellicle beneath the plaque calcify, making removal of the calculus via periodontal debridement very difficult. Additionally, calculus binds to tooth surface irregularities, making mechanical calculus removal difficult. Calculus is not firmly attached to dental implants because the titanium surface is nonporous, which is just the opposite of natural teeth. Thus,

calculus can actually be "chipped" off from dental implants (Lang, Mombelli, & Attström, 2003; Matarasso et al., 1996).

ANATOMIC FACTORS

Dental **anatomic factors** of importance to the accumulation of dental plaque include root morphology (size and shape) and position of teeth in the arch.

Root Morphology

Knowledge of dental morphology, supplemented by radiographs and the patient's dental history, is needed to identify dental anomalies. An anomaly is defined as a deviation from normal tooth development or function. Examples of dental anomalies include cervical enamel projections (CEPs), enamel pearls, and palatogingival grooves.

Several deviations in the shape or form of the tooth root can occur and often contribute to increased plaque accumulation and more severe periodontal disease. Palatal grooves (also called **palatogingival grooves** or lingual grooves) are present on about 5 to 8% of maxillary incisors, tend to accumulate plaque, and can become the focus of a narrow, deep pocket (Hou & Tsai, 1993; see also Figure 5–5 ■). Likewise, plaque may accumulate undisturbed in the deep mesial groove of the upper first premolars.

Enamel in the furcation area of the root surface may manifest as cervical enamel projections (CEPs) (Figure 5–6a ■) or enamel pearls (Figure 5–6b). These ridges of enamel may allow increased plaque accumulation. Essentially, a CEP is an extension of enamel from the cementoenamel junction apically to the entrance of the furcation, which may predispose periodontal destruction within the furcation. It may be difficult to detect a CEP clinically because the area is covered by gingiva. The highest incidence of CEPs is on the buccal aspect of the mandibular second molars. An enamel pearl is similar to a CEP except that it consists of a clump of enamel most commonly located in the bifurcation of molar roots just apical to the cementoenamel junction. It is often mistaken for calculus.

Furcation involvements create a complication because they form a cul-de-sac that creates a plaque trap. Difficult access in this protected area fosters increased bacterial deposits and often leads to more severe periodontal disease. Proximal furcations on maxillary molars present particular problems because of even more limited access (Figure 5–7 ■).

(a)   (b)

■ **FIGURE 5–5** Clinical photographs of (a) a palatogingival groove with a deep pocket associated with it, and (b) an extracted lateral incisor exhibiting a deep palatal groove.

(a)   (b)

■ **FIGURE 5–6** (a) Clinical photograph of a cervical enamel projection (CEP) at the furcation entrance. (b) Enamel pearl located at the lingual bifurcation on the mandibular first molar resembles a pearl. It is a potential plaque trap.

(a)

(b)

■ **FIGURE 5–7** Clinical photographs of calculus within furcations: (a) dark calculus evident on all internal surfaces of maxillary molar furcations; (b) more veneerlike calculus in internal groove of mesial root of the mandibular molar.

Tooth Position

Tooth position may influence plaque accumulation and access for oral hygiene and therapy. Most studies that have evaluated the influence of crowding, tilting, rotations, and so on, have found that such tooth position anomalies lead to increased plaque accumulation (and more tissue inflammation), especially in patients who do not have excellent oral hygiene practices (Figure 5–8 ■). Open contacts allow for food impaction, which may contribute to plaque-induced inflammation.

IATROGENIC FACTORS

There are a number of procedures, techniques, and materials used in dentistry that indirectly, and on occasion directly, contribute to the initiation and/or progress of periodontal disease. These are termed **iatrogenic factors.**

Restorative Dentistry

Rough-surfaced and overcontoured amalgams, composites, crowns, bridges, and other types of restorations have been associated with increased gingival inflammation and periodontal disease. Plaque accumulation is enhanced by subgingival placement of restorations because of problems with greater surface roughness of the materials, fit of the margin to the remaining tooth structure, and contour of the restoration. Subgingival restorations that invade the biologic width and restorations with defective or overhanging margins may have a profound effect on periodontal health (Figure 5–9 ■).

Injuries to the gingiva can occur during restorative dentistry procedures. For example, a large portion of the

■ **FIGURE 5–8** Crowded teeth with inflammation of the gingiva.

(a)

(b)

■ **FIGURE 5–9** Overhanging restorations contributing to more advanced periodontitis: (a) clinical photograph of deficient crown margins exposed at surgery; (b) radiograph of large overhang on mandibular molar resulting in more advanced bone loss on that tooth surface.

interdental papilla can be destroyed by the careless use of a wedge during matrix stabilization. Also, retraction cord, impression material, and temporary restorations may result in irreversible damage to the periodontium.

Fixed crowns and bridges must be designed such that the patient can clean all surfaces of the restoration, including the pontic area. If removable partial dentures are designed so that they impinge on the soft tissue or they exert torque on the teeth, traumatic injury to the periodontium can occur. In the presence of dental plaque, these insults can result in more rapid, more severe destruction of periodontal structures.

Exodontics

Extractions can adversely affect adjacent teeth if their attachment apparatus is damaged. The soft tissue and bone supporting an adjacent tooth can be irreversibly destroyed. Failure to remove calculus from adjacent tooth surfaces during the extraction may negate the chance for proper healing on the adjacent teeth. An environment may be set up that actually fosters plaque accumulation. Frequently, patients stop eating on the side where teeth have been extracted. In addition to the decrease in masticatory (chewing) stimulation to the periodontium, plaque begins to form on those teeth, and patients avoid brushing the area.

Orthodontics

Orthodontic appliances have long been associated with increased plaque accumulation, gingivitis, and caries. Fixed appliances (bands, brackets, and wires) present excellent retentive areas for bacterial growth and can contribute significantly to inflammation. Special attention needs to be paid to these orthodontic plaque-retentive areas. More frequent recalls may be indicated for patients undergoing orthodontic therapy, especially adults (Figure 5–10 ■).

■ **FIGURE 5–10** Clinical photograph of orthodontic bands and brackets with increased plaque and inflammation.

TRAUMATIC FACTORS

Trauma to the periodontium from several sources can result in the loss of the attachment apparatus, changes in the local anatomy, and increased plaque accumulation and can contribute to the initiation and progression of periodontal diseases.

Toothbrush Trauma

Toothbrush trauma can completely destroy a narrow band of attached gingiva and result in extensive recession. In fact, toothbrush abrasion is one of the two most common factors associated with recession, the other being permanent tooth position. Such abrasion also results in extensive grooving of the root surfaces, creating plaque traps and causing cleaning problems for the patient (Figure 5–11 ■).

> #### Did You Know?
>
> An average American spends 38.5 total days brushing teeth over a lifetime. The majority of these people may not be brushing correctly.

Factitious Disease

Occasionally, patients may persistently gouge or "scratch" their gingiva with their fingernails or other devices (factitious disease). This action usually results in extensive exposure of the root surface and localized in-

■ **FIGURE 5–12** Clinical photograph of a factitious habit; recession area on the mandibular right central incisor.

flammation. Although relatively rare, whenever isolated areas of recession are noted and a thorough evaluation fails to identify the etiology of the condition, factitious disease should be considered. The change in the local gingival anatomy often leads to greater plaque accumulation and inflammation (Figure 5–12 ■).

Food Impaction

Food impaction is one of the more common local factors that may contribute to the initiation and progression of inflammatory periodontal disease. Open contacts, uneven marginal ridges, irregular positions of teeth, and

(a)

(b)

■ **FIGURE 5–11** Examples of trauma to tissues from home-care procedures due to overzealous use of devices: (a) dental floss lesions between maxillary molars; (b) toothbrush abrasion in cervical area of teeth.

■ **FIGURE 5-13** Example of uneven marginal ridges that can cause food impaction. Lower panel shows condition after reshaping of marginal ridges.

■ **FIGURE 5-14** Clinical photograph of local cocaine application mimicking an aspirin burn.

nonphysiologic contours of teeth and restorations can result in the impaction of food on the gingiva and into the gingival sulcus (Figure 5–13 ■). The cause of the initial breakdown in an area of food impaction or food retention is not clear. Forceful wedging of food beneath the gingival tissues may produce inflammation from physical trauma, and/or food retention leads to food degradation and chemical irritation that affords an excellent breeding ground for bacteria that can initiate and perpetuate the disease process.

Chemical Injury

Indiscriminate use of topically applied aspirin tablets, dental bleaching materials, strong mouthwashes, and various other topical drugs (including cocaine) may result in ulceration/burning of the gingival tissue. Injuries of this nature are usually transient, but may temporarily interfere with plaque control and contribute to periodontal inflammation (Figure 5–14 ■).

In-office dental bleaching commonly uses high concentration of hydrogen/carbamide peroxide (up to 37%) than home bleaching systems (10% carbamide peroxide). Gingival irritation is a common adverse effect.

Usually, these burns show up as a white lesion followed by a red rim. If patients feel burning or tingling of the gingiva during bleaching, the procedure should be stopped and the area rinsed with water. Gingival protection with rubber dams or soft tissue protectors should be used with high peroxide concentrations. Good fitting bleaching trays will also minimize gingival problems.

RDH Rapid Dental Hint

When your patient says that she takes aspirin for a toothache, make sure that she doesn't apply the tablet directly to the gingiva around the tooth—it is acidic and can "burn" the tissue.

Occlusion

In the past, occlusal trauma was considered to be a major factor in the initiation of periodontal diseases. It has been conclusively proven that occlusal trauma does not initiate gingival or periodontal inflammation or pocket formation. Heavy occlusal forces can, however, cause clinical tooth mobility and the radiographic appearance of bone loss. However, these changes involve the periodontal ligament and bone, not the marginal gingival surface tissues.

Occlusal trauma may increase the rate of progression of periodontitis if plaque-induced inflammation is also present. In this regard, trauma from occlusion acts

(a)

(b)

■ **FIGURE 5–15** Examples of tongue piercings (a) Dorsoventral median tongue piercing. (b) Dorsolateral lingual tongue piercing.

as a contributing local factor in the presence of inflammation, but is not a primary etiologic factor by itself.

Oral Piercings

Oral piercing is frequently seen in patients today. Lip piercing may cause dental/periodontal injury on the facial aspect of the mandibular incisors (Chambrone & Chambrone, 2003), while tongue piercing affects the lingual aspect of the mandibular incisors (Figure 5–15 ■). Dental complications from oral piercing include tooth chipping or fracture, gingival recession, bone loss, interference with speech and swallowing, and increased salivary flow with calculus formation (Choc, Almas, & Schoor, 2005). Insertion of jewelry into oral structures is usually done by individuals not familiar with oral anatomy.

DENTAL HYGIENE NOTES

The dental hygienist must be able to recognize other factors that may contribute to a patient's periodontal condition. Oral biofilms are a primary risk factor for periodontal diseases. Other than the primary risk factors, contributory or secondary factors to periodontal diseases include calculus, which is "dead" bacteria with a porous surface that harbors biofilms, tooth aberrations, and occlusion. It is important to recognize these contributory factors. When possible, they should be eliminated.

KEY POINTS

- Inflammatory periodontal diseases are infections caused by bacteria.
- Certain secondary local and systemic contributing factors influence the initiation and progression of the disease.

- Dental calculus is not a cause for the periodontal diseases, but a LOCAL contributing factor.

SELF-QUIZ

1. Which one of the following sources accounts for the mineralization of subgingival calculus? (pp. 84–85)
   a. Salivary proteins
   b. Crevicular fluid
   c. Dental plaque
   d. Acquired pellicle
2. Which one of the following reasons explains the finding of supragingival calculus on the lingual surfaces of the mandibular incisors? (p. 84)
   a. Difficulty in cleaning the area with a toothbrush
   b. Inability of efficient salivary flow to that area
   c. Presence of the parotid duct
   d. Presence of Warton's duct
3. Which one of the following reasons makes calculus an important local etiologic factor for periodontal diseases? (pp. 82–85)
   a. It is porous and can provide a reservoir for bacteria.
   b. It directly irritates the epithelial lining of the pocket.
   c. Minerals cause a breakdown in the epithelial attachment.
   d. The presence of lipooligosaccharides causes the tissues to erode.
4. All of the following anatomic factors may predispose a site to periodontal disease except one. Which one is the exception? (pp. 85–87)
   a. Tooth position
   b. Furcation area
   c. Crown surface
   d. Root surface

5. On which of the following surfaces do palatogingival grooves usually appear? (p. 85)
   a. Lingual surface of mandibular lateral incisor
   b. Lingual surface of mandibular central incisor
   c. Palatal surface of maxillary lateral incisor
   d. Palatal surface of maxillary central incisor
   e. Palatal surface of maxillary canine

REFERENCES

Carranza, F. A., Jr. 1996. Dental calculus. In eds. F. A. Carranza, Jr., and M. G. Newman, *Clinical periodontology,* 9th ed., 150–160. Philadelphia: W. B. Saunders.

Chambrone, L., and L. A. Chambrone. 2003. Gingival recessions caused by lip piercing: case report. *J Can Dent Assoc* 69(8):505–508.

Choe, J., K. Almas, and R. Schoor 2005. Tongue piercing risk factor to periodontal health. *NY Dental J.* 71(5):40–43.

Douglass, C. 1998. Risk assessment for periodontal disease in adults. *Oral Care Report* 8:1–11.

Ellwood, D., J. Melling, and P. Rutter. 1979. The accumulation of organisms on the teeth. In ed. Society for General Microbiology, *Adhesion of micro-organisms to surfaces,* 137–164. New York: Academic Press.

Hou, G. L., and C. C. Tsai. 1993. Relationship between palatoradicular grooves and localized periodontitis. *J. Clin. Periodontol.* 20:668–682.

Lang, N. P., A. Mombelli, and R. Attström. 2003. Dental plaque and calculus. In: Linde, J., Karring, T., Lang, N. P. *Clinical periodontology and implant dentistry,* 4th ed., 81–105. Oxford, UK: Blackwell Publishing.

Mandel, I. D. 1990. Dental calculus (calcified dental plaque). In eds., R. J. Genco, H. M. Goldman, and D. W. Cohen, *Contemporary periodontics,* 135–146. St. Louis, MO: Mosby.

Mandel, I. D. 1995. Calculus update: Prevalence, pathogenicity and prevention. *J. Am. Dent. Assoc.* 126:573–580.

Matarasso, S., Quaremba, G. F. Coraggio, E. Vaia, E. Cafiero, and N. P. Lang. 1996. Maintenance of implants: An *in vitro* study of titanium implant surface modifications subsequent to the application of different prophylaxis procedures. *Clinical Oral Implants Research* 7:64–72.

Pihlstrom, B. L., R. B. McHugh, T. H. Oliphant, and C. Ortiz-Campos. 1983. Comparison of surgical and nonsurgical treatment of periodontal disease. A review of current studies and additional results after 6 1/2 years. *J. Clin. Periodontol.* 10:524–541.

Zander, H. 1953. The attachment of calculus to root surfaces. *J. Periodontol.* 24:16–19.

Chapter 6

Oral-Systemic Disease Connection

Raymond A. Yukna

John D. Mason

OUTLINE
Introduction
Systemic Risk Factors for Periodontal Diseases
Periodontal Diseases as Risk Factors for
  Systemic Conditions
Dental Hygiene Notes
Key Points
Self-Quiz
References

EDUCATIONAL OBJECTIVES

Upon completion of this chapter, the reader should be able to:

• List and discuss possible systemic risk factors for periodontal diseases.
• Discuss periodontal diseases as a risk factor for specific disease entities such as diabetes mellitus, cardiovascular disease, and preterm low-birth-weight babies.
• Describe the role of diabetes mellitus as a risk factor for periodontal diseases.
• Discuss the importance of smoking as a risk factor for periodontal diseases.
• Discuss the association of hormones and periodontal diseases.
• Discuss the adverse effect of osteonecrosis of the jaws in dental patients taking bisphosphonates.

GOAL: To introduce the concept of risk factors for periodontal diseases and the relationship of periodontal diseases as a risk factor for other medical diseases.

KEY WORDS
bisphosphonate 97
C-reactive protein 103
osteonecrosis of the
  jaw (ONJ) 97
risk factors 94
systemic diseases 102

INTRODUCTION

The oral-systemic disease connection is a rapidly advancing area of research. Many published research articles have found a potential link between oral (periodontal) disease and coronary heart disease, adverse pregnancy outcomes, diabetes, bacterial pneumonia, and Alzheimer's disease. More research is still needed to find a definitive connection.

SYSTEMIC RISK FACTORS FOR PERIODONTAL DISEASES

While it must be assumed that general health affects a patient's resistance to the development of periodontal diseases, no specific systemic disease has been shown to produce periodontal diseases in the absence of local irritating factors. In fact, the presence of certain systemic conditions may actually enhance or intensify the response to the oral biofilms beyond what would occur if the systemic condition were not present.

While it is not possible to include every systemic disorder that has an impact on periodontal disease progression, numerous conditions potentially modify biofilm accumulation and disease progression.

Periodontal diseases are no longer regarded as infections to which everyone is equally susceptible. Research is trying to determine why some patients are more at risk than others for destructive periodontal diseases. Although bacteria are essential for the development of periodontitis, they are insufficient by themselves. A susceptible host is also necessary, so host factors play a substantial role. Advances in the understanding of the pathogenesis of many chronic systemic diseases have increased awareness of the significant interactions and association that can occur between oral diseases such as periodontal diseases and systemic diseases (Barnett, 2003). A rather large number of genetic and environmental or acquired factors place individuals at risk for periodontitis (Box 6–1).

Box 6–1   **Social Factors Contributing to Periodontal Disease**
• Tobacco • Stress • Alcohol • Drugs

Genetics

It is now known that host susceptibility factors play an important role in high-risk periodontal patients. Evidence for genetic control of **risk factors** for some forms of periodontal disease includes the following:

- A consistent association of periodontitis with certain genetically transmitted traits.
- Studies of separated twins with chronic onset forms of periodontitis.
- Genetic studies of aggressive forms of periodontitis.

Periodontal diseases can no longer be thought of as a prevalent condition for which all people are at equal risk if they fail to practice good oral hygiene. It appears that microbial and host factors are both important to disease susceptibility, but neither, independently, accounts for all degrees of periodontal disease. Because periodontal diseases are more than likely diverse in etiology, any thought of a universal host risk factor is probably also inappropriate. An association has been found between the susceptibility and severity to periodontitis and the presence of a substance called *interleukin-1* (IL-1). IL-1 is a cytokine that is released from inflammatory cells in the body for the purpose of altering either its own function or those of adjacent cells. An IL-1 gene-positive patient is about seven times more likely to develop or have advanced periodontal disease than a gene-negative patient, and this genotype occurs in approximately 30% of the population (Newman, 1998).

As with many other diseases, susceptibility to periodontal diseases may, to some extent, be genetically determined. Several congenital diseases with periodontal manifestations have been identified, such as hereditary gingival fibromatosis, cyclic neutropenia, Down syndrome, Papillon-Lefévre syndrome, Chediak-Higashi disease, and hypophosphatasia, among others.

It is now clear that genetic factors that act on and modify host responses to the microbial challenge are major determinants of susceptibility to periodontitis, as well as determinants of the rates and extent of disease progression and disease severity. Roughly 50% of the enhanced risk for severe periodontitis can be accounted for by heredity alone. Studies of families with aggressive periodontitis and groups of individuals with chronic periodontitis have shown that certain chromosomes and, in some cases, specific gene loci are linked to enhanced susceptibility for periodontitis (Newman, 1998).

Periodontal findings in twins who were reared together or apart have shown a significant genetic component for probing depth, attachment loss, and plaque that could not be explained by differences in family environment such as oral hygiene practices and frequency of dental visits (Michalowicz et al., 1991).

Age, Gender, and Race

Epidemiologic studies have shown that the incidence (rate of occurrence) of periodontal diseases increases with age (Abdellatif & Burt, 1987). This is likely the result of the cumulative effects of bacterial irritation of the tissues over many years, rather than a reduction in host resistance as a function of the aging process. Evidence strongly suggests that periodontal health can be maintained throughout life if local etiologic factors are controlled.

The National Institute of Dental and Craniofacial Research Survey of Oral Health of Adults in the United States shows that males have a greater incidence and severity of periodontal diseases.

No firm evidence documents that race is a significant risk factor in destructive forms of periodontitis other than as it may be related genetically within particular families.

Stress

Being under long-term physical and psychological stress seems to increase susceptibility to periodontal infection. Stress (along with depression, financial problems, social isolation, and other psychosocial factors) is another systemic risk factor for periodontitis because it may depress the immune response to periodontal pathogens, thereby increasing the severity of periodontal disease (Genco, Ho, et al., 1998; Peruzzo, Benatti, et al., 2007). Stressful life events such as divorce, joblessness, and lifestyle factors have been correlated with increased severity of periodontal disease (Kloostra, Eber, & Inglehart, 2007). Stress works in two ways. People under stress change their behavior and may pay less attention to oral hygiene. Also, their bodies increase the production of glucocorticosteroids (hormones made in the body that have anti-inflammatory actions and protect against stress) and cortisone, a type of glucocorticosteroid, which results in immunosuppression and a reduced resistance to infection. Stress variables also seem to have an effect on healing.

Endocrine System

Diabetes

Diabetes mellitus is a group of diseases that results in hypgerglycemia (high blood sugar or glucose). Diabetes mellitus is classified into type 1 diabetes and type 2 diabetes. Type 1 is caused by a severe insulin deficiency resulting from a destruction of beta-cells of the pancreas, which produce and secrete the hormone called insulin. Insulin is needed to control blood glucose levels since it helps bring blood glucose from the diet and that produced in the liver into the cells. The cells utilize glucose for energy. These patients are treated with insulin injections.

In type 2 diabetes, which is more common than type 1, insulin is being secreted from the pancreas, but not in sufficient amounts. Most probably, the insulin receptors on the cells surface of the tissues are not sensitive enough for the insulin to bind to the cell and allow for glucose uptake into the cell. This is referred to as insulin resistance.

Diabetes is associated with a reduced ability to cope with infections and with impaired wound healing. The balance of evidence suggests that both type 1 diabetes and type 2 diabetes carry an increased risk of severe gingivitis and periodontitis (Moritz & Mealey, 2006; Page & Beck, 1997). Diabetics may be more susceptible to developing periodontal disease. The relationship between diabetes and periodontal diseases is more likely to be observed in poorly controlled individuals (Nishimura, Takahashi, Kurihara, Takashiba, & Murayama, 1998; Ryan, Carnu, & Tenzler, 2006; Taylor et al., 1996). Patients with chronic, poorly controlled diabetes appear to have more attachment loss and bone loss than diabetics with good metabolic control (Safkan-Seppälä & Ainamo, 1992) (Figure 6–1 ■).

Epidemiologic studies on type 1 and type 2 diabetic patients indicate that although persons on optimal control are at equal risk for developing periodontal disease, too few diabetics are optimally controlled, and maintaining strict control is difficult in the long term.

Elevated blood sugar levels (hyperglycemia) may suppress the host's immune response and lead to poor wound healing and recurrent infections such as multiple or recurrent periodontal abscesses. Impaired polymorphonuclear leukocyte chemotaxis (Manouchehr-Pour, Spagnuolo, Rodman, & Bissada, 1981; McMullen, Van Dyke, Horoszewicz, & Genco, 1981), and phagocytosis (Cutler, Eke, Arnold, & Van Dyke, 1991) have been implicated as factors in the predisposition of patients to

■ **FIGURE 6–1**   56-year-old patient with type 2 diabetes mellitus. Note the clinical appearance of the gingiva.

■ **FIGURE 6–2**   Example of pregnancy gingivitis exhibiting proximal puffiness and easy bleeding on probing, reflecting an exaggerated response to local irritants due to hormonal factors.

severe periodontal destruction. Women with a family history of type 2 diabetes or diagnosed as prediabetic may be at higher risk for gestational diabetes. Close periodontal supervision would seem prudent and early intervention vital. Recent evidence indicates that *meticulous control* of the diabetic state is associated with periodontal health (Grossi & Genco, 1998).

It has been concluded that poor metabolic control of type 1 diabetes together with smoking is extremely detrimental for clinical attachment loss (Syrjala, Ylostalo, Niskanen, & Knuuttila, 2003).

Hormones

Gingivitis and periodontitis have been noticed clinically to be more severe in some patients during periods of change or imbalance in estrogen/progestin levels (Amar & Chung, 1994). In pregnant, pubertal, and postmenopausal patients, an exaggerated inflammatory response to local irritation may be evident. Hormonal status in general does have an influence on the inflammatory response.

Pregnancy   While evidence suggests that pregnancy itself may not be associated with an increased risk of periodontitis, pregnant patients often exhibit exaggerated gingival inflammatory changes in the second and third trimesters, sometimes called pregnancy gingivitis (Figure 6–2 ■). Teeth often become more mobile during pregnancy due to changes in the periodontal ligament, but return to normal after delivery.

Oral Contraceptives   Oral contraceptives act by elevating hormonal levels simulating pregnancy to prevent ovulation. Thus, it is expected that the same gingi-

val changes seen during pregnancy will also be seen in women taking oral contraceptives. Gingival changes may include inflammation and enlargement with increased amount of fluid flow into the tissue. As with pregnancy-associated gingivitis, gingival inflammation in women on oral contraceptives occurs in the presence of very little plaque. The most profound gingival changes are seen in the first few months of initially taking the contraceptive. If the condition worsens, a different formulation may be tried. Maintenance of meticulous oral hygiene is important. Once the woman discontinues the contraceptive, the gingival condition usually reverses.

Since the inception of oral contraceptives, the newer formulations contain a lower concentration of hormones. Unfortunately, most of the clinical studies investigating oral contraceptive usage were done in the 1960s. One report suggests that because of the lower concentrations in the current oral contraceptive formulations, the inflammatory response of the gingiva to dental plaque was not affected, so no gingival changes were found (Preshaw, Knutson, & Mariotti, 2001). A more recent study failed to validate the theory that earlier high- or current low-dose oral contraceptive use is associated with increased levels of gingivitis or periodontitis and suggests an important reexamination of the perceived association between OC use and periodontal diseases (Taichman, 2005).

Puberty   Hormonal imbalance is also felt to contribute to the increased severity of gingivitis seen at puberty, when there is an exaggerated response to plaque. The mechanisms are probably similar to those present in pregnancy. Gingival inflammation and enlargement can occur in both males and females, but it is more prevalent in females. Changes in hormonal levels (estrogen and progesterone) and gingival inflammatory changes are transitory and will revert to normal levels post circumpubertal period.

Menopause/Osteoporosis Osteoporosis as a result of estrogen depletion causes bone to become more porous, with less trabeculation and decreased thickness of the cortical plate (Jeffcoat, 1998). Under sufficient dental plaque stimulus, this can lead to more severe periodontal disease, including tooth loss. A correlation has been found between osteoporosis and both periodontal disease and tooth loss in postmenopausal women (Bando, Nitta, Matsubara, & Ishikawa, 1998; Jeffcoat, 1998; Oh, Bashutski, & Giannobile, 2007), but it is not considered a definitive risk factor.

Certain risk factors associated with osteoporosis include age, calcium intake (e.g., through the consumption of milk, yogurt, cheese, fish, and calcium supplements), physical activity (e.g., walking, tennis), body build, and smoking status. In a recent study, Bando and colleagues (1998) found that normal masticatory function in periodontally healthy postmenopausal women might inhibit or delay the progress of osteoporotic changes in skeletal bone.

A study by Jeffcoat (1998) related systemic osteoporosis to oral bone loss, and Kribbs (1990) and Nitta and coworkers (Nitta, Bando, Matsubara, & Ishikawa, 1997) discussed the impact of periodontal health on osteoporosis in postmenopausal women. In the latter study, twelve edentulous postmenopausal women were compared with fourteen periodontally healthy postmenopausal women: "The edentulous patients had less bone mineral density of the lumbar spine and less occlusal force." Preliminary evidence suggests that supplementation with biphosphonates, such as alendrolate (Fosamax®, Merck & Co., West Point, PA), may be helpful in stabilizing dental supporting bone because it helps improve total bone mineralization. Calibrating dental radiographs (i.e., subtraction radiography) as a diagnostic tool for systemic osteoporosis may help in early detection of both oral and systemic bone loss (Jeffcoat, 1998).

Bisphosphonates

Many dental patients with osteoporosis (reduction in bone mass due to loss of calcium), Paget's disease, or bone metastasis (with or without hypercalcemia) associ-

ated with breast and prostate cancer are taking a **bisphosphonate** (Gross, 2008). Bisphosphonates are drugs that inhibit bone resorption and reduce increased levels of blood calcium caused by cancer. Bisphosphonates inhibit bone removal or resorption by osteoclasts (cells that resorb bone), thereby allowing the buildup of new bone. This will then help to prevent fractures of the hip and spine. Normally, an equilibrium exists between osteoblasts (cells that lay down new bone) and osteoclasts. The problem arising in patients taking bisphosphonates is that there are no more osteoclasts to resorb or "eat" necrotic (dead) bone, so the new bone is laid down with the diseased bone. If necrotic bone cannot be resorbed by the osteoclasts using normal healing, then the necrotic bone will inhibit healing and affect blood supply to the area, resulting in **osteonecrosis of the jaw (ONJ)** (also referred to as bisphosphonate-related osteonecrosis of the jaw [BRONJ]) (Ruggiero, 2008). Many invasive dental procedures may precipitate the development of ONJ.

Although first observed in 2004 in patients taking intravenous bisphosphonates, cases of ONJ are being seen in patients taking oral bisphosphonates. Patients are considered to be at risk for ONJ if they are currently taking or previously were taking a bisphosphonate. Bisphosphonates, once taken into the body, bind to bone and stay there for long periods of time, even if discontinued. This long half-life of about ten years or more is of concern because even if the drug is discontinued before dental procedures, it is still in the body.

There are two subclasses of bisphosphonates: nonnitrogenous and nitrogenous bisphosphonates (Table 6–1 ■). The non-nitrogenous or first-generation bisphosphonates are not as potent as the nitrogenous, second- and third-generation or bisphosphonates, which contain nitrogen and appear to be implicated in causing ONJ. Bisphosphonates remain in the bone indefinitely even after the drug is discontinued.

Osteonecrosis of the jaw occurs after precipitating causes such as extractions or periodontal and implant procedures where there is poor or delayed wound healing in the mouth. Clinically, ONJ is characterized by exposed, necrotic bone in the maxillofacial region (more common in the mandible than maxilla) that has persisted for more than eight weeks (Figures 6–3 ■ and 6–4 ■) (Marx, 2007). Osteonecrosis of the jaws can occur after extractions (highest incidence), implant placement, periodontal procedures, endodontic therapy, orthodontic therapy, and even spontaneously without any treatment

Table 6–1   Bisphosphonates

Subclass of Bisphosphonate	Trade Name	Generic Name	Route of Administration	Indication	Potency
Non-nitrogenous	Didronel	etidronate	oral	Paget's disease	1
Non-nitrogenous	Bonefos	clodronate	oral	bone metastasis	10
Nitrogenous	Skelid	tiludronate	oral	Paget's disease	10
Nitrogenous	Aredia	pamidronate	oral, IV	Paget's disease and hypercalcemia (inhibits release of calcium from bone in cancer)	100
Nitrogenous	Fosamax	alendronate	oral	osteoporosis	500
Nitrogenous	Boniva	ibandronate	oral, IV	osteoporosis	1,000
Nitrogenous	Actonel	risedronate	oral	osteoporosis	2,000
Nitrogenous	Zometa, Reclast	zoledronate	IV	Zometa for hypercalcemia; mutiple myeloma (cancer of the body's plasma cells); Reclast for osteoporosis (once a year injection)	10,000

(Otomo-Corgel, 2007). The following factors are thought to be risk factors for ONJ: (1) corticosteroid therapy, (2) diabetes, (3) smoking, (4) alcohol use, (5) poor oral hygiene, and (6) chemotherapeutic drugs.

Prior to treatment with bisphosphonates, the patient should have a thorough oral examination and all invasive dental procedures including extractions and restorative, endodontic, and periodontal therapies (American Association of Oral and Maxillofacial Surgeons, 2007; Wade & Suzuki, 2007). Patients should be encouraged to practice good oral hygiene.

Once a patient has been taking an oral bisphosphonate for more than three years, the risk of developing ONJ increases (Zak, Spina, Spinazze, Perkinson, & Spinazze, 2007a, 2007b). *Although the risk of developing ONJ is low in patients taking oral bisphosphonates* (Migliorati et al., 2005; Edwards BJ et al., 2008), dental treatment may need to be altered. There is currently no data from clinical trials evaluating dental management of patients on oral bisphosphonate therapy. Preventive care is extremely important to reduce the incidence of ONJ. Recommendations focus on conservative surgical procedures, proper

■ **FIGURE 6–3**   Edentulous patient had pieces of bone that became necrotic and continued to slough off after tooth extractions. (Courtesy of Jacqueline Plemons, DDS, Baylor College of Dentistry)

■ **FIGURE 6–4**   Case of ONJ that occurred spontaneously. Note the white area, which is exposed necrotic bone. (Courtesy of Jacqueline Plemons, DDS, Baylor College of Dentistry)

sterile technique, appropriate use of oral disinfectants, and the dentist's clinical and professional judgment (American Dental Association of Scientific Affairs, 2006). Consultation with the patient's physician is necessary.

Patients taking oral bisphosphonates for less than three years can have invasive dental treatment, but if the patient has been taking bisphosphonates for more than three years, the C-terminal cross-linked telopetide (CTx) blood test can be performed to determine the amount of bone resorption. The CTx test is performed by Quest Diagnostics and sent to its lab in California (http://www.questdiagnostic.com). If the results of the CTx blood test are greater than 150 pg/ml, then dental procedures can be performed. Values less than 100 pg/ml are associated with a high risk of developing ONJ (Fugazzotto et al., 2007; Grant et al., 2008; Marx 2007). It is recommended to discontinue the drug for 3 months prior to the planned procedure and send for CTx testing. Once treatment is done, extend the "drug holiday" for an additional 3 months (Cartsos et al., 2008; Marx, 2007; Marx et al., 2005). Thus, patients on long-term oral bisphosphonates should be treated with caution (Wang, Weber, & McCauley, 2007).

On the other hand, while patients are taking IV bisphosphonates any invasive dental procedures should be avoided. Dentists need to exercise their professional judgment, perhaps after consultation with the patient's physician, in deciding whether invasive treatment is needed under the particular clinical situations (American Dental Association Council on Scientific Affairs, 2006).

Hematologic System

Several blood dyscrasias have been associated with uncommon, unusual, extreme forms of periodontal diseases. Agranulocytosis and neutropenia (including cyclic neutropenia) are associated with an increased severity of gingivitis and periodontitis as well as necrotic ulcerations. Acute leukemia is characterized by purple-colored gingival enlargement, ulceration, inflammation, and spontaneous severe bleeding. These changes are attributable to infiltration of malignant cells, neutropenia, impaired phagocytosis, platelet deficiency, and decreased effectiveness of associated immune mechanisms. Patients with these medical problems require special attention.

HIV/AIDS

Human immunodeficiency virus (HIV) seropositive individuals appear to be vulnerable to aggressive necrotizing periodontal diseases, including necrotizing ulcerative gingivitis (NUG) and necrotizing ulcerative periodontitis (NUP) (Murray, 1994). The development of severe forms of gingivitis and periodontitis is focused on an impairment of the host response (i.e., functional defects in the host's neutrophils) to combat infections. It appears that the degree of immunodeficiency influences the prevalence and severity of these periodontal diseases in the HIV-infected population and may also influence treatment expectations and prognosis (Figure 6–5 ■).

(a)

(b)

■ **FIGURE 6–5**   Periodontal lesions associated with HIV infection: (a) Inflammation of the gingiva with characteristic lesions; (b) more advanced lesions that resemble necrotizing ulcerative periodontitis (NUP) and that are nonresponsive to typical therapy. (Figure 6–5a courtesy of Proctor & Gamble, Cincinnati, OH)

Nutritional Status

Nutritional deficiencies have not been shown to cause periodontal diseases. Nutrition studies are commonly done by inducing a deprivation state of a single nutrient or a group of related nutrients in laboratory animals that result in decreased formation of the periodontal ligament, bone, and cementum. Very few patients have a diet that is totally lacking in a single nutrient or group of related nutrients; therefore, the information gained from these experimental laboratory studies in animals may not apply to the human clinical situation.

Vitamin deficiencies are probably given more significance in the etiology of periodontal diseases from a clinical standpoint than other nutritional substances. The vitamin most often studied is ascorbic acid (vitamin C), which plays an important role in the normal functions of fibroblasts, osteoblasts, and odontoblasts. When vitamin C levels are greatly reduced (i.e., scurvy), wound healing is impaired.

Some other considerations concerning the diet may be important in the overall dental problems of some patients. Tough or coarse foods do not provide functional stimulation to the gingiva, nor do they help to remove plaque below the contact points or cervical bulge on the teeth.

Patients who regularly eat between meals present a problem in that they constantly provide a food source for the bacteria and may have difficulty in maintaining good oral hygiene.

Drug Use Status

Tobacco Products

Cigarette smoking is a major (and may be the most significant) risk factor for severe periodontal diseases. Smokers are about two to six times more likely to have periodontal destruction than nonsmokers, yet they can exhibit less gingival bleeding on probing (Heasman et al., 2006; Jansson & Lavstedt, 2002; Krall, Hayes, Garvey, & Garcia, 1997; Tonetti, 1998). Multiple studies report that smokers are at greater risk for loss of attachment, alveolar bone loss, and tooth loss compared to nonsmokers (Papantonopoulos, 2004). They also may respond less favorable to surgical and nonsurgical periodontal therapy (Fisher et al., 2008).

A study by Krall and colleagues (1997) found that current male cigarette smokers had significantly fewer teeth than those men who reported never smoking. The number of missing teeth was positively related to pack/years of cigarette use, age, and coffee consumption and inversely related to level of education. It is more accurate to use the term "pack/years" rather than "pack/day" because it describes the exposure to toxins in a cumulative way. The study also found that current smokers had higher levels of tooth mobility, calculus deposition, and probing depth than men who had never smoked. Former cigarette smokers and men who smoked pipes or cigars were similar to men who never smoked in regard to tooth loss.

Generally, the periodontal status of former smokers has been found to be intermediate between that of never smokers and current smokers (Haber & Kent, 1992; Haber et al., 1993). It has been suggested that the past effects of smoking on the periodontium cannot be reversed, but that smoking cessation is beneficial to periodontal health (American Academy of Periodontology, 1999). The inflammatory function in the periodontal tissues of smokers who quit reverts back to normal (Nair et al., 2008).

Although smoking does not dramatically affect the oral microbiota, studies have shown that smoking and tobacco products directly modulate the subgingival microflora by favoring colonization with periodontal pathogens (Grossi et al., 1996). Additionally, smoking may suppress the host-defense system, which may promote periodontal disease progression (Kibayashi et al., 2007). Thus, smoking increases the risk for periodontal diseases and interferes with the ability of the gingiva and bone to respond to treatment (Gunsolley et al., 1998; Tonetti, 1998). This mechanism is probably through an altered host response. Effects of smoking seem to be related not only to the local effects in the oral cavity (heat, dryness, and increased plaque and calculus deposits), but also to a suppression of the immune system altering the host response to periodontal pathogens. To adequately deal with bacterial infections, functioning neutrophils are necessary. It has been well documented that cigarette smoke can have harmful effects on various neutrophil functions (Kenny, Kraal, Saxe, & Jones, 1977). For example, tobacco smoke can impair the chemotaxis and phagocytosis of neutrophils (Lannan et al., 1992). Thus, the PMNs do not function properly in eliminating invasive, pathogenic bacteria. Individuals with alterations in their host-defense system would then be more susceptible to periodontal infections by preexisting pathogenic bacteria.

Another problem associated with smoking is that products of cigarette smoke remain on the root surfaces and in the gingival crevicular fluid, thereby providing a reservoir of irritants for the soft tissue and preventing tissue attachment.

Research has found that the presence of a specific gene (interleukin-1 beta) has been associated with risk for periodontal disease severity. It has also been reported that in heavy cigarette smokers, carriage of interleukin-1 gene complex was associated with an increased risk for peri-implant (around the implant) bone loss (Feloutzis et al., 2003).

Smokeless tobacco for some may be an alternative to cigarette smoking. However, research has shown that smokeless tobacco may also contribute to periodontal diseases and may eventually lead to cancerous changes in the soft tissues (Figure 6–6 ■). A common finding is gingival recession adjacent to the site of tobacco placement. More research is needed to determine whether smokeless tobacco use is associated with an increased level of plaque-associated gingivitis. New studies have found that cigar and pipe smoking may be as harmful to periodontal tissues as cigarette smoking (Krall, Garvey, & Garcia, 1999).

Strict supragingival plaque control has been documented to reduce indicators of subgingival inflammation and destruction to a similar extent in smokers and never-smokers (Gomes et al., 2007).

Cannabis (marijuana) smoking may be a risk factor for periodontal disease that is independent of the use of tobacco. An article in *Journal of the American Medical Association* (JAMA) documented that although tobacco smoking was strongly associated with increased incidence of periodontal disease, there was no interaction between cannabis use and tobacco smoking in predicting the condition's occurrence (Thomson et al., 2008).

Alcohol

Alcohol abuse may also contribute to periodontal diseases. Chronic alcohol intake presents an increased risk for periodontitis because of poor oral hygiene due to overall neglect and a tendency to malnutrition. Alcohol consumption is related to increased incidence (Drake, Hunt, & Koch, 1995) and prevalence of tooth loss, especially in men (Krall et al., 1997; Kranzler, Babor, Goldstein, & Gold, 1990).

Xerostomia Due to Drugs

Several medications, such as diuretics (antihypertensive drugs) and psychotropic drugs (i.e., anti-anxiety drugs such as Valium; antidepressants such as Elavil; and antipsychotic drugs such as Clozaril and Risperdal) can cause xerostomia or dry mouth, which can be uncomfortable for the patient, interfere with plaque control, and thereby increase periodontal inflammation. The reduced salivary flow has also been associated with increased caries.

Gingival Overgrowth Due to Drugs

Gingival enlargement or overgrowth in response to plaque accumulation can be exaggerated by medications such as phenytoin (used for seizures), calcium channel blockers such as nifedipine or diltiazem (for cardiovascular problems and hypertension), and cyclosporine (in transplant patients). The alveolar bone and attachment apparatus are not affected by these drugs (Ciancio, 1996; Figure 6–7 ■).

The areas of enlargement generally begin interproximally and slowly grow to form triangular tissue masses that eventually unite in a continuous curtain of firm gingival tissue across facial and lingual surfaces. The enlarged tissue interferes with oral hygiene and is often inflamed. Gingival overgrowth has been reported to occur in about 50% of patients receiving phenytoin (Ciancio, Yaffe, & Catz, 1972), 15% of patients receiving nifedipine (Barak, Engelberg, & Hiss, 1987), and 25% of patients receiving cyclosporine (Daley, Wysocki, & May, 1986).

Steroids   According to the American Academy of Periodontology, there is a lack of influence of steroids on periodontal disease (Kinane, 1999). Systemic steroids are

■ **FIGURE 6–6**   Clinical example of smokeless tobacco lesions damaging the periodontium.

■ **FIGURE 6–7**   Example of drug-induced gingival overgrowth related to the use of cyclosporine.

used in the management of asthma and other inflammatory conditions including skin conditions and ear problems.

PERIODONTAL DISEASES AS RISK FACTORS FOR SYSTEMIC CONDITIONS

Although inflammatory periodontal diseases are local infections of the gingiva and bone, it has been shown that the presence of periodontitis may itself be a risk factor for other infections in the body, **systemic diseases,** and pregnancy-related problems (American Academy of Periodontology, 1998; Costerton & Keller, 2007; Kim & Amar, 2006). This means that although a relationship may have been found, it is not yet known that it is a cause-and-effect relationship; risk factors are not causative. Risk factors may predict disease, but it does not necessarily follow that they will cause disease. Examples of systemic conditions with such a relationship include cardiovascular disease and stroke (Gapski & Cobb, 2006), type 2 diabetes mellitus (Moritz & Mealey, 2006), respiratory conditions (Scannapieco & Ho, 2001), adverse pregnancy outcomes (Paquette, 2006) and possible Alzheimer's disease (Stein et al. 2006). Additionally,

Did You Know?

The U.S. Surgeon General stated that the oral cavity may be the initial site of disease that can serve as the portal of entry of microorganisms into the general circulation, which can have an adverse effect on your patient's general health status.

in 2007, pancreatic cancer may be shown to be linked to periodontal disease (Michaud et al., 2007).

Diabetes

A conference on oral health and systemic health that was held in Switzerland in December 2002 (Barnett, 2003) concluded that evidence showed that untreated periodontitis can complicate glycemic control of patients with diabetes (Saremi et al., 2005). Diabetics may be *more susceptible* to developing periodontal disease, but diabetes does not cause it. Of all the systemic diseases, diabetes and periodontal diseases have been the most extensively studied. It has been shown that periodontal diseases may be responsible for higher levels of blood glucose in diabetics (Grossi & Genco, 1998). A study that evaluated periodontitis in diabetics with different interleukin (IL-1) genotypes concluded that the prevalence of severe attachment loss increased with decreasing diabetic control (Guzman, Karima, Wang, & Van Dyke, 2003) When these infections are controlled or eliminated in diabetic patients, their insulin requirements can often be reduced (Ryan et al., 2006). Effective treatment of periodontal diseases can result in a reduced need to gear up tissue metabolism to fight the infection and lower blood sugar levels, thereby reducing insulin requirements and helping in diabetic control with an additional benefit of reducing other complications (e.g., blindness, renal failure, neuropathy, and coronary artery disease) of diabetes. According to the American Academy of Periodontology, control of infections, including periodontal diseases, may be essential to the establishment of good metabolic control in diabetics (American Academy of Periodontology, 1998). However, it is really not conclusive because it cannot be predicted with certainty that the treatment of a patient's periodontal condition will have any effect on blood sugar.

 Rapid Dental Hint

When evaluating your patient, screen for symptoms and signs of diabetes.

Cardiovascular Disease

In the late 1990s, researchers found a possible link between periodontal diseases and coronary heart disease (CHD) with an increased risk for atherosclerosis and thromboembolisms, independent of other risk factors for these cardiovascular diseases (Genco, Glurich, Haraszthy, Zambon, & DeNardin, 1998). This link may have been explained by the systemic inflammatory burden caused by inflammatory periodontal diseases (Nakib et al., 2004). However, as with all of the other systemic diseases mentioned in this chapter, the studies are not conclusive of cause and effect. Men with periodontitis, especially those under age 50, are 25% more likely to develop CHD (American Academy of Periodontology, 1998; Beck, 1996). Two different surveys have shown that heart disease is the most common condition shared by periodontitis patients (Umino & Nagao, 1993).

In the late 1990s, the connection between heart attacks and periodontal disease was felt to be so convincing that proper plaque control might actually be an exercise that saves a patient's life. Although it may seem unlikely that an infection in the mouth may result in heart disease, there are several possible links that might explain this association. For example, it is well known that if a person has periodontal disease, oral bacteria will enter the blood stream even after chewing or tooth brushing. When bacteria from the inflamed gingival tissue enter the blood stream, they trigger platelets to gather around them in a clump, possibly infecting and obstructing the blood vessels in the heart and the brain (Shanies & Hein, 2006). Forty percent of those bacteria, especially *Streptococcus sanguis* and *Porphyromonas gingivalis,* have been traced to the mouth (Genco, Glurich, et al. 1998). Patients have a 50% increased risk for heart disease (DeStefano, Andda, Kahn, Williamson, & Russell, 1993) and 30% increased risk for stroke if they also have periodontitis.

Periodontitis and cardiovascular diseases are both associated with a systemic inflammatory response that contributes to elevated levels of serum **C-reactive protein.** C-reactive protein (CRP) is an inflammatory serum marker or a predictor of increased risk for cardiovascular disease (Gapski & Cobb, 2006). A study by D'Aiuto, Ready, and Tonetti in 2004 found that periodontitis may result in an increased cardiovascular risk based on serum CRP levels and that successful periodontal therapy could decrease these serum inflammatory markers.

Did You Know?

Ninety-one percent of patients with coronary artery disease suffered from moderate to severe periodontitis, compared to 66% in non-cardiac patients.

In 2004 Nakib and colleagues reported on a study that was performed between 1996 and 1998 on 6,931 subjects. Results found that compared to subjects with no or mild periodontitis, subjects with moderate or severe periodontitis were more likely to have coronary artery calcification (CAC), but the difference was not statistically significant. Thus, these researchers suggested that periodontitis may not be strongly associated with CAC (Nakib et al., 2004). Future studies need to be conducted on this subject. Recommending periodontal treatment for the prevention of artherosclerotic cardiovascular disease is not warranted based on present scientific evidence (Demmer & Desvarieux, 2006). Periodontal treatment is recommended because it will benefit the patient's oral health.

Adverse Pregnancy Outcomes

Women with periodontal disease may be seven to eight times more predisposed to deliver premature (< 37 weeks) infants with low birth weight (< 5.5 lb) (Davenport et al., 1998). Periodontal disease in the mother may be responsible for many of the low-birth-weight, premature births (PLBW). Current data suggest a relationship between elevated prostaglandin E_2 (PGE_2) levels in the gingival crevicular fluid (GCF) as a marker of current periodontal disease activity and decreasing birth weight (Offenbacher et al., 1998). Also, the elevated levels of PGE_2 stimulate labor contractions (Doheny, O'Reilly, Sexton, & Morrison, 2007). The increased production of PGE_2 by the mother is due to a response to the anaerobic periodontal infection (e.g., *Porphyromonas gingivalis, Tannerella forsythensis,* and *Camplytobacter rectus*). This twofold elevation in PGE_2, which is seen in the GCF and amniotic sac, was observed in PLBW compared with normal-birth-weight mothers (Hill, 1998), One-hundred and twenty-four pregnant or postpartum mothers were examined for periodontitis at the University of North Carolina (Offenbacher et al., 1996). Mothers with a defined preterm low-birth-weight delivery demonstrated that periodontal disease was a "statistically significant risk factor for PLBW." PLBW status is defined as a birth weight of less than 2500 g (5.51 lbs) and/or a gestational age of less than 37 weeks at delivery or premature rupture of membranes. "PLBW cases had significantly worse periodontal disease than respective normal birth weight (NBW) controls." PLBW is a major health problem because it occurs in 1 in 10 deliveries and results in infant mortality, long-term morbidity, and 5 million neonatal intensive care unit hospital stays per year. The emotional, social, and financial burdens on families are extraordinary (Dasanayake, 1998).

A clinical pilot study published in 2003 was conducted to determine whether treatment of periodontitis reduces the risk of spontaneous preterm birth. This study concluded that although this pilot study found that performing scaling and root planing in pregnant women with periodontitis might reduce spontaneous preterm birth, larger trials need to be done (Jeffcoat et al., 2003) to confirm that periodontal therapy decreases the frequency of preterm delivery and neonatal complications.

Fetal exposures to periodontal pathogens also may increase the risk for maternal vaginal bleeding during pregnancy, preeclampsia (hypertension occurring during pregnancy; can affect both mother and fetus) and intrauterine fetal growth restriction (Paquette, 2006).

Rapid Dental Hint

If your patient is pregnant, stress the importance of periodontal treatments to reduce the risk of adverse pregnancy outcomes.

Respiratory Diseases

Patients with periodontal disease may be at risk for respiratory diseases (Hayes, Sparrow, Cohen, Vokonas, & Garcia, 1998). Periodontal disease is added to the list of other risk factors for this problem, including the elderly, people who smoke, and individuals confined to nursing homes or hospitals. Examples of respiratory diseases include pneumonia (Azarpazhooh & Leake, 2006), bronchitis, and emphysema. Pneumonia may be the result of infection by anaerobic bacteria, which is a component of dental plaque (American Academy of Periodontology, 1998; Scannapieco & Mylotte, 1996).

Bacteria (oral biofilms) found in the oral cavity can be taken up into the lung to cause respiratory diseases. Many bacteria present in aspirated saliva are anaerobic, including *Porphyromonas gingivalis, Fusobacterium nucleatum,* and *Bacteroides oralis* (Terpenning, 2006). Recent hypotheses relate to the presence in saliva of enzymes and cytokines associated with oral pathogens, and that could alter the colonization of the respiratory tract or promote infection by respiratory pathogens (Mojon, 2003). Oral hygiene and frequent professional oral healthcare are useful in reducing the development of pneumonia in high-risk elderly people in nursing homes and hospitals

(Azarpazhooh & Leake, 2006; Scannapieco, Wang, & Shiau, 2001). It is important to emphasize oral care in patients in hospital and nursing home environments.

Alzheimer's Disease

Early exposure to inflammatory diseases, including periodontal disease, may increase the risk for developing Alzheimer's disease later in life (Stein et al., 2006). Possible ways that oral bacteria are involved include spreading of Gram-negative pathogens from the oral cavity to the brain, genetic predisposition, and injury to brain tissue due to the production of inflammatory mediators in response to periodontal bacteria (Stein et al., 2006). Research is currently being conducted delving into this relationship.

DENTAL HYGIENE NOTES

Oral conditions can significantly influence events elsewhere in the body. Periodontal disease is a risk factor for certain systemic conditions; certain systemic conditions are also a risk factor for periodontal disease. It is well known that medical conditions such as diabetes mellitus may modify the reaction to dental plaque, which may make the individual more susceptible to periodontal disease. Additionally, periodontal diseases have been documented to cause some medical conditions including coronary heart disease, diabetes mellitus, low-birth-weight babies, and respiratory diseases. It then becomes apparent that periodontal clinicians are treating the "whole" patient and attempting to control both periodontal diseases and medical conditions.

KEY POINTS

- Currently, evidence-based dentistry supports the use of risk assessment techniques to guide clinical decisions in the treatment of periodontal diseases.
- Although a relationship may have been found between certain medical conditions and periodontal disease, it is not yet known that it is a cause-and-effect relationship; risk factors are not causative.
- Other risk factors not strongly related but still associated with increased probability of periodontal diseases include aging, gender, genetic predisposition, stress, nutrition, and systemic diseases including immunosuppression.
- Not only do certain medical conditions predispose individuals to periodontal diseases, but also peri-

odontal diseases predispose people to certain medical conditions.

- Patients taking oral bisphosphonates for osteoporosis must be assessed and monitored for osteonecrosis of the jaws (ONJ). Patients taking intravenous bisphosphonates should not have any elective dentistry performed on them.
- Attempts to manage risk factors are important in the prevention and treatment of periodontal diseases.

SELF-QUIZ

1. Which one of the following concerns should the dental hygienist be aware of in patients taking bisphosphonates? (pp. 97–98)
   a. Diabetes
   b. Osteonecrosis of the jaw
   c. Stroke
   d. Hypertension
   e. Respiratory diseases

2. Which one of the following evidence exists to support the concept of a genetic predisposition to periodontal diseases? (p. 94)
   a. Presence of a specific type of bacteria
   b. Increased levels of bacterial enzymes in the blood
   c. Association of periodontitis with certain transmitted traits
   d. Transmission of bacteria through saliva from mother to child

3. Which one of the following mechanisms explains how increased stress adversely affects the periodontium? (p. 95)
   a. Increases in subgingival pathogenic bacteria
   b. Increases in estrogen levels results in gingivitis
   c. Less compliance with home care of teeth and gums
   d. Shifts in the concentration of available endotoxins

4. The hormonal changes associated with pregnancy cause an increased incidence of gingival disease because these changes are associated with an increase in sex hormone levels. (p. 96)
   a. Both the statement and the reason are correct and related.
   b. Both the statement and the reason are correct but not related.
   c. The statement is correct, but the reason is not.
   d. The statement is not correct, but the reason is correct.
   e. Neither the statement nor the reason is correct.

5. Smoking affects the periodontium by which one of the following mechanisms? (pp. 100–101)
   a. Decreasing the number of melanocytes
   b. Suppressing of the immune system
   c. Altering the metabolism of fibroblasts
   d. Increasing the amount of fibrotic tissue
   e. Decreasing the number of periodontal pathogens

6. Periodontal diseases may be important risk factor for all of the following medical conditions except one. Which one is the exception? (pp. 102–104)
   a. Stroke
   b. Hypertension
   c. Diabetes mellitus
   d. Low-birth-weight babies
   e. Kidney failure

7. Which of the following statements about smoking and periodontal diseases is true? (pp. 100–101)
   a. Smoking dramatically affects the oral microflora.
   b. Smoking cessation is beneficial to periodontal health.
   c. Past effects of smoking on the periodontium are usually reversible.
   d. Current smokers have a low level of tooth mobility.
   e. Smokeless tobacco does not increase the incidence of periodontal disease.

8. Which of the following substances may be related to periodontal disease activity and low birth weight babies? (p. 103)
   a. Blood
   b. Suppuration
   c. Gingival crevicular fluid
   d. Prostaglandin E_2
   e. Saliva

9. Which of the following bacterium in the mouth has been found to possibly infect and obstruct blood vessels in the heart and the brain? (pp. 102–103)
   a. *Prevotella intermedia*
   b. *Fuscobacterium nucleatum*
   c. *Porphyromonas gingivalis*
   d. *Campylobacter rectus*
   e. *Tannerella forsythensis*

10. Which of the following explains why patients with periodontal disease may be at risk for respiratory diseases especially in hospitals and nursing homes? (p. 104)
   a. neglected oral hygiene
   b. decayed teeth
   c. collapsed circulatory system
   d. increased risk for heart failure
   e. increased risk for other systemic diseases

REFERENCES

Abdellatif, H. M., and B. A. Burt. 1987. An epidemiological investigation into the relative importance of age and oral hygiene status as determinants of periodontitis. *J. Periodontol.* 66:16–33.

Amar, S., and K. M. Chung. 1994. Influence of hormonal variation on the periodontium in women. *Periodontology* 6:79–87.

American Academy of Periodontology. 1998. Periodontal disease as a potential risk factor for systemic disease (Position Paper). *J. Periodontol.* 69:841–850.

American Academy of Periodontology. 1999. Tobacco use and the periodontal patient (position paper). *J. Periodontol.* 70:1419–1427.

American Dental Association Council on Scientific Affairs. 2006. Dental management of patients receiving oral bisphosphonate therapy. JADA 137(8): 1144-1150.

Azarpazhooh, A., and J. L. Leake 2006. Systematic review of the association between respiratory diseases and oral health. *J Periodontol.* 77:1465–1482.

Bando, K., H. Nitta, M. Matsubara, and I. Ishikawa. 1998. Bone mineral density in periodontally healthy and edentulous postmenopausal women. *Ann. Periodontol.* 3:322–326.

Barak, S., I. S. Engelberg, and J. Hiss. 1987. Gingival hyperplasia caused by nifedipine—histopathologic findings. *J. Periodontol.* 58:639–642.

Barnett, M. L. 2003. Coordination Meeting on Oral Health and Systemic Health Periodontal Medicine: Health Policy Implications. Geneva, Switzerland. *J. Periodontol.* 74:1081–1086.

Beck, J. D. 1996. Periodontal implications: Older adults. *Ann. Periodontol.* 1:322–457.

Cartsos, V. M., Zhu, S., Zavras, A. I. 2008. Bisphosphonate use and the risk of adverse jaw outcomes: A medical claims study of 714,217 people. J Am Dent Assoc. 139:23–30.

Ciancio, S. G. 1996. Medications as risk factors for periodontal disease. *J. Periodontol.* 67:1055–1059.

Ciancio, S. G., S. J. Yaffe, and C. C. Catz. 1972. Gingival hyperplasia and diphenylhydantoin. *J. Periodontol.* 43:411–414.

Costerton, J. and D. Keller. 2007. Oral periopathogens and systemic effects. *Gen Dent* 55:210–215.

Cutler, C. W., P. Eke, R. R. Arnold, and T. E. Van Dyke. 1991. Defective neutrophil function in an insulin-dependent diabetic patient. A case report. *J. Periodontol.* 62:394–401.

D'Aiuto F., D. Ready, and M.S. Tonetti. 2004. Periodontal disease and C-reactive protein-associated cardiovascular risk. *J. Periodontol. Res.* 39:236–241.

Daley, T. D., G. P. Wysocki, and C. May. 1986. Clinical and pharmacological correlations in cyclosporin-induced gingival hyperplasia. *Oral Surg. Oral Med. Oral Patho.* 62:417–421.

Dasanayake, A. P. 1998. Periodontal disease as a risk factor in pregnancy. *Ann. Periodontol.* 3:206–212.

Davenport, E. S., C. E. C. S. Williams, J. A. C. Sterne, V. Sivapathasundram, J. M. Fearne, and M. A. Curtis. 1998. The East London study of maternal chronic periodontal disease and preterm low birth weight infants: Study design and prevalence data. *Ann Periodontol.* 3:213–221.

Demmer, R.T., and M. Desvarieux. 2006. Periodontal infections and cardiovascular disease. *JADA* 137(10 supplement):14S–20S.

DeStefano, F., R. F. Andda, H. S. Kahn, D. F. Williamson, and C. M. Russell. 1993. Dental disease and risk of coronary heart disease and mortality. *Br. Med. J.* 306:688–691.

Doheny, H. C., M. J. O'Reilly, D. J. Sexton, and J. J. Morrison. 2007. THG113.31, a specific PGF2 alpha receptor antagonist, induces human myometrial relaxation and BKCa channel activation. *Reprod. Biol. Endocrinol.* 5: 10. Published online 2007 March 16. doi: 10.1186/1477-7827-5-10.

Drake, C. W., R. J. Hunt, and G. G. Koch. 1995. Three-year tooth loss among black and white older adults in North Carolina. *J. Dent. Res.* 74:675–680.

Edwards, B. J., J. W. Hellstein, and P. L. Jacobson. Updated recommendations for managing the care of patients receiving oral bisphosphonate therapy: An advisory statement from the American Dental Association Council on Scientific Affairs. *J Am Dent Assoc.* 2008; 139; 1674–1677.

Feloutzis A., N. P. Lang, M. S. Tonetti, W. Burgin, U. Bragger, et al. 2003. Il-1 gene polymorphism and smoking as risk factors for peri-implant bone loss in a well-maintained population. *Clin. Oral Implants Res.* 14:10–17.

Fisher, S., L. Kells, J. P. Picard, S. C. Gelskey, et al. Tobacco smoking and periodontal health in a Saudi Arabian population. *J Periodontol* 2008; 79(3): 461–468.

Fugazzotto, P. A., Lightfoot, W. S., Jaffin, R., Kumar, A. 2007. Implant placement with or without simultaneous tooth extraction in patients taking oral bisphosphonates: Postoperative healing, early follow up, and the incidence of complications in two private practices. *J Periodontol.* 7819: 1664–1669.

Gapski, R., and C. M. Cobb. 2006. Chronic inflammatory periodontal disease. A risk factor for cardiovascular disease and ischemic stroke? *Grand Rounds in Oral-Sys.Med.* 1:14–22.

Genco, R. J., I. Glurich, V. Haraszthy, J. Zambon, and E. DeNardin. 1998. Overview of risk factors for periodontal disease and implications for diabetes and cardiovascular disease. *Compendium* (special issue) 19:40–45.

Genco, R. J., A. W. Ho, J. Kopman, S. G. Grossi, R. G. Dunford, and L. A. Tedesco. 1998. Models to evaluate the role of stress in periodontal diseases. *Ann. Periodontol.* 3:288–302.

Gomes, S. C., I. B. Piccini, C. Susin, et al. 2007. Effect of supragingival plaque control in smokers and never-smokers: 6 month evaluation of patients with periodontitis. *J. Periodontol.* 78(8):1515-1521.

Grant, B. T., C. Amenedo, K. Freeman, R. A. Kraut. 2008. Outcomes of placing dental implants in patients taking oral bisphosphonates: A review of its cases. *J Oral Maxillofac Surg*; 66:223–230.

Gross, H.B. 2008. Bisphosphonate-induced osteonecrosis: Dental considerations. *Compendium* 29(2):112–113.

Grossi, S. G., and R. J. Genco. 1998. Periodontal disease and diabetes mellitus: A two-way relationship. *Ann. Periodontol.* 3:51–61.

Grossi, S. G., F. B. Skrepcinski, T. DeCaro, J. J. Zambon, D. Cummins, and R. J. Genco. 1996. Responses to periodontal therapy in diabetics and smokers. *J. Periodontol.* 67(Suppl.):1094–1102.

Gunsolley, J. C., S. M. Quinn, J. Tew, C. M. Gooss, C. N. Brooks, and H. A. Schenkein. 1998. The effect of smoking on individuals with minimal periodontal destruction. *J. Periodontol.* 69:165–170.

Guzman S., M. Karima, H. Y. Wang, and T. E. Van Dyke. 2003. Association between interleukin-1 genotype and periodontal disease in a diabetic population. *J. Periodontol.* 74:1183–1190.

Haber, J., and R. L. Kent. 1992. Cigarette smoking in periodontal practice. *J. Periodontol.* 63:100–106.

Haber, J., J. Wattles, M. Crowley, R. Mandell, K. Joshipura, and R. L. Kent. 1993. Evidence for cigarette smoking as a major risk factor for periodontitis. *J. Periodontol.* 64:16–23.

Hayes, C., D. Sparrow, M. Cohen, P. S. Vokonas, and R. I. Garcia. 1998. The association between alveolar bone loss and pulmonary function: The VA dental longitudinal study. *Ann. Periodontol.* 3:257–261.

Heasman, L, F. Stacey, P. M. Preshaw, G. I. McCracken, S. Hepburn, and P. A. Heasman. 2006. The effect of smoking on periodontal treatment response: A review of clinical evidence. *J. Clin. Periodontol.* 33:241–253.

Hill, G. B. 1998. Preterm birth: Associations with genital and oral microflora. *Ann. Periodontol.* 3:222–232.

Jansson, L., and S. Lavstedt. 2002. Influence of smoking on marginal bone loss and tooth loss – A prospective study over 20 years. *J. Clin. Periodontol.* 29:750–756.

Jeffcoat, M. K. 1998. Osteoporosis: A possible modifying factor in oral bone loss. *Ann. Periodontol.* 3:312–321.

Jeffcoat, M.K., J.C. Hauth, N.C. Geurs, M. S. Reddy, S. P. Cliver, et al. 2003. Periodontal disease and preterm birth: Results of a pilot intervention study. *J. Periodontol.* 74:1214–1218.

Kenny, E. G., J. H. Kraal, S. R. Saxe, and J. Jones. 1977. The effect of cigarette smoke on human oral polymorphonuclear leukocytes. *J. Periodont. Res.* 12:227–234.

Kibayashi, M., M. Tanaka, N. Nishida, et al. 2007. Longitudinal study of the association between smoking as a periodontitis risk and salivary biomarkers related to periodontitis. *J. Periodontol.* 78:859–867.

Kim, J, and S. Amar. 2006. Periodontal disease and systemic conditions: A bidirectional relationship. *Odontology* 94:10-21.

Kinane, D. F. 1999. Periodontitis modified by systemic factors. *Ann. Periodontol.* 4:54–63.

Kloostra, P. W., R. M. Eber, and M. R. Inglehart. 2007. Anxiety, stress, depression and patient's responses to periodontal treatment: Periodontists' knowledge and professional behavior. *J. Periodontol.* 78:64–71.

Krall, E., A. Garvey, and R. Garcia. 1999. Alveolar bone loss and tooth loss in male cigar and pipe smokers. *J. American Dent. Assoc.* 130:57–64.

Krall, E., C. Hayes, A. J. Garvey, and R. I. Garcia. 1997. Study finds a correlation between smoking and tooth loss. *J. Mass. Dent. Soc.* 46:20–23.

Kranzler, H. R., T. F. Babor, L. Goldstein, and J. Gold. 1990. Dental pathology and alcohol-related indicators in an outpatient clinic sample. *Community Dent. Oral Epidemiol.* 18:204–207.

Kribbs, P. J. Comparison of mandibular bone in normal and osteoporotic women. *J Prosthet Dent* 1990; 63 218–222

Lannan, S., A. McLean, E. Drost, M. Gillooly, K. Donaldson, et al. 1992. Changes in neutrophil morphology and morphometry following exposure to cigarette smoke. *Int. J. Exp. Pathol.* 73:183–191.

Manouchehr-Pour, M., P. J. Spagnuolo, H. M. Rodman, and N. F. Bissada. 1981. Comparison of neutrophil chemotactic response in diabetic patients with mild and severe periodontal disease. *J. Periodontol.* 52:410–414.

Marx, R. E. 2007. *Oral and Intravenous Bisphosphonate-Induced Osteonecrosis of the Jaws: History, Etiology, Prevention, and Treatment.* Chicago, Il: *Quintessence*: 15.

Marx, R. E., Y. Sawatari, M. Fortin, V. Broumand. 2005. Bisphosphonate-induced exposed bone (osteonecrosis/osteopetrosis) of the jaws: risk factors, recognition, prevention, and treatment. *J oral maxillofae Surg* 63:1567–1575.

Marx, R. E. 2007. Oral and intravenous bisphosphonates. Induced osteonecrosis of the jaws. 1st ed. Hanover Park, IL: *Quintessence.* 64–66.

McMullen, J. A., T. E. Van Dyke, H. U. Horoszewicz, and R. J. Genco. 1981. Neutrophil chemotaxis in individuals with advanced periodontal disease and a genetic predisposition to diabetes mellitus. *J. Periodontol.* 52:167–173.

Michalowicz, B. S., D. P. Aeppli, R. K. Kuba, J. E. Bereuter, J. P. Conry, et al. 1991. A twin study of genetic variation in proportional radiographic alveolar bone height. *J. Dent. Res.* 70:1431–1435.

Michaud, D. S., K. Joshipura, E. Giovannucci, et al. 2007. A prospective study of periodontal disease and pancreatic cancer in U.S. male health professionals. *Journal of the National Cancer Institute* 99:171–175.

Migliorati, C. A., J. Casiglia, J. Epstein, P. L. Jacobsen, M. A. Siegel, and S-B. Woo. 2005. Managing the care of patients with bisphosphonate-associated osteonecrosis: An American Academy of Oral Medicine position paper. *JADA* 136:1658–1668.

Mojon, P. 2003. Respiratory infection: How important is oral health? *Current Opinion in Pulmonary Medicine* 9(3): 166–170.

Moritz, A. J., and B. L. Mealey. 2006. Periodontal disease, insulin resistance, and diabetic mellitus. *Grand Rounds Oral-Sys. Med.* 2:13–20.

Murray, P. 1994. Periodontal diseases in patients infected by human immunodeficiency virus. *Periodontology 2000* 6:50–67.

Nair, P., G. Sutherland, R. M. Palmer, R. F. Wilson, and D. A. Scott. 2003. Gingival bleeding on probing increases after quitting smoking. *J. Clin. Periodontol.* 30:435–437.

Nakib, S.A., J.S. Pankow, J.D. Beck, S. Offenbacher, G. W. Evans, et al. 2004. Periodontitis and coronary artery calcification: The Atherosclerosis Risk in Communities (ARIC) study. *J. Periodontol.* 75(4):505–510.

Newman, M. 1998. Genetic, environmental, and behavioral influences on periodontal infections. *Compendium* (special issue) 19:25–31.

Nishimura, F., K. Takahashi, M. Kurihara, S. Takashiba, and Y. Murayama. 1998. Periodontal disease as a complication of diabetes mellitus. *Ann. Periodontol.* 3:20–29.

Nitta, H., K. Bando, M. Matsubara, and I. Ishikawa. 1997. *Impact of periodontal health on osteoporosis in postmenopausal women.* Periodontal Diseases and Human Health: New Directions in Periodontal Medicine. Sunstar–Chapel Hill, Chapel Hill, NC, March 24–25.

Offenbacher, S., H. L. Jared, P. G. O'Reilly, S. R. Wells, G. E. Salvi, et al. 1998. Potential pathogenic mechanisms of periodontitis-associated pregnancy complication. *Ann. Periodontol.* 3(1): 233–250.

Offenbacher, S., B. Katz, G. Fertik, J. Collins, D. Boyd, et al. 1996. Periodontal infection as a possible risk factor for preterm low birth weight. *J. Periodontol.* 67: 1103–1113.

Oh, T. J., J. Bashutski, and W. V. Giannobile. 2007. The interrelationship between osteoporosis and oral bone loss. *Grand Rounds Oral-Sys Med.* 2:10–21.

Otomo-Corgel, J. 2007. Implants and oral bisphosphonates: Risky business? *J. Periodontol.* 78:373–376.

Page, R. C., and J. D. Beck. 1997. Risk assessment for periodontal diseases. *Int. Dent. J.* 47:61–87.

Papantonopoulos, G. H. 2004. Effect of periodontal therapy in smokers and non-smokers with advanced periodontal disease: Results after maintenance therapy for a minimum of 5 years. *J. Periodontol.* 75:839–843.

Paquette, D. W. 2006. Periodontal disease and the risk for adverse pregnancy outcomes. *Grand Rounds in Oral-Sys. Med.* 4:14-25a.

Peruzzo, D. C., B. B. Benatti, G. M. D. Ambrosano, et al. 2007. A systematic review of stress and psychological factors as possible risk factors for periodontal disease. *J. Periodontol.* 78(8):1491–1504.

Preshaw P. M., M. A. Knutsen, and A. Mariotti. 2001. Experimental gingivitis in women using oral contraceptives. *J Dent Res* 80:2011–2015.

Ruggiero, S. L. 2008. Bisphosphonate-related osteonecrosis of the jaws. *Compendium* 29(2):97–105.

Ryan, M. E., O. Carnu, and R. Tenzler. 2006. The impact of periodontitis on metabolic control and risk for diabetic complications. *Grand Rounds Oral-Sys. Med.* 2:24–34.

Safkan-Seppälä, B., and J. Ainamo. 1992. Periodontal conditions in insulin-dependent diabetes mellitus. *J. Clin. Periodontol.* 19:24–29.

Saremi, A., R. G. Nelson, M. Tulloch-Reid, et al. 2005. Periodontal disease and mortality in type 2 diabetes. *Diabetes Care* 28:27–32.

Scannapieco, F. A., B. Wang, and H. J. Shiau. 2001. Oral bacteria and respiratory infection: Effects on respiratory pathogen adhesion and epithelial cell proinflammatory cytokine production. *Ann. Periodontol.* 6(1): 78–86.

Scannapieco, F. A., and A.W. Ho. 2001. Potential associations between chronic respiratory disease and periodontal disease: Analysis of National Health and Nutrition Examination Survey III. *J. Periodontol.* 72:50–56.

Scannapieco, R. A., and J. M. Mylotte. 1996. Relationships between periodontal disease and bacterial pneumonia. *J. Periodontol.* 67:1114–1122.

Shanies S., and C. Hein. 2006. The significance of periodontal infection in cardiology. *Grand Rounds Oral-Sys. Med.* 1:24–33.

Stein, P. S., S. Scheff, D. R. Dawson, III. Alzheimer's disease and periodontal disease; mechanisms underlying a potential bidirectional relationship. Grand Rounds Oral-sys med. 2006, 1:14–240.

Syrjala. A.M., P. Ylostalo, M.C. Niskanen, and M.L. Knuutila. 2003. Role of smoking and HbA1c level in periodontitis among insulin-dependent diabetic patients. *J. Clin. Periodontol.* 30:871–875.

Taichman, S. L. 2005. Oral contraceptives and periodontal diseases: Rethinking the association based upon analysis of National Health and Nutrition Examination Survey Data. *Periodontol.* 76:1374–1385.

Taylor, G. W., B. A. Burt, M. P. Becker, R. J. Genco, M. Shlossman, et al. 1996. Severe periodontitis and risk for poor glycemic control in patients with noninsulin-dependent diabetes mellitus. *J. Periodontol.* 67: 1085–1093.

Terpenning, M. S. 2006. The relationship between infections and chronic respiratory diseases: An overview. *J. Periodontol.* 6:66–70.

Thomson, W. M., R. Poulton, J. M. Broadbent, et al. 2008. Cannabis smoking and periodontal disease among young adults. *JAMA* 299(5):525–531.

Tonetti, M. S. 1998. Cigarette smoking and periodontal diseases: Etiology and management of the disease. *Ann. Periodontol.* 3:88–101.

Umino, M., and M. Nagao. 1993. Systemic disease in elderly dental patients. *Int. Dent. J.* 43:213–218.

Wade, M. L., and J. B. Suzuki. 2007. Issues related to diagnosis and treatment of bisphosphonate-induced osteonecrosis of the jaws. *Grand Rounds Oral-Sys. Med.* 2:46–53b.

Wang, H. L., D. Weber, and L. K. McCauley. 2007. Effect of long-term oral bisphosphonates on implant wound healing: Literature review and a case report. *J. Periodontol.* 78:584–594.

Zak, M., A. N. Spina, R.P. Spinazze, W. L. Perkinson, and D. J. Spinazze. 2007a. Bisphosphonates and the dental patient: Part 1. *Compendium* 28(9):510–516.

Zak, M., A. N. Spina, R. P. Spinazze, W. L. Perkinson, and D. J. Spinazze. 2007b. Bisphosphonates and the dental patient: Part 1. *Compendium* 28(9):510–516.

Part II

Periodontal Diseases: Classification

Chapter **7**
Gingival Diseases

Chapter **8**
Periodontitis and Other Periodontal Conditions

Chapter **9**
Necrotizing Periodontal Diseases

Chapter **10**
Occlusal Trauma

Chapter **11**
Abscesses of the Periodontium

Gingival Diseases

Surendra Singh

OUTLINE
Introduction
Gingival Diseases
Histopathogenesis of Gingivitis
Pathogenesis of Gingivitis
Classification of the Periodontal Diseases
Dental Hygiene Notes
Key Points
Self-Quiz
References

GOAL: To provide an understanding of the clinical features and histopathogenesis of gingival diseases.

EDUCATIONAL OBJECTIVES

Upon completion of this chapter, the reader should be able to:

- Recognize and distinguish the two main forms of inflammatory periodontal diseases (1999 Classification of Periodontal Diseases).
- List and compare the plaque-induced gingival diseases and non-plaque-induced gingival diseases.
- List and describe the different stages in the histopathogenesis of gingivitis.
- Explain the host response to the presence of microorganisms within dental plaque.
- Explain the relationship of hormones and medications with periodontal diseases.
- Describe the clinical and histologic features of gingival inflammation.
- Discuss the clinical and histological relationship of the inflammatory and immune host responses to inflammatory periodontal diseases.

KEY WORDS

gingivitis 113
gingival pocket 116
histopathogenesis 113

non-plaque
   associated gingival
   diseases 124
plaque-associated
   gingival
   diseases 117

INTRODUCTION

Periodontal diseases are not a single disease entity, but a group of lesions affecting the tissues that form the attachment apparatus of a tooth or teeth. Periodontal diseases, which consist of gingivitis and periodontitis, are microbial infections wherein the microorganisms act in concert with a host's reduced capacity to resist disease. To successfully treat periodontal diseases, it is essential that one is able to recognize different types of the diseases. When classifying inflammatory periodontal diseases, it is important to include not only diseases that have primary manifestation and etiology in the periodontium, but also periodontal manifestations of systemic diseases. In this chapter a comprehensive classification of the gingival diseases or conditions affecting gingival tissues is presented.

GINGIVAL DISEASES

Gingivitis is defined as an inflammatory lesion, mediated by host/microorganism interactions, which remains limited to the gingival tissues and does not involve the underlying periodontal ligament, cementum, or alveolar and supporting bone (American Academy of Periodontology, 2003). In this broad condition, the apical extent of the junctional epithelium and the coronal gingival connective tissue attachment remain at the cementoenamel junction; hence, there is no attachment loss. Gingivitis can affect children, adolescents, and adults.

Gingivitis has been further defined based on clinical manifestations, duration of the disease, and association with either dental plaque or systemic factors such as medical conditions or medications (Gurenlian, 2007; Page, 1986).

Some professionals question whether gingivitis should be considered a periodontal disease, since it does not cause loss of significant amounts of periodontal support or tooth mortality (loss). However, most researchers have concluded otherwise (Page, 1986; Ranney, 1986, 1993).

HISTOPATHOGENESIS OF GINGIVITIS

Stages in the Histopathogenesis

As discussed in previous chapters, the reaction of the host to the presence of dental plaque (biofilm) is inflammatory in nature, initially developing into inflammation of the gingival unit. Inflammation confined to the gingiva (epithelium and lamina propria) results in gingivitis.

The **histopathogenesis,** or the events that occur in the *periodontal tissues* that lead to the development of gingivitis and periodontitis, is best explained by reviewing the different stages occurring in the initiation and progression of the periodontal disease as it relates to clinical signs. In a previous chapter, the role of the host immune system in the inflammatory process and periodontal disease progression was reviewed. In this section, the *microscopic tissue changes* seen as a result of periodontal diseases are discussed. It is important to remember that all of these inflammatory and immunological events that occur during the time frame in the development of periodontal lesions are intermingled and must not be considered as separate entities.

Page and Schroeder (1976) described the development of periodontal diseases as a progression of inflammation through four different stages: *initial lesion, early lesion, established lesion,* and *advanced lesion* (Table 7–1 ■; Figure 7–1 ■). The initial and early lesions are

Table 7–1	Page and Schroeder's Stages of Pathogenesis of Periodontal Disease		
Stage	*Onset Time After Plaque Accumulation*	*Histopathological Signs*	*Features*
Initial	2 to 4 days	Acute inflammation; PMNs, machrophages; vasculitis	Subclinical; no signs of gingivitis; increased flow of GCF
Early	4 to 7 days	T-cell lesion	Clinical signs of gingivitis first seen (redness, bleeding on probing, edema)
Established	2 to 3 weeks	B-cell lesion; plasma cells	Chronic gingivitis (gingiva may appear bluish-red with increased probing depths)
Advanced	Undetermined	Alveolar bone loss, periodontal pocket formation; B-cell lesion	Periodontitis

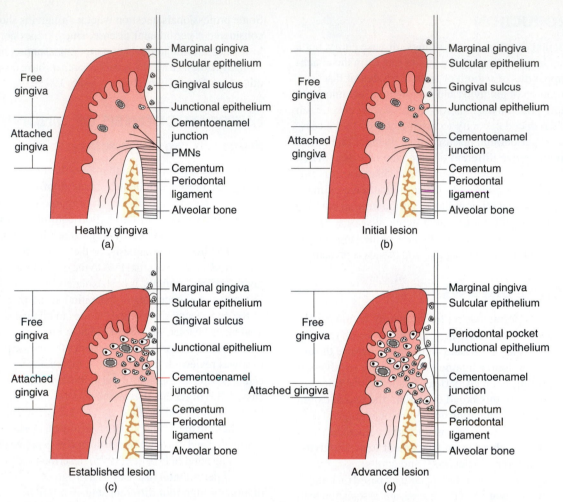

■ FIGURE 7–1 Page and Schroeder's histopathologic periodontal lesions. (a) Healthy gingiva: Little supragingival plaque accumulation; a few defense cells, primarily PMNs, migrate through the junctional epithelium into the gingival crevice and out into the oral cavity. (b) Initial lesion: This develops two to four days after plaque accumulation at the gingival margin. Vasodilation results in an increased emigration of PMNs from the blood vessels into the connective tissue and entering the gingival crevice. This is gingivitis but the lesion is not clinically visible. Early lesion: This lesion appears at the site of the initial lesion within four to seven days following plaque accumulation. The same features seen in the initial lesion appear in the early lesion but they are accentuated with an increased number of PMNs and macrophages. T-lymphocytes begin to migrate into the tissue and gingival crevice. A greater area of gingival connective tissue is affected. About 60 to 70% of collagen is destroyed. Acute inflammation features continue in the early lesion. This is still gingivitis. (c) Established lesion: This is characterized by the presence of PMNs, macrophages, and antibody-producing plasma cells (B lymphocytes), which comprise 10 to 30% of the infiltrate. More collagen has been destroyed. The bulk of plaque bacteria and cells in the gingival crevice cause the junctional epithelium to detach from the tooth. The pocket epithelium is mostly derived from junctional epithelium with the formation of epithelial ridges and microulcerations. This is chronic gingivitis and is still reversible if oral hygiene is reinstated. (d) Advanced lesion: This is periodontitis. Plasma cells (> 50%) are the primary cells involved in periodontitis. There is clinical attachment loss with loss of clinical connective tissue attachment to the tooth and apical migration of the junctional (pocket) epithelium, resulting in a periodontal pocket. In addition, the alveolar and supporting bone has been destroyed.

representative of acute inflammation, while the established lesion is considered to be chronic gingivitis and the advanced lesion is periodontitis and will be discussed in the following chapter (Page & Schroeder, 1976). The information from the research by Page and Schroeder was obtained from animal specimens and a few human juvenile tissue samples. Also, since there are many factors involved in the initiation and progression of periodontal diseases, it is difficult to exactly pinpoint a clear delineation between the different stages, especially in humans. Also, it is unclear when and if an established lesion develops into an advanced lesion. Thus, even though this classic work by Page and Schroeder is primarily with nonhuman tissues, it is still the foundation from which the histopathogenesis of inflammatory periodontal diseases can be studied. The inflammatory and immune changes discussed above are involved in the histopathogenesis of periodontal diseases.

Initial Lesion (PMN Dominated)

The initial lesion develops after two to four days of plaque accumulation (Löe, Theilade, & Jensen, 1965; Page & Schroeder, 1976). Dental plaque accumulates on the tooth surface at the free gingival margin level (Figure 7-1b). The protective wall of PMNs (leukocyte wall) between the plaque mass and the junctional and sulculur epithelium becomes compromised (Miyasaki, 1991). Bacterial antigens cross the permeable junctional epithelium and enter the gingival connective tissue. The response of the tissue to the antigens is acute inflammation, developing within minutes of the insult. It is characterized by a dilation of blood vessels within the connective tissue subjacent to the junctional epithelium (Page & Schroeder, 1976). There is an increased flow of gingival crevicular fluid (GCF) into the crevice and migration of PMNs from the connective tissue into the junctional epithelium (Payne, Page, Ogilvie, & Hall, 1975) and gingival crevice in response to chemotactic factors released by bacteria and inflammatory cells. There is some loss of collagen in the lamina propria because of the action of collagenase that is replaced with inflammatory cells such as PMNs. This lesion is not clinically seen and is reversible with appropriate oral hygiene (Löe et al., 1965).

Early Lesion (T-Cell Dominated)

The early lesion evolves from the initial lesion after approximately seven days of plaque accumulation and can continue for up to fourteen days. Clinically, this lesion is observable as gingivitis. The presence and accentuation

of the features in the initial lesion characterize the early lesion (see Figure 7–1b). PMNs continually migrate from the blood vessels through the junctional epithelium into the gingival crevice, and there is increased gingival crevicular flow. T-lymphocytes accumulate immediately subjacent to the junctional epithelium. There is no apparent dividing line between the initial and early lesions. Approximately 60 to 70% of collagen is lost in the connective tissue. Changes start to occur in the junctional epithelium. As a result of the downgrowth of accumulating plaque, the gingival sulcus begins to deepen. This is still an acute gingivitis without clinical connective tissue attachment loss and no bone loss as yet. This lesion is reversible with adequate oral hygiene, healing without adverse consequences.

Bleeding on probing occurs when there are ulcerations in the epithelium lining the soft tissue wall of the pocket, and the engorged blood vessels from the underlying connective tissue protrude through the epithelium.

Established Lesion (Few B Cells/Plasma Cells)

As adverse clinical conditions progress, the early lesion develops into the chronic or established gingivitis lesion (Page & Schroeder, 1976). The gingiva responds to massive accumulations of plaque, which affects a greater area of tissue (see Figure 7–1c). The time period for the initiation of the established lesion has not actually been determined, but it can start within two to three weeks after plaque accumulation (Page & Schroeder, 1976). The manifestations of acute inflammation still persist. Established lesions may persist for months or years without progressing into periodontitis (Page, 1986; Zappa, 1995). As gingivitis becomes clinically more severe, the proportion of T-cells decreases, and B-cells and plasma cells increase within the lamina propria (Zappa, 1995). More collagen is lost and replaced by an inflammatory cell infiltrate. The gingival fibers are still attached to the root surface; there is no clinical connective tissue attachment loss at this stage. Because of the massive amounts of subgingival plaque that advance in an apical direction, the junctional epithelium detaches laterally from the tooth surface to become pocket epithelium with elongation of epithelial ridges deeper into the connective tissue in an attempt to maintain epithelial integrity (Kinane & Lindhe, 1998); this leads to the formation of microulcerations, which may increase the permeability of the epithelium to bacteria and their by-products.

The gingival margin becomes swollen and enlarged, and the gingival margin can be separated easily from the tooth surface, forming a **gingival pocket** or pseudopocket. No alveolar bone loss occurs at this stage. Clinical signs are present and more severe than in the early lesion. Most of the changes that occur in the established lesion are still reversible. The advanced lesion (Figure 7-1d) is periodontitis and is discussed in the following chapter.

PATHOGENESIS OF GINGIVITIS

The Gingival Pocket

In early periodontal lesions a gingival pocket (Figure 7–2 ■) is formed by gingival enlargement and coronal migration of the gingival margin. There is no loss of clinical connective tissue attachment (the gingival fibers remain attached to the root surface and the junctional epithelium has not migrated apically onto the root surface). Additionally, there is no alveolar and supporting bone loss. Gingival pockets are not true pockets, they are false or "pseudo," which means that the increased height of the gingiva creates an impression that a deep pocket has been formed when probing instruments are used around a tooth (Ranney, 1986). There is no attachment of gingival connective tissue above the cementoenamel junction, and since there is no loss of clinical connective tissue attachment to the root surface, it is not a true pocket. The pocket epithelium extends laterally and detaches from the tooth surface, permitting apical movement of the bacteria in plaque between the tooth and epithelium. A pseudopocket is often seen in drug-induced gingivitis (e.g., gingivitis produced by the use of phenytoin, cyclosporine, and certain calcium channel blockers), severe gingival inflammation, and hormone-induced gingivitis (e.g., during pregnancy or puberty).

Host Response to Gingival Inflammation

The gingiva reacts to the presence of microorganisms within dental plaque by alterations in the gingival vascular (blood) supply. The initial response from the gingival tissue is vasodilation of the blood vessels in the lamina propria (gingival connective tissue) in close proximity to the junctional epithelium. With this, there is an increased permeability (increased opening) of the vessels allowing the exchange of fluid and cells between the blood and lamina propria. This allows for the increased migration of neutrophils (leukocytes) from the blood vessels into the lamina propria and junctional epithelium.

These changes in the underlying lamina propria and epithelium cause the clinical features of edema (fluid filled) and redness in the gingival tissues. Gingival redness occurs due to the increased vascularity at inflamed sites. Inflamed gingival is edematous because of the increased vascular permeability of blood vessels in the inflamed connective tissue. Fluid "leaks" out of blood vessels into the tissue, resulting in edema. The ulceration of the epithelium (due to the vascular changes) allows for a communication into the underlying lamina propria where there are an increased number of blood vessels. Thus, when a periodontal probe is placed in the gingival sulcus of inflamed gingiva, bleeding occurs.

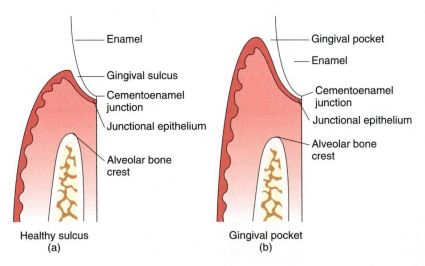

Enamel

Gingival sulcus

Cementoenamel junction

Junctional epithelium

Alveolar bone crest

Healthy sulcus
(a)

Gingival pocket

Enamel

Cementoenamel junction

Junctional epithelium

Alveolar bone crest

Gingival pocket
(b)

■ **FIGURE 7–2** (a) Physiologic periodontium. (b) A gingival pocket. The gingival margin has migrated coronally, but there is no attachment loss or bone loss. There is a deepened pocket, but it is not a true pocket because the depth is due to the coronal position of the gingiva. This type of pocket is seen in gingivitis.

There is no loss of gingival connective tissue attachment (gingival fibers) and no alveolar and supporting bone loss. Gingivitis is reversible if the irritant is removed below the threshold of causing a host response.

CLASSIFICATION OF THE PERIODONTAL DISEASES

Over the years a number of classification systems have been developed to organize and name various disease entities or conditions affecting the periodontium. In 1989, the American Academy of Periodontology (AAP) recommended a classification based on the data from periodontal research that was used by the dental community to describe different forms of periodontal diseases. This was modified in 1992 (American Academy of Periodontology) in a position paper published by the Academy to include gingival diseases. In 1999 at the International Workshop for a Classification of Periodontal Diseases and Conditions the American Academy of Periodontology proposed a new classification system (Armitage, 1999) (Table 7–2 ■). *This new classification system is not based on the age of the patient at the time of presentation but rather describes distinct forms of periodontal diseases based on clinical, radiographic, and historical data.* Please note that the 1999 Classification lists both gingival diseases and periodontitis and other conditions relating to the periodontium. Box 7–1 lists the entire classification, not just gingival diseases (Holmstrup, 1999). Note that all periodontal diseases and conditions are listed, but only gingival diseases will be discussed in this chapter.

Dental Plaque-Induced Gingival Diseases

Gingivitis Associated with Dental Plaque

Gingivitis is a reaction of the host (body) to the bacteria present in the dental biofilm (plaque). Gingivitis, which exemplifies itself as inflammation of the gingiva, is the most common of the periodontal diseases (Page, 1985). Dental biofilms as the etiology or cause of gingivitis have been confirmed in Löe's classic "Experimental Gingivitis in Man" study (Löe, Theilade, & Jensen, 1965). **Plaque-associated gingivitis** begins at the gingival margin and can spread throughout the remaining gingival unit. Plaque-induced gingivitis will not develop unless there are bacteria present (American Academy of Periodontology, 1992); however, the composition of the required oral microbiota is not specific (Moore, Moore, &

Cato, 1987). Gingivitis is reversible following the removal of dental biofilms and maintenance of good oral hygiene self-care (Watt & Marinho, 2005). However, if oral hygiene procedures are discontinued and the level of oral hygiene is not adequate, allowing the accumulation of biofilms, clinical signs of acute gingivitis develop within one to three weeks. This classic model of gingivitis induction is used in clinical trials to test anti-gingivitis oral rinses.

Since the bacteria associated with chronic, long-standing, plaque-induced gingivitis are not very specific, recognition of gingivitis is primarily made clinically. However, the earliest changes may not be seen clinically and only histologically under the microscope. With the development of gingivitis, the healthy gingiva changes in color, contour, consistency, and surface texture. Plaque-associated gingivitis starts within the interdental papilla and is clinically characterized by gingival redness, gingival bleeding, swelling, and gingival sensitivity and tenderness (Löe et al., 1965; Suzuki, 1988). The features of dental plaque-induced gingivitis can be summarized in Box 7–2 (Mariotti, 1999).

Treatment of gingivitis includes maintenance of adequate oral hygiene self-care and regular professional mechanical debridement.

Gingival Diseases Modified by Systemic Factors

Gingivitis Associated with the Endocrine System Altered hormonal balances elicit an apparent exaggerated response to dental plaque. Hormonal-influenced gingivitis manifests as puberty-associated gingivitis, menstrual cycle-associated gingivitis, and pregnancy-associated gingivitis. Additionally, poorly controlled plasma glucose levels resulting in a diabetes-associated gingivitis may aggravate the inflammatory response of the gingiva to plaque.

Puberty Gingivitis During puberty, the dramatic elevation in steroid hormones often can cause a gingival response that is similar to what has been described for pregnancy gingivitis. In addition to a rise in hormones (estrogen and progesterone), the incidence and severity

Rapid Dental Hint

Gingivitis may develop without the patient even knowing. A patient may not recognize that he or she has periodontal disease. It is important for you to inform the patient of the signs and symptoms.

Table 7–2   Common Gingival Diseases

Disease	Patient Population	Clinical Features	Causes of the Disease	Microbiologic Features	Figure
Gingivitis associated with dental plaque (Figure 7–3 ■)	Adolescents, adults	Gingival redness, bleeding, and enlargement Absence of clinical attachment loss and bone loss	Inadequate oral hygiene	No specific bacteria are demonstrated although high levels of *Streptococcus sanguis, S. mitis, Fusobacterium nucleatum, Actinomyces viscosus,* and *Veillonella parvula* have been detected	 ■ **FIGURE 7–3** Plaque-induced gingivitis
Gingival diseases associated with the endocrine system (Figure 7–4 to 7–5 ■)	Pregnant patients, adolescents, diabetics	Intense gingival inflammation Absence of clinical attachment loss and bone loss	Changes in sex hormone level; exaggerated response to plaque	*Prevotella intermedia* (pregnancy gingivitis and puberty gingivitis)	 ■ **FIGURE 7–4** Puberty gingivitis
Gingival diseases associated with blood dyscrasias	Leukemia	Intense gingival inflammation, petechiae, mucosal ulcers, gingival bleeding	Abnormal proliferation and development of leukocyte	None	 ■ **FIGURE 7–5** Diabetes mellitus–associated gingivitis

■ FIGURE 7–6 Phenytoin-related gingivitis

■ FIGURE 7–7 Nifedipine-related gingivitis

■ FIGURE 7–8 Cyclosporine-related gingivitis

■ FIGURE 7–9 Herpes simplex infection

Gingival diseases modified by medications (Figures 7–6 to 7–8 ■)	Patients taking phenytoin, calcium channel blockers, cyclosporine	Gingival enlargement or overgrowth Absence of clinical attachment loss and bone loss	Medications and dental plaque	No specific bacteria demonstrated
Gingival diseases of viral origin (Figure 7–9 ■)	Herpes virus infections (primary herpetic gingivostomatitis, recurrent oral herpes, varicella-zoster infections)	Movable oral mucosa appears as vesicles that easily rupture to form painful ulcers affecting the gingiva	Herpes simplex viruses type 1 and 2, varicella-zoster virus	Viral, not bacterial

Gingival diseases of fungal origin (Figure 7–10a, b ■)	Linear gingival erythema, antibiotic use, corticosteroid use	Candida-species (Candida albicans)	Denture sore mouth appears as red gingiva underlying a denture; may also show a whitish patches that can be wiped off the mucosa leaving a slightly bleeding surface	Fungal, not bacteria
Gingival manifestations of systemic conditions, mucocutaneous disorders (Figure 7–11a, b ■)	These include skin disease such as pemphigus, lichen planus, benign mucous membrane pemphigoid (BMMP), and others	Abnormality in the immune system	Gingiva may appear blotchy red, have blisters or vesicles, or slough (peel) off from the underlying connective tissue	None

(a)
(b)
■ FIGURE 7–10
(a) Chronic atrophic candidiasis (denture sore mouth)
(b) Linear gingival erythema

(a)
(b)
■ FIGURE 7–11
(a) Erosive lichen planus
(b) pemphigus vulgaris

Box 7–1   Classification of Periodontal Diseases and Conditions

I. Gingival diseases
  A. Dental plaque–induced gingival diseases*
    1. Gingivitis associated with dental plaque only
      a. Without other local contributing factors
      b. With local contributing factors (see VIIIA)
    2. Gingival diseases modified by systemic factors
      a. Associated with the endocrine system
        (1) Puberty-associated gingivitis
        (2) Menstrual cycle–associated gingivitis
        (3) Pregnancy-associated
          (a) Gingivitis
          (b) Pyogenic granuloma
        (4) Diabetes mellitus–associated gingivitis
      b. Associated with blood dyscrasias
        (1) Leukemia-associated gingivitis
        (2) Other
    3. Gingival diseases modified by medications
      a. Drug-influenced gingival diseases
        (1) Drug-influenced gingival enlargements
        (2) Drug-influenced gingivitis
          (a) Oral contraceptive–associated gingivitis
          (b) Other
    4. Gingival diseases modified by malnutrition
      a. Ascorbic acid–deficiency gingivitis
      b. Other
  B. Non-plaque-induced gingival lesions
    1. Gingival diseases of specific bacterial origin
      a. *Neisseria gonorrhea*–associated lesions
      b. *Treponema pallidum*–associated lesions
      c. *Streptococcal* species–associated lesions
      d. Other
    2. Gingival diseases of viral origin
      a. Herpes virus infections
        (1) Primary herpetic gingivostomatitis
        (2) Recurrent oral herpes
        (3) Varicella-zoster infections
      b. Other
    3. Gingival diseases of fungal origin
      a. Candida species infections
        (1) Generalized gingival candidiasis
      b. Linear gingival erythema
      c. Histoplasmosis
      d. Other
    4. Gingival lesions of genetic origin
      a. Hereditary gingival fibromatosis
      b. Other
    5. Gingival manifestations of systemic conditions
      a. Mucocutaneous disorders
        (1) Lichen planus
        (2) Pemphigoid
        (3) Pemphigus vulgaris
        (4) Erythema multiforme
        (5) Lupus erythematosus
        (6) Drug-induced
        (7) Other
      b. Allergic reactions
        (1) Dental restorative materials
          (a) Mercury
          (b) Nickel
          (c) Acrylic
          (d) Other
        (2) Reactions attributable to
          (a) Toothpastes/dentifrices
          (b) Mouthrinses/mouthwashes
          (c) Chewing gum additives
          (d) Foods and additives
        (3) Other
    6. Traumatic lesions (factitious, iatrogenic, accidental)
      a. Chemical injury
      b. Physical injury
      c. Thermal injury
    7. Foreign-body reactions
    8. Not otherwise specified

*A section on gingival diseases (1A) was added to the current 1999 system. This includes plaque-induced gingivitis and non-plaque-induced diseases (1B). Also included in this classification system are gingival diseases that can be modified by systemic factors such as medications or diabetes mellitus.

Box 7-2   **Clinical Features of Gingival Diseases**

- Caused by nonspecific bacteria (although certain types of bacteria are associated with gingivitis, the condition is currently still considered of nonspecific bacterial origin)
- Dental plaque present at the marginal gingiva
- Clinical signs of inflammation are limited to the gingiva
- No clinical attachment loss
- It is reversible to health following the removal of the dental plaque causing it
- Even though bacteria are the primary risk factors, secondary factors apparently modify the clinical characteristics of the disease. This has resulted in many subclassifications.

of gingivitis in adolescents are influenced by a number of factors, including plaque levels, dental caries, mouth breathing, tooth crowding, and tooth eruption (Stamm, 1986). The distinguishing feature between plaque-induced gingivitis and puberty gingivitis is the development of gingival inflammation in the presence of a small amount of dental plaque. Meticulous oral hygiene is the recommended treatment.

Menstrual-Cycle Gingivitis   During the menstrual cycle there are increased levels of estrogen and progesterone. These changes in hormone levels cause gingival inflammation characterized as enlarged, red interdental papilla. Connective tissue attachment loss and alveolar and supporting bone loss are not evident. All gingival changes are reversible after ovulation. It is important to note that gingival changes primarily are seen when plaque is present. Also, not every female patient will have this inflammatory response during menstruation.

Pregnancy Gingivitis   Pregnancy gingivitis is inflammation of the gingiva associated with pregnancy. The incidence of gingivitis during pregnancy ranges between 30 and 100%. The effects of pregnancy on preexisting gingivitis are seen by the second month of gestation and are most severe in the eighth month at the time of peak hormone levels (American Academy of Periodontology, 1992; Silness & Löe, 1963). Pregnant patients with healthy gingiva usually do not develop gingivitis, but, if gingivitis or periodontitis is present, the course of the disease is aggravated by pregnancy.

The degree of gingival inflammation is related to the state of oral hygiene of the patient. Accumulation of dental plaque parallels the gingival changes. The severity of the gingivitis is greater in pregnant than in nonpregnant women (Löe, 1965) but is not associated with more destructive periodontitis (Cohen, Shapiro, Friedman, Kyle, & Franklin, 1971). The condition regresses postpartum (Silness & Löe, 1963). However, gingivitis during pregnancy can be prevented or be resolved by adequate plaque control starting early in the pregnancy.

Dental plaque present at the gingival margin results in an *exaggerated inflammatory response* of the gingiva. Tissue inflammation and enlargement seen in pregnancy is not caused by the pregnancy itself but rather by the shifts in the hormonal levels, which aggravate the inflammation. Hormonal changes during pregnancy are due to elevated progesterone and estrogen levels, which in the final gestational month are ten to thirty times greater than that seen during the normal menstrual cycle (Amar & Chung, 1994). Elevations in these steroids, especially progesterone, cause an increased permeability of the blood vessels (microvasculature) (Lindhe & Bränemark, 1968) within the lamina propria, resulting in gingival redness, edema, and increased flow of gingival crevicular fluid (Amar & Chung, 1994; Lindhe, Lindhe, Attström, & Björn, 1968). Subgingival growth of *Prevotella intermedia* is enhanced because this bacterium can substitute progesterone, as well as testosterone and estradiol, as growth factors. Elevated levels of *Prevotella intermedia* are also seen in puberty gingivitis (Kornman & Loesche, 1980).

Pregnancy gingivitis is not synonymous with a pregnancy tumor. A pregnancy tumor is a non-neoplasm, pyogenic granuloma occurring in a pregnant patient. It arises from an analogue of a dormant (inactive) tumor and is stimulated during pregnancy. Clinically, it presents as a painless protuberant, mushroom-like exophytic mass that is attached to a base at the gingival margin. It will regress or completely disappear postpartum.

Treatment of pregnancy gingivitis consists of periodontal debridement and oral home care instruction. The gingiva may be erythematous and painful. Meticulous plaque control is important. The gingival condition will resolve postpartum.

Diabetes Mellitus–Associated Gingivitis   Diabetes mellitus is one of the important risk factors for periodontal diseases. Type 1 diabetes is not as common as type 2 diabetes, which is caused by the development of either resistance to insulin in muscle (insulin is not working to bring glucose into cells), impaired secretion of insulin from the pancreas, or increased glucose production by the liver. All causes result in an elevation of blood glucose levels or hyperglycemia, which causes complications related to accelerated artherosclerosis, retinopathy (blindness), renal (kidney) failure, neuropathy (diseases of the nervous system), altered wound healing, and periodontal conditions.

Diabetes mellitus–associated gingivitis is characterized by inflammation of the gingiva, especially where plaque is present without clinical attachment loss or bone loss. It is similar to plaque-induced gingivitis and is more commonly seen in children with poorly controlled type 1 diabetes.

Gingivitis Associated with Blood Dyscrasias

Leukemia-Associated Gingivitis   Leukemia is a disease characterized by an abnormal proliferation of leukocytes (white blood cells) in the blood and bone marrow. Oral manifestations are seen as gingival bleeding and enlargement starting at the interdental papilla and spreading to the attached gingiva.

Treatment of patients with gingival diseases modified by systemic factors first involves getting the systemic disease under control followed by professional periodontal debridement and maintenance of oral home care.

Gingival Diseases Modified by Medications

Drug-Influenced Enlargements   Commonly used drugs can lead to the appearance of gingivitis (American Academy of Periodontology, 2004; Dongari et al. 1993). There are many types of medications (Box 7–3) that can cause gingival overgrowth or enlargement (Kanno et al., 2008).

There are no specific bacteria associated with this type of gingivitis and no specific risk factors other than poor oral hygiene and use of the medication.

Based on current histological and ultrastructural findings, drug-influenced gingival changes are more accurately referred to as "gingival overgrowth" or "enlargement," rather than "gingival hypertrophy," which is defined as an increase in connective tissue volume, or gingival hyperplasia, which is defined as an abnormal increase in the number of fibroblasts (Hallmon & Rossmann, 1999).

The etiology of drug-induced gingival overgrowth is not exactly known. Either there is an excessive production of collagen by gingival fibroblasts, making the gingiva appear thickened or enlarged (Brown, Beaver, & Bottomley, 1991), or the action of collagenase, which breaks down collagen, is reduced (Hallmon & Rossmann,

---

> **Box 7–3   Classification of Medications Associated with Gingival Enlargement**
>
> - Phenytoin (incidence 50%): Used to control convulsive or seizure disorders (Angelopoulos & Goaz, 1972; Dongari, McDonnell, & Langlais, 1993; Steinberg & Steinberg, 1982)
> - Cyclosporine (incidence about 30%): Used for immunosuppressive or antirejection therapy when an individual receives an organ transplant (Greenberg, Armitage, & Shiboski, 2008; Seymour & Jacobs, 1992; Thomason et al., 1995)
> - Calcium channel blockers (nifedipine, amlodipine, diltiazem): Used for the treatment of cardiovascular conditions such as hypertension, angina, and arrhythmias. Although nifedipine was the first calcium channel blocker (Barclay, Thomson, Idle, & Seymour, 1992) and is the one most frequently associated with gingival enlargement (incidence about 15%), the condition can occur with any drug in this class (Nishikawa et al., 1991)
> - Sodium valproate: Used as an antidepressant and anticonvulsant (rare occurrence)

1999). The highly active fibroblasts become sensitive to these medications in the presence of inflammation (Brown et al., 1991).

Enlargement often occurs within one to three months after the start of the medication (Nishikawa et al., 1991). Although the amount of the drug used daily and duration of use may be related to the severity of the overgrowth (Addy, McElnay, Eyre, Campbell, & D'Arcy, 1982), several studies have failed to see any relationship between these factors (Hassell & Hefti, 1991).

While some clinical studies have shown the level of plaque accumulation affects the severity of the overgrowth, others have shown that, although plaque control and the removal of local irritants is of some benefit for gingival health, these measures alone do not prevent gingival overgrowth (Hefti, Eshenaur, Hassell, & Stone, 1994; Seymour & Smith, 1991). It is often difficult to determine whether the increased plaque accumulation preceded the gingival overgrowth or occurred because of ineffective oral hygiene in the presence of enlarged gingiva (Rees, 1998). Since hypertension is an adverse effect of cyclosporine, patients may also be taking a calcium channel blocker such as nifedipine, which may also induce gingival overgrowth. Other calcium channel blockers associated with gingival enlargement include diltiazem, verampamil, and amlodipine. Thus, it is difficult to assess the actual frequency of gingival overgrowth related to the use of cyclosporine (Lundergan, 1989).

If there is only gingival enlargement without bone loss, periodontal debridement with oral home care instruction is the mainstay. These procedures may be difficult because of the tissue contours. Surgical intervention (e.g., gingivectomy) may be necessary; however, as long as the patient is taking the medication, the gingiva will revert back to the original form. Thus, surgery may need to be done frequently.

Drug-Influenced Gingivitis

Oral Contraceptive–Associated Gingivitis   The etiology of oral contraceptive-induced gingival inflammation is similar to that seen in pregnancy (Pearlman, 1974), since the drugs used contain combinations of estrogen and progesterone that simulate pregnancy. Therefore, the same gingival changes observed during pregnancy are seen with oral contraceptive use (Mealey, 1996). *However, much lower concentrations of hormones are used in today's oral contraceptive pills, thus reducing the incidence of gingival diseases* (Preshaw, Knutsen, & Mariotti, 2001).

Non-Plaque-Induced Gingival Diseases

Gingival Diseases of Specific Bacteria Origin

This category includes gingival lesions caused by infections with *Neisseria gonorrhea, Treponema pallidum, Streptococci,* or other microorganisms. The gingival lesions appear as either erythematous (red), edematous (fluid-filled) ulcers, or inflamed, nonulcerated gingiva.

Gingival Diseases of Viral Origin

This section is associated with gingivitis caused by viral infections such as herpes viruses (herpes simplex virus type 1 and 2, primary herpetic gingivostomatitis [Slots, 2005] and varicella-zoster virus). These viruses primarily affect babies and then become latent or dormant until adulthood at which time they appears as recurrent herpes

 Rapid Dental Hint

Inflammation of a patient's gingival tissue can be due to many factors including plaque, medications, systemic diseases. Do a careful assessment of every patient.

labialis. Primary gingivostomatitis may also be seen during adolescence or adulthood.

Gingival Diseases of Fungal Origin

This section is associated with gingivitis caused by fungal infections such as candidiasis, coccidioidomycosis, cryptococcosis, histoplasmosis, and others. Oral candidiasis (*C. albicans*) is usually seen in HIV-seropositive and other immunocompromised patients. The lesions appear as a band of erythema of the attached gingiva, which is termed linear gingival erythema (LGE). The prevalence of LGE in HIV-infected populations is relatively unknown since the stage of HIV disease varies among the population (Mealey, 1996) and more structured studies need to be conducted.

Gingival Lesions of Genetic Origin

Hereditary gingival fibromatosis clinically appears as a fibrotic gingival enlargement that is genetically derived and occurs rarely. The enlargement of the gingiva may cover the entire tooth surface.

Gingival Manifestations of Systemic Conditions

Mucocutaneous diseases are lesions involving the mucous membranes including the mouth and/or the skin. Oral manifestations of mucocutaneous diseases are seen in erosive lichen planus (Figure 7–11a ■) (Endo et al., 2008), benign mucous membrane pemphigoid, bullous pemphigoid, and pemphigus vulgaris (Figure 7–11b). More adult women than men have been documented with the disease. Oral lesions may involve all or part of the gingiva and other mucous membranes of the oral cavity. Gingival involvement may manifest as desquamative gingivitis characterized by desquamation or sloughing (peeling) of the epithelium, leaving a red, painful underlying connective tissue surface. No specific bacteria have been identified. The cause of these mucocutaneous diseases is multifactoral, with some of the diseases being autoimmune in nature whereby the body attacks and destroys its own tissue (Weinberg, Insler, & Campen, 1997).

Allergic reactions due to ingredients or contents of dentifrices, mouthrinses, chewing gum are relatively rare and are usually attributed to chemical additives.

Traumatic Lesions

Physical injury to the gingival tissues may be due to thermal (e.g., burns from hot beverages), chemical (e.g., chemical products such as sloughing of tissues from oral rinses or dentifrices, aspirin burn), or physical (e.g., aggressive tooth brushing, incorrect use of dental floss, fingernails, or toothpicks) injury.

DENTAL HYGIENE NOTES

Gingivitis is a type of inflammatory periodontal disease that is defined as a microbial infection that is confined to the gingival unit. Gingivitis is the result of the outcome of host-bacterial interactions and are modified by systemic factors including medical conditions and medications. Gingivitis is characterized by the presence of a gingival pocket in which there is neither loss of attachment nor bone loss.

The dental hygienist must be familiar with the clinical and histological features of gingivitis so that a distinction between the different gingival diseases can be made. This will allow for a more comprehensive treatment plan and definitive treatment for the patient.

KEY POINTS

- Inflammatory periodontal diseases are broadly classified into gingivitis and periodontitis.
- Gingivitis is defined as inflammation confined to the gingiva.
- Gingivitis is reversible.
- Dental plaque (biofilm) is the major risk factor for gingivitis; there are other contributory risk factors such as medications, hormones, and systemic diseases.

SELF-QUIZ

1. Which one of the following features describes gingivitis? (p. 113)
   a. Occurs primarily in children
   b. Extensive attachment loss
   c. Bone loss does not occur
   d. Primary risk factors include pathogenic bacteria and calculus
2. All of the following medications are contributing risk factors in causing gingival enlargement except one. Which one is the exception? (pp. 119, 123, 124)
   a. Phenytoin
   b. Cyclosporine
   c. Ibuprofen
   d. Nifedipine
   e. Valproate
3. Which one of the following periodontal diseases is described by having inflammation of the gingiva without loss of clinical connective tissue attachment? (pp. 114–116)
   a. Dental plaque-induced gingivitis
   b. Chronic periodontitis
   c. Aggressive periodontitis
   d. Refractory periodontitis
   e. Necrotizing ulcerative periodontitis
4. Which one of the following bacteria is found in high numbers in pregnancy gingivitis? (p. 122)
   a. *Porphyromonas gingivalis*
   b. *Prevotella intermedia*
   c. *Actinomyces viscosus*
   d. *Actinobacillus actinomycetemcomitans*
   e. *Streptococcus sanguis*
5. Which periodontal lesion, according to the classification of Page and Schroeder (1976), is characterized by chronic gingival inflammation and the presence of plasma cells? (pp. 113–114)
   a. Initial
   b. Early
   c. Established
   d. Advanced
6. Today most oral contraceptives do not cause gingival inflammation because of the lower levels of hormones used. (p. 124)
   a. Statement and reason are correct.
   b. Statement and reason are false.
   c. Statement is true but reason is false.
   d. Statement is false but reason is true.
7. Which periodontal lesion, according to the classification of Page and Schroeder (1976) is characterized by chronic gingival inflammation and the initial presence of PMNs? (pp. 113–115)
   a. Initial
   b. Early
   c. Established
   d. Advanced
8. During the disease process, the junctional epithelium transforms into (p. 115)
   a. alveolar bone.
   b. periodontal ligament.
   c. pocket epithelium.
   d. sulcular epithelium.
   e. oral epithelium.

9. Which of the following lesions does clinical inflammation first appear? (pp. 113, 115)
   a. Initial
   b. Early
   c. Established
   d. Advanced
10. Which of the following features occurs first after two to four days of plaque accumulation? (p. 115)
    a. Dilation of blood vessels in the lamina propria
    b. Destruction of connective tissue by collagenase
    c. Influx of plasma cells
    d. Phagocytosis of bacteria by macrophages

REFERENCES

Addy, V., J. McElnay, D. Eyre, N. Campbell, and P. D'Arcy. 1982. Risk factors in phenytoin-induced gingival overgrowth. *J. Periodontol.* 54:373–377.

Amar, S., and K. M. Chung. 1994. Influence of hormonal variation on the periodontium in women. *Periodontology 2000* 6:79–87.

American Academy of Periodontology. 1992. *The etiology and pathogenesis of periodontal diseases* (Position Paper), 1–9. Chicago: Author.

American Academy of Periodontology. 2003. *Glossary of periodontal terms* (4th ed.). Chicago: Author.

American Academy of Periodontology. 2004. Drug-associated gingival enlargement. *J. Periodontol.*, 75:1424–1431.

Angelopoulos, A. P., and P. W. Goaz. 1972. Incidence of diphenylhydantoin gingival hyperplasia. *Oral Surg. Oral Med. Oral Path.* 34:898–906.

Armitage, G. C. 1999. Development of a classification system for periodontal diseases and conditions. *Ann. Periodontol.* 84: 1–6.

Barclay, S., J. M. Thomason, J. R. Idle, and R. A. Seymour. 1992. The incidence and severity of nifedipine-induced gingival overgrowth. *J. Clin. Periodontol.* 19:311–314.

Brown, R. S., W. T. Beaver, and W. K. Bottomley. 1991. On the mechanisms of drug-induced gingival hyperplasia. *J. Oral Pathol. Med.* 20:201–209.

Cohen, D. W., J. Shapiro, L. Friedman, G. C. Kyle, and S. Franklin. 1971. A longitudinal investigation of the periodontal changes during pregnancy and fifteen months post-partum. Part III. *J. Periodontol.* 42:653–657.

Dongari, A., H. T. McDonnell, and R. P. Langlais. 1993. Drug-induced gingival overgrowth. *Oral Surg. Oral Med. Oral Pathol.* 76:543–548.

Endo, H., T. D. Rees, W. W. Hallmon, et al. 2008. Disease progression from mucosal to mucocutaneous involvement in a patient with desquamative gingivitis associated with permphigus vulgaris. *J. Periodontol.* 79:369–375.

Greenberg, K. V., G. C. Armitage, and C. H. Shiboski. 2008. Gingival enlargement among renal transplant recipients in the era of new-generation immunosuppressants. *J. Periodontol.* 79(3):453–460.

Gurenlian, J. R. 2007. The role of dental plaque biofilm in oral health. *J. Dent. Hyg.* 81(5):116.

Hallmon, W. W., and J. A. Rossmann. 1999. The role of drugs in the pathogenesis of gingival overgrowth. *Periodontology 2000* 21:176–196.

Hassell, T., and A. F. Hefti. 1991. Drug-induced gingival overgrowth: Old problem, new problem. *Crit. Rev. Oral Pathol. Med.* 2:103–137.

Hefti, A. F., A. E. Eshenaur, T. M. Hassell, and C. Stone. 1994. Gingival overgrowth in cyclosporine A treated multiple sclerosis patients. *J. Periodontol.* 65:744–749.

Holmstrup, P. 1999. Non-plaque-induced gingival lesions. *Ann. Periodontol.* 4:20–29.

Kanno, C. M., J. A. Oliverira, J. F. Garcia, et al. 2008. Effects of cyclosporine, phenytoin, and nifedipine on the synthesis and degradation of gingival collagen in tufted capuchin monkey (*Cebus paella*):L Histochemical and MMP-q and -2 and collagen I gene expression analysis. *J. Periodontol.* 79(1):114–122.

Kinane, D. F., and J. Lindhe. 1998. Pathogenesis of periodontitis. In eds. J. Lindhe, T. Karring, and N. P. Lang, *Clinical periodontology and implant dentistry,* 189–225. Copenhagen: Munksgaard.

Kornman, K. S., and W. J. Loesche. 1980. The subgingival microflora during pregnancy. *J. Periodontol. Res.* 5:111–122.

Lindhe, J., and P. I. Bränemark. 1968. Experimental studies on the etiology of pregnancy gingivitis. *Perio. Abst.* 16:50–51.

Lindhe, J., J. Lindhe, R. Attström, and A. Björn. 1968. Influence of sex hormones on gingival exudation in dogs with chronic gingivitis. *J. Periodont. Res.* 3:279–283.

Löe, H. 1965. Periodontological changes in pregnancy. *J. Periodontol.* 36:209–217.

Löe, H., E. Theilade, and S. B. Jensen. 1965. Experimental gingivitis in man. *J. Periodontol.* 36:177–187.

Lundergan, W. P. 1989. Drug-induced gingival enlargements. Dilantin hyperplasia and beyond. *J. Calif. Dent. Assoc.* 17:48–52.

Mariotti, A. 1999. Dental plaque-induced gingival diseases. *Annals of Periodontology* 4:7–19.

Mealey, B. L. 1996. Periodontal implications: Medically compromised patients. *Ann. Periodontol.* 1:256–321.

Miyasaki, K. T. 1991. The neutrophil: Mechanisms of controlling periodontal bacteria. *J Periodontol.* 62: 761–774.

Moore, L. V. H., W. E. C. Moore, and E. P. Cato. 1987. Bacteriology of gingivitis. *J. Dent. Res.* 66:989–995.

Nishikawa, S., H. Tada, A. Hamasaki, S. Kasahara, J. Kido, et al. 1991. Nifedipine-induced gingival hyperplasia: A clinical and in vitro study. *J. Periodontol.* 62:30–35.

Page, R. C. 1985. Oral health status in the United States. Prevalence of inflammatory periodontal diseases. *J. Dent. Educ.* 49:354–364.

Page, R. C. 1986. Gingivitis. *J. Clin. Periodontol.* 13:245–255.

Page, R. C., and H. E. Schroeder. 1976. Pathogenesis of inflammatory periodontal disease. A summary of current work. *Lab Investigations* 33:235–249.

Payne, W. A., R. C. Page, A. L. Ogilvie, and W. B. Hall. 1975. Histopathologic features of the initial and early stages of experimental gingivitis in man. *J. Periodont. Res.* 10:51–64.

Pearlman, B. A. 1974. An oral contraceptive drug and gingival enlargement: The relationship between local and systemic factors. *J. Clin. Periodontol.* 1:47–57.

Preshaw P. M., M. A. Knutsen, and A. Mariotti 2001. Experimental gingivitis in women using oral contraceptives. *J. Dent. Res.* 80:2011–2015.

Ranney, R. R. 1986. Discussion: Pathogenesis of gingivitis. *J. Clin. Periodontol.* 13:356–359.

Ranney, R. R. 1993. Classification of periodontal diseases. *Periodontology 2000* 2:13–25.

Rees, T. D. 1998. Drugs and oral disorders. *Periodontology 2000* 18:21–36.

Seymour, R. A., and D. J. Jacobs. 1992. Cyclosporin and the gingival tissues. *J. Clin. Periodontol.* 19:1–11.

Seymour, R. A., and D. G. Smith. 1991. The effect of a plaque control programme on the incidence and severity of cyclosporin-induced gingival changes. *J. Clin. Periodontol.* 18:107–110.

Silness, J., and H. Löe. 1963. Periodontal disease in pregnancy. *Acta Odontol. Scand.* 21:533–551.

Slots, J. 2005. Herpes viruses in periodontal disease. *Periodontology 2000* 38(1):33–62.

Stamm, J. W. 1986. Epidemiology of gingivitis. *J. Clin. Periodontol.* 13:360–370.

Steinberg, S. C., and A. D. Steinberg. 1982. Phenytoin-induced gingival overgrowth in severely retarded children. *J. Periodontol.* 53:429–433.

Suzuki, J. B. 1988. Diagnosis and classification of periodontal diseases. *Dent. Clin. North America* 32:195–216.

Thomason, J. M., R. A. Seymour, J. S. Ellis, P. J. Kelly, G. Parry, et al. 1995. Iatrogenic gingival overgrowth in cardiac transplantation. *J. Periodontol.* 66:742–746.

Watt, R. G., and V. C. Marinho. 2005. Does oral health promotion improve oral hygiene and gingival health? *Periodontology 2000* 37(1):35–47.

Weinberg, M. A., M. S. Insler, and R. B. Campen. 1997. Mucocutaneous features of autoimmune blistering diseases. *Oral Surg. Oral Med. Oral Pathol. Oral Radiol. Endod.* 84:517–534.

Zappa, U. 1995. Histology of the periodontal lesion: Implications for diagnosis. *Periodontology 2000* 7:22–38.

Chapter 8

Periodontitis and Other Periodontal Conditions

Surendra Singh

OUTLINE

Introduction
Pathogenesis of the Periodontitis Lesion
Classification of Periodontitis and Other Conditions
Peri-Implant Diseases
Treatment of Periodontitis
Dental Hygiene Notes
Key Points
Self-Quiz
References

GOAL: To provide an understanding of the features of periodontitis.

EDUCATIONAL OBJECTIVES

Upon completion of this chapter, the reader should be able to:

- Define the course of the progression of periodontitis.
- Explain the pathogenesis of periodontitis.
- Explain changes in the 1999 classification of periodontitis.
- Explain the different features of the various types of periodontitis.
- Discuss periodontitis as a risk factor for systemic diseases.

KEY WORDS

aggressive
  peridontitis **137**
bone loss **129**
chronic
  periodontitis **137**
connective tissue
  attachment loss **129**
infrabony defects **135**
peri-implant disease
  143
periodontal pocket
  129
periodontitis **129**

INTRODUCTION

Periodontitis is widespread in the population, afflicting children and adults. **Periodontitis** is defined as clinical attachment loss with subsequent bone loss. According to the 1999 classification of the periodontal diseases, periodontitis is categorized into chronic and aggressive forms. Diagnosis of periodontitis is not based on the age of the patient but rather on clinical and radiographic findings. Dental biofilms are the primary risk factor for periodontitis. Modifying contributory factors such as systemic diseases are also involved in the development and progression of the periodontitis lesion.

Histopathogenesis of Periodontitis

Initiation of Inflammatory Periodontal Diseases

If gingivitis is not resolved, the inflammatory reaction may spread into the gingival connective tissue attachment, alveolar and supporting bone, and the principal fibers. At this stage, the disease is periodontitis.

This chapter deals primarily with the tissue changes that occur during the initiation and development of gingivitis and periodontitis. When these tissue changes occur within the periodontal tissues, the inflammatory and immune responses are also triggered. Thus, the features that are reviewed in this chapter occur as part of the entire inflammatory and immunological events.

These histological lesions presented in this chapter were initially classified and published in 1976 by Page and Schroeder. Page and Schroeder classified gingivitis and periodontitis according to histopathology from animal and some human adolescent specimens. This classi-

Did You Know?

The periodontal ligament fibers are the most resistant to destruction and thus are the last structures to be lost during disease activity.

fication is still used in periodontic literature; however, it is not a realistic, up-to-date classification. The initial early and established lesions reflected the histopathology of clinically early and chronic gingivitis and were discussed in the previous chapter. The advanced lesion reflected the histopathology of the progression of gingivitis into periodontitis (Table 8–1 ■).

Advanced Lesion (Plasma Cell/ Antibody Dominated)

The advanced lesion is characteristic of periodontitis. The inflammatory infiltrate extends into the alveolar and supporting bone and periodontal ligament (see Figure 8–1d ■). **Periodontal pocket** formation occurs with the clinical **connective tissue attachment loss** to the root surface and the apical migration of the apical aspect of the junctional epithelium along the root surface that was previously occupied by connective tissue; attachment loss occurs. Subsequently, there is alveolar and supporting **bone loss.** The apical and lateral migration of the junctional or pocket epithelium permits extension of subgingival plaque on the root surface. The lymphocytic infiltrate in the subjacent connective tissues is primarily B-cells. The advanced lesion may become stable or progress continuously (Goodson, 1992).

Table 8–1   Page and Schroeder's Stages of Pathogenesis of Periodontal Disease

Stage	Onset Time after Plaque Accumulation	Histopathological Signs	Features
Initial	2 to 4 days	Acute inflammation; PMNs, machrophages; vasculitis	Subclinical; no signs of gingivitis; increased flow of GCF
Early	4 to 7 days	T-cell lesion	Clinical signs of gingivitis first seen (redness, bleeding on probing, edema)
Established	2 to 3 weeks	B-cell lesion; plasma cells	Chronic gingivitis
Advanced	Undetermined	Alveolar bone loss, periodontal pocket formation; B-cell lesion	Periodontitis

(a) Healthy gingiva
- Marginal gingiva
- Sulcular epithelium
- Gingival sulcus
- Junctional epithelium
- Cementoenamel junction
- PMNs
- Cementum
- Periodontal ligament
- Alveolar bone
- Free gingiva
- Attached gingiva

(b) Initial lesion
- Marginal gingiva
- Sulcular epithelium
- Gingival sulcus
- Junctional epithelium
- Cementoenamel junction
- Cementum
- Periodontal ligament
- Alveolar bone
- Free gingiva
- Attached gingiva

(c) Established lesion
- Marginal gingiva
- Sulcular epithelium
- Gingival sulcus
- Junctional epithelium
- Cementoenamel junction
- Cementum
- Periodontal ligament
- Alveolar bone
- Free gingiva
- Attached gingiva

(d) Advanced lesion
- Marginal gingiva
- Sulcular epithelium
- Periodontal pocket
- Junctional epithelium
- Cementoenamel junction
- Cementum
- Periodontal ligament
- Alveolar bone
- Free gingiva
- Attached gingiva

■ **FIGURE 8–1**   Page and Schroeder's histopathologic periodontal lesions. (a) Healthy gingiva: Little supragingival plaque accumulation; a few defense cells, primarily PMNs, migrate through the junctional epithelium into the gingival crevice and out into the oral cavity. (b) Initial lesion: This develops two to four days after plaque accumulation at the gingival margin. Vasodilation results in an increased emigration of PMNs from the blood vessels into the connective tissue and entering the gingival crevice. This is gingivitis, but the lesion is not clinically visible. Early lesion: This lesion appears at the site of the initial lesion within four to seven days following plaque accumulation. The same features seen in the initial lesion appear in the early lesion, but they are accentuated with an increased number of PMNs and macrophages. T-lymphocytes begin to migrate into the tissue and gingival crevice. A greater area of gingival connective tissue is affected. About 60 to 70% of collagen is destroyed. Acute inflammation features continue in the early lesion. This is still gingivitis. (c) Established lesion: This is characterized by the presence of PMNs, macrophages, and antibody-producing plasma cells (B-lymphocytes), which comprise 10 to 30% of the infiltrate. More collagen has been destroyed. The bulk of plaque bacteria and cells in the gingival crevice cause the junctional epithelium to detach from the tooth. The pocket epithelium is mostly derived from junctional epithelium with the formation of epithelial ridges and microulcerations. This is chronic gingivitis and is still reversible if oral hygiene is reinstated. (d) Advanced lesion: This is periodontitis. Plasma cells (> 50%) are the primary cells involved in periodontitis. There is clinical attachment loss with loss of clinical connective tissue attachment to the tooth and apical migration of the junctional (pocket) epithelium, resulting in a periodontal pocket. In addition, the alveolar and supporting bone has been destroyed.

PATHOGENESIS OF THE PERIODONTITIS LESION

Sequence of Events in Pocket Formation

A pocket is defined as a pathologically deepened gingival sulcus (American Academy of Periodontology, 2001). The development of a periodontal pocket between the root surface and the gingiva includes the transformation of a thin junctional epithelium into a pocket epithelium with the development of microulcerations and epithelial ridges (Müller-Glauser & Schroeder, 1982) (Figure 8–2 ■).

The Periodontal Pocket

As the inflammatory infiltrate progresses from the coronal gingival connective tissue subjacent to the junctional epithelium into the underlying connective tissue, an extensive amount of collagen is destroyed. The detachment of the gingival clinical connective tissue attachment (gingival fibers) to the tooth allows apical migration of the junctional epithelium onto the root surface. Apical and lateral migration of the junctional epithelium continues, and as this epithelium separates from the root surface, a periodontal pocket is formed. The junctional epithelium migrates apically only as a result of the destruction of

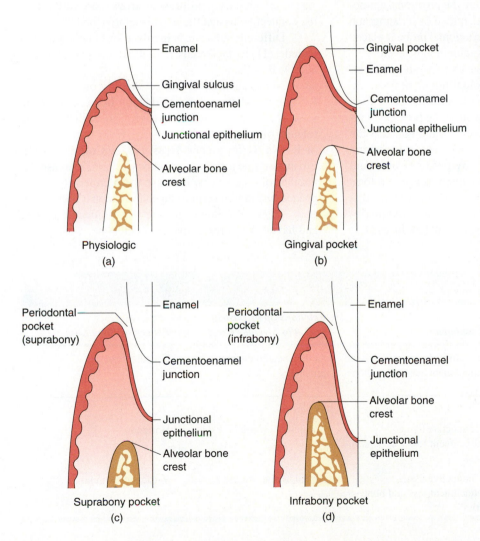

Physiologic
(a)

Enamel
Gingival sulcus
Cementoenamel junction
Junctional epithelium
Alveolar bone crest

Gingival pocket
(b)

Gingival pocket
Enamel
Cementoenamel junction
Junctional epithelium
Alveolar bone crest

Suprabony pocket
(c)

Periodontal pocket (suprabony)
Enamel
Cementoenamel junction
Junctional epithelium
Alveolar bone crest

Infrabony pocket
(d)

Periodontal pocket (infrabony)
Enamel
Cementoenamel junction
Alveolar bone crest
Junctional epithelium

■ **FIGURE 8–2** (a) Healthy periodontium. (b) Gingivitis pocket seen in gingivitis. Note that the junctional epithelium is located at the CEJ. (c) A suprabony pocket is a type of periodontal pocket. The deepened pocket is caused by attachment loss. There is also bone loss. The base of the pocket is coronal to the crest of alveolar bone. This type of pocket is a result of the tissue destruction that occurs in periodontitis. (d) An infrabony pocket is another type of periodontal pocket. The base of the pocket is apical to the crest of bone. This type of pocket is seen in periodontitis.

the gingival collagen fibers. With increasing periodontal pocket depths, it becomes an ideal environment for plaque accumulation, making it difficult to clean.

There are two types of periodontal pockets: suprabony and infrabony. The difference between the two kinds of pockets lies in the relationship of the base of the pocket or the coronal extent of the junctional epithelium to the alveolar crest and the type of bone destruction (Table 8–2 ■). Bone destruction occurs as the inflammatory infiltrate extends into the alveolar crest and then into the trabecular bone.

The base of a suprabony pocket (junctional epithelium) is coronal to the crest of bone (see Figure 8–2c), while the base of an infrabony pocket (junctional epithelium) is apical to the crest of bone (see Figure 8–2d). This is in contrast to the healthy periodontium (Figure 8–2a) and gingivitis (Figure 8–2b) where the junctional epithelium is at the CEJ. This can be identified on a radiograph when a dense object such as a periodontal probe is placed at the base of the pocket as the radiograph is taken.

Root Surface The areas of cementum that no longer have gingival or periodontal ligament fibers attached undergo changes. The surface of the cementum is rough because of the detachment of the previously inserting connective tissue. It was once thought that the surface of cementum becomes rough, easily absorbing endotoxins, bacteria, and their by-products onto and slightly into its surface. This cementum is referred to as necrotic cementum. However, current theory states that the influence of root surface roughness and endotoxin-contaminated cementum was overestimated. In 1987, it

was documented that extensive root planing may not be warranted because the endotoxins were found to be very superficial and not embedded deeply into the cementum. They are weakly adherent to the cementum (Nakib, Bissada, Simmenlink, & Golstine, 1982). Excessive cementum removal to provide, a smooth, glass-like root surface is unnecessary (Greenstein, 1992, Hughes, Augr, & Smales, 1988).

Bone Resorbing Factors

The inflammatory process causes the resorption of alveolar and supporting bone. A consequence of pocket formation and loss of clinical connective tissue attachment is bone resorption. The process of bone loss involves the inflammatory cells including PMNs and macrophages. As the inflammatory infiltrate destroys more collagen in the connective tissue, the bone is approached.

Different substances involved in bone resorption include: (1) prostaglandins, (2) endotoxins, (3) cytokines, and (4) B-cells.

Numerous factors can act directly on osteoclasts to stimulate their activity to destroy bone. One of the main mechanisms of bone resorption is through the release of prostaglandins (PGE_2) from macrophages or PMNs (Offenbacher, Heasman, & Collins, 1993). Prostaglandins activate resting osteoclasts, increase the number of osteoclasts, increase the number of macrophages, and inhibit bone collagen formation (Offenbacher et al., 1993). Prostaglandins are also produced in bone and have a direct resorptive effect on bone.

Table 8–2	**Classification of Pockets**		
Type of Pocket	*Pathogenesis*	*Relationship of Base of Pocket to Alveolar Crest*	*Pattern of Bone Loss*
Gingival (pseudopocket) pocket	No clinical connective tissue attachment loss and no bone loss	At the cementoenamel junction	No bone loss
Periodontal pockets:			
Suprabony pocket	Connective tissue attachment loss and bone loss	Coronal to alveolar crest	Horizontal
Infrabony pocket	Connective tissue attachment loss and bone loss	Apical to alveolar crest	Vertical or angular

Did You Know?

In fact, on extracted teeth, endotoxins can be brushed away.

Bone resorption can also occur when bacteria release endotoxins, which activate inflammatory cells such as macrophages resulting in the production and release of cytokines such as IL-1 (Schwartz, Goultschin, Dean, & Boyan, 1997). IL-1 is most important in periodontal destruction (Ishikawa, Nakashima, Koseki, et al., 1997). IL-1 can also stimulate PGE_2 production. Another theory of bone resorption is explained by the role of cytokines and prostaglandins in stimulating collagenase production by PMNs (Reynolds & Meikle, 1997). Collagenase is an enzyme that destroys collagen, which is a component of bone.

Site Specificity

An important feature of inflammatory periodontal diseases is the site-specific localization of periodontal destruction. Pocket formation and bone loss does not occur in all areas of the dentition at the same time, but it could occur on a few teeth at a time or even on only some aspects of some teeth at any given time, while other teeth are healthy. The composition of subgingival plaque samples from different sites in the oral cavity of the same mouth has been shown to be different. These differences have presented a problem for research analysis and treatment response to therapy (Socransky & Haffajee, 1997).

Did You Know?

Look at a patient's radiographs. In some cases only one or two sites have bone loss (with deep probing depths). Isn't that strange? Yes, this is the concept of site specificity. It may be related to the width and quality of the bone or the type of bacteria present in the pocket or the host response.

Relationship of Bone Loss and Pocket Formation

Alveolar and supporting bone is destroyed as the pocket develops. Since the level of bone corresponds to previous periodontal destruction and changes in the soft tissue of the pocket wall reflect the present inflammatory condition, the degree of bone loss is not necessarily correlated with the depth of periodontal pockets. Radiographically, extensive bone loss can be associated with shallow pocket depths and vice versa. For example, a patient may have had severe periodontitis at one time but had periodontal treatment that stopped the progression of the disease. Clinically, the probing depths are shallow, but radiographically bone loss is evident.

Pattern of Bone Loss

The types of pockets that form and the pattern of bone loss depend on the route the inflammation takes from the gingiva to the underlying supporting structures. The route of extension of the inflammatory infiltrate from the gingiva into the interdental bone is by way of the blood vessels. The interdental bone is resorbed more rapidly than the bundle bone because it is more vascular and less resistant to resorption. Interproximally (between adjacent teeth), inflammation usually spreads along the interdental blood vessels from the gingiva through the crestal bone into the bone marrow spaces extending out to the periodontal ligament fibers (Figure 8–3a ■). On the facial

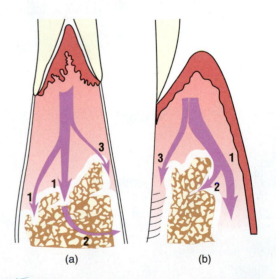

(a)   (b)

■ **FIGURE 8–3**   (a) The inflammatory infiltrate spreads from the gingiva through the lamina propria into the bone following the most vascular pathway, which is where most of the blood vessels are located. Sometimes the most vascular area (larger blood vessels) is on the side of the alveolar crest, allowing the inflammation to directly enter the periodontal ligament. (b) On the direct facial surface, inflammation extends along the supraperiosteal artery before entering bone.

and lingual surfaces of teeth, the inflammatory infiltrate follows along the supraperiosteal blood vessels located in the periosteum on the outer surface of the bone (Figure 8–3b). Usually, the principal fibers are the most resistant to destruction and are the last to be resorbed.

The penetration of the inflammatory infiltrate into the marrow spaces and on the bone surfaces is associated with a loss of the equilibrium (balance) between bone formation and bone resorption, leading to loss of alveolar bone. The pattern of bone loss varies among individual teeth and on different surfaces of the same tooth. Bone destruction can occur on any surface of the tooth. The pattern of bone loss can occur in two different ways:

1. Horizontal bone loss when bone resorption occurs from its outer aspect buccal and lingual walls. Bone is lost equally on the surfaces of two adjacent teeth with the interproximal bone level remaining flat (Figure 8–4a ■), and the deepest portion of the pocket is located coronal to the alveolar crest.
2. Vertical or angular bone loss occurs when the inflammation travels directly from the gingiva into the periodontal ligament and then the bone. The interproximal bone level is not flat and even as in horizontal bone loss. Bone loss occurs at different rates around the tooth and is more rapid on one side of the tooth than the other. The base or the

(a)

(b)

(c)

■ **FIGURE 8–4** (a) Horizontal pattern of bone loss between the premolars and second premolar and first molar. Interproximal bone (arrows) is destroyed on both sides of adjacent teeth equally. (b) *Left side:* Dry skull specimen showing furcation involvement (F) and vertical pattern of bone loss on the mesial aspect of the first molar (arrow). Note that the interproximal bone is not flat as with horizontal bone loss. (c) *Right side:* After the gingiva has been reflected from the tooth and bone, a vertical defect is seen on the mesial aspect of the first molar.

■ **FIGURE 8–5**   Note vertical bone loss on the distal of the premolar. A gutta percha point placed in the peri-odontal pocket before the radiograph was taken to show the origin of the abscess was the base of the pocket. This tooth had a hopeless prognosis and treatment was planned for extraction.

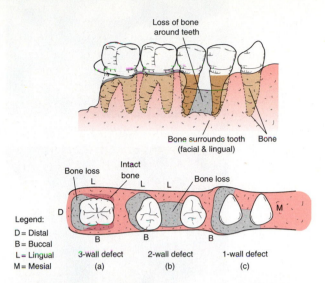

■ **FIGURE 8–6**   Vertical bone destruction is classified according to the number of bony walls surrounding the defect. In health there are four bony walls surrounding a tooth: mesial (M), buccal (B) or facial, distal (D), and lin-gual (L). In periodontitis one or more of the bony walls is destroyed. If three bony walls remain, it is called a three-wall defect (a). If the buccal and lingual bony walls re-main, it is called a two-wall defect or crater (b). If one bony wall remains (e.g., buccal/lingual cortical plate or proximal [mesial, distal] wall of bone), it is called a one-wall defect or hemiseptum (c).

deepest portion of the bony defect is apical to the alveolar bone crest, creating an infrabony defect (Figure 8–4b, c). If a sinus tract is present, a gutta percha point (it is radiopaque and will show up on an X-ray) is carefully inserted into the tract. The point will "trace" the tract to the site of origin. In Figure 8–5 ■ a patient came in with an abscess. To determine the origin of this infection, a point was placed and then an X-ray taken.

The terms *infrabony* and *intrabony* have been used interchangeably to describe all vertical bony defects; however, these terms are frequently misused in the peri-odontal literature (Weinberg & Eskow, 2000). The term *intra-* translates to mean "within or inside the bone" and *infra-* to mean "below the crest of bone." An infrabony defect is a "generic" term to describe any periodontal vertical bony defect.

Periodontal **infrabony defects** are classified ac-cording to the number of osseous (bony) walls surround-ing the pocket (Figures 8–6 ■ and 8–7 ■). There are four bony interproximal walls surrounding the tooth: the

mesial, facial (buccal), distal, and lingual. Most vertical bone loss occurs interproximally, although vertical bone loss does occur on the direct facial and lingual walls. Types of defects include the following:

- Three-wall bony defect. The three-wall defect has three bony walls remaining interproximally or fa-cially or lingually, with the tooth forming the fourth wall. An intrabony defect is a type of three-wall bony defect with specific characteristics (Prichard, 1979). As a result of the disease process, the bone lining the infrabony defect is usually composed of cortical bone. In an intrabony defect, the walls have cancellous bone behind them. The only way to de-termine if the defect is intrabony is during the sur-gical procedure when the bone is exposed. Thus, it is incorrect to refer to all infrabony defects as in-trabony. A three-wall defect that wraps around the tooth and involves two or more adjacent root sur-faces is referred to as a circumferential defect.

(a)

(b)

(c)

(d)

■ **FIGURE 8–7** (a-b) X-ray of three-wall defect on the mesial of the mandibular molar; surgical entry exposes the three-wall defect. Note that the distal bony wall against the molar is resorbed. Thus, three walls remain: buccal, lingual, and mesial. (c) Surgical entry of a two-wall defect—the buccal and lingual walls remain. (d) Surgical entry of a one-wall defect—the buccal wall remains.

- Two-wall bony defect. The two-wall defect has two bony walls remaining. An interdental crater is the most common angular bony defect. It is a two-wall osseous defect with a buccal and lingual wall remaining.
- One-wall bony defect. The one-wall defect has one bony wall remaining and usually occurs interdentally. If the remaining wall is the proximal wall, the defect is referred to as a hemiseptum.

Factors Related to Pattern of Bone Loss

The bone destructive process radiates from the plaque mass, at the base of the periodontal pocket, 1.5 to 2.5 mm circumferentially (Tal, 1984) (Figure 8–8 ■). Within this 2 mm "circle," bone destruction does not occur. Outside this 2 mm "circle," bone destruction occurs. Thus, the width and thickness of the interdental septum primarily determines if the pattern of bone destruction is horizontal or vertical. Bone destruction occurring where there is a wide interdental septum (> 2 mm in width) will most likely not occur across the entire septum and results in a vertical pattern of bone loss. Bone destruction occurring where the interdental septum is narrow (< 2 mm) can be total and results in a horizontal pattern of bone loss.

Teeth such as lower incisors, which have thin facial or lingual cortical plates of bone with little to no cancellous bone between the alveolar bone proper and the outer plate, will usually show a horizontal pattern of

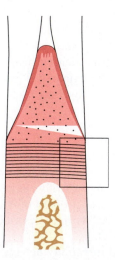

■ **FIGURE 8–8** The range of bone destruction determines the pattern of bone loss. The area of bone destruction radiates from the plaque mass about 2 mm.

■ **FIGURE 8–9** This panoramic radiograph show the teeth of the lower left quadrant, exhibiting generalized severe bone loss of 30 to 80%. The **red line** depicts the existing bone level, whereas the **green line** depicts where the bone was originally, prior to the patient developing periodontal disease. The **orange arrows** point to *furcation involvement,* or the loss of enough bone to reveal the location at which the individual roots of a molar begin to branch from the single root trunk; this is a sign of advanced periodontal disease. The **blue arrow** shows up to 80% bone loss on tooth #21, and clinically, this tooth exhibited gross mobility. Finally, the **peach oval** highlights the aggressive nature with which periodontal disease generally affects mandibular incisors. Because their roots are generally situated very close to each other, with minimal interproximal bone, and because of their location in the mouth, where plaque and calculus accumulation is greatest because of the pooling of saliva, mandibular anteriors suffer excessively.

bone loss. Molars that have a thick facial cortical plate of bone will usually show a vertical pattern of bone loss. Figure 8–9 ■ is a panoramic radiograph showing different levels of bone loss.

CLASSIFICATION OF PERIODONTITIS AND OTHER CONDITIONS

Box 8–1 lists all periodontal diseases and conditions so that the student can see all diseases and conditions together. However, only periodontitis is discussed in this chapter.

Periodontitis is an inflammatory lesion mediated by host/microorganism interactions, and results in clinical attachment loss and alveolar and supporting bone loss. Adolescents as well as adults can develop periodontitis. One of the changes that was made in the periodontitis classification was replacing the term "adult periodontitis" with "chronic periodontitis." **Chronic periodontitis** is subdivided as localized (≤ 30% of the sites affected) and generalized (> 30% of the sites affected). Disease severity is divided into three groups, which are based on the amount of clinical attachment loss (CAL): slight = 1–2 mm CAL; moderate = 3–4 mm

CAL; and severe = ≥ 5 mm CAL. The Academy decided that adults as well as adolescents could develop periodontitis and "adult" was too restrictive. Thus, the age factor is eliminated from the criteria for periodontal diseases.

The term "early-onset periodontitis" was replaced with "**aggressive periodontitis.**" Again, the age-dependent nature of the patient was a factor in changing the terms. The older term "early-onset periodontitis" included prepubertal periodontitis, juvenile periodontitis (localized or LJP and generalized), and rapidly progressive periodontitis. Localized juvenile periodontitis is now termed localized aggressive periodontitis, and generalized juvenile periodontitis is now referred to as generalized aggressive periodontitis. Prepubertal periodontitis with complicating systemic involvement is now included under the heading of periodontitis as a manifestation of systemic diseases (IV).

Refractory periodontitis will no longer have a separate disease classification because any periodontal case can be considered refractory (e.g., localized aggressive periodontitis can be a refractory periodontitis case) or unresponsive to periodontal treatment (e.g., refractory chronic periodontitis).

Box 8–1   **Current Classification of Periodontal Diseases and Conditions**

I. Gingival diseases (reviewed in Chapter 7)
  A. Dental plaque–induced gingival diseases*
  B. Non-plaque-induced gingival lesions
II. Chronic periodontitis[†]
  A. Localized
  B. Generalized
III. Aggressive periodontitis[†]
  A. Localized
  B. Generalized
IV. Periodontitis as a manifestation of systemic diseases
  A. Associated with hematologic disorders
    1. Acquired neutropenia
    2. Leukemias
    3. Other
  B. Associated with genetic disorders
    1. Familial and cyclic neutropenia
    2. Down syndrome
    3. Leukocyte adhesion deficiency syndromes
    4. Papillon-Lefèvre syndrome
    5. Chediak-Higashi syndromes
    6. Histiocytosis syndromes
    7. Glycogen storage disease
    8. Infantile genetic agranulocytosis
    9. Cohen syndrome
    10. Ehlers-Danlos syndrome (Types IV and VIIIAD)
    11. Hypophosphatasia
    12. Other
  C. Not otherwise specified (NOS)
V. Necrotizing periodontal diseases
  A. Necrotizing ulcerative gingivitis (NUG)
  B. Necrotizing ulcerative periodontitis (NUP)
VI. Abscesses of the periodontium
  A. Gingival abscess
  B. Periodontal abscess
  C. Pericoronal abscess

VII. Periodontitis associated with endodontic lesions
  A. Combined periodontal–endodontic lesions
VIII. Developmental or acquired deformities and conditions
  A. Localized tooth-related factors that modify or predispose to plaque-induced gingival diseases/periodontitis
    1. Tooth anatomic factors
    2. Dental restorations/appliances
    3. Root fractures
    4. Cervical root resorption and cemental tears
  B. Mucogingival deformities and conditions around teeth
    1. Gingival/soft tissue recession
      a. Facial or lingual surfaces
      b. Interproximal (papillary)
    2. Lack of keratinized gingiva
    3. Decreased vestibular depth
    4. Aberrant frenum/muscle position
    5. Gingival excess
      a. Pseudopocket
      b. Inconsistent gingival margin
      c. Excessive gingival display
      d. Gingival enlargement (see IA3 and IB4)
    6. Abnormal color
  C. Mucogingival deformities and conditions on edentulous ridges
    1. Vertical and/or horizontal ridge deficiency
    2. Lack of gingiva/keratinized tissue
    3. Gingival/soft tissue enlargement
    4. Aberrant frenum/muscle position
    5. Decreased vestibular depth
    6. Abnormal color
  D. Occlusal trauma
    1. Primary occlusal trauma
    2. Secondary occlusal trauma

*Can occur on a periodontium with no attachment loss or on a periodontium with attachment loss that is not progressing.
[†]Can be further classified on the basis of extent and severity. As a general guide, extent can be characterized as localized ≤ 30% of sites involved and generalized > 30% of sites involved. Severity can be characterized on the basis of the amount of clinical attachment loss (CAL) as follows: slight = 1–2 mm CAL; moderate = 3–4 mm CAL; and severe = ≥ 5 mm CAL.
Source: Armitage, G.C. 1999. Development of a classification system for periodontal diseases and conditions. *Ann Periodontal* 4:1–6.

Did You Know?

Domestic animals (dogs, cats, ferrets) as well as wild animals can develop periodontitis.

Chronic Periodontitis

The current classification system of periodontitis (Table 8–1) does not rely on the age of the patient to make a diagnosis. Chronic periodontitis is the most common form of periodontal disease affecting both adults and adolescents and has a slow rate of progression (Löe, Anerud, Boysen, & Morrison, 1986). It is directly related to the presence of plaque. Recently, researchers have documented that genetics may play an important noncontrollable risk factor linked to periodontitis (Newman, 1998). Chronic periodontitis may be modified by and/or associated with systemic diseases (e.g., diabetes mellitus, HIV infection). Also, other nonsystemic factors such as smoking and stress may modify the progression of periodontitis. Table 8–2 reviews common features of different types of periodontitis.

In order for a person to develop periodontitis, gingivitis must have been present. Even though specific bacteria have been identified as related to the disease, it is still considered a nonspecific bacterial infection. Detection of *Porphyromonas gingivalis* indicates a high probability that periodontitis is present (Christersson, Zambon, Dunford, Grossi, & Genco, 1989). Other local risk factors include calculus, overhanging restorations and other retentive conditions that favor microbial growth, smoking, systemic conditions, hormonal factors, and stress (American Academy of Periodontology, 1992).

Chronic periodontitis is classified according to the extent and severity of the disease. Extent is defined as the number of sites affected and is divided into localized and generalized (Table 8–3 ■): *localized* when ≤ 30% of the sites are affected and *generalized* if > 30% of the sites are affected. Severity is defined as how much disease has occurred and is based on the amount of attachment loss (measurement from the cementoenamel junction to wherever the base of the probe is. This is the clinical attachment level, which is used to determine the amount of attachment loss. Essentially, it is the amount of gingival recession plus the probing depth. If there is no gingival recession, then the attachment level is equal to the probing depth). Severity is classified into mild (or slight), moderate, and severe. *Mild* = 1 to 2 mm clinical attachment loss; *moderate* = 3 to 4 mm clinical attachment loss; and *severe* = ≥ 5 mm clinical attachment loss. When recognizing that the patient has chronic periodontitis, the extent and severity should also be noted. Figure 8–10 shows a case of generalized moderate to localized severe chronic periodontitis. Table 8–4 ■ lists common features of periodontitis.

Features of chronic periodontitis include pocket formation and alveolar and supporting bone destruction (see Figure 8–10). Tooth mobility may not necessarily be evident.

Established risk factors for chronic periodontitis include bacteria within dental plaque, smoking, and diabetes mellitus. Clinical features seen in smokers with periodontitis include deeper probing depths, enhanced gingival recession, more supragingival dental plaque, and more bone loss and attachment loss. There is little clinical gingival inflammation and bleeding because the tissues become less vascular and more fibrotic (thicker

Table 8–3 Definitions of the Extent and Severity of Chronic Periodontitis

EXTENT	
Localized	when ≤ 30% of the sites are affected
Generalized	when > 30% of the sites are affected
SEVERITY	
Mild	1 to 2 mm clinical attachment loss (CAL)
Moderate	3 to 4 mm CAL
Severe	> 5 mm CAL

Table 8–4 Common Features of the Periodontitis

Disease	Patient Population	Clinical Features	Causes of the Disease	Microbiologic Features
Chronic periodontitis (Figure 8–10 ■)	Most prevalent in adults but can occur in children and adolescents	Pocket information; bone loss; inflammation	Primary etiologic factor is dental plaque (poor oral hygiene); many other risk factors (e.g., smoking, systemic diseases)	High numbers of *Porphyromonas gingivalis*, *Tannerella forsythensis*, *Prevotella intermedia*, and *Eikenella corrodens*
Generalized aggressive periodontitis (Figure 8–11 ■)	Usually affects persons under 30 years of age but patients may be older	Generalized: Severe gingival inflammation rapid bone destruction affecting at least three permanent teeth other than first molars and incisors	Defect in polymorphonuclear (PMN) and/or macrophage function	Some predominant bacteria include *Prevotella intermedia*, *Actinobacillus actinomycetemcomitans*
Localized aggressive periodontitis (Figure 8–12 ■)	Except for the presence of periodontitis, patients are otherwise clinically healthy; puberty onset	Sparse amount of plaque and calculus; little inflammation Localized: Incisor and first molar sites	Defect in PMN chemotaxis	*Actinobacillus actinomycetemcomitans*, *Capnocytophaga* species

■ FIGURE 8–10 Chronic periodontitis.

■ FIGURE 8–11 Aggressive periodontitis in an adolescent (Courtesy of Procter & Gamble, Cincinnati, OH)

■ FIGURE 8–12 Localized aggressive periodontitis (Courtesy of Procter & Gamble, Cincinnati, OH) gingival tissue), which in a way masks the clinical appearance of inflammation. The nicotine present in tobacco appears to cause constriction of the blood vessels. Smokers also appear to have a decreased PMN migration into the oral cavity and depressed phagocytic function, resulting in a diminished immune host response to bacteria and impaired healing response.

Aggressive Periodontitis

At the 1999 International Workshop for a Classification of Periodontal Diseases and Conditions, the American Academy of Periodontology suggested to eliminate the old term "early-onset periodontitis" because it was too restrictive in terms of age. Early-onset periodontitis included prepubertal periodontitis, juvenile periodontitis, and rapidly progressive periodontitis. Aggressive periodontitis (AgP) can occur at any age and the disease is not necessarily confined to individuals under age 35. The term "aggressive periodontitis" was chosen since it is a rapidly progressive form of periodontitis and is less dependent on the age of the individual than "early-onset periodontitis" (Tonetti & Mombelli, 1999) (see Figures 8–12, 8–13).

Aggressive periodontitis (AgP) is divided into localized and generalized. Localized aggressive periodontitis (LAP) replaces the older term localized juvenile periodontitis (LJP), and generalized aggressive periodontitis (GAP) replaces the older term generalized juvenile periodontitis (GLP). Individuals with aggressive periodontitis have specific clinical and laboratory findings that make it distinctively different from chronic periodontitis. The common features of localized and generalized aggressive periodontitis are the following (Tonetti & Mombelli, 1999):

- Except for the presence of periodontitis, patients are otherwise clinically healthy.
- Rapid attachment loss and bone destruction.
- Familial disposition.

Secondary features that may be present include the following:

- Amounts of microbial deposits are inconsistent with the severity of the periodontal tissue destruction.
- Elevated levels of *Actinobacillus actinomycetemcomitans* and, in some populations, *Porphyromonas gingivalis.*
- Progression of attachment loss and bone loss may be self-arresting.
- Phagocyte abnormalities.

Features of localized aggressive periodontitis include the following:

- Circumpubertal onset.
- Serum antibody response to the bacteria.
- Localized first molar/incisor presentation with interproximal attachment loss on at least two permanent teeth, one of which is a first molar, and involving no more than two teeth other than first molars and incisors.

Features of generalized aggressive periodontitis include the following:

- Usually affecting individuals under 30 years of age, but can be older.
- Pronounced episodic nature of the destruction of attachment and bone.
- Poor antibody response to the bacteria.
- Generalized interproximal attachment loss and bone destruction affecting at least three permanent teeth other than first molars and incisors.

It should be noted that not all characteristics listed above must be present to assign a diagnosis or classify the disease. The diagnosis may be based on clinical, radiographic, and historical data (Tonetti & Mombelli, 1999). Adjunctive lab testing may be used to help with the diagnosis.

To these primary classifications, secondary descriptors may be added. For example, risk factors that modify the disease progression include cigarette smoking, emotional stress, drugs, and sex hormones.

Rapid Dental Hint

How do you determine if an aggressive case is localized or generalized? Remember that generalized disease affects at least three permanent teeth other than first molars and incisors, and localized affects at least two permanent teeth, one a first molar, and involving no more than two teeth other than first molars and incisors.

Etiology

A distinguishing feature found in AgP that is not seen in chronic periodontitis is the presence of polymorphonuclear (PMN) and macrophage defects (Page et al., 1983). These white blood cells do not function properly in eliminating the bacteria. Thus, there is a strong genetic or heredity component to this disease, which means that

Rapid Dental Hint

Remember, periodontitis can be linked to heart attacks, diabetes mellitus, and low-birth-weight babies. That is why it is important to do appropriate patient assessments.

genetic factors may be important in the development of AgP. Children with GAgP are more prone to ear, skin, and upper respiratory tract infections (Suzuki, 1988).

Plaque accumulation is minimal in LAgP, there is slight gingival inflammation, and bone loss is not as rapid as in the generalized form. There is usually no accompanying infection. Patients may have either defective PMNs or macrophages, but not both. There is a defect in PMN chemotaxis and impaired phagocytosis in 70 to 80% of patients (Suzuki, Collison, Falkner, & Nauman, 1984). The PMNs are not working properly and arrive late to the diseased site (depressed chemotaxis), so they cannot properly devour the foreign material including bacteria (impaired phagocytosis).

Predominant bacteria in LAP include *Actinobacillus actinomycetemcomitans, Prevotella intermedia, Eikenella corrodens, Campylobacter rectus,* and *Capnocytophaga* species (American Academy of Periodontology, 1989). High numbers of *Actinobacillus actinomycetemcomitans* in the subgingival pocket are associated with the localized form, and they may invade the soft tissue (epithelium and connective tissue) rather than just staying in the pocket (Saglie et al. 1982).

Rapid Dental Hint

Since about 90% of LAP have high counts of *Actinobacillus actinomycetemcomitans,* these patients will require a systemic antibiotic because this periodontal pathogen does not stay in the pocket area and invades the soft tissues. Root debridement and surgery cannot reach the bacteria in the soft tissue.

Refractory and Recurrent Periodontitis

Refractory periodontitis is a type of periodontitis wherein periodontitis patients previously treated conventionally (periodontal debridement, periodontal surgery, oral hygiene instructions) do not respond favorably to therapy and are considered resistant to treatment. Per-

sistent periodontitis in patients with poor compliance with home care or heavy tobacco use precludes the use of the term refractory. These patients more likely have recurrent periodontitis. High numbers of *Prevotella intermedia, Tannerella forsythensis, Fusobacterium nucleatum,* and *Porphyromonas gingivalis* are found in subgingival refractory sites. Recurrent periodontitis is periodontitis that recurs.

Under the new classification system (Armitage, 1999), periodontitis associated with refractory and recurrent conditions has been eliminated as a separate disease category. It was concluded that only a small percentage of periodontitis cases are actually nonresponsive to treatment. Instead, the refractory designation could be applied to all forms of periodontitis (e.g., refractory chronic periodontitis, refractory aggressive periodontitis).

Periodontitis Associated with Endodontic Lesions

Lesions of the periodontal ligament and adjacent alveolar bone may originate from interactions of the periodontium or tissues of the dental pulp (Meng, 1999). Infections coming from the pulp can cause tissue destruction that proceeds from the apical region (apical foramen) of a tooth coronally toward the gingival margin. Thus, there may be communication between endodontic and periodontal lesions (Figure 8–13 ■).

Periodontitis as a Manifestation of Systemic Diseases

Dental plaque initiates periodontal diseases but the form of disease and its progression is dependent on the host defenses to this challenge. Systemic conditions and environmental exposures may modify the normal defenses and influence the outcome of periodontal disease (Kinane, 1999). A reduction in the number of function of polymorphonuclear leukocytes (PMNs) usually results in increased rate and severity of periodontal tissue destruction. Additionally, numerous drugs such as phenytoin, nifedipine, and cyclosporine predispose to gingival overgrowth in response to plaque and thus may be an effect in modifying preexisting periodontitis (Kinane, 1999). Several systemic diseases such as diabetes mellitus (Lalla, 2007; Mealey & Ocampo, 2007), Down syndrome, Papillon-Lefévre syndrome, hyphophosphatasia, Chediak-Higashi syndrome, and HIV infection also appear to predispose individuals to periodontitis. These patients also have compromised host responses. Certain environmental con-

■ **FIGURE 8–13** Radiograph of an endodontic-periodontic lesion. Mandibular first molar: The infection originated in the pulp and spread from the apex (periapical pathology) coronally into the periodontal ligament creating a probable pocket on the distal. Not only is there an endodontic infection but there is deep probing depths with bone loss on the distal. The premolar has an endodontic lesion.

ditions or exposures including cigarette smoking and emotional stress may modify periodontitis.

Periodontitis as a Risk Factor for Systemic Conditions

This topic is not included in the 1999 AAP classification of periodontal diseases and is discussed thoroughly in Chapter 6. There is strong evidence relating periodontal disease, and diabetes, cardiovascular disease, respiratory diseases, and adverse pregnancy outcomes.

PERI-IMPLANT DISEASES

Inflammatory conditions surrounding dental implants are becoming more common today, as more implants are being placed. Periodontal disease around implants is not listed in the original or new classification from the American Academy of Periodontology; however, inflammation and periodontal destruction around implants is clinically recognized. Loss of an implant after successful placement is often due to a bacterial infection. Gram-negative anaerobes, primarily the *Fusobacterium* species and *Prevotella intermedia,* are found in the subgingival pockets. **Peri-implant disease** is a collective term for soft-tissue inflammation surrounding an implant. Peri-implant mucositis is the term used to describe reversible

inflammation in the gingiva around a functioning implant (Albrektsson & Isidor, 1994). Peri-implantitis is the term used for inflammatory changes in the soft tissues leading to loss of supporting bone around a functioning implant (Albrektsson & Isidor, 1994) (Figure 8–14 ■). The primary risk factor for peri-implant diseases is the presence of certain bacteria (Mombelli & Lang, 1998).

Treatment of peri-implant diseases is based on proper clinical and radiographic assessment. It may include periodontal debridement, oral hygiene instruction, mouthrinses, systemic antibiotics, periodontal surgery, or removal of the implant.

(a)

(b)

■ **FIGURE 8–14** A case of peri-implantitis. (a) The gingiva was bleeding, red, and had significant probing depth. (b) A gingival flap was reflected. Note bone loss is approximately to the sixth thread. Bone loss to the first thread is considered normal.

TREATMENT OF PERIODONTITIS

The treatment for all types of periodontal diseases begins with oral hygiene care and nonsurgical therapy (scaling and root planing). Smoking cessation is also included in the treatment plan. Reevaluation of initial therapy at four to eight weeks (Segelnick & Weinberg, 2006) will determine further treatment needs. Periodontal surgery may be required for pocket elimination or reduction. All patients will be placed on a maintenance schedule. Patients with chronic periodontitis do not require any systemic antibiotics. However, in selected cases, if the patient is having a difficult time with home care, a mouthrinse such as chlorhexidine may be recommended as an adjunct to periodontal debridement procedures. Patients with aggressive periodontitis will require a systemic antibiotic during scaling and root planing and periodontal surgery because *Actinobacillus actinomycetemcomitans,* which is found in more than 90% of LAP, have invaded the epithelium and connective tissue, making root debridement and periodontal surgery ineffective in bacterial elimination (Renvert et al., 1990, Saglie et al., 1982).

Periodontal patients with diabetes who show poor oral health should be placed in a monitored oral health program that will take care of both the patient's dental and general health (Bakhshandeh et al., 2007).

DENTAL HYGIENE NOTES

Periodontitis is classified based on clinical presentation rather than age, as was done in previous classification systems. Periodontitis is a microbial infection that is the result of host–bacteria interactions. Periodontitis is characterized by attachment loss with subsequent bone loss. Different patterns of bone loss are evident on radiographs. Periodontitis can be modified by systemic factors wherein the host has a reduced capacity to resist infection.

The dental hygienist must differentiate between gingivitis and periodontitis because treatment options will differ. In order to treat a clinical case of periodontal disease, the dental hygienist must have an understanding of the the histogenesis and pathogenesis of the disease.

KEY POINTS

- Periodontitis is inflammation that extends from the gingiva into the supporting periodontal structures.
- Periodontitis is most common in adults, although it does occur in a smaller number of children and adolescents.
- Dental plaque (biofilms) is the major risk factor for periodontal diseases; there are other contributory risk factors such as medications, hormones, and systemic diseases.
- Inflammatory periodontal disease is also seen around dental implants.

SELF-QUIZ

1. Which one of the following features describes chronic periodontitis? (p. 139)
   a. Occurs primarily in children
   b. No connective tissue attachment loss occurs
   c. Bone loss does not occur
   d. Risk factors include pathogenic bacteria and smoking
2. The latest classification of periodontitis is based on all of the following factors except one. Which one is the exception? (p. 137)
   a. Age of patient
   b. Clinical presentation
   c. Radiographic survey
   d. Historical data
   e. Microbial profile
3. Which one of the following forms of periodontitis is associated with a chemotactic defect in the polymorphonuclear leukocytes or machrophages? (p. 142)
   a. Dental plaque-induced gingivitis
   b. Chronic periodontitis
   c. Puberty gingivitis
   d. Localized aggressive periodontitis
   e. Drug-influenced gingivitis
4. Which one of the following bacteria is found in high numbers in localized aggressive periodontitis? (p. 142)
   a. *Prophyromonas gingivalis*
   b. *Prevotella intermedia*
   c. *Actinomyces viscosus*
   d. *Actinobacillus actinomycetemcomitans*
   e. *Streptococcus sanguis*
5. Which one of the following types of pocket has its base located apical to the alveolar crest as evidenced on a radiograph? (p. 132)
   a. Gingival
   b. Pseudo
   c. Suprabony
   d. Infrabony

6. Which one of the following features differentiates periodontitis from gingivitis? (p. 129)
   a. Dilation of blood vessels in the lamina propria
   b. Redness of the gingival
   c. Loss of connective tissue attachment
   d. Number of bacteria present in the pocket
7. Which periodontal lesion, according to Page and Schroeder (1976), is characterized by attachment loss and bone resorption? (pp. 129–130)
   a. Initial
   b. Early
   c. Established
   d. Advanced
8. A periodontal pocket forms when (pp. 131–132)
   a. the junctional epithelium migrates apically and laterally from the tooth surface.
   b. gingival fibers proliferate.
   c. bacteria multiply in the pocket.
   d. alveolar bone loss occurs.
9. All of the following factors are responsible for bone loss except one. Which one is the exception? (pp. 132–133)
   a. Prostaglandins
   b. Endotoxins
   c. B-cells
   d. Hyaluronidase
10. Which of the following periodontal disease classifications is characterized by localized vertical bone loss in the first molars in a 13 year-old patient with little plaque accumulation? (p. 141)
    a. Chronic periodontitis
    b. Generalized gingivitis
    c. Localized aggressive periodontitis
    d. Ulcerative periodontitis

REFERENCES

Albrektsson, T., and F. Isidor. 1994. Consensus report of session IV. In eds. N. P. Lang and T. Karring, *Proceedings of the First European Workshop on Periodontology*, 365–369. London: Quintessence.

American Academy of Periodontology. 1989. *Proceedings of the World Workshop in Clinical Periodontics*, I-2–I-4. Chicago: Author.

American Academy of Periodontology. 1992. *The etiology and pathogenesis of periodontal diseases* (Position Paper), 1–9. Chicago: Author.

American Academy of Periodontology. 2001. *Glossary of periodontal terms* (4th ed.). Chicago: Author.

Armitage, G. C. 1999. Development of a classification system for periodontal diseases and conditions. *Ann. Periodontol.* 4:1–6.

Bakhshandeh, S., H. Murtomaa, R. Mofid, M. M. Vehkalahti, and K. Suomalainen. 2007. Periodontal treatment needs of diabetic adults. *J Clin Periodontol* 34:53–57.

Christersson, L. A., J. J. Zambon, R. G. Dunford, S. G. Grossi, and R. J. Genco. 1989. Specific subgingival bacteria and diagnosis of gingivitis and periodontitis. *J. Dent. Res.* 68:1633–1639.

Goodson, J.M. 1992. Diagnosis of periodontitis by physical measurement: Interpretation from episodic disease hypothesis. *J. Periodontol.* 63:373–382.

Greenstein, G. 1992. Periodontal response to mechanical non-surgical therapy. *J. Periodontol.* 63:118–130.

Hughes, F. J., D. W. Augr, and F. C. Smales. 1988. Investigation of the distribution of cementum-associated lipopolysaccharides in periodontal disease by scanning electron microscope immunohistochemistry. *J. Periodont. Res.* 23:100–102.

Ishikawa, I., K. Nakashima, T. Koseki, et al. 1997. Induction of the immune response to periodontopathic bacteria and its role in the pathogenesis of periodontitis. *Periodontology 2000* 14:79–111.

Kinane, D. F. 1999. Periodontitis modified by systemic factors. *Ann. Periodontal.* 4:54–63.

Lalla, E. 2007. Periodontal infections and diabetes mellitus: When will the puzzle be complete? *J. Clin. Periodontol.* 34:913–916.

Löe, H., A. Anerud, H. Boysen, and E. Morrison. 1986. Natural history of periodontal disease in man. Rapid, moderate and no loss of attachment in Sri Lankan laborers 14 to 46 years of age. *J. Clin. Periodontol.* 13:431–440.

Mealey, B. L., and G. L. Ocampo. 2007. Diabetes and periodontal disease. *Periodontology 2000* 44(1):127–153.

Meng, H. X. 1999. Periodontic-endodontic lesions. *Ann. Periodontol.* 4:84–89.

Mombelli, A., and N. P. Lang. 1998. The diagnosis and treatment of periimplantitis. *Periodontology 2000* 17:63–76.

Müller-Glauser, W., and H. H. Schroeder. 1982. The pocket epithelium: A light- and electron-microscopic study. *J. Periodontol.* 53:133–144.

Nakib, N. M., N. F. Bissada, J. W. Simmenlink, and S. N. Golstine. 1982. Endotoxin penetration into root cementum of periodontally healthy and diseased human teeth. *J. Periodontol.* 53:638–678.

Newman, M. 1998. Genetic, environmental, and behavioral influences on periodontal infections. *Compendium* (special issue) 19:25–31.

Offenbacher, S., P. A. Heasman, and J. G. Collins. 1993. Modulation of host PGE_2 secretion as a determinant of periodontal disease expression. *J. Periodontol.* 64: 432–444.

Page, R. C., T. Bowen, L. Altman, E. Vandesteen, H. Ochs, et al. 1983. Prepubertal periodontitis I. Definition of a clinical disease entity. *J. Periodontol.* 54:257–271.

Page, R. C., and H. E. Schroeder. 1976. Pathogenesis of inflammatory periodontal disease. A summary of current work. *Lab Investigations* 33:235–249.

Prichard, J. F. 1979. Management of intrabony defects. In ed. J. F. Prichard, *The diagnosis and treatment of periodontal disease,* 358–361. Philadelphia: W. B. Saunders.

Renvert, S., M. Wikström, G. Dahlèn, and J. Slots, and J. Egelberg. 1990. On the inability of root debridement and periodontal surgery to eliminate *Actinobacillus actinomycetemocomitans* from periodontal pockets. *J. Clin. Periodontol.* 17:351–355.

Reynolds, J. J., and M. C. Meikle. 1997. Mechanisms of connective tissue matrix destruction in periodontitis. *Periodontology 2000* 14:144–157.

Saglie, R. F., F. A. Carranza, Jr., M. G. Newman, L. Cheng, and K. J. Lewin. 1982. Identification of tissue-invading bacteria in human periodontal disease. *J. Periodontol. Res.* 17:452–455.

Schwartz, Z., J. Goultschin, D. D. Dean, and B. D. Boyan. 1997. Mechanisms of alveolar bone destruction in periodontitis. *Periodontology 2000* 14:158–172.

Segelnick, S. L., and M. A. Weinberg. 2006. Reevaluation of initial therapy: When is the appropriate time? *J. Periodontol.* 77:1598–1601.

Seymour, G. J., R. N. Powell, and W. I. R. Davies. 1979. Conversion of a stable T cell lesion to a progressive B cell lesion in the pathogenesis of chronic inflammatory periodontal disease: A hypothesis. *J. Clin. Periodontol.* 6:267–277.

Socransky, S. S., and A. D. Haffajee. 1997. The nature of periodontal diseases. *Ann. Periodontol.* 2:3–10.

Suzuki, J. B. 1988. Diagnosis and classification of periodontal diseases. *Dent. Clin. North America* 32:195–216.

Suzuki, J. B., B. C. Collison, W. A. Falkler, and R. R. Nauman. 1984. Immunologic profile of juvenile periodontitis. II. Neutrophil chemotaxis, phagocytosis and spore germination. *J. Periodontol.* 55:461–467.

Tal, H. 1984. Relationship between the interproximal distance of roots and the prevalence of intrabony pockets. *J. Periodontol.* 55:604–607.

Tonetti, M. S., and A. Mombelli. 1999. Early-onset periodontitis. *Ann. Periodontol.* 4:39–52.

Weinberg, M.A., and R.N. Eskow. 2000. Osseous effects: Proper terminology revisited. *J. Periodontol.* 71:1928.

Chapter 9

Necrotizing Periodontal Diseases

Surendra Singh

OUTLINE

Introduction
Dental Hygiene Notes
Key Points
Self-Quiz
References

EDUCATIONAL OBJECTIVES

Upon completion of this chapter, the reader should be able to:

- Explain the current classification of ulcerative periodontal diseases.
- Describe the features of periodontal ulcerative gingivitis.
- Describe the features of periodontal ulcerative periodontitis.

GOAL: To provide an understanding of ulcerative periodontal diseases.

KEY WORDS

necrotizing periodontal diseases 148

necrotizing ulcerative gingivitis 148

necrotizing ulcerative periodontitis 148

INTRODUCTION

Necrotizing periodontal diseases are unique from other periodontal diseases. Necrotizing periodontal diseases include **necrotizing ulcerative gingivitis** (NUG) and **necrotizing ulcerative periodontitis** (NUP). The term acute necrotizing ulcerative gingivitis (ANUG) was changed to necrotizing ulcerative gingivitis (NUG). The Academy decided that the term "acute" was a clinical descriptive term and should not be used as a diagnostic classification since there is no chronic form of NUG.

Even though necrotizing periodontal diseases are classified as a separate entity, these conditions may actually be manifestations of underlying systemic problems (e.g., HIV infection). Additionally, other risk factors include tobacco smoking, preexisting periodontal disease, and trauma.

Necrotizing Ulcerative Gingivitis (NUG)

Clinical features of necrotizing ulcerative gingivitis (NUG) are different from other periodontal diseases (e.g., gingivitis). Necrotizing ulcerative gingivitis is a rapidly destructive, recurring, noncommunicable gingival infection. Under the new classification (Armitage, 1999), NUG is considered a type of necrotizing periodontal disease limited to the gingival tissues. Additionally, the term "acute" in ANUG is a clinical descriptive term and should not be used as a diagnostic classification (Rowland, 1999). NUG is relatively uncommon (incidence 0.1 to 10%) and mostly affects young adults 18 to 30 years old. It has also been known as "trench mouth" or "Vincent's infection." During World War I, NUG reached very high levels of incidence and was called "trench mouth," referring to the trenches soldiers inhabited during the war. In addition to bacteria, other predisposing factors are emotional stress, cigarette smoking, or decreased nutritional intake. During stressful periods, oral hygiene measures may decrease, smoking may increase, and the immune function may be suppressed.

Did You Know?

Necrotizing periodontal disease used to be called "trench mouth" because of its prevalence among soldiers who were stuck in the trenches during World War I without the means to properly take care of their teeth.

NUG is clinically characterized by small, gray, ulcerative lesions that begin at the tips of the interdental papillae and spread to the gingival margin to form punched-out or cratered lesions. A grayish-white pseudomembrane covering the affected areas may be present. A prominent sign of NUG is punched-out, ulcerated (necrotic) interdental papillae, which are caused by ulcer formation on the tip of the papillae. The marginal gingiva is bright red, inflamed, and extremely painful. Patients complain of difficulty eating and a burning sensation in the mouth. There is spontaneous gingival bleeding (i.e., the gingiva bleeds when touched or during eating). There are usually heavy deposits of plaque. These signs and symptoms are sudden in onset, localized, and recurrent. If left untreated, the infection may spread to the underlying periodontal structures. Lymphadenopathy (lymph nodes that are abnormal in size, consistency, or number), fever, and fetid oral odor (foul mouth odor) are variable findings and not always present. The signs and symptoms of NUG usually resolve a few days after adequate treatment, however. (Table 9–1 ■ Figure 9–1 ■). Three criteria must be present for a diagnosis, of NUG: 1) pain, 2) bleeding and 3) interproximal necrosis.

This condition is usually recognized on the basis of clinical signs and symptoms. It has a bacterial origin and is confirmed to be an infectious disease because reduction of dental biofilms either by mechanical debridement or the use of antibiotics will resolve clinical signs and symptoms. Microbiological samples of the affected areas show specific bacteria. High numbers of *Prevotella intermedia,* spirochetes (*Treponema* sp.), and *Fusobacterium* sp. have been isolated (Loesche, Syed, Laughon, & Stoll, 1982). Spirochetes have been shown to penetrate deep into the connective tissue (Listgarten & Lewis, 1967). Normally, bacteria stay in the pocket and do not invade the underlying tissues. Thus, NUG is a manifestation of a mixed bacterial infection modified by particular systemic determinants.

A complete laboratory workup is indicated in the management of patients with NUG, especially if a systemic disease is suspected or if the patient does not respond to conventional therapy (Murayama et al., 1994).

Differential diagnosis of NUG includes primary herpetic gingivostomatitis, recurrent aphthous ulcer (canker sores), desquamatous gingivitis, acute leukemia, and infectious mononucleosis. Primary herpetic gingivostomatitis occurs in a much younger patient; an elevated temperature is more common, and the patient appears

Table 9–1	Common Features of Necrotizing Periodontal Diseases				
Disease	*Patient Population*	*Clinical Features*	*Causes of the Disease*	*Microbiologic Features*	
Necrotizing ulcerative gingivitis (NUG)	Usually young adults	Punched-out interdental papillae, pain, and bleeding	Inadequate oral hygiene; stress; cigarette smoking; immunosuppression	Specific bacteria: spirochetes, *Prevotella intermedia*, *Fusobacterium nucleatum*	See Figure 9–1
Necrotizing ulcerative periodontitis (NUP)	HIV-infected individuals	Periodontal involvement of deeper structures; rapid loss of bone and spontaneous gingival bleeding	Immunodeficiency	Similar to adult periodontitis; bacteria: *Porphyromonas gingivalis*, *P. intermedia*, *F. nucleatum*. Also *Candida albicans*	See Figure 9–2

more ill and shows a general malaise. The oral lesions in primary herpes are vesicles that coalesce into ulcers, which occur on the attached gingival and oral mucosa. The papillae are not punched out as in NUG.

Thus, primary herpetic gingivostomatitis is a differential diagnosis of necrotizing ulcerative gingivitis. Actually, NUG can be easily recognized when interproximal papillae necrosis, bleeding, and pain are all seen. If these three features are not present, a diagnosis of NUG cannot be made.

■ **FIGURE 9–1**   NUG (Courtesy of Procter & Gamble, Cincinnati, OH)

The patient is in a lot of pain, so it may be impossible to perform any type of periodontal debridement on the first office visit. If debridement is started, gentle ultrasonic or sonic instrumentation is the best choice. A systemic analgesic and antibiotic such as metronidazole may be prescribed. After a few days, when the pain has reduced, the patient should return to the office for periodontal debridement.

Immunosuppression

Depressed PMN function (chemotactic, phagocytic) is suppressed in patients with NUG. NUG may also be the first sign of HIV infection. HIV-infected patients may present with severe forms of periodontal diseases. These patients are immunodeficient with a specific decrease in CD4+ lymphocytes. Conflicting reports concerning the classification system of HIV-associated periodontal lesions exist. New terminology was proposed in the early 1990s that is recognized by the United States and the rest of the world (EEC-Clearinghouse, 1993).

Necrotizing ulcerative gingivitis in HIV-infected patients is characterized by the destruction of one or more interdental papillae that became ulcerated, cratered, and necrotic (Murray, 1994), but there is no bone loss. NUG may represent an early form of NUP (Mealey, 1996).

These oral findings do not seem to correspond to supragingival plaque accumulation (Mealey, 1996) since removal of dental plaque does not improve the gingival condition as typically seen in chronic, plaque-associated gingivitis. The lesion is confined to the gingiva and does not involve bone loss. Pain is the hallmark of NUG (Rowland, 1999). It is important for dental practitioners to recognize soft tissue lesions early, since they may be the first signs of HIV infection (Mealey, 1996; Winkler, Grassi, & Murray, 1988; Winkler & Robertson, 1992).

The microorganisms present in the gingival lesions of HIV-positive patients are not similar to the microorganisms found in the gingival lesions of HIV-negative individuals but may be similar to those found in HIV-negative individuals who have chronic periodontitis (Mealey, 1996; Murray, Winkler, Peros, French, & Lippke, 1991). Implicating pathogens include *Porphyromonas gingivalis* (Pg), *Prevotella intermedia* (Pi), *Actinobacillus actinomycetemcomitans* (Aa), *Fusobacterium nucleatum*, spirochetes, and *Candida albicans* (fungus) (American Academy of Periodontology, 1992).

Necrotizing Ulcerative Periodontitis (NUP)

Necrotizing ulcerative periodontitis may also be the first clinical sign of underlying systemic disease, such as in human immunodeficiency virus (HIV) infection (Murayama, Kurihara, Nagai, Dompkowski, & Van Dyke, 1994). Necrotizing ulcerative periodontitis is not limited to HIV infections and is often seen in patients who have severe malnutrition and who are immunosuppressed (Armitage, 1999). However, this form of periodontal disease in the HIV-positive patient may coexist with other forms of periodontitis such as aggressive or chronic periodontitis. NUP is characterized by the extensive necrosis of the gingiva with exposure and rapid destruction of the underlying bone extending past the mucogingival junction (Figure 9–2 ■). If not successfully treated, NUP can spread into the adjacent maxilla and mandible (Mealey, 1996). Essentially, all NUP sites bleed on probing, and about 50% of sites show spontaneous bleeding (American Academy of Periodontology, 1992). Extensive clinical attachment loss is common, but deep periodontal

■ **FIGURE 9–2**   NUP (Courtesy of Procter & Gamble, Cincinnati, OH)

pocket formation is not evident (American Academy of Periodontology, 1992).

The microbial population of subgingival sites with NUP is similar to that of chronic periodontitis, which is also similar to NUG. This may prove that NUG may be a precursor to the tissue and bone destruction seen in NUP (Murray, 1994).

DENTAL HYGIENE NOTES

The American Academy of Periodontology refers collectively to necrotizing ulcerative gingivitis (NUG) and necrotizing ulcerative periodontitis (NUP) as ulcerative periodontal diseases (Rowland, 1999). The reason for this is that both NUG and NUP may be considered the same disease but at different stages. Thus, they may not be separate diseases but named under the necrotizing ulcerative diseases. Both NUG and NUP are diseases related to a decreased systemic resistance, as seen in HIV-infected patients, to bacteria present in the periodontal tissues. NUG is confined to the gingival unit and NUP involves gingiva and the attachment apparatus (bone, cementum, periodontal ligament). Three criteria (pain, bleeding, and papillae necrosis) must be present for a diagnosis of NUG.

KEY POINTS

- NUG and NUP are ulcerative inflammatory periodontal diseases.
- Three criteria must be present for a diagnosis of NUG: pain, bleeding, and papillary necrosis.

Rapid Dental Hint

Necrotizing gingivitis affects the gingiva. Necrotizing periodontitis is a more advanced condition involving the underlying bone.

- NUG involves the gingival unit.
- NUP involves the attachment apparatus.
- *Prevotella intermedia* and spirochetes are associated with gingival lesions.

SELF-QUIZ

1. Which one of the following statements describes a patient with necrotizing periodontal disease? (p. 148)
   a. Higher prevalence in females than males
   b. Higher incidence of skin lesions
   c. Pain is a prominent feature
   d. Geographic distribution shows a higher prevalence in the eastern United States

2. Which of the following bacterium present in NUG patients may penetrate periodontal tissues? (p. 148)
   a. *Treponema denticola*
   b. *Prevotella intermedia*
   c. *Fusobacterium species*
   d. *Streptococcus sanguis*

3. Both necrotizing ulcerative gingivitis and necrotizing ulcerative periodontitis are currently categorized under the classification of (p. 148)
   a. acute necrotizing diseases.
   b. necrotizing ulcerative diseases.
   c. chronic periodontitis.
   d. aggressive periodontitis.

4. Necrotizing ulcerative gingivitis may be the first clinical sign of an underlying systemic disease such as (p. 149)
   a. human immunodeficiency virus infection.
   b. diabetes mellitus.
   c. osteoporosis.
   d. kidney failure.

5. Which of the following diseases must be differentiated from NUG? (pp. 148–149)
   a. Herpes simplex type 2
   b. Primary herpetic gingivostomatitis
   c. Canker sores
   d. Acquired immunodeficiency syndrome

6. All of the following are criteria that define NUG except one. Which one is the exception? (p. 148)
   a. Pain
   b. Bleeding
   c. Papillary necrosis
   d. Fever

7. The distinguishing feature between NUP and NUG is (p. 150)
   a. amount of gingival bleeding.
   b. alveolar bone loss.
   c. number of bacteria present in pocket.
   d. intensity of pain.

8. Which of the following conditions is a concern in immunosuppressed necrotizing ulcerative disease patients? (pp. 149–150)
   a. Fungal infection
   b. Heart problems
   c. Stunting of growth
   d. Protozoa infection

9. A prominent sign of NUG is (p. 148)
   a. high fever.
   b. punched-out interdental papillae.
   c. gingival abscess formation.
   d. alveolar bone loss.

10. The "older" term for NUG is (p. 148)
    a. oral gingivitis.
    b. atypical gingivitis.
    c. trench mouth.
    d. aphthous ulcer.

REFERENCES

American Academy of Periodontology. 1992. *The etiology and pathogenesis of periodontal diseases* (Position Paper), 1–9. Chicago: Author.

Armitage, G. C. 1999. Development of a classification system for periodontal diseases and conditions. *Ann. Periodontol.* 4:1–6.

EEC-Clearinghouse on Oral Problems Related to HIV Infections and WHO Collaborating Centre on Oral Manifestations for the Human Immunodeficiency Virus. 1993. Classification and diagnostic criteria for oral lesions in HIV infection. *J. Oral Pathol. Med.* 22: 289–291.

Listgarten, M. A., and D. W. Lewis. 1967. The distribution of spirochetes in the lesion of acute necrotizing ulcerative gingivitis: An electron microscopic and statistical survey. *J. Periodontol.* 38:379–386.

Loesche, W. J., S. A. Syed, B. E. Laughon, and J. Stoll. 1982. The bacteriology of acute necrotizing ulcerative gingivitis. *J. Periodontol.* 53:223–230.

Mealey, B. L. 1996. Periodontal implications: Medically compromised patients. *Ann. Periodontol.* 1:256–321.

Murayama, Y., H. Kurihara, A. Nagai, D. Dompkowski, and T. Van Dyke. 1994. Acute necrotizing ulcerative gingivitis: Risk factors involving host defense mechanisms. *Periodontology 2000* 6:116–124.

Murray, P. A. 1994. Periodontal diseases in patients infected by human immunodeficiency virus. *Periodontology 2000* 6:50–67.

Murray, P. A., J. R. Winkler, W. J. Peros, C. K. French, and J. A. Lippke. 1991. DNA probe detection of periodontal pathogens in HIV-associated periodontal lesions. *Oral Microbiol. Immunol.* 6:34–40.

Rowland, R. W. 1999. Necrotizing ulcerative gingivitis. *Ann Periodontol.* 4:65–73.

Winkler, J. R., M. Grassi, and P. A. Murray. 1988. Clinical description and etiology of HIV-associated periodontal diseases. In eds. P. B. Robertson and J. S. Greenspan, *Perspectives on oral manifestations of AIDS,* 49–70. Littleton, MA: PSG Publishing.

Winkler, J. R., and P. B. Robertson. 1992. Periodontal disease associated with HIV infection. *Oral Surg. Oral Med. Oral Pathol.* 73:145–150.

Chapter 10

Occlusal Trauma

Mea A. Weinberg

Stuart J. Froum

OUTLINE
Introduction
Occlusion
Pathogenesis of Occlusal Trauma
Classification of Occlusal Trauma
Clinical Findings in Occlusal Trauma
Radiographic Findings in Occlusal Trauma
Outcomes of Treatment of Occlusal Trauma
Occlusal Therapy
Dental Hygiene Notes
Key Points
Self-Quiz
References

EDUCATIONAL OBJECTIVES

Upon completion of this chapter, the reader should be able to:

- List the classification of malocclusion.
- Identify and distinguish between the two types of occlusal trauma.
- Identify and describe the clinical and radiographic signs of occlusal trauma.
- Define the interrelationship between occlusal trauma and periodontitis.

GOAL: To provide information about the etiology, clinical manifestations, and therapy of occlusal trauma.

KEY WORDS

bruxism 157
codestructive 158
malocclusion 154
occlusion 154
occlusal therapy 165
occlusal trauma 156

parafunctional habits 157
primary occlusal trauma 160
secondary occlusal trauma 161
tooth mobility 161

INTRODUCTION

Soon after the identification of microorganisms as a risk factor for periodontitis, the role of occlusion in periodontal diseases was considered. Although numerous studies using human and animal models have been published on this subject, it still remains a controversial issue.

OCCLUSION

Occlusion describes the contact relationship of teeth in function and dysfunction and is defined as any contact between the incisal or occlusal surfaces of the maxillary and mandibular teeth. It consists of all tooth contacts during swallowing and chewing. Centric occlusion (CO) is defined as maximal intercuspation or contact of the maxillary and mandibular teeth. The centric relation (CR) is the most retruded (posterior) position of the mandibule in relation to the maxilla from which lateral movements of the jaw can be made.

An "ideal" or normal occlusion occurs where the arrangement of teeth is considered to be most correct. This is to say, upon closing the mouth, all upper and lower teeth come together at the same time and there are no crowded, malpositioned, or tipped teeth. Few patients have an ideal or normal occlusion. Usually, there are deviations from normal. Any deviation from the ideal or normal occlusion, for example, crowding, malpositioned, or tipped teeth, is referred to as **malocclusion.** However, malocclusion does not necessarily indicate occlusal disease. Classification of the various forms of malocclusion is done with Edward H. Angle's principles of defining occlusion. This classification is based on the interdigitation of the maxillary and mandibular teeth. Malpositioning is described in terms of crowding of individual teeth or groups of teeth. Figure 10–1 ■ describes the three classes of malocclusion. If the maxillary first molar is missing, the maxillary canine is used. The use of study casts to provide a better indication of occlusion is sometimes required. The main purpose for using this classification is for diagnostic consistency and treatment planning because malocclusion is a contributing risk factor for inflammatory periodontal diseases.

Functional occlusion consists of teeth that are in function when the mandible moves in lateral and protrusive excursions or movements. Lateral movements are defined by the direction in which the mandible is moving (Figure 10–2 ■). If the mandible moves to the left, the movement is called a left working movement, and the left side of the arch is known as the working side. In a left working movement, the right side is known as the nonworking (balancing) side. If the mandible moves to the right, the movement is called a right working movement, and the right side of the arch is then referred to as the working side. The left side is referred to as the nonworking (balancing) side. For some patients, a lateral movement results in contacts between the posterior teeth on the working side. This is called group function (Figure 10–3 ■). For other patients, a lateral movement results in contact only between the maxillary and mandibular canines on the working side. This is called canine protection or canine guidance (see Figure 10–3). It is generally believed that during lateral movements there should be no tooth contact on the nonworking side. However, balancing side contacts are probably prevalent in most patients. Denture wearers need tooth-to-tooth contacts on both the working and nonworking sides for the dentures to function effectively.

Protrusive occlusion is movement of the mandible in a direction anterior to centric occlusion (Figure 10–4 ■). Guidance for this movement should be on the anterior teeth, and edge-to-edge contact of the incisors should be possible. Any posterior contact during protrusive occlusion is considered undesirable. Posterior interference is seen frequently with an extruded or tipped tooth. A classic example of a prematurity occurs when an amalgam filling is too high (placed above the line of occlusion), and upon biting down, the patient feels as though that particular area is touching first. Therefore, in this situation, one or more teeth are touching the occlusal surface rather than all the teeth touching simultaneously.

Cases where patients have occlusions that are not ideal but are symptom-free and their dentition "survives" or "adapts" to this deviated occlusion are referred to as physiologic occlusion. Pathologic occlusion occurs when

> **Did You Know?**
>
> Back in the nineteenth century there were strong overtones of religious belief in the concept of occlusion.

> **Did You Know?**
>
> Buck teeth is a type of Class II malocclusion present in about 45% of the population.

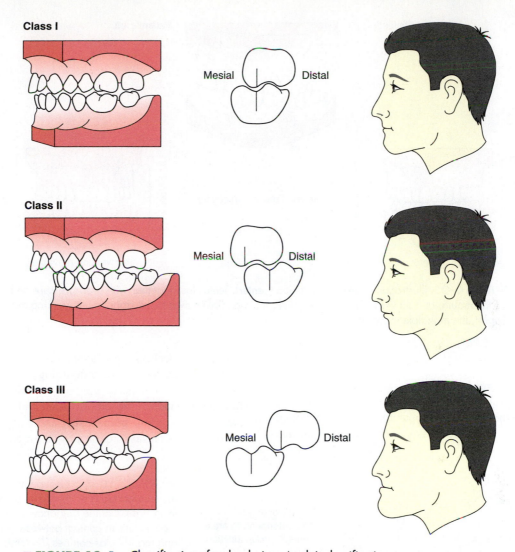

FIGURE 10–1   Classification of malocclusion: Angle's classification.

patients show evidence or signs and have symptoms of occlusal disease (Goldman & Cohen, 1980).

Overbite (amount of vertical overlap of anterior teeth) and overjet (horizontal protrusion of upper teeth

Did You Know?

At a meeting of the Philadelphia Academy of Stomatology in 1898, Edward H. Angle proposed that orthodontics be based on the science of dental occlusion and offered a definition of normal occlusion as the ideal to be attained in the treatment of malocclusion.

beyond the lower) are measured with a periodontal probe. Normally, the incisal edges of the lower incisors and the cingulum of the upper incisors establish the stops necessary to maintain tooth position. A deep overbite can occur as a result of skeletal relationship, extrusion or migration of teeth, or if posterior teeth are missing, causing the anterior teeth to handle the occlusal load. Overclosure of anterior teeth can cause trauma to the gingiva of the maxillary and/or mandibular anterior teeth (Figure 10–5 ■). This is referred to as a traumatic overbite. An open bite occurs when anterior and/or posterior maxillary and mandibular teeth do not occlude.

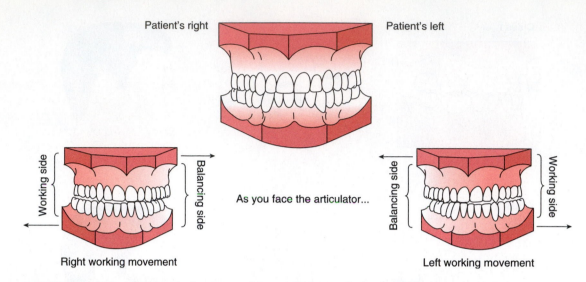

■ **FIGURE 10–2** Illustration of centric occlusion (*center*). Teeth close together with even pressure on both sides of the mouth. In right working movement (*left*), the mandible moves to the right. In left working movement (*right*), the mandible moves to the left.

Terminology

Occlusal trauma (also termed trauma from occlusion, periodontal traumatism, or occlusal disease) is defined as injury to the attachment apparatus (bone, periodontal ligament, and cementum) as a consequence of normal or excessive occlusal force(s) applied to a tooth or teeth (American Academy of Periodontology, 2001). In addition to periodontal tissue damage, excessive occlusal force also can affect the temporomandibular joint, muscles of mastication, pulp tissue, and integrity of the restoration. Occlusal force is a force (or energy) trans-

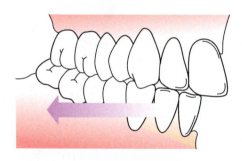

Right working movement
All posterior teeth are in contact: group function

■ **FIGURE 10–3** Group function: Lateral movement results in contact of all posterior teeth (*top*). Canine guidance: Lateral movement results in contact between the maxillary and mandibular canines (*bottom*).

Right working movement
Only the canines are in contact: canine protection

■ FIGURE 10–4 Protrusive occlusion (movement): Mandible moves forward from centric occlusion so that there is contact of the incisors.

mitted to the teeth and their supporting structures by tooth-to-tooth contacts or through food substances or any other intervening material. When the magnitude (size), direction, frequency, and/or duration of these forces exceeds the reparative capacity of the attachment apparatus, the result is occlusal disease. This is determined clinically by signs and symptoms. Traumatogenic occlusion is defined as any occlusion that produces forces that directly or indirectly cause injury to the attachment apparatus.

Premature occlusal contact (also called occlusal interference) occurs when there are interferences to closure of opposing teeth (Figure 10–6 ■); that is, a tooth that occludes with an opposing tooth before full closure is achieved in centric occlusion. This premature contact prevents the other teeth in the arch from achieving contact simultaneously. Premature contacts also can occur during lateral movements when the mandible moves from one side to the other. In addition, an extruded (also termed supererupted) or a tipped tooth may cause posterior occlusal interferences. Premature contacts should be eliminated if there is evidence of damage to the attachment apparatus or increasing tooth mobility.

Parafunctional habits are activities of the masticatory (chewing) system that are beyond the normal range of function. Chewing and swallowing are normal, whereas grinding and clenching are abnormal or parafunctional activities. Parafunctional activities often occur during sleep or stressful situations. Premature contacts also may predispose to parafunctional habits. *Physiologic occlusion* is defined as survival of the dentition despite its deviation from a preconceived hypothetical normal. Most people have some occlusal discrepancies, but in most cases, the dentition has "adapted" to the discrepancies and shows no signs of occlusal trauma. On the other hand, the dentition in a pathologic occlusion generally shows evidence of occlusal disease.

Occlusal therapy is designed to control the forces generated by tooth-to-tooth contact so they are tolerated by the attachment apparatus.

Parafunctional Habits

Bruxism, a type of parafunctional habit, is the unconscious grinding and/or clenching of the teeth when the

■ FIGURE 10–5 A deep overbite causes the mandibular incisors to touch the palatal gingiva of the maxillary anterior area.

■ FIGURE 10–6 In protrusion (anterior teeth edge to edge), note that the initial interference is on the maxillary incisors, which prevents the right lateral incisor from occluding.

Rapid Dental Hint

A quick and easy way to see if a patient is a tongue thruster is to ask the patient to swallow. The mentalis (chin) muscle will contract (easily seen) if the patient is a thruster. Also, you can see the tongue up against the palatal surface of the incisors.

patient is not swallowing or chewing. During sleep, it is called nocturnal bruxism and is often associated with stressful situations. While most patients show signs of bruxism, only 5 to 20% are consciously aware of it (Hallmon, 1999). The early signs of bruxism may go undetected, but with increased duration, intensity, and direction of the habit, wear facets will be visible on tooth surfaces and tooth mobility may be seen. Initially, this increase in functional demand will be accommodated by the periodontium. Other changes include cusp fractures, increased thermal sensitivity, and increased tooth mobility, which can resolve when the parafunctional action is discontinued. Other examples of parafunctional habits include nail biting, tongue thrusting, and chewing of foreign objects between the teeth such as bobby pins, nails, pipes, and pencils.

Tongue thrusting or thumb sucking often creates a class II, division I malocclusion with an anterior and posterior open bite (Figure 10–7 ■). During swallowing, the tongue is placed between the maxillary and mandibular anterior teeth and on the sides rather than on the hard palate near the rugae. The lips and chin muscles contract, visualized as a massive grimace. Tongue thrusting eventually

■ **FIGURE 10–7** An anterior open bite caused by tongue thrusting.

Did You Know?

The prevalence of digit sucking decreases steadily from the age of 2 years to approximately 10% by the age of 5.

tually can lead to a mouth-breathing habit, which may cause a localized gingival inflammation of the maxillary and mandibular incisor region that is unrelated to plaque accumulation. In addition, the lips will be dry and parted at rest. Parafunctional activity can produce symptoms from the musculature or TMJ. Palpation of the muscles of mastication can detect muscle spasms or pain. Parafunctional habits may lead to occlusal trauma. Occlusal trauma is defined as injury to the attachment apparatus as a result of excessive occlusal force.

Rapid Dental Hint

Do not forget to do an occlusal exam when performing a patient evaluation. Check for any occlusal interferences using articulating paper or floss.

The Role of Occlusal Trauma in the Initiation and Progression of Periodontal Diseases

Research has concluded that occlusal trauma alone does not cause gingivitis, periodontitis, pocket formation, or gingival recession (Ramfjord & Ash, 1981; Svanberg, King, & Gibbs, 1995; Harrel & Nunn, 2004). The gingival unit is independent, having its own blood supply, and is not affected by occlusal trauma (Keller & Cohen, 1955). In healthy conditions, the structure and adaptive nature of the attachment apparatus to occlusal forces permit a certain degree of physiologic mobility. Adaptation refers to alterations or adjustments that the body develops to accommodate to its environment. However, when occlusal forces are excessive, beyond the capability of the attachment apparatus to repair itself, tissue injury occurs, resulting in occlusal trauma.

A more complex and controversial issue is the interrelationship between periodontal inflammation and trauma from occlusion. Is the presence of inflammation **codestructive** and accelerated when occlusal trauma is also present? Numerous human and animal models were developed to determine the effects of occlusal forces on the progression of periodontitis. According to the codestructive theory, occlusal forces will accelerate the rate of periodontal destruction and result in connective tissue attachment loss, in the presence of preexisting inflammation. This concept is still controversial. It is also debatable whether these factors interfere with wound healing in the treatment of periodontal diseases. The conflicting results of different studies may be due to differences in animal species, the procedures used for producing occlusal trauma, and inherent measurement inaccuracies.

Human Studies

Glickman (1963) introduced the concept of codestruction, whereby inflammation and trauma from occlusion are synergistic factors in periodontal destruction. He suggested that while occlusion does not cause gingival inflammation or pocket formation, inflammation of the supporting tissues in the presence of occlusal trauma alters the pathway of inflammation. Subsequently, the inflammatory infiltrate will spread more rapidly through tissue damaged by excessive occlusal forces and move directly into the periodontal ligament space, causing the development of angular bone defects and infrabony pockets. Thus, according to Glickman, inflammation and occlusal trauma become codestructive, whereby the progression of periodontitis is accelerated by the presence of occlusal trauma.

However, other investigators (Shefter & McFall, 1984) reported no relationship between occlusal disharmonies and pathoses associated with inflammatory periodontal disease in patients with mild to moderate periodontitis.

Animal Studies

In an attempt to reproduce the kind of occlusal trauma that might occur in the human dentition, early studies placed high restorations on teeth to reproduce the jiggling forces caused by premature tooth contacts. Jiggling or reciprocating forces were applied in opposite directions on a tooth at the same time. This prevented the tooth from moving away from the force. Unilateral forces would have allowed the traumatized teeth to migrate away from the occlusal forces. In many studies, tissue inflammation was induced using silk ligatures placed around the teeth near the gingival margin to enhance plaque retention.

Primate Model   Meitner (1975) examined the effects of jiggling forces on marginal periodontitis in squirrel monkeys by forcing wedges into the embrasure between teeth. The wedges were moved every 48 hours, allowing the teeth to be subjected to reciprocating forces every other day. Although this type of trauma is quite different from that caused by premature contacts, there was no accelerated loss of connective tissue attachment.

Polson (1974) also found that there was no difference in loss of connective tissue attachment and bone destruction in periodontally involved teeth of squirrel monkeys subjected to a single episode of trauma.

Beagle Model   The results of several beagle dog studies (Ericsson & Lindhe, 1982; Lindhe & Svanberg, 1974) showed that when heavy occlusal forces were combined with plaque-induced periodontitis, the rate of clinical attachment loss was accelerated; but this model system also showed that trauma from occlusion does not aggravate gingival inflammation or cause loss of clinical attachment in chronic gingivitis (Ericsson & Lindhe, 1977). In the beagle, when jiggling forces were applied to a periodontally healthy tooth or a tooth with chronic gingivitis, the tooth became hypermobile.

PATHOGENESIS OF OCCLUSAL TRAUMA

The pathologic features of occlusal trauma are different from those of inflammation. With occlusal trauma, healing of traumatized tissue need not be considered an inflammatory process because no inflammatory/immune cells such as leukocytes, lymphocytes, or plasma cells are present. Thus repair is initiated after the trauma is removed, without the tissue exhibiting the classic signs of inflammation. The lesion of occlusal trauma in the normal, healthy periodontium usually develops following compression and tension of the periodontal ligament (PDL) fibers and resorption and deposition of bone. Compression of the PDL fibers results in obstruction of blood flow to the fibers, which in turn results in bone resorption. If the destructive process is greater than the repair potential of the periodontal tissue, injury may result. The alveolar bone undergoes osteoclastic resorption in areas of pressure, which results in the widening of the periodontal ligament space (Svanberg et al., 1995). Clinically, increased tooth mobility may result to accommodate for the widened PDL. Regardless of the status of the original attachment apparatus, there will be increasing tooth mobility until the PDL can adapt to the applied force. When adaptation is complete, new lamina dura may be seen radiographically, even though the increased

PDL space of hypermobile teeth will remain. When the occlusal trauma is eliminated, bone repair will occur, and a functional width of the PDL will be reestablished. If, however, the trauma continues, excessive widening of the PDL results to accommodate the bone loss. This results in increasing tooth mobility.

The gingival connective tissue attachment is not affected, nor is there apical migration of the junctional epithelium. This same tissue reaction that occurs in a patient with a healthy periodontium also occurs in a patient with a reduced bony support who also has a healthy periodontium.

If the codestructive theory was correct, then the pathway of inflammation would be seen as proceeding not from the gingiva to the bone and finally to the PDL but rather from the gingiva directly into the PDL, inducing the formation of an infrabony pocket with associated vertical bone loss (Glickman & Smulow, 1965). Removal of the trauma but not the inflammation does not decrease tooth mobility, and the crestal bone does not repair (Polson, Meitner, & Zander, 1976). Kantor, Polson, and Zander (1976) removed both jiggling forces and inflammation, resulting in new bone formation without an increase in alveolar bone height. Collectively, these studies show that occlusal trauma does not initiate gingivitis or periodontitis. Although the importance of the role of dental plaque in inflammatory peri-odontal diseases is undisputed, the influence of occlusal trauma on the attachment level remains controversial (Hallmon, 1999).

CLASSIFICATION OF OCCLUSAL TRAUMA

Occusal trauma can be classified as either primary or secondary and either can be localized to a single tooth or generalized, affecting several teeth (Table 10–1 ■).

Primary occlusal trauma is defined as injury to the supporting structures (PDL, cementum, and bone) caused by excessive occlusal forces (forces greater than experienced during normal chewing function) placed on a tooth or teeth with normal periodontal tissue support (Figure 10–8 ■). Examples of causes of primary occlusal trauma include the following:

- A "high" restoration, where, on biting, the restored tooth creates a premature contact with the opposing tooth.
- Parafunctional habits involving tooth-to-tooth contact such as bruxism, clenching, or object-to-tooth contact such as biting on pencils or nail biting.
- A malpositioned or maligned tooth, including teeth that are extruded (moved occlusally) or tipped.
- A periapical (around the apex of the root) abscess or infection causing a tooth to be extruded.
- Physical "blow" to a tooth or teeth.

Table 10–1	Periodontal Occlusal Traumatic Lesions				
Type of Occlusal Trauma	*Etiology*	*Pocket Formation*	*Bone Height*	*Mobility*	*Treatment Options*
Primary	Excessive occlusal force(s)	No	Normal height or slight bone loss	Adapted	Selective grinding, appliances, monitoring without treatment
Secondary	Normal or excessive occlusal force(s)	No/Yes. Periodontal pockets may be present, but due to periodontal destruction rather than the occlusal trauma	Reduced height (moderate/severe)	Progressive	Splinting if necessary, selective grinding, extraction, orthodontic movement, appliances, monitoring

■ **FIGURE 10–8**   Primary occlusal trauma. A tooth with normal periodontal tissues is exposed to excessive occlusal load (arrow). As a result of bone resorption, the periodontal ligament space gradually increases in size on both sides of the teeth as well as in the periapical region.

■ **FIGURE 10–9**   Secondary occlusal trauma. If a tooth with reduced periodontal tissue support has been exposed to excessive occlusal forces, a widened periodontal ligament space and increased mobility result.

- A removable partial denture clasp around an abutment tooth.
- Orthodontic movement of teeth.

Parafunctional activity may result in primary occlusal trauma. This occurs when a tooth is subjected to greater forces over a longer period of time than what normally occurs in chewing and swallowing. Food chewing is not a cause of primary occlusal trauma because the forces are most likely not long-standing or severe enough to affect the attachment apparatus.

When the forces generated during bruxism exceed the adaptive capacity of the periodontium on a regular basis, occlusal trauma is initiated (Caffesse & Fleszar, 1992).

Secondary occlusal trauma occurs when normal (e.g., chewing) or excessive occlusal forces cause injury in a periodontium with reduced bone support (Figure 10–9 ■). Bone levels around the tooth are inadequate to support these forces, and the tooth is less resistant to occlusal loading. In other words, a tooth in secondary occlusal trauma has insufficient bone support, and normal

chewing and swallowing forces are excessive, causing injury to the attachment apparatus. This can occur even when the periodontal tissues are healthy, but there is a reduced bone height. Therefore, the distinguishing feature between primary and secondary occlusal trauma is the amount of bony support surrounding the tooth.

Other parafunctional habits such as lip, nail, or cheek biting, tongue thrusting, or the placement of foreign objects between the teeth (e.g., pipe clenching and chewing, pencil biting, playing a wind musical instrument, and clenching fingernails or bobby pins) may affect the attachment apparatus. However, these do not appear to occur as frequently as tooth-to-tooth contact habits. A less common cause of primary occlusal trauma is occupational bruxism, which occurs in certain stressful occupations.

CLINICAL FINDINGS IN OCCLUSAL TRAUMA

Tooth Mobility

The most common sign of occlusal trauma is increasing **tooth mobility** over a period of time. However, excessive occlusal forces may not always cause tooth hypermobility (Svanberg et al., 1995). Since mobility due to occlusal trauma is an adaptive function, it may not be considered pathologic (resulting in disease). A tooth with excessive occlusal load may adapt to the forces by exhibiting increased but not increasing mobility. However, if there is progressive tooth mobility over a period of several days or weeks, it may then be considered pathologic (Green & Levine, 1996). Consequently, for the proper recognition of occlusal disease, tooth mobility has to be assessed on two or more separate occasions (Svanberg et al., 1995).

A tooth in primary occlusal trauma may show mobility. In this case, the tooth becomes mobile so that it can adapt to the abnormal force placed on it. Thus the mobility of the tooth could be classified as an adapted mobility (Tarnow & Fletcher, 1986). For example, mobility of a tooth caused by a high restoration will come to a plateau and no longer increase; this is adapted mobility. Tooth mobility in absence of supporting alveolar bone may be characteristic of a parafunctional habit. However, tooth mobility does not occur in all patients who grind and clench their teeth. In some cases, tooth wear accommodates for the bruxing habit.

Tooth hypermobility, produced by excessive occlusal forces, does not cause gingival inflammation, worsen the severity of chronic gingivitis, or act as a primary cause for connective tissue attachment loss (Svanberg et al., 1995).

Besides excessive occlusal forces, tooth mobility may result from severe gingival inflammation extending into the connective tissue attachment, the loss of supporting alveolar bone, pregnancy, and orthodontic movement, or may occur following surgical therapy. Tooth mobility will usually decrease by the fourth week after surgery. The cause and progression of the mobility must be determined because treatment options differ.

Fremitus

Fremitus is the vibrational movement of a tooth under occlusal function. Fremitus is detected by placing the index finger on the gingival-tooth interfaces (Figure 10–10 ■) of the maxillary teeth and asking the patient to tap the teeth up and down, grind from side to side, and move the jaw into an edge-to-edge (protrusive) occlusion. Centric prematurities are detected by the presence of fremitus.

Pain

Pain from percussion, pain upon biting, and the pain of tooth hypersensitivity are symptoms of primary and secondary occlusal trauma. For example, after receiving a

■ **FIGURE 10–10** A technique for detecting fremitus. The index finger is placed partly on the facial tooth surfaces and the gingiva. Tooth movements can be detected when the patient taps the teeth together and grinds side to side.

restoration, a patient may call to report tooth pain. An evaluation will reveal that the restoration is high, causing pain and mobility upon biting or chewing. Once the restoration is reduced in height, the pain and mobility will disappear.

Tooth Migration

Pathologic tooth migration usually is indicative of moderate to severe periodontitis and secondary occlusal trauma (Towfighi et al., 1997). Pathologic migration is defined as a change in tooth position resulting from disruption of the forces that maintain teeth in a normal position (Chasens, 1979). Excessive occlusal forces, which include the normal forces of chewing or swallowing applied to teeth, and extensive bone loss may cause teeth to migrate (Towfighi et al., 1997). Clinically, pathologic tooth migration results in widened spaces between teeth (diastemas), flaring or fanning of anterior teeth, and/or extrusion of teeth (Figure 10–11 ■). Although it is a common sign of secondary occlusal trauma, pathologic tooth migration may be caused by periodontal surgery or extensive inflammation extending into the PDL.

Attrition and Abfraction

Forces generated during bruxism frequently are greater than the adaptive capacity of the periodontium. Consequently, the contoured surface of a tooth may be ground flat, to the point where the dentin may be exposed (Figure

■ **FIGURE 10–11**   A 45-year-old patient with advanced periodontitis. Patient complaints of recently widened spaces, flaring of the maxillary incisors, and extrusion of the maxillary right central incisor are often an indication that the reduced attachment apparatus is reacting to occlusal forces.

10–12 ■). Cracks and pits form on the worn edges and may become plaque traps. Clinical features of attrition include flattened occlusal or incisal surfaces of teeth. The canines and central and lateral incisors most commonly receive the heaviest and earliest lateral wear (Lytle, 1990). Exposed dentin may cause a tooth to become sensitive. Wear facets frequently are seen as a flat, shiny, worn spot on the side of a cusp of a tooth (Figure 10–13 ■). The presence of attrition and wear facets does not necessarily indicate occlusal habits. Wear on teeth also may be due to the patient's age or diet. Once a facet has developed,

■ **FIGURE 10–12**   Anterior view of a 55-year-old patient who was unaware he was a bruxer. Note the generalized heavy wear such that all teeth appear flat and on the same plane. (Courtesy of Dr. Xiu Yan Li)

■ **FIGURE 10–13**   Showing a mandibular anterior teeth wear facet on the mandibular canine. (Courtesy of John Eum, DDS, New York University College of Dentistry)

it remains. If a patient has wear facets for many years with no changes, it is probably not an active process. Abfraction lesions are small cracks or notches in the enamel (cervical area) of a tooth which occur with clenching/bruxing (e.g. occlusal loading).

Muscle/Temporomandibular Joint

Occlusal trauma may cause the muscles that work the jaw, the largest being the temporalis and the masseter, to become chronically sore, resulting in headaches and muscle pain. Pain usually occurs during chewing or upon waking in the morning. This type of pain may be emanating from the temporomandibular joint (TMJ). The patient may report muscle spasms in the head, neck, and ear area. Pathology must be ruled out when a patient complains of any type of facial pain, including TMJ pain.

Tooth Structure

Tooth fractures and long-term chipping of enamel are additional signs of occlusal trauma related to the magnitude of forces that the teeth endure.

RADIOGRAPHIC FINDINGS IN OCCLUSAL TRAUMA

Along with the clinical examination, radiographs are useful for recognizing the signs of occlusal trauma and/or the signs of adaptation to significant occlusal forces (Caffesse & Fleszar, 1992).

Widening of the PDL occurs as an adaptation response to accommodate excessive occlusal loading and also may result in the resorption of alveolar bone. Radiographically, when the PDL space is wider at the coronal third of the root, it is referred to as crestal funneling.

Radiographically, a tooth in primary occlusal trauma may or may not show vertical bone loss as a result of widening of the PDL space. However, this should not be confused with bone loss related to periodontitis (Ricchetti, 1998; Figures 10–14 ■ and 10–15 ■) because primary occlusal trauma does not show loss of connective tissue attachment, increased probing depth, and related infrabony pockets (Polson & Zander, 1983). The presence of angular bony defects is not necessarily a sign of occlusal trauma. If a widened PDL space is present but no tooth mobility exists, occlusal trauma is not necessarily present. The findings may be a functional adaptation to the occlusal forces. Additionally, an increase in the density, referred to as osteoporosis, of the alveolar bone and the excessive deposition of cementum, referred to as hypercementosis, around the apical part of the root may be evident (Figure 10–16 ■).

Radiographically, a tooth in secondary occlusal trauma shows reduced bone levels that are inadequate to support the tooth under a normal load without increasing mobility, migration, or fremitus (Ricchetti, 1998). Vertical bone loss is accompanied by widening of the PDL. Occasionally, root resorption may occur.

■ **FIGURE 10–15**   A radiograph showing a typical lesion of secondary occlusal trauma. The tooth has a reduced bony support and increasing tooth mobility. The tooth has an adverse crown-to-root ratio.

OUTCOMES OF TREATMENT OF OCCLUSAL TRAUMA

The desired outcome of treatment of occlusal trauma is that the patient remains comfortable during chewing and is able to maintain the dentition in a state of health. The dental hygienist can determine if the reversal of signs and symptoms of occlusal trauma has achieved the following outcomes (American Academy of Periodontology, 1996). These include the following:

■ **FIGURE 10–14**   A radiograph showing a typical lesion of primary occlusal trauma. Widening of the periodontal ligament space has occurred due to a heavy occlusal force placed on the premolar. Note that there are no increased probing depths.

■ **FIGURE 10–16**   Hypercementosis (excessive deposition of cementum) seen on the root may be indicative of occlusal trauma.

- Elimination or significant reduction of tooth mobility (the patient should be comfortable when in function).
- Elimination of occlusal prematurities and fremitus.
- Elimination of parafunctional habits.
- Prevention of further tooth migration.
- Decrease or stability of radiographic changes.

Inadequate resolution of occlusal trauma is identified by

- Increasing tooth mobility.
- Progressive tooth migration.
- Patient continuing to complain of discomfort with pain and tooth mobility.
- Premature contacts remaining.
- Radiographic signs remaining, including widening of the PDL space.
- Parafunctional habits continuing.
- TMJ problems remaining or worsening.

OCCLUSAL THERAPY

The objective of **occlusal therapy** is to control the direction, duration, magnitude, and/or frequency of excessive occlusal forces. Practitioners have different views as to whether occlusal therapy is necessary in the overall periodontal treatment plan.

Box 10–1 lists the most common approaches to treating trauma from occlusion. The key to treatment of occlusal trauma lies in the ability to determine if physiologic or pathologic occlusion exists. Physiologic occlusion does not need to be treated, whereas pathologic occlusion that shows signs and symptoms of occlusal problems requires treatment. Occlusal treatment has been shown to significantly reduce the progression of periodontal disease and be an important adjunct therapy in the comprehensive treatment of periodontal disease (Harrel & Nunn, 2001)

Since primary occlusal trauma is caused by excessive occlusal forces, treatment is aimed at eliminating or reducing the forces. Treatment options include selective grinding, control of habits, orthodontic movement, or monitoring of the condition without treatment.

In contrast to the primary occlusal traumatic lesion, the secondary occlusal traumatic lesion is not re-

---

> **Box 10–1   Approaches to Treating Occlusal Trauma**
>
> - Selective grinding
> - Control of habits
> - Orthodontic tooth movement
> - Splinting
> - Restorative procedures
> - Monitoring without treatment

---

versible, since its cause is loss of bony support around a tooth or teeth. Treatment options for secondary occlusal trauma include splinting, selective grinding, orthodontic movement, extraction, or monitoring of the condition without treatment. Reductions in tooth mobility are limited, because the mobility is due to a reduced periodontal support rather than to excessive occlusal force. Premature contacts on mobile teeth are detected and eliminated by selective grinding.

Selective Grinding

Selective grinding or occlusal equilibration is defined as the reshaping of the occlusal or incisal surfaces of teeth to create harmonious contacts between the upper and lower dentition. The goal of selective grinding is to eliminate premature contacts in primary or secondary occlusal trauma. Correction of prematurities should be done in centric occlusion, centric relation, and protrusive and lateral movements so that a traumatic contact of teeth occurs during movements of the mandible (Burgett, 1995). Prematurities are detected by the use of wax, articulating paper, or dental floss.

Selective grinding always should be completed after inflammation has been controlled. Once the inflammation is eliminated by periodontal debridement and oral hygiene self-care, the tooth mobility may decrease because the fibers of the connective tissue attachment repair and a tooth with an intact connective tissue attachment has additional rigidity. Once periodontal health is reestablished, the occlusal condition is reevaluated. A decision to perform selective grinding depends on the degree of patient discomfort and function rather than on the assumption that selective grinding is necessary to halt the progression of disease (Gher, 1996).

Primary occlusal trauma caused by a high restoration is treated by selective grinding. However, severe discrepancies may be resolved best by replacing the restoration. Selective grinding reshapes the occlusal surfaces of teeth to create harmonious contact relationships between the opposing teeth. This is accomplished with hand instruments or a high-speed handpiece and a bur. Tooth surfaces should be smooth so that patients do not develop secondary occlusal habits by "playing" with a rough surface. Selective grinding also can be performed on teeth in secondary occlusal trauma.

Control of Parafunctional Habits

Appliances

If the cause of the occlusal trauma is bruxism, selective grinding usually will not correct the problem; however, counseling the patient may alleviate the psychological component of clenching and grinding. Because such problems are difficult to resolve, a bite plane or Hawley appliance may be fabricated from an orthodontic resin material that disoccludes the posterior teeth. This does not allow the opposing arches to contact and permit the attachment apparatus to heal. The appliance also can be used as an adjunct to selective grinding to stabilize the occlusion and allow the attachment apparatus to rest.

During sleep, a night guard can be worn to control occlusal habits. A night guard serves to protect the teeth from abnormal occlusal wear due to bruxism. Occlusal contacts between the upper and lower teeth are eliminated, thus stabilizing the occlusion and negating the effects of grinding and clenching at night (Chasens, 1990). The night guard is made of either hard or soft acrylic, usually covering the occlusal surfaces of all teeth in the maxillary arch (Figure 10–17 ■). The night guard is adjusted so that all mandibular teeth make simultaneous contact in centric occlusion.

Exercise

Besides using appliances to alter or control occlusal habits, exercise is important as well, especially if the patient clenches. An exercise to follow includes clenching for 5 seconds, then releasing, and repeating this five times in a row (for a total of 60 seconds). This should be done five times a day for 14 consecutive days. If one day is missed, the exercise must be started again.

■ **FIGURE 10–17**   A hard acrylic night guard was made for this 35-year-old bruxer. It is used to protect the teeth during the night and help eliminate the habit. Night guards have full occlusal coverage and usually are made for the maxillary arch.

Orthodontics

Orthodontic treatment may be indicated in periodontal patients exhibiting drifting, migration, extrusion, or flared anterior teeth. The goal is to move a tooth or teeth into a more functional, less traumatic position.

Restorative Procedures

To establish a stable posterior occlusion, restorations may be placed if other treatment options, including orthodontics or selective grinding, are not possible. For example, if a patient has anterior teeth and some or all of the posterior teeth on both sides are missing, the anterior teeth may become overloaded. Thus, restorations (e.g., removable partial dentures [RPDs] or crowns) will restore the posterior occlusion and distribute the load to protect the anterior teeth.

Splinting

Splinting of teeth is considered the treatment of choice for patients who complain of discomfort or if the examination reveals that the mobility interferes with chewing (mastication). Although tooth mobility that develops after periodontal surgery usually will subside within a few months, temporary splinting may be necessary to prevent secondary occlusal trauma. Splinting is also done on teeth in primary occlusal trauma if the mobility was caused by avulsion of the tooth or if the patient received a blow to the mouth resulting in loosening of a tooth or teeth.

Splinting permits healing of the attachment apparatus by holding a tooth in a totally fixed position. This allows the PDL to become narrower and the mobility to be reduced (Ricchetti, 1998). Instead of one tooth experiencing the brunt of forces, the forces are distributed and spread over several teeth, which are better able to absorb the trauma. If mobility is not increasing over time, it may not be necessary to splint. The attachment apparatus may have adapted to the excessive forces and is in a stage of repair (Chasens, 1990). Unfortunately, it is difficult to determine at any given point in time if a patient's attachment apparatus is in a state of repair. That is why monitoring mobility is so important.

Temporary splinting uses wires and composite material, acid etching nylon mesh, or fixed bridges or crowns that are joined or soldered together (Figures 10–18 ■, 10–19 ■). A night guard is considered a type of occlusal splint.

Disadvantages of splinting include compromised aesthetics, reduced plaque-control efficacy, and a changed stable occlusion. Because of these disadvantages, splinting is not done routinely, and if it is selected, it should be considered with the preceding problems in mind.

DENTAL HYGIENE NOTES

Overall, the periodontal response to occlusal trauma can be considered a physiologic adaptation. This adaptation can result in permanently increased tooth mobility if the trauma continues. However, if plaque control is adequate, connective tissue attachment loss should not occur. Removal of the injurious occlusal forces allows the lesion to

■ **FIGURE 10–18** The fixed prosthesis consists of multiple crowns on the maxillary teeth that have been soldered. This represents a form of permanent splinting.

■ **FIGURE 10–19** The incisors were splinted with wire and composite due to increasing mobility on these teeth that made the patient uncomfortable. This type of splinting is referred to as extracoronal because no channel was prepared in the tooth.

repair itself, but this may be compromised by the presence of dental plaque. Therefore, maintenance of adequate plaque control is of utmost importance in preventing and reversing the problem. The question of increased periodontal tissue destruction when periodontitis coexists with occlusal trauma remains unresolved.

Occlusal trauma alone does not cause gingivitis, loss of connective tissue attachment, or pocket formation. Unless there is compromised periodontal support, there is little or no damage to the teeth or the attachment apparatus from normal masticatory (chewing) forces. Normal forces are only traumatogenic in secondary occlusal trauma, when the periodontal support is reduced by disease.

The role of the dental hygienist in the identification of occlusal trauma is important for the overall treatment of the patient. Treatment differs depending on the type of occlusal trauma and its etiology. To help distinguish between primary and secondary occlusal trauma, the dental hygienist can use radiographs and present and past dental history. The occlusal forces required to produce occlusal trauma generally are related to the remaining bony support for a given tooth.

KEY POINTS

• Occlusal trauma does not initiate gingivitis or periodontitis, but in the presence of inflammation periodontal destruction may be accelerated.

- Parafunctional habits may cause occlusal trauma.
- The most common clinical sign of occlusal trauma is increasing tooth mobility.
- Pathologic tooth migration is usually indicative of moderate to severe periodontitis and secondary occlusal trauma.
- Different treatments are available for occlusal trauma.

SELF-QUIZ

1. All the following parts of the periodontium are affected by occlusal trauma except one. Which one is the exception? (pp. 159–160)
   a. Periodontal ligament
   b. Alveolar bone
   c. Gingiva
   d. Cementum
2. Which one of the following definitions pertains to primary occlusal trauma? (p. 160)

Type of Occlusal Force	Bone Support
a. Normal	Adequate
b. Excessive	Adequate
c. Normal	Reduced
d. Excessive	Reduced

3. All the following signs and symptoms are found in occlusal trauma except one. Which one is the exception? (pp. 160–163)
   a. Tooth mobility
   b. Tooth migration
   c. Pain upon chewing
   d. Occlusal erosion
4. Which one of the following radiographic signs is evident in occlusal trauma? (pp. 163–164)
   a. Widening of the periodontal ligament space
   b. Deposition of acellular cementum
   c. Deposition of alveolar bone
   d. Receding pulp tissue
5. Occlusal trauma in combination with chronic inflammatory periodontitis may result in greater tooth mobility and alveolar bone loss because occlusal trauma causes periodontal pocket formation. (p. 160)
   a. Both the statement and the reason are correct and related.
   b. Both the statement and the reason are correct but not related.
   c. The statement is correct, but the reason is not.
   d. The statement is not correct, but the reason is correct.
   e. Neither the statement nor the reason is correct.

6. Two days after a patient receives an amalgam restoration, he reports back to the office complaining of pain and looseness of the tooth. Which one of the following treatments would be most appropriate? (p. 160)
   a. Replace the amalgam with composite.
   b. Reduce the height of the restoration.
   c. Polish the restoration.
   d. Maintain the restoration as is.
7. Which one of the following factors is the primary cause of secondary occlusal trauma? (p. 161)
   a. Tooth with severe bone loss
   b. Night and daytime bruxism
   c. Tongue thrusting
   d. Pipe chewing
8. A patient complains of soreness in the jaw upon waking in the morning. She is having stressful problems at work. She complains that some of her lower teeth are "wearing down." Which one of the following conditions does this patient most likely have? (pp. 157–158)
   a. Fractured jaw
   b. Parafunctional habit
   c. Severe periodontitis
   d. Necrotizing ulcerative gingivitis
9. A patient has returned for a two-week followup visit after periodontal surgery complaining of tooth mobility. There was no mobility before the surgery was done. Which one of the following should be explained to the patient? (p. 162)
   a. Teeth must be splinted immediately.
   b. Mobility will decrease in time.
   c. Additional surgery will be needed.
   d. Systemic antibiotics are indicated.
10. Which one of the following conditions is best treated with a night guard? (p. 166)
    a. Tooth with severe bone loss
    b. Tongue-thrusting habit
    c. Teeth with severe abrasion
    d. Clenching and grinding

REFERENCES

American Academy of Periodontology. 1996. *Parameters of care.* Chicago: American Academy of Periodontology, Scientific and Educational Affairs Department.

American Academy of Periodontology. 2001. *Glossary of periodontal terms* (4th ed.). Chicago: Author.

Burgett, F. G. 1995. Trauma from occlusion. *Dent. Clin. North Am.* 39:301–311.

Caffesse, R. G., and T. J. Fleszar. 1992. Occlusal trauma. In eds. T. G. Wilson, K. S. Komman, and M. G. Newman, *Advances in periodontics,* 205–225. Chicago: Quintessence.

Chasens, A. I. 1979. Periodontal disease, pathologic tooth migration and adult orthodontics. *N.Y. J. Dent.* 49:40–43.

Chasens, A. I. 1990. Controversies in occlusion. *Dent. Clin. North Am.* 34:11–123.

Ericsson, I., and J. Lindhe. 1977. Lack of effect of trauma from occlusion on the recurrence of experimental periodontitis. *J. Clin. Periodontol.* 4:115–127.

Ericsson, I., and J. Lindhe. 1982. Effect of long-standing jiggling on experimental marginal periodontitis in the beagle dog. *J. Clin. Periodontol.* 9:497–503.

Gher, M. E. 1996. Nonsurgical pocket therapy: Dental occlusion. *Ann. Periodontol.* 1:567–580.

Glickman, I. 1963. Inflammation and trauma from occlusion: Codestructive factors in chronic periodontal disease. *J. Periodontol.* 34:5–10.

Glickman, I., and J. B. Smulow. 1965. Effect of excessive occlusal forces upon the pathway of gingival inflammation in humans. *J. Periodontol.* 36:141–147.

Goldman, H. M., and W. D. Cohen (eds.). 1980. Occlusal adjustment. In *Periodontal therapy,* 6th ed., 1065–1111. St. Louis, MO: Mosby.

Green, M. S., and D. F. Levine. 1996. Occlusion and the periodontium: A review and rationale for treatment. *J. Calif. Dent. Assoc.* 24:19–27.

Hallmon, W. W. 1999. Occlusal trauma: Effect and impact on the periodontium. *Ann. Periodontol.* 4:102–107.

Harrel S. K., and M.E. Nunn. 2004.The effect of occlusal discrepancies on gingival width. *J Periodontol.* 75(1): 98–105.

Harrel, S. K., and M. E. Nunn. 2001. The effect of occlusal discrepancies on periodontitis. II. Relationship of occlusal treatment to the progression of periodontal disease. *J Periodontol.* 72(4): 495–505.

Kantor, J., A. M. Polson, and H. A. Zander. 1976. Alveolar bone regeneration after removal of inflammatory and traumatic factors. *J. Periodontol.* 47:687–695.

Keller, G., and W. Cohen. 1955. India ink perfusions of the vascular plexus of oral tissues. *Oral Surg.* 8:539–542.

Lindhe, J., and G. Svanberg. 1974. Influence of trauma from occlusion on progression of experimental periodontitis in the beagle dog. *J. Clin. Periodontol.* 1:3–14.

Lytle, J. D. 1990. The clinician's index of occlusal disease: Definition, recognition, and management. *Int. J. Periodontic Restorative Dent.* 10:103–123.

Meitner, S. 1975. Codestructive factors of marginal periodontitis and repetitive mechanical injury. *J. Dent. Res.* 54:78–85.

Owens, B. M., and G. S. Gallien. 1995. Noncarious dental "abfraction" lesions in an aging population. *Compend. Contin. Educ. Dent.* 16(6):552–554.

Polson, A. M. 1974. Trauma and progression of marginal periodontitis in squirrel monkeys. II. Codestructive factors of periodontitis and mechanically produced injury. *J. Periodontol. Res.* 9:108–113.

Polson, A. M., S. W. Meitner, and H. A. Zander. 1976. Trauma and progression of marginal periodontitis in squirrel monkeys: IV. Reversibility of bone loss due to trauma alone and trauma superimposed upon periodontitis. *J. Periodontol. Res.* 11:290–298.

Polson, A. M., and H. A. Zander. 1983. Effect of periodontal trauma upon intrabony pockets. *J. Periodontol.* 54:586–591.

Ramfjord, S. P., and M. M. Ash. 1981. Significance of occlusion in the etiology and treatment of early, moderate and advanced periodontitis. *J. Periodontol.* 52:511–517.

Ricchetti, P. A. 1998. Treatment of the periodontium affected by occlusal traumatism. In eds. M. Nevins and J. T. Mellonig, *Periodontal therapy: Clinical approaches and evidence of success,* Vol. 1, 132–133. Chicago. Quintessence.

Shefter, G. J., and W. T. McFall. 1984. Occlusal relations and periodontal status in human adults. *J. Periodontol.* 55:368–374.

Svanberg, G. K., G. J. King, and C. H. Gibbs. 1995. Occlusal considerations in periodontology. *Periodontology 2000* 9:106–117.

Tarnow, D. P., and P. Fletcher. 1986. Splinting of periodontally involved teeth: Indications and contraindications. *N.Y. State Dent. J.* (May):24–25.

Towfighi, P. P., M. A. Brunsvold, A. T. Storey, B. M. Arnold, D. E. Willman, and C. A. McMahan. 1997. Pathologic migration of anterior teeth in patients with moderate to severe periodontitis. *J. Periodontol.* 68:967–972.

Chapter **11**

Abscesses of the Periodontium

Surendra Singh

OUTLINE

Introduction
Gingival Abscess
Periodontal Abscess
Pericoronal Abscess
Dental Hygiene Notes
Key Points
Self-Quiz
References

EDUCATIONAL OBJECTIVES

Upon completion of this chapter, the reader should be able to:

• List the classification of abscesses of the periodontium.
• Identify and describe the clinical and radiographic findings of three types of abscesses of the periodontium.

GOAL: To educate about the etiology, clinical manifestations, and therapy of different types of abscesses of the periodontium.

KEY WORDS

gingival abscess 171
pericoronal abscess
   173
periodontal abscess
   171

INTRODUCTION

An abscess is defined as an infection originating from the tooth or periodontium. Pain and swelling from an abscess usually brings the patient into the dental office as an emergency visit. Classification of abscesses is based upon the location of the infection. For example, a gingival abscess is an infection located in the gingival unit, usually the free (marginal) gingiva; a periodontal abscess is an infection located within the tissues adjacent to the periodontal pocket; and a pericoronal abscess is an infection located within the tissue around the crown of a partially erupted tooth, usually the last tooth in the arch.

The 1999 American Academy of Periodontology Classification of Periodontal Diseases added abscesses of the periodontium. It was a consensus that gingival/periodontal abscesses are part of the clinical course of gingivitis and periodontitis and thus a specific diagnosis and treatment challenges are required (Armitage, 1999). This chapter reviews the classification, and definitions of abscesses of the periodontium and treatment of these abscesses will be discussed in Chapter 27.

GINGIVAL ABSCESS

A **gingival abscess** is an acute infection characterized by a localized, painful edema at the free gingival margin or interdental papilla. Usually, there are no signs of periodontitis in the patient's mouth. Foreign objects such as popcorn kernels, fish bones, or seeds that become lodged in the gingival crevice are responsible for many gingival abscesses. Calculus is usually not the cause. Since the abscess develops fairly rapidly, the patient often will know the cause. The infection usually is rapidly expanding from the gingival margin or interdental papilla. Within 24 to 48 hours, the lesion will appear fluctuant (soft and movable). Purulent exudate (pus) may be exuding from the surface. If treatment is not immediately given, the abscess will usually rupture on its own. Pus is a collection of white blood cells (neutrophils), dead (necrotic) tissue, and bacteria in tissue fluid. Before treatment is started, it is necessary to determine the origin of the abscess.

Rapid Dental Hint

When a patient presents with an abscess it is important to determine if the "origin" of the abscess is periodontal or endodontic.

PERIODONTAL ABSCESS

Features

A **periodontal abscess,** also called a lateral periodontal abscess, is the most common type of abscess involving the periodontium. It is a localized purulent nidus of acute inflammation as a result of invasion of bacteria into the periodontal tissues, specifically within the gingival wall of a periodontal pocket (Figures 11–1 ■, 11–2 ■). Periodontal abscess formation usually occurs with pre-existing advanced periodontitis. Patients with diabetes mellitus are also more susceptible to periodontal abscess formation. A periodontal abscess often causes destruction of the periodontal ligament and alveolar and supporting bone (Meng, 1999).

A periodontal abscess usually occurs around teeth with deep periodontal pockets and in furcation sites because of anatomical limitations, which makes oral hygiene and professional instrumentation difficult. The opening of the periodontal pocket often is occluded because either there is healing at the coronal tissue area or there may be a foreign body (e.g., food), resulting in a buildup of pus.

Microbiology

Microorganisms found in the periodontal/gingival abscess resemble the microbiota of chronic periodontitic lesions. Microorganisms that colonize and are found in the exudate of the periodontal abscesses are primarily

■ **FIGURE 11–1**   Periodontal abscess involving the mandibular molar. The buccal probed 10 mm. The pocket was occluded. Drainage was established after anesthesia was administered and the orifice of the pocket was opened with a curet. (Courtesy of John Eum, DDS, New York University College of Dentistry)

■ **FIGURE 11–2** Periodontal abscess on the buccal surface of the mandibular premolar. 10 mm probing depths were recorded.

Gram-negative anaerobic rods (Meng, 1999). Other bacteria associated with and found with high frequency in periodontal abscesses include *Porphyromonas gingivalis, Prevotella intermedia, Fusobacterium nucleatum, Campylobacter retus,* and *Capnocytophaga* sp. The eradication of *Porphyromonas gingivalis* from abscessed sites after treatment indicates that this bacterium is highly associated with abscess formation. *Actinobacillus actinomycetemocomitans* is usually not found in the exudate.

Acute Versus Chronic

Periodontal abscesses can present as acute or chronic (long-standing). An abscess occurs if the acute abscess is not resolved or treated. A common chief complaint when

Did You Know?

Pus is generally a viscous, yellowish-white fluid formed in infected tissue, consisting of white blood cells, cellular debris, and necrotic tissue.

a periodontal abscess is developing is that "I have pressure in my gums." The acute periodontal abscess presents as a shiny, swollen, discolored mass on the gingiva or mucosa at the lateral aspect of the root, but not at the free gingival margin as is the gingival abscess. It is usually located on the lateral aspect of the tooth surface where the periodontal pocket is. Finger pressure may produce purulent drainage. The involved tooth may be tender to percussion (especially upon chewing or mastication), mobile, with deep probing depths, and edematous gingiva. Occasionally, patients may demonstrate localized lymphadenopathy (palpable lymph nodes) and fever. If the abscess is present on the lateral aspect of the tooth, there will be a radiolucent area, but if the abscess is formed on the facial or lingual part of the tooth, it will not show up on the radiograph. The patient does not usually display symptoms as in an acute periodontal abscess, but some symptoms, such as a deep, dull pain or elevation of the tooth, may be present.

Differential Diagnosis

A differential diagnosis of a periodontal abscess is a periapical (endodontic) abscess (Figures 11–3 ■, 11–4 ■, 11–5 ■). Clinicians often must be able to differentiate

(a)

(b)

■ **FIGURE 11–3** (a) A sinus tract is present on the maxillary central incisor. (b) To determine the origin of the infection, a gutta percha point is inserted into the fistula. Temperature testing revealed this tooth was nonvital and an X-ray confirmed the gutta percha point ended at the apical region of the tooth.

■ FIGURE 11–4   X-ray showing a previously endodontically treated tooth that still had a chronic infection. An apicoectomy was performed whereby the apical part of the root was excised, and a retrograde amalgam was placed.

the origin of the infection, which is sometimes challenging. An endodontic abscess usually occurs adjacent to the apex of a necrotic tooth and often heals following endodontic therapy. There may be a sinus tract draining the abscess. The sinus tract originates from deep within the periodontal tissues and opens and drains onto the gingiva (Figure 11–3). Table 11–1 ■ shows the common features of periapical and periodontal abscesses. Often there is a combined lesion: endo-perio lesion where the tooth is nonvital with a periodontal defect and deep pocket.

> **Did You Know?**
>
> A gingival abscess occurs by the gingival margin. A periodontal abscess occurs where there is a deep pocket.

Treatment

The initial objective of treatment is to perform an incision and drainage. Since the pocket may be occluded, opening the pocket (incision) to drain the pus may be difficult. After obtaining profound anesthesia, the pocket should be carefully opened with a probe or curet to drain the pus. The tissue is very friable. Once the pocket is open, curette the soft tissue pocket wall with the cutting edge of the curet, pus will usually just exude out into the oral cavity. In the majority of cases, an antibiotic is not necessary. Only if there is systemic involvement (e.g., fever, lymphadenopathy), an antibiotic is necessary, and this is not very often necessary. After drainage is achieved, periodontal debridement is performed to remove the plaque and calculus from the root surface. The patient should then be referred to a periodontist for further treatment.

PERICORONAL ABSCESS

Pericoronal abscess, also referred to as pericoronitis, is a localized infection involving the gingiva adjacent to a partially erupted tooth, usually the mandibular third molar

(a)   (b)

■ FIGURE 11–5   (a) Periapical pathology (PAP) on the premolar. The tooth tested nonvital. Endodontic therapy is indicated. (b) X-ray showing periapical pathology (PAP) on the central incisor. Root canal therapy was performed and final post and crown were fabricated.

Table 11–1   Differences Between a Gingival, Periodontal, Periapical, and Pericoronal Abscess

	Gingival Abscess	*Periodontal Abscess*	*Periapical Abscess*	*Periocoronitis (Pericoronal Abscess)*
Symptoms	Swelling, warmth, redness, fluctuant mass near the gingival margin on the buccal aspect, pain	Swelling, warmth, redness, fluctuant mass on the lateral aspect of the tooth, may or may not have pain (Figures 11–1, 11–2)	Tender to percussion (tap the occlusal/incisal edge of tooth with a mirror handle); tender when chewing/biting; pressure tenderness; tooth is extruded; maybe lymphadenopathy (Figures 11–3, 11–4, 11–5)	Trismus, difficulty in swallowing, facial swelling, lymphadenopathy (Figure 11–6)
Origin of infection	Gingiva	Periodontal ligament, bone	Pulp	Gingiva
Vital	Yes	Yes	Nonvital	Yes
Caries	No caries	No caries	Caries present	No
Periodontal status	Deep pocket	Deep pocket	No pocket – not probable except when the lesion extends into the periodontal ligament resulting in deep pocket. This lesion becomes an endodontic-periodontic lesion. Remember the lesion has an pulpal origin.	Good
Tooth mobility	No tooth mobility	May or may not have tooth mobility	Yes	No
Location of abscess	Abscess located by the gingival margin	Abscess usually located at lateral aspect of tooth	Sinus tract usually located in apical area	Partially erupted third molar
X-ray findings	No radiolucency	Lateral radiolucency	Apical radiolucency	Impacted third molar
Differentiation	Periodontal abscess	Endodontic abscess	Periodontal abscess	None
Treatment	Incision and drainage through pocket opening. Periodontal debridement.	Incision and drainage through pocket. Periodontal debridement. Definitive treatment may include extraction of the tooth or periodontal surgery. Antibiotics are not required if there is no systemic involvement (e.g., fever, lymphadenopathy)	Root canal. Antibiotics are not needed if the tooth is nonvital. Antibiotics are required if the tooth is vital and there is swelling and lymphadenopathy.	Antibiotics are usually needed (penicillin drug of choice). Extraction of the third molar. Surgical removal of the operculum

■ FIGURE 11–6   Pericorontitis. The third molar is partially covered by an operculum. (Courtesy of Dr. Michael Turner, New York University College of Dentistry)

region (Figure 11–6 ■). The gingival flap (or operculum) overlying the erupting tooth is usually red and edematous with food and debris collecting under the operculum. The operculum will disappear once the tooth fully erupts, but many of these teeth remain partially erupted indefinitely because of inadequate arch space for complete eruption or when the tooth is extracted. The offending microorganisms are Gram-negative anaerobes. The infection may spread posteriorly into the oropharyngeal area and medially to the base of the tongue and involve the regional lymph nodes (Meng, 1999). Patients may experience difficulty in swallowing, complain of a dull ache, and may demonstrate limited jaw opening (trismus).

DENTAL HYGIENE NOTES

An abscess is an infection originating from the tooth or periodontium. It is important to determine the point of origin so that proper treatment is given. The patient's chief complaint and a review of the dental history will help to determine the type of abscess. For instance, the patient should be asked if he or she recently had anything to eat that would cause a gingival abscess. The gingival abscess is confined to the marginal gingival or interdental papilla. If the patient has moderate to advanced periodontitis, then most likely it will be a periodontal abscess. Periodontal abscesses are part of the clinical course of the progression of periodontitis. Upon probing these sites, pus will usually come out of the pocket. The microbiota of a periodontal abscess is Gram-negative anaerobic rods, which are similar to that found in deep periodontal pockets (Meng, 1999) This is a form of drainage that is necessary to eliminate the infection. A periapical abscess differs from a periodontal abscess in that the abscessed tooth is usually nonvital and will require endodontics therapy.

Oral examination of a patient complaining of pain and trouble opening his/her mouth will most likely reveal an operculum around a partially erupted mandibular third molar.

The location of the infection will give a good indication on the type of abscess.

KEY POINTS

- Periodontal abscesses are bacterial infections.
- It is important to determine the origin of the abscess.
- The location of the abscess is important.

SELF-QUIZ

1. Which of the following is the most common bacterium found in the purulent exudate of a tooth with a periodontal abscess? (p. 172)
   a. *Porphyromas gingivalis*
   b. *Candida albicans*
   c. *Staphlococcus sp.*
   b. *Actinobacillus actinomycetemcomitans (Aa)*
2. A gingival abscess is localized to the (p. 171)
   a. periapical area.
   b. interdental papilla.
   c. periodontal pocket.
   d. pericoronal area.
3. Which of the following is a clinical feature of a periodontal abscess? (pp. 171–172)
   a. Fibrotic gingiva
   b. Edematous gingiva
   c. Gingival recession
   d. Firm gingiva
4. Which of the following is a complication from a pericoronal abscess? (pp. 173–175)
   a. Gingival recession
   b. Trismus
   c. Attrition
   d. Furcation defect
   e. Fibrotic gingiva

5. Which of the following is occurring when a pocket entrance is "opened" with a probe or curet on a tooth with an acute periodontal abscess? (p. 173)
   a. Transformation of the epithelium into connective tissue
   b. Conversion of the acute abscess into a gingival abscess
   c. Incision and drainage
   d. Laceration of the fistula tract

REFERENCES

Armitage, G. C. 1999. Development of a classification system for periodontal diseases and conditions. *Ann. Periodontol.* 4:1–6.
Meng, H. X. 1999. Periodontal abscess. *Ann. Periodontol.* 4:79–82.

Part III

Periodontal Diseases: The Assessment Phase

Chapter **12**
Dental Hygiene Process of Care for the Patient with Periodontal Disease

Chapter **13**
Patient History

Chapter **14**
Clinical Examination: Extraoral/Intraoral Examination and Dental Evaluation

Chapter **15**
Clinical Examination: Gingival Assessment

Chapter **16**
Clinical Examination: Periodontal Assessment

Chapter **17**
Radiographic Assessment

Chapter **18**
Advances in Detecting and Monitoring the Periodontal Diseases

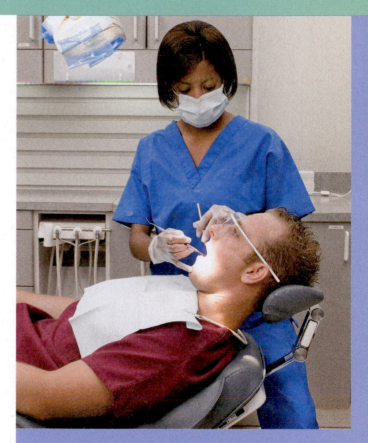

Dental Hygiene Process of Care for the Patient with Periodontal Disease

Cheryl Westphal

OUTLINE
Introduction
Assessment
Dental Hygiene Diagnosis
Planning
Implementation
Evaulation
Dental Hygiene Notes
Key Points
Self-Quiz
References

GOAL: To provide information on the procedures of patient care.

EDUCATIONAL OBJECTIVES

Upon completion of this chapter, the reader should be able to:

- List and explain five phases of the dental hygiene process for periodontal patient care.
- Explain the importance of stating the goals for periodontal patient care.
- Understand the differences between a dental diagnosis and a dental hygiene diagnosis.

KEY WORDS

assessment 179
dental hygiene
    diagnosis 180
documentation 179
evaluation 180

implementation 180
objective data 179
subjective data 179
treatment plan 180

INTRODUCTION

The purpose of the dental hygiene process of care is to provide a framework within which the individualized needs of the patient can be met. The dental hygiene process of care is an assessment process involving five phases (Mueller-Joseph & Petersen, 1995) of a search for clues leading up to the identification and classification of the nature of the disease and the steps in patient care needed to alleviate the problem (Bates, Bickley, & Hoekelman, 1995; DeGowin, 1994):

- Assessment
- Dental hygiene diagnosis
- Planning
- Implementation
- Evaluation

ASSESSMENT

Assessment is the gathering of all relevant information concerning the patient including medical/dental history, vital signs, extraoral and intraoral examination, periodontal and dental examination, radiographs, indices, and risk assessments (e.g., patient use of tobacco, presence of systemic disease). In the patient history assessment, clues are symptoms, which are abnormalities experienced by the patient. Information obtained by observations of and statements made by the patient are termed **subjective data.** In the clinical examination, on the other hand, clues are signs, which are abnormalities perceived by the practitioner. Information obtained from observations of the patient and statements made by the practitioner are termed **objective data.**

Data collection starts with taking down the medical/dental history, followed by the extra/intraoral examination, restorative charting, gingival assessment, periodontal assessment, oral hygiene evaluation, radiographs, and additional diagnostic laboratory tests if required.

From the moment the patient enters the care cycle within the practice, the whole person is assessed to understand aspects such as his or her health background, health beliefs, cultural background, social and economic background, educational background, and work-related issues. These factors play an important role when determining a home-care regime for the person that will yield compliance.

Social, Economic, and Cultural Considerations

A review of the patient's dental and medical history from the viewpoint of social and economic concerns provides insight as to the patient's ability to afford subsequent dental followup home-care regimes. Often factors such as people's beliefs about the role they should play in their own healthcare and the part their bad habits play in causing periodontal disease will impact upon their desire to maintain their oral health after surgery or other extensive dental care. A complete discussion with the patient is crucial to elicit the information instead of a nonverbal form of the medical history questionnaire often done without any review of these factors.

Technology and Documentation

Since data collection is an ongoing process, an appropriate method of written and visual **documentation** is required. The intraoral camera is a recent technological advance that can be used to document various findings before and after the treatment procedure. The practitioner is able to view and record such conditions as plaque retention sites, gingival conditions, faulty margins or caries, and stain or other deposits. The recordings can then be utilized to explain the condition and create a historical record that can be placed in the patient's file and used to show the patient any progress or degeneration of the periodontal condition being treated at subsequent appointments. Many different manufacturers exist that offer systems of computers and cameras available for chairside use. The intraoral camera can be employed during the charting, oral soft tissue exam, or oral hygiene evaluation to involve the patient in the process and discuss the findings. Currently, the great majority of practitioners who use intraoral video cameras do not have those cameras integrated with their computer systems, although the number who do is growing. This involves converting the images to a digital format using specialized software. Although some practitioners do not feel the need to permanently save images after case presentation, doing so is a valuable tool in terms of educating patients and increasing the likelihood that the recommended treatment procedures will be performed.

Computer technology is becoming essential for the treatment record, appointment planning, recare visit booking, and patient documentation parts of running a dental practice. Oral hygiene evaluations as part of the computer record of the patient offer an array of visual presentations that can enhance treatment planning and patient compliance with the recommended procedures. Patients can be shown a pictorial display of their probing depths, caries, gum and tooth recession, other gingival involvement, or potential treatment outcomes of surgery or prosthetic replacements.

DENTAL HYGIENE DIAGNOSIS

After the data are collected, the dental hygienist reviews and analyzes the information. A **dental hygiene diagnosis** differs from a dental diagnosis, since a dental diagnosis gives a name to the disease and the dental hygiene diagnosis identifies the patient's actual or potential response to the disease process (Mueller-Joseph & Petersen, 1995). The purpose of a dental hygiene diagnosis is to keep the planning of patient care centered on problems or conditions that are responsive to dental hygiene intervention (Mueller-Joseph & Petersen, 1995). For example, a patient has inflamed gingiva, but no bone loss is shown on the radiographs. The dental hygienist should also understand the need to disrupt the pathogenic bacteria so that a more beneficial microflora will populate the tooth/soft tissue area.

After the disease is diagnosed, the practitioner should determine the cause so that a treatment plan can be established that will eliminate or control the condition. The dental hygienist should know why the patient developed the condition in order for appropriate treatment to be rendered. For example, a patient complains of tooth pain. The dental hygienist assesses the situation and asks questions of the patient to determine whether the pain occurs with cold or hot foods or liquids. The dental hygienist can then determine the etiologic factor for this condition and develop a plan to eliminate the pain.

PLANNING

Planning is the establishment of realistic goals and treatment strategies to facilitate optimal oral health. A **treatment plan** involves the development of a written treatment plan for the patient's individual needs based on data collection and assessment. Alternative options should be included in the plan that may be implemented instead of the ideal plan if the patient is in poor health, if the patient is not compliant or motivated to follow the ideal plan, or if the patient cannot afford the ideal treatment. The treatment plan must be presented to the patient and agreed upon before any treatment is started. An appropriate sequence of treatments must be stated. Developing a plan involves knowledge from a variety of disciplines besides dental hygiene, including behavioral sciences, pharmacology, anatomy and physiology, chemistry, and microbiology. Critical thinking and decision-making skills are necessary to provide effective and efficient dental hygiene services.

When developing a dental care plan, the goal or end result of treatment must be stated (Mueller-Joseph & Petersen, 1995). The goal is a statement that addresses and identifies the purpose for implementing dental care. The individualized plan also identifies the interventions necessary to meet the healthcare goals of the patient. Interventions are procedures carried out by the dental hygienist to help the patient reach the desired goal. For example, let us say that a dental diagnosis is pregnancy gingivitis. The dental hygiene diagnosis is gingival inflammation related to the elevated hormonal levels and inadequate home care of the teeth and gums by the patient. The aims of dental hygiene treatment are to reduce plaque levels by oral hygiene instruction and educate the patient about the influence of plaque and hormones on overall dental health. Dental hygiene intervention deals with the disruption of plaque by mechanical debridement.

IMPLEMENTATION

Once the care plan is presented to the patient and an informed consent form is signed by the patient and dentist, treatment commences. This **implementation** phase includes (1) preparing the operatory for the patient, (2) using proper infection control procedures, (3) carrying out periodontal debridement procedures, (4) implementing pain management procedures, (5) applying chemotherapeutic agents, (6) carrying out fluoride therapy, (7) undertaking coronal polishing, (8) teaching the patient proper care of oral prostheses, (9) teaching the patient proper care and maintenance of restorations, (10) providing the patient with health education and preventive counseling, (11) providing the patient with nutritional counseling, and (12) documenting the process properly.

The dentist will make a dental diagnosis of gingivitis, whereas the dental hygiene diagnosis focuses on educating the patient on the need and benefit (Mueller-Joseph & Petersen, 1995) of proper plaque control to reduce supragingival plaque accumulation. Thus, the dental hygiene diagnosis might be "gingival inflammation related to biofilm accumulation."

EVALUATION

The **evaluation** phase of therapy deals with feedback on the effectiveness of the treatment and procedures. This phase occurs after treatment has been completed, when the patient returns for a followup visit a few weeks after the nonsurgical periodontal therapy (initial therapy or

Phase I therapy) or surgical therapy has been completed, or for periodontal maintenance (recall) procedures.

DENTAL HYGIENE NOTES

The dental hygiene diagnosis provides the foundation for the development, implementation, and evaluation of the dental hygiene treatment plan (American Dental Hygienist Association, 2005). It is a key element in identifying an existing or potential periodontal/oral problem.

KEY POINTS

- Five components of the dental hygiene process enable the dental hygienist to identify the patient's periodontal problem, to determine the cause of the problem, and then to treat the problem.
- An intraoral camera can be useful to point out areas of recession, plaque-retentive sites, bleeding points, and restorations.
- Documentation is an integral part of the dental hygiene process; good documentation in the patient's chart is of utmost importance.

SELF-QUIZ

1. All of the following are components of the dental hygiene process except one. Which one is the exception? (pp. 179–180)
   a. Assessment
   b. Dental diagnosis
   c. Treatment planning
   d. Implementation
   e. Evaluation
2. Which one of the following reasons is important for determining the individual goals for periodontal patient care? (pp. 179–180)
   a. Establishes a rapport with the patient
   b. Emphasizes the need for prevention in the care of the patient
   c. Identifies the purpose for treating the patient
   d. Evaluates for treatment needs after the first appointment

3. Which one of the following statements explains the purpose of a dental hygiene diagnosis? (p. 180)
   a. Keeps the planning of patient care centered on problems or conditions that are responsive to dental hygiene intervention
   b. Helps the dental hygienist determine the need for additional radiographs
   c. Identifies the type of periodontal disease
   d. Anticipates the effectiveness in achieving the desired outcome of therapy
4. Before undergoing any periodontal treatment, every patient should have his or her mouth and dentition photographed with an intraoral camera because the intraoral camera is an important part of documentation. (p. 179)
   a. Both the statement and the reason are correct and related.
   b. Both the statement and the reason are correct but not related.
   c. The statement is correct, but the reason is not.
   d. The statement is not correct, but the reason is correct.
   e. Neither the statement nor the reason is correct.
5. Which of the following reasons best explains the purpose of evaluation of periodontal therapy? (p. 180)
   a. Determines the need for additional periodontal intervention
   b. Deals with the feedback on the effectiveness of treatment
   c. Identifies the type of disease present
   d. Allows the dental hygienist to introduce oral hygiene care products for home use

REFERENCES

American Dental Hygienist's Association. Dental Hygiene Diagnosis Position Paper. June 2005. American Dental Hygienist Association. Chicago, IL.

Bates, B., L. S. Bickley, and R. A. Hoekelman. 1995. *A pocket guide to physical examination and history taking,* 2nd ed. Philadelphia: Lippincott.

DeGowin, R. L. 1994. *DeGowin & DeGowin's diagnostic examination,* 3–4. New York: McGraw-Hill.

Mueller-Joseph, L., and M. Petersen. 1995. The dental hygiene process of care. In eds. L. Mueller-Joseph and M. Petersen, *Dental hygiene process: Diagnosis and care planning,* 1–19. Albany, NY: Delmar.

Chapter 13

Patient History

Ann M. Goodwin

Rosemary DeRosa Hays

OUTLINE
Introduction
The Interview
Dental Hygiene Notes
Key Points
Self-Quiz
References

EDUCATIONAL OBJECTIVES

Upon completion of this chapter, the reader should be able to:

- Explain the importance of data collection.
- Illustrate the importance of total health assessment in providing periodontal services.

GOAL: To provide information on the patient history-taking process.

KEY WORDS
chief complaint 183
dental/medical history
    183
interview process 183

INTRODUCTION

The patient's first visit is the time to collect subjective data. A complete **dental/medical history** is an essential aspect of the initial evaluation. It is here that the dental hygienist becomes an advantageous partner in the healthcare evaluation process. The hygienist interviews the patient for his or her history, which is divided into the personal profile, social history, chief complaint, history of the present illness, medical history, family history, and dental history. The collective diagnostic information developed through this interview provides a basis for future comparisons to evaluate the progress of disease, the efficacy of treatment, and the appearance of new findings. Therefore, taking the patient history is a mandatory first step in the treatment process.

THE INTERVIEW

The **interview process,** so critical to the successful completion of the dental and medical history, demands a high level of communication between the patient and the dental hygienist. If done properly, an interview helps establish a rapport between the dental hygienist and the patient. History taking can be accomplished through a questionnaire, a patient interview, or a combination of both. The most practical and successful method for assessing the health status of a patient is a combination questionnaire and interview.

During the interview, open-ended questions such as "What changes in your health or medications have occurred since your last dental visit?" or "What in your mouth bothers you?" open doors to gaining more pertinent information. If good rapport develops, the patient will feel more comfortable, and as the interview progresses, he or she will volunteer more information. Open-ended questions put patients more at ease. Nevertheless, closed-ended questions also are necessary, such as "When was your last dental visit?" These types of questions do not require much responding from the patient; rather, they can be answered usually in one sentence.

Did You Know?

Seventy-three percent of Americans would rather go grocery shopping than floss.

Personal Profile

The obvious place to begin the interview is by asking questions concerning the patient's identity. This personal profile consists of the patient's name, age, address, occupation, and telephone number. Some of this information is needed for identification purposes, while the patient's age and sex may be useful in the classification of the periodontal disease. Document the name, address, and telephone number of the patient's physician, which will be useful if consultation is necessary.

Social History

The social history includes the patient's occupation, lifestyle, marital status, diet, and use of alcohol and tobacco, both smoking and chewing tobacco. Habits such as cigarette smoking or use of smokeless tobacco should be noted because they are potential risk factors for periodontal diseases.

Cigarette smoking is reported in pack-years, which is determined by multiplying the number of packs of cigarettes smoked per day by the number of years the patient has smoked. Documenting the amount of smoking in pack-years gives a better understanding of the total exposure of nicotine during the lifetime of an individual. For example, if a person smoked one pack every day for ten years, this is ten pack-years.

The patient's lifestyle, including family and social structure, attitudes, and behaviors, is part of the social history. A patient's social perceptions, priorities, amount of stress, and ideas on aesthetics provide clues to compliance with dental care. A dental hygienist can work toward changing a patient's attitudes and behaviors by understanding the patient's cultural differences, motivation, patience, education, and expectations.

Chief Complaint

The next step is to ask the patient to identify his or her **chief complaint** (CC). The patient should state in his or her own words why he or she is seeking treatment. Determination of the CC assists in the identification of any ongoing disease process. Symptoms of periodontal problems include pressure in the gingiva or jaw or itchy gingiva. Signs of periodontal disease include bleeding, halitosis (bad breath), and/or tooth mobility. Given the insidious nature of periodontal diseases, many patients have no idea there is a problem. If the patient's CC involves something

Rapid Dental Hint

The patient's chief complaint is very important. Ask him or her, "Why did you come to the dental office today?" You must treat the chief complaint first before any other procedures are performed.

other than periodontal disease, that must be treated first before any other dental treatment is rendered.

History of Present Illness

The history of the CC expands on the patient's awareness of the problem and is also referred to as the history of present illness. The dental hygienist should inquire how long the patient's problem has existed, any previous treatment(s), and if this problem has occurred before. For instance, if the patient's CC is "bleeding from the gums," the dental hygienist should ask about the onset, cause, location, and duration of the bleeding.

Medical History

The current and past status of the patient's general health, or medical history, should be the next area of investigation. A questionnaire, an interview, or a combination of questionnaire and interview can be used to accomplish this. Sometimes, however, a simple telephone call to the patient prior to the first appointment may screen for potential medical problems. A written questionnaire provides a baseline for treatment, whereas an interview provides both personal contact with the patient and supplementary information that may contribute to a more comprehensive evaluation. It is important to listen closely to the patient and have a genuine interest in what is said in order to provide insight, accuracy, and clarity in the history (McDaniel, Miller, Jones, & Davis, 1995). Allowing the patient to describe symptoms or complaints at length encourages trust and fosters a sympathetic professional relationship, but it is only necessary to record the relevant facts and details. A high percentage of dental patients have medical conditions that can have an effect on a clinician's therapeutic decisions (Peacock & Carson, 1995).

Questions concerning current medication use and drug allergies are crucial because the answers may have a direct effect on any treatment the dentist eventually prescribes. Both prescription and over-the-counter medications the patient is taking should be recorded. The name,

dosage, and indications also should be written on the form. The hygienist should look especially for any potential drug–drug or drug–food interactions. Adverse side effects (undesirable effects of the drug on the body) of certain medications may be the source of dental problems. For example, antidepressant and antihypertensive medications may cause xerostomia, or dry mouth. Some medications for hypertension or epileptic seizures may cause enlargement of the gingiva, which can result in plaque-control problems. Absorption from the intestines of certain antibiotics such as tetracycline is delayed with food and calcium-containing products including milk and other dairy products. Consultation with the patient's physician may be necessary. If the patient does not know the names of the medications, ask him or her to bring the containers to the next office visit. If a patient is regularly taking medication for diabetes or hypertension, it is extremely important to ask if he or she took the medication as prescribed on that day; if so, the dosage and frequency of usage should be noted on the form. Sometimes a patient may forget to take high blood pressure (antihypertensive) medication and present with uncontrolled blood pressure. If this is the case, the hygienist should contact the patient's physician.

The medical history may uncover other conditions that can have an effect on periodontal health or treatment, such as diabetes mellitus, leukemia, or acquired immunodeficiency syndrome (AIDS) (Neff, 1997). At this time a link between periodontal disease and certain discussed medical conditions that the patient has can be made. If the patient is suspected of being medically compromised, consultation with the patient's physician is indicated, and a written release should be obtained from the patient before treatment begins.

Infective endocarditis is of particular concern in dental care. Infective endocarditis is an infection of the tissue lining of the heart that can result in damage to the heart valves. Any dental procedure that causes bleeding could allow bacteria to enter the bloodstream, resulting in bacteremia. Before initiating any dental treatment that may cause bleeding in patients who are susceptible to developing infective endocarditis, proper antibiotic protection should be administered. The American Heart Association (AHA) recommends a prophylactic antibiotic regimen for such patients (see Chapter 28). Because specific recommendations vary depending on the individual patient's condition, the dental hygienist should collaborate with the dentist and/or patient's physician to determine the appropriate premedication therapy. It is the responsibility of the dental hygienist, however, to screen for susceptible patients by taking a complete health history.

The medical history form is a legal document that provides a past and present profile of the patient's health. After the medical history is complete, the document must be dated and signed by the patient and the dentist, and at each future visit, the form should be updated. The patient should review this information and sign the form again. A new form should be filled out yearly. Indelible ink, preferably black (because it will copy better than blue), should be used. If the patient is a minor, a parent or legal guardian should date and sign the form.

 Rapid Dental Hint

If a patient does not know the name of drugs he or she is taking, ask him or her to bring in the pill containers.

Family History

The family history consists of the present and past medical illnesses of family members. Such a record may help to identify disease trends in the family that are risk factors for dental/periodontal diseases such as diabetes and ischemic heart disease.

Dental History

The dental history includes past and present dental treatments, past dental problems, oral habits, nutritional profile, past response to treatment, and oral hygiene status. This information is collected by way of a written form and an interview with the patient.

The past dental history often provides insight into previous dental experiences, pleasant or unpleasant, in all areas of dentistry, including oral surgery, periodontics, restorative dentistry, endodontics, and orthodontics. Experiences with local anesthetics and nitrous oxide should be recorded. Questions especially pertinent to the dental hygiene visit include those regarding the patient's last dental visit, what was done, and how long since the last prophylaxis.

A nutritional or diet profile of the patient is helpful in assisting the dental hygienist in recognizing a caries-prone diet. During the interview, the dental hygienist can suggest ways in which the patient can alter his or her diet to promote better dental health.

Past dental history also provides information on the patient's dental health values. The periodontal history may be significant. For example, a patient should be asked if previous periodontal surgery was performed (make sure he or she understands what periodontal surgery is). The patient may respond that he or she has had periodontal surgery twice in the past year. Upon further questioning, it may become apparent that the patient returned to the dental office only once for a periodontal maintenance appointment. This information suggests that the patient is noncompliant with oral hygiene self-care and dental visits.

Other areas to explore include the patient's attitude toward dental care and the present surroundings and the level of desire for treatment. Question the patient on what specific oral hygiene regimen he or she follows, including the types of products used. Question the patient on what kind of toothbrush (e.g., soft, medium, or hard bristled), electric brushes, dental floss, and mouthrinse he or she uses. The frequency of product use should be documented, as well as compliance with recommended periodontal maintenance appointments.

Did You Know?

A survey shows that 83% of U.S. adults are very satisfied with the services they get from their dentists. This survey was done by Louis Harris and Associates in an effort to study U.S. attitude toward dentists.

DENTAL HYGIENE NOTES

The initial step performed on a periodontal patient is to obtain a complete dental/medical, social, and family history. Determination and recording of medications the patient is taking is important since certain drugs affect the periodontium, and severe drug interactions can occur. Other factors, such as the number of cigarettes smoked, should also be recorded.

KEY POINTS

- The interviewing process establishes rapport with the patient.
- Medical diseases and medications can affect conditions in the mouth.
- Update a patient's dental/medical history at every appointment.

SELF-QUIZ

1. Which one of the following information collected from the patient is subjective? (pp. 183–184)
   a. Medical history
   b. Dental examination
   c. Periodontal examination
   d. Radiographic survey
   e. Oral hygiene evaluation

2. Which one of the following statements explains the importance of patient information collected during the interview? (p. 183)
   a. Anticipates patient's attitude about periodontal care.
   b. Determines the number of visits for the patient.
   c. Allows the patient to voice his or her opinions about treatment.
   d. Provides a basis for future comparison.
   e. Establishes a rapport between patient and hygienist.

3. Which one of the following actions should a dental hygienist take before periodontal treatment is started if the patient cannot remember the names of the medications he or she is taking? (p. 184)
   a. Call the patient's pharmacist to confirm the medications.
   b. Call the patient's physician to confirm the medications.
   c. Tell the patient to bring the containers to the next appointment.
   d. Tell the patient to call home.

4. On which one of the following parts of the interview does the history of present illness expand? (p. 184)
   a. Chief complaint
   b. Dietary profile
   c. Medical history
   d. Social history
   e. Dental history

5. All the following types of communications are most appropriate to determine the medical history of a patient except one. Which one is the exception? (p. 184)
   a. Telephone
   b. Questionnaire
   c. Interview
   d. Computer

REFERENCES

McDaniel, T. F., D. Miller, R. Jones, and M. Davis. 1995. Assessing patient willingness to reveal health history information. *J. Am. Dent. Assoc.* 126:375–379.

Neff, L. 1997. Oral health and systemic disease. *Access* 11(3):29–34.

Peacock, M. E., and R. E. Carson. 1995. Frequency of self-reported medical conditions in periodontal patients. *J. Periodontol.* 66:1004–1007.

Chapter 14

Clinical Examination: Extraoral/Intraoral Examination and Dental Evaluation

Ann M. Goodwin

Rosemary DeRosa Hays

Cheryl M. Westphal

OUTLINE

Introduction
Extraoral/Intraoral Examination
Dental Evaluation
Tooth Stain Evaluation
Dentinal Hypersensitivity
Dental Hygiene Notes
Key Points
Self-Quiz
References

EDUCATIONAL OBJECTIVES

Upon completion of this chapter, the reader should be able to:

- Discuss the role of the dental hygienist in evaluating the dental and oral hygiene status of a patient.
- Describe the importance of performing an intraoral and extraoral examination.
- Describe the components of the dental examination.
- Explain how the findings of the dental evaluation relate to the recognition of periodontal diseases.
- Discuss the different types of tooth stains and their clinical significance.

GOAL: To explain the clinical components of a dental examination and how it relates to the periodontal condition.

KEY WORDS

caries 189	oral cancer 188
dental charting 188	tooth wear 191
dental implants 189	
dentinal hypersensitivity 195	

INTRODUCTION

After completing the patient history, the next aspect of patient assessment involves the collection of objective data by means of a physical examination of the patient. The dental hygienist's tools for this task include the extraoral/intraoral examination, the dental evaluation, the oral hygiene evaluation, the gingival assessment, and the periodontal examination. This section focuses on the extraoral/intraoral examination and the dental evaluation. The section concludes with a brief discussion of dental hypersensitivity.

EXTRAORAL/INTRAORAL EXAMINATION

There are five steps to an extraoral and intraoral examination: (1) inspection, (2) palpation, (3) percussion, (4) auscultation, and (5) olfaction. Inspection involves using the eyes to observe the patient. Palpation is the action of feeling by the sense of touch. Auscultation is the act of listening to sounds from different parts of the body (e.g., using the stethoscope to hear temporomandibular joint [TMJ] sounds upon opening). Percussion is the process of striking a part of the body (e.g., detection of the source of a painful tooth) to give off a sound. Olfaction involves using the nose to smell odors on the breath such as alcohol or the fruity breath of diabetes mellitus.

In the overall appraisal, the dental hygienist should examine the patient's gait, eyes, lips, skin, and head and neck area. Check for lymphadenopathy or lymph nodes that are abnormal in size, consistency, or number. The TMJ also should be examined.

The overall assessment also includes determination of the patient's vital signs. Vital signs include blood pressure, pulse rate, and respiration rate and provide immediate evidence of the patient's basic physiologic functions. Vital signs should be taken at every dental appointment.

The intraoral examination involves screening for **oral cancer** by examining the tongue, gingiva, lining mucosa, and hard palate for color, bleeding, enlargements, and the presence of pain. It is not within the scope of this textbook to thoroughly discuss the components of the extraoral/intraoral examination.

Did You Know?

Just like fingerprints, everyone's tongue print is different.

DENTAL EVALUATION

Dental evaluation begins with a general assessment of the dentition. **Dental charting** is done and analyzed not only for existing restorations, periodontal factors, and needed care but also for the impact of each finding on gingival health. The dental hygienist must examine overhangs, food impaction sites, crown contours, bridge abutments (a tooth or implant used for support and retention of a crown or removable partial denture), and pontics (a missing tooth that is replaced with a restoration and for which there are no roots) as possible plaque-retention sites and evaluate the success of the patient in cleansing these areas. Box 14–1 lists the components of the dental evaluation. Identification of these areas and any resulting dental needs will allow for sequential planning, proper instrumentation, and continual recording and updating of the patient's clinical services.

Box 14–1 **Components of the Dental Evaluation**

- Number of teeth present or absent
- Evaluation of the teeth for dental and root caries
- Restorative status: presence and condition of existing restorations
- Dental implants
- Malpositioning and proximal contact relationships
- Occlusion/parafunctional habits
- Conditions of tooth wear
- Intraoral appliances
- Dental anomalies
- Dentinal hypersensitivity

Evaluate the Number of Teeth

The dental hygienist should begin by determining which teeth are present or missing in the dentition and charting the findings. Information provided by the past dental history, patient interview, and radiographic findings will enable the dental hygienist to determine whether missing teeth were missing at birth, are impacted, or have been extracted due to periodontal, endodontic, or restorative problems. The history of extractions should be discussed to determine the patient's attitude toward dental health and the incidence of dental disease.

Caries

Clinical evidence of dental **caries** may be detected first visually, through a change in tooth color, and then by tactile instrumentation and radiographs, fiberoptics, or other transilluminating devices. The standard method for classifying dental caries is G. V. Black's classification system. Types of dental caries are described by location. Pit and fissure caries frequently is found in the grooves and crevices of occlusal, lingual, and buccal surfaces. Smooth-surface caries is found on the facial, lingual, and interproximal surfaces of teeth.

Root-surface caries is found on the roots of teeth. This is of particular concern in periodontal therapy because of an increased accumulation of plaque due to loss of anatomic tooth structure and difficulty in removing tooth-accumulated materials (e.g., bacterial plaque, calculus, and stains) from that location. Several risk factors predispose to root caries: (1) gingival recession, which exposes the cementum to the oral environment (causes of gingival recession include periodontal disease and postperiodontal surgery; the number of teeth with gingival recession increases with age only because the teeth have been in the mouth longer); (2) xerostomia, particularly in the elderly due to systemic medication, which may decrease salivary flow; (3) head and neck radiation, resulting in xerostomia; (4) advanced age, because of age-related reduction in salivary gland function; (5) lack of fluoride; and (6) smoking and poor general health status or multiple medication use (smokers and patients on multiple medications had a significantly higher prevalence of root caries than nonsmokers and patients in good health) (Page, 1998; Ravald & Birkhed, 1992).

Root caries is detected clinically by visual inspection and/or use of an explorer or periodontal probe. There are two classifications of root caries. Root caries either can be apparent on an exposed root surface (Figure 14–1 ■), where the gingival margin has receded onto the root surface below the caries, or has developed in a pocket, with the gingival tissue covering the root area in a way that makes detection of the caries more difficult.

Rapid Dental Hint

Patients with rampant caries should be evaluated further for the cause. These caries may be due to methamphetamine use.

Did You Know?

Seventy-eight percent of Americans have had at least one cavity by age 17.

Root caries is preventable with rigorous oral self-care and professional care.

Restorative Status

Existing dental restorations should be evaluated for defective or undercontoured surfaces, overhanging margins, and proximal contacts. Ill-fitting removable prosthetic appliances, including clasps, also should be noted. Patients' complaints of floss breaking or shredding may indicate a defective restorative margin. Noting any inadequacies is of particular concern in the periodontal assessment. Any dental restoration should follow the contour of the original tooth, and there should be a tight, firm contact point between the restoration and the adjacent tooth. Overhangs and open margins are conducive to plaque retention, impede oral hygiene, hinder proper scaling and root planing, affect probing accuracy, and can contribute to gingival inflammation and periodontal breakdown. At each appointment, the dental hygienist should update and record any changes that will influence ongoing treatment and continuity of care.

Rapid Dental Hint

When root caries is recognized, determine the cause. Is it xerostomia due to medications?

■ FIGURE 14–1   Gingival recession allows for visibility of root caries on the palatal surface of the maxillary first molar.

Dental Implants

Dental implants and their prosthetic suprastructures present a vast array of dental configurations conducive to plaque retention. Patient complaints about an implant should be addressed as soon as possible (Wilson, 1996). Methods of examination of dental implants and peri-implant tissues (Figure 14–2 ■) are reviewed later in the textbook.

Malpositioning and Proximal Contact Relationships

Evaluation of malposed teeth should include teeth that are in facial or lingual version when compared with the normal alignment of existing dentition. Malpositioning can have an effect on oral hygiene and the integrity of a sound periodontium. Tooth crowding can occur anywhere in the dentition. Crowding of teeth may encourage food impaction and plaque accumulation by compromising oral hygiene and consequently exacerbating gingival inflammation (Figure 14–3 ■). Crowding of teeth per se does not cause or accelerate periodontal tissue destruction, but crowding does make oral hygiene difficult, resulting in the accumulation of bacterial plaque and calculus, and this can then start the process of tissue destruction.

Often a missing tooth may cause the adjacent tooth to tip mesially. When the crown tips or tilts into the edentulous space, causing the gingival on the mesial surface

■ FIGURE 14–3 Crowding of the mandibular incisors decreases the efficiency of oral hygiene practices.

to bunch up, a plaque trap is created. When proximal contact is lost, for example, after an extraction, teeth can drift or shift physiologically (both crown and root movement) into the edentulous space. Tipped (just the crown moves, whereas the root is stationary) and drifted teeth (the entire tooth has moved) can lead to uneven marginal ridges. If a tooth is missing, the opposing tooth may extrude into the edentulous space (Figure 14–4 ■). In such a situation, the tooth will be coronal to the line of occlusion. When

■ FIGURE 14–2 Dental implants replacing the maxillary left central and lateral incisor, canine, and first premolar. Note the tissues around the implants. Gingival recession is present on these teeth.

■ FIGURE 14–4 The maxillary first molar is ankylosed and never fully erupted. This tooth is intruded. The mandibular first molar is extruded above the occlusal plane. Uneven marginal ridges result from this occlusal problem.

a tooth is apical to the occlusal plane, it is considered to be intruded. Frequently, a tilted or extruded tooth is associated with a plunger cusp, which is a pronounced cusp with steep inclined planes that causes a wedging effect on the interproximal area of the opposite arch. This may lead to food impaction and inflamed tissues.

Contacts between teeth should be checked using dental floss. The patient may complain of food impaction where there is an open contact or disastema between two adjacent teeth. Open contacts develop because of (1) congenital tooth abnormalities, (2) teeth that are extruded beyond the occlusal plane, (3) loss of support from an adjacent tooth, and (4) loss of bone support around a tooth (causing the tooth to move and lose adjacent tooth contact; Figure 14–5 ■).

■ **FIGURE 14–5** Numerous diastemas in the maxillary arch were caused by loss of bony support.

Adjacent marginal ridges should be at the same level. Uneven marginal ridges due to extrusion or intrusion of a tooth produce a poor tooth contact relationship, which results in loss of protection of the interdental papillae from food impaction or trauma.

Conditions of Tooth Wear

Conditions and situations that may account for loss of tooth structure include dental attrition, abrasion, and erosion. Usually, the intraoral examination coupled with a patient interview will reveal the type of **tooth wear** and its causes.

Attrition is the loss of tooth structure as a result of tooth-to-tooth contact. Causes include unconscious clenching or grinding of teeth, constant chewing of abrasive foods, the normal wear of tooth structure by physiologic masticatory (chewing) forces, or the mesial drifting of teeth due to the normal aging process. It is important to recognize a bruxing habit in patients who are undergoing restorative care. Contact between a natural tooth and a porcelain crown surface results in rapid wear of the tooth because porcelain is a very hard material. It is best to have tooth-to-artificial-crown contacts on a metallic surface or a highly polished porcelain surface. Attrition is found most often on the incisal/occlusal surfaces of teeth (Figure 14–6 ■) but also is found on proximal tooth surfaces that are flat, as seen with mesial drifting. Attrition also occurs as wear facets, which are small, smooth, polished, flat surfaces on the enamel where there is heavy tooth contact. Usually, wear facets are seen on the side of a tooth cusp.

(a)

(b)

■ **FIGURE 14–6** (a) Attrition of the maxillary teeth due to bruxism. (b) Note that the brownish dentin is exposed as a result of enamel loss.

Abrasion is the abnormal mechanical wearing away of tooth structure for reasons other than mastication. Frequently, it is evident on exposed cementum as a notch apical to the cementoenamel junction (Figure 14–7 ■). Examples of abrasion include excessive force from improper toothbrushing techniques (Dyer, Addy, & Newcombe, 2000), use of a hard-bristle toothbrush, and very abrasive dentifrices. Abrasion also can occur on the incisal/occlusal surfaces when an object such as a pin or pipe is held between the teeth for many years.

Abfractions are classified as a noncarious dental lesion. Numerous theories are found in dental literature concerning the etiology of abfraction including tooth fatigue, flexure (stress), and biomechanical loading of the tooth especially at the cervical area of the tooth. These lesions are usually wedge shaped with sharp line angles. Dental abfractions can occur alone or associated with toothbrush abrasion. Treatment involves observation or placement of a restoration (Owens & Gallien, 1995).

Rapid Dental Hint

When abrasion is recognized, first determine if it is localized or generalized. Generally, the patient's brushing technique, toothbrush, or dentifrice should be changed.

Erosion is the chemical wearing away of tooth structure, usually enamel (Figure 14–8 ■). It is caused by dietary acids (e.g., acidic beverages, lemons) and gastric juices coming from regurgitation or vomiting, as seen in bulimia. Location of the erosion cannot be considered pathognomonic (a direct cause) for certain etiologic factors, although if erosion is present on the palatal surfaces of maxillary incisors, it is most likely due to gastric juices. Traditionally, erosion is proportionally greater in younger patients, but erosion may increase with age as the salivary flow rate decreases.

Intraoral Appliances

Orthodontics, retainers, and splinting wires often present difficulty in cleansing the areas through normal toothbrushing and flossing techniques. Once plaque builds around such appliances and the gingival tissue response occurs with edema and gingival overgrowth, the condition becomes even more difficult to manage. Determining the need for altered home care through a complete oral hygiene analysis can prevent future inflammatory responses.

TOOTH STAIN EVALUATION

Development and Significance

Tooth stains are discolorations on or within tooth surfaces. Depending on its origin, the stain can be classified as exogenous or endogenous. Depending on its location, the stain can be intrinsic if it is internal to the hard tissue or extrinsic if it is external to the surface. Exogenous stains are derived from external sources and often are thought to reside on the outer surface of the

■ **FIGURE 14–7**   V- or U-shaped notching at the exposed cervical root surface just apical to the cementoenamel junction.

■ **FIGURE 14–8**   Erosion in a 35-year-old woman who was bulimic. Chronic vomiting wore away the enamel on the palatal surfaces of the maxillary anterior teeth, creating a shiny, smooth surface.

tooth. They come from chromogenic (producing color or pigment) bacteria, foods, or chemicals. Endogenous stains are incorporated into the structure of the tooth and cannot be removed by surface polishing. Combinations of these classifications can exist, so stains can be exogenous and extrinsic or endogenous and intrinsic (Table 14–1 ■).

Types of Intrinsic Stains

Endogenous stains are always intrinsic because they come from within the tooth and therefore are incorporated into the tooth structure. Examples include (Goldstein & Garber, 1995):

- A nonvital tooth where the pulpal contents have discolored the enamel (this could have resulted from deep dental caries).
- An older patient in whom the teeth appear "yellowish brown" from dentin exposure (with aging, the enamel becomes thinner, exposing the darker color of the underlying dentin).
- Ingestion of excessive fluoride (fluorosis) between the third month of pregnancy and 8 years of age (the teeth appear as whitish opaque to brownish).
- Ingestion of the antibiotic tetracycline during calcification of the developing teeth.

Women should not take tetracycline after the second trimester of pregnancy, and children up to 8 years of age also should not be given tetracycline. Minocycline, a semisynthetic derivative of tetracycline, can cause discoloration in adult teeth. Discoloration depends on concentration (the more tetracycline ingested, the more discoloration). Initially, a yellow fluorescent color is seen that changes to a nonfluorescent grayish brown color.

Extrinsic stains may become intrinsic if they are incorporated into the enamel or dentin, as in amalgam leakage or tobacco stain embedded into the enamel surface.

Rapid Dental Hint

Removing a tetracycline stain is tough. Bleaching the teeth may help somewhat. The best treatment for tetracycline stains, however, especially if they are severe, is porcelain veneers.

Types of Extrinsic Stains

Yellow stain can cause the tooth to appear yellowish or dull. It is associated with the color of the underlying plaque and can be removed by plaque removal. Brown-black stain can be seen in coffee or tea drinkers who do not brush enough to remove the tannin. Plaque does not have to be present, since the pellicle may take on the brown staining alone. Increasing brushing frequency or changing the toothpaste to a more abrasive one may be all that is needed to control the staining. Chewing tobacco often penetrates microcracks in the enamel, resulting in a dark brown-black stain.

Smoking tobacco can produce a stain that is light to dark brown and leathery. It will follow the distribution of the plaque or lodge on the tooth surface most exposed to the tar products of combustion. The stain can cover the cervical third of the tooth or expand to cover the central third as well. It is mostly on the lingual surfaces but can be in the pits and fissures as well. Some tobacco staining can be so severe that it will incorporate in the irregular surfaces of the enamel or exposed dentin. The exogenous, extrinsic stain becomes subsurface and intrinsic, and it increases with neglect. After removal of the extrinsic stain by polishing, increased frequency of plaque removal is required for maintenance. Intrinsic stains may require bleaching for removal.

Black-line stain is a black line that follows in continuous fashion, the facial and lingual gingival margin. It has virtually no thickness and is only 1 mm wide. It usually traverses 1 mm above the gingival margin. This stain is associated with the gram-positive rod of *Actinomyces* species (Slots, 1974). Even though this bacterium is present, the stain is not associated with poor oral hygiene. The microorganisms embed in an adherent matrix and attach to the pellicle. The stain is common in women and children and occurs naturally. Meticulous home care is required to reduce the quantity or frequency of black stain.

Green stain is light or yellowish green to very dark green. The composition comes from chromogenic bacteria and fungi, decomposed hemoglobin (blood), and some inorganic elements. The stain is common in children, occurring on the gingival half of the facial surfaces of the maxillary anterior teeth and extending to the proximal surfaces. The stain can occur as a small curved line following the gingival margin or become a diffused smear covering the facial surface. The enamel under the stain is often rough and demineralized, which encourages plaque retention. Plaque and stain removal through polishing is

Table 14–1	**Classification of Common Tooth Stain**		
Stain	*Origin*	*Treatment*	*Figure*
Intrinsic stains			
Brownish red, bluish black	Nonvital pulp	Root canal treatment, tooth leaching	
Grayish brown	Tetracycline	Vital tooth bleaching	
Whitish brown Localized	Decalcification	Restore with a restoration; use sodium fluoride (0.05%) rinse	
Generalized	Excessive fluoride ingestion during enamel formation (fluorosis)	Restorative care or no treatment necessary	
Yellowish brown	Dentin exposure	No treatment necessary	
Extrinsic stains			
Brown	Tobacco (nicotine)	Remove with scaling and tooth polishing	
	Coffee or tea (tannins)	Remove with scaling and tooth polishing	
	Chlorhexidine oral rinse, stannous fluoride dentifrice or rinse	Remove with scaling and tooth polishing Brush dorsal surface of tongue	

Stain	Origin	Treatment	Figure
Black-line	Gram-positive rods	Remove with scaling and tooth polishing	
Green stain	Chromogenic bacteria	No scaling, polish with mild abrasive	

necessary, yet prevention of recurrence depends on meticulous home care.

Chlorhexidine, used in oral rinses to control plaque and gingivitis, discolors the teeth with a yellow-brown stain on the proximal surfaces, on restorations, and on the tongue (Löe & Schlott, 1970). In approximately 50% of patients, staining occurs within a few days after starting the rinse. The cause of the staining is unclear, but it may be the result of a reaction with foods containing aldehydes or ketones. Although the staining is not permanent, it is a significant side effect that may deter routine compliance. Polishing the enamel or exposed root surfaces removes the stain. Often a patient will have staining only interproximally and not on the direct facial or lingual surfaces. This indicates that the patient practices good oral self-care.

Rapid Dental Hint

Determine if the stain is intrinsic or extrinsic because the treatment options will vary.

Significance of Stains

The significance of stains relates to the rough surfaces they may create and the resulting plaque retention sites. Stains can adhere directly to a tooth, discolor the pellicle and plaque, or become part of the tooth.

If either of the first two occurs, the tooth surface could have an overlay of stain. This is cosmetic at first until it increases in thickness. If plaque adheres to the stain, the same gingival response occurs. The stain needs to be removed in order to promote oral cleanliness and eliminate possible plaque retention sites.

The key to choosing a removal process is identification of the stain by source and location. Analysis of the color is not always the only determinant of source. Some colors, such as brown, may represent poor hygiene, tobacco use, tea or coffee consumption, or dental fluorosis. The analysis also must determine if the stain resides on the surface and can be removed by polishing or is intrinsic and must be removed by tooth bleaching.

DENTINAL HYPERSENSITIVITY

Many patients experience **dentinal hypersensitivity** as a painful response to an irritation where roots are exposed. Dentinal hypersensitivity is a transient, sharp pain arising from exposed dentin in response to a stimulus; it does not last very long. Hypersensitivity will vary in intensity from very mild to excruciatingly painful. Some patients can tolerate the pain, whereas others simply cannot endure it.

Etiology of Dentinal Hypersensitivity

Although not all patients with exposed dentin experience dentinal or root surface hypersensitivity, an estimated 10 to 25% of people in the United States complain of some type of acute or chronic dentinal hypersensitivity resulting from vigorous toothbrushing, tooth whitening, thermal stimulus, mechanical periodontal debridement, or periodontal surgery that exposes the root surfaces.

While there are numerous theories explaining the etiology of hypersensitive tooth surfaces, the most prevalent theory is the hydrodynamic explanation (Paine, Slots, & Rich, 1998). This theory states that the fluid in the exposed dentinal tubules contracts or expands when an external stimulus is applied. The pain experienced is due to this minute fluid movement within the tubules.

The most common situation in which hypersensitivity occurs is as follows: Initially, gingival recession occurs, in which the gingival margin migrates apically as a result of trauma or forceful toothbrushing, and this exposes the underlying cementum. The thin cementum can be worn away easily by the abrasive agents in dentifrices or from mechanical root debridement, which exposes the underlying dentin and the open dentinal tubules. Usually, the pain is instigated by thermal changes such as cold air or cold foods (ice cream or a cold drink), a mechanical stimulus such as toothbrushing or touch with an instrument or other object, or a chemical stimulus such as sweets.

Identification

It is important to rule out any dental pathology. The dental hygienist can be among the first practitioners to recognize dentinal hypersensitivity. A patient usually complains of a tooth that hurts but will not say, "I have a hypersensitive tooth." If a patient cannot identify a specific tooth, then the problem probably is not a hypersensitive tooth but rather a root or crown fracture, leaking restorations, or teeth in hyperfunction. If the patient points to a tooth, the dental hygienist should ask further questions pertaining to various risk factors.

Testing for sensitivity should be a part of the initial examination and should include something that can be used as a baseline measurement of sensitivity. The air-blast test is one method of assessing hypersensitivity. The area should be dried before using the air syringe. Most patients who have gingival recession should have sensitivity tests. It also may be important to do pretreatment sensitivity tests before periodontal therapy (e.g., instrumentation, periodontal surgery) so that it can be determined if any posttherapy sensitivity was present before treatment or has resulted from the treatment (Zapletalová, Perina, Novotný, & Chmelíčková, 2007). Management of hypersensitivity is discussed in Chapter 20.

DENTAL HYGIENE NOTES

The dental examination follows the medical/dental history and is an intricate step in assessing baseline data and dental care of the patient. With a thorough and systematic approach to the dental examination, risk factors can be identified that will aid in the appropriate treatment planning needs of the patient.

KEY POINTS

- The dental examination involves identification of contributory local risk factors for periodontal diseases.
- Individual teeth and the entire dentition are examined for deviations.
- Dentinal hypersensitivity is a common complaint; identification causes will help in its treatment.

SELF-QUIZ

1. Which one of the following risk factors is characteristic for root caries? (p. 189)
   a. Chlorhexidine
   b. Xerostomia
   c. Parafunctional habit
   d. Alcohol consumption
2. Which one of the following methods best detects root caries? (p. 189)
   a. Explorer #23
   b. Radiographs
   c. Rinsing with a disclosing agent
   d. Brushing with an abrasive dentifrice
3. Which of the following terms describes loss of tooth structure due to occlusion on an opposing porcelain crown? (p. 191)
   a. Abrasion
   b. Attrition
   c. Erosion
   d. Wear facet
4. Which one of the following extrinsic stains is related to chromogenic bacteria? (p. 193, Table 14–1)
   a. Black
   b. Brown
   c. Green
   d. Yellow
5. All visible stains have to be removed from the tooth surfaces because stains are harmful to the teeth. (p. 195)
   a. Both the statement and the reason are correct and related.
   b. Both the statement and the reason are correct but not related.
   c. The statement is correct, but the reason is not.
   d. The statement is not correct, but the reason is correct.
   e. Neither the statement nor the reason is correct.

REFERENCES

Dyer D., M. Addy, and R. Newcombe. 2000. Studies in vitro of abrasion by different manual toothbrush heads and a standard toothpaste. *J Clin. Periodontal.* 27:99–103.

Goldstein, R. E., and D. A. Garber. 1995. *Complete dental bleaching,* 2–13. Chicago: Quintessence.

Löe, H., and C. Schlott. 1970. The effect of mouthrinses and topical application of chlorhexidine on the development of dental plaque and gingivitis in man. *J. Periodont. Res.* 5:79–83.

Page, R. 1998. Risk assessment for root caries in adults. *Oral Care Rep.* 8:7.

Paine, M. L., J. Slots, and S. K. Rich. 1998. Fluoride use in periodontal therapy: A review of the literature. *J. Am. Dent. Assoc.* 129:66–69.

Ravald, N., and D. Birkhed. 1992. Prediction of root caries in periodontally treated patients maintained with different fluoride programmes. *Caries Res.* 26:450–458.

Slots, J. 1974. The microflora of black stain on human primary teeth. *Scand. J. Dent. Res.* 82:484.

Wilson, T. G. 1996. A typical maintenance visit for patients with dental implants. *Periodontology 2000* 12:29.

Zapletalová, Z., J. Perina, R. Novotný, and H. Chmelíčková. 2007. Suitable conditions for sealing of open dentinal tubules using a pulsed Nd:YAG laser. *Photomed Laser Surg.* (December) (6):495–9.

Chapter 15

Clinical Examination: Gingival Assessment

Eva M. Lupovici

OUTLINE

Introduction
Objectives of a Gingival Assessment
Risk Factors for Gingival Diseases
Clinical Assessment Procedures
Dental Hygiene Notes
Key Points
Self-Quiz
References

EDUCATIONAL OBJECTIVES

Upon completion of this chapter, the reader should be able to:

- Describe the rationale for performing a gingival assessment as part of the patient evaluation.
- Describe the clinical features of the gingiva in health and disease.
- Evaluate the procedures used in performing a gingival assessment.
- Differentiate bleeding at the gingival margin from bleeding on probing.
- Recognize and discuss factors found in gingival assessment procedures that may be predictors of future disease activity.

GOAL: To provide knowledge of the clinical and histologic features of gingival changes in disease.

KEY WORDS

bleeding on probing 205	inflammatory periodontal diseases 199
gingival assessment 199	

INTRODUCTION

Traditional diagnostic procedures are divided into two components: detection of inflammation and assessment of damage to periodontal tissues (Armitage, 1996). Detection of inflammation will be discussed in this subsection, and the next subsection addresses the resulting damage to the periodontium.

In considering the status of the periodontium, practitioners frequently state that the tissue is either "normal" or "diseased," with no in-between stage. In medicine as well as in dentistry, however, there is a range of normality. Slight deviations from the healthy norm can fall within the range of normality for an individual.

OBJECTIVES OF A GINGIVAL ASSESSMENT

The purpose of performing a **gingival assessment** is to evaluate the condition of the gingival tissues and to determine inflammatory and noninflammatory changes. Gingival assessment is one of the essential steps in identifying **inflammatory periodontal diseases.** The accurate recording of initial examination findings is essential in formulating an appropriate treatment plan, as a baseline comparison with future clinical findings after the initial phase of therapy is completed, and in subsequent periodontal maintenance visits.

RISK FACTORS FOR GINGIVAL DISEASES

The inflammatory process occurs in response to the presence of irritation to the tissues caused by dental plaque. Inflammation is the host's response to the irritation, which stimulates tissue repair. However, as noted in previous chapters, additional risk factors predispose a host to gingival or periodontal diseases. Host susceptibility to periodontal diseases should be considered if inflammation is not resolved after treatment. Having knowledge of all the potential risk factors is important in providing the appropriate treatment.

Risk factors for gingival inflammation or gingival enlargement include the following:

- Poor home care.
- Changes in hormone levels, as seen in pregnancy, menopause, puberty, or use of oral contraceptives.
- Systemic diseases, such as diabetes mellitus, leukemia, or human immunodeficiency virus (HIV) infection.
- Eruption of the permanent dentition.
- Certain drugs, including phenytoin, valproate, cyclosporine, and calcium channel blockers.

CLINICAL ASSESSMENT PROCEDURES

When examining the interdental papillae and gingival margin, the dental hygienist should compare them with adjacent areas. These are the first areas that are affected clinically by inflammation. In the presence of inflammation, gingival tissue manifests some or all of the following five cardinal signs: redness (rubor), swelling (tumor), and heat (calor). Pain (dolor) and loss of function (functio laesa) may not be present until the advanced stages of periodontal disease. If inflammation is not resolved, then the inflammatory infiltrate progresses into the attached gingiva and alveolar mucosa. Since the alveolar mucosa is composed of loose connective tissue, the inflammatory infiltrate travels through it more quickly than through the attached gingiva, which is composed of dense connective tissue.

Color

The entire mouth should be examined visually, not just the anterior portions of the oral cavity. In health, the color of the gingiva is salmon pink. Color is determined by the degree of vascularity, epithelial keratinization, presence of melanin, and thickness of the epithelium. In the presence of inflammation, the color of the tissues can be various shades of red (erythema) or light to whitish pink, depending on the chronicity of the lesion. Initially, there is a bright red color, which can change to deeper red or bluish red (cyanotic) or pale white in severe periodontal disease. Tissue redness should not be used as the sole indicator of inflammation, nor is it strongly associated with or a predictor for future periodontal disease activity (PDA) (Halazonetis, Haffajee, & Socransky 1989). However, the absence of gingival redness is more indicative of the absence of disease (Lang, Adler, Joss, & Nyman, 1990).

Gingiva color may appear to be healthy superficially at clinical examination and still be diseased because the site of inflammation is deep within the tissues and not seen at the gingival margin until after the disease progresses. Conversely, individuals with thin oral epithelium may have a healthy gingiva that is red in color.

Within the normal range, healthy gingiva varies in color. In certain dark-skinned individuals such as Asians, African descendants, and Mediterranean people, the gingiva will appear to have a light brown to black pigmentation due to the presence of melanin (Table 15–1 ■).

Table 15–1   Clinical and Histologic Changes Seen in Health and Gingivitis

Clinical Features	Histologic Features	Figure
	Color	
In *health,* the gingiva is salmon pink.	Presence of keratin.	salmon pink gingiva
Pigmentation	Indicates the production of melanin by melanocytes; this does not indicate the presence of inflammation or disease.	pigmented gingiva
In *acute inflammation,* the tissues exhibit various shades of red (fiery red); in *chronic inflammation,* the gingiva may be a bluish red (cyanotic or magenta), or pale white.	Redness is due to increased vasodilation (engorged blood vessels) resulting in locally increased blood flow. As the condition worsens, the bluish red color is due to stagnation of blood in the vessels. The pale white color is due to the repair process with excessive collagen formation.	inflamed gingiva
Free gingival margin	**Contour**	
Knife-edged	Intact gingiva fibers brace the gingiva to the tooth.	knife-edged free gingival margins
Rolled or rounded	Destruction of gingival fibers.	rolled free gingival margins

Gingival cleft	Narrow slit in the gingiva starting at the gingival margin; probably associated with tooth position in the arch or the beginning of pocket formation; not related to occlusal forces, as once thought.	 gingival cleft
Interdental papillae		
Pyramidal or pointed (flatter in posterior)	Papillae completely fill in gingival embrasure; no tissue destruction.	 pyramidal papillae
Bulbous	Enlarged papillae due to accumulation of fluid in the tissue; the papilla is not tucked in the gingival embrasure but partly covers the enamel.	 bulbous papillae
Blunted	Destruction of the tip of the papilla.	 blunted papillae
Absent	Destruction of the entire papilla; occurs where there is a diastema.	 absent papillae
Cratered	Destruction of the tissue between the papillae; a "concavity."	 cratered papillae

Consistency		
Firm and resilient	Intact collagen fibers in the lamina propria give the gingiva its firm consistency. Tissues are easily compressed with a blunt instrument.	 firm gingiva
Edematous	Loss of collagen and vascular permeability resulting in fluid accumulation in the surrounding tissue.	 edematous gingiva
Fibrotic	Reparative process whereby the fibroblasts in tissue in an attempt to heal produce and secrete excessive collagen. Tissue becomes hard and nonresilient. Tissue is not compressible.	 fibrotic gingiva
Retractable	Loss of collagen fibers. Papillae and margins are easily retracted by a blast of air.	 retractable gingiva
Surface Texture		
Stippling	Stippling results from the intersecting epithelial ridges on the undersurface of the epithelium. An excessive amount of stippling is seen in chronic inflammation.	 stippling
Shiny and smooth	Can occur in health or disease. In disease, loss of stippling occurs because of accumulation of fluid in the underlying gingival connective tissue.	 loss of stippling

Another cause for variation in gingival color may be an amalgam restoration. The metals from an amalgam restoration may absorb into the gingiva, causing a bluish-gray color. This is termed an amalgam tattoo. This condition causes discoloration of the gingiva (Figure 15–1 ■) but is not inflammatory in nature, and the gingiva is considered to be healthy.

Rapid Dental Hint

When assessing the color of the gingival tissues, compare these tissues with adjacent areas.

Contour

Examining the contour of the gingiva is the next phase of the gingival assessment. Gingival contour is determined by the shapes and positions of the teeth, alignment of the teeth, location and size of the contact area, size of the gingival embrasure, and soft-tissue inflammation. Therefore, the contour of the gingiva will vary from anterior to posterior areas and between individual teeth.

Marginal Gingiva and Interdental Papillae

In health, the marginal gingiva (or free gingival margin) is knife-edged in contour. In disease, the margins become rolled or rounded due to destruction of the circular fibers.

Interdental papillae in healthy gingiva are tightly tucked into the gingival embrasures. Papillae of anterior teeth are pyramidal in shape because they follow the cementoenamel junction (CEJ) and contact areas, which are narrow. Papillae of posterior teeth are flatter because the CEJ is flatter and the contact areas are wider. In disease, the papillae become bulbous or enlarged because of edema. The papillae may be cratered where there is a depression between the facial and lingual papillae or blunted where the tip of the papilla is absent and there is an open gingival embrasure. Blunting of the gingiva also may be due to noninflammatory causes such as overuse or misuse of interdental cleaning aids. It may be caused in response to the use of an interdental brush in areas where the interdental papilla completely fills the gingi-

■ **FIGURE 15–1**   An amalgam tattoo is seen on the lingual surface near the second premolar. This is healthy gingiva.

val embrasure. Changes in the contour of the gingiva can reflect current or past periodontal tissue destruction.

Gingival Clefts

In examining gingival contour, the dental hygienist may observe a gingival cleft or a pseudocleft. A gingival cleft is a V-shaped slit that extends apically from the gingival margin. A gingival cleft may be caused by many factors, such as incorrect toothbrushing, improper flossing (flossing cleft), or a break through the gingiva around a tooth as a result of pocket formation. Gingival clefts can resolve spontaneously or may require periodontal surgery.

A pseudocleft is a gingival cleft that occurs when adjacent papillae become enlarged to the point that they join each other at the center of the tooth (see Table 15–1). This is not a true cleft because there is no marginal tissue destruction. Pseudocleft is seen commonly in patients with crowding of teeth or in patients with severely enlarged gingiva who are taking certain medications such as phenytoin, cyclosporine, or nifedipine. Additionally, coronal migration of the gingival margin caused by the gingival overgrowth results in the formation of a pseudopocket or gingival pocket.

Consistency

The consistency of the gingiva is examined by lightly pressing the side of the periodontal probe against the marginal and interdental gingiva. Consistency refers to the firmness of the underlying connective tissue. In health, the gingiva is firm and resilient when pressed. As stated earlier, inflammatory changes occur within the vascular connective tissue of the gingiva, and when edema is present, the tissue will "pit" and not rebound quickly when the periodontal probe is applied lightly. Edema causes gingival enlargement, resulting in the formation of a gingival pocket or pseudopocket. Firm, resilient gingiva may not be an indicator of health, however, as seen with fibrotic gingiva. Upon examination, fibrotic gingiva will be hard and will not show a "pit" when tested with a periodontal probe.

Recent studies have found that smokers have the same or less gingival inflammation than nonsmokers (American Academy of Periodontology, 1996; Stafne, 1997). However, the gingival consistency in smokers tends to be fibrotic with rolled gingival margins. Smoking or smokeless tobacco chewing causes the tissue to become hyperkeratinized with an abnormal whitish thickening of the keratin layer of the epithelium. Following smoking cessation, the gingiva returns to its condition prior to smoking (Haber, 1994).

During the disease process, the collagen fibers are destroyed, causing the gingiva to be retractable or flaccid (see Table 15–1). Once the inflammation is eliminated and controlled, the collagen fibers may reform and unite the gingiva to the tooth.

Surface Texture

Surface texture is assessed by drying the attached gingiva with gauze and observing the surface for stippling. Clinically, stippling is described as having an appearance similar to the outside peel of an orange. The presence or absence of stippling does not necessarily indicate the health status of the gingiva. Stippling is present in health and in chronic inflammation when the gingiva becomes fibrotic. In chronic inflammation, the presence of stippling represents tissue scarring. Edematous gingival tissue may retain stippling. In the absence of stippling, the gingiva is described as being smooth or shiny.

Size: Gingival Enlargement

The size of the gingiva is influenced by several factors, such as cellular and intercellular elements and vascular supply. In gingival overgrowth or enlargement, the free gingival margin is located coronal to its normal position at or slightly coronal to the CEJ. Gingival enlargement can be the result of a tissue response to inflammation caused by dental plaque, hormonal imbalance in pregnancy and puberty, side effects of certain medications,

mouth breathing, and iatrogenic dentistry such as poorly contoured crowns.

The alternative drying and wetting of the gingiva during mouth breathing promotes an inflammatory response causing gingival enlargement from the maxillary canine to the canine. The appearance of the gingiva, especially the palatal surface, is usually shiny and red in color.

Gingival enlargement of the maxillary tuberosity is not considered to be a disease state. The enlargement is developmental in origin.

Hereditary gingival fibromatosis is a rare form of severe gingival enlargement seen commonly in children beginning with the eruption of either the primary or permanent dentition. The etiology is unknown, but heredity is most likely involved. Gingival enlargement is generalized throughout the mouth, involving both the papillae and the marginal gingiva. The teeth may be completely covered by tissue overgrowth, preventing eruption.

Hormonal and Drug-Influenced Gingivitis

Hormonal Changes

Clinically, gingivitis in pregnancy is characterized by either generalized or localized inflammation to the gingival papillae, which show a sharp demarcation from the attached gingiva. The inflammation or swelling can spread to involve the marginal gingiva. The gingiva is bright red and edematous, with a shiny, smooth surface. The molars show the most inflammation, followed by the premolars and the incisors (Silness & Löe, 1963).

In more severe cases, pregnancy tumors also may occur, but these are not considered a true neoplasm; they are an inflammatory reaction to the dental plaque. Actually, a pyogenicgranuloma occurring in a pregnant patient is called a pregnancy tumor. This swelling appears mainly in the anterior facial areas of the mouth. It is a mass of tissue that protrudes outward. It is deep red and edematous.

Postpartum, these gingival conditions usually regress to their status during the second month of pregnancy. Most of the gingival changes seen during pregnancy can be prevented by removal of plaque and meticulous home care.

Gingival inflammation during pregnancy is not exclusive to pregnancy. Similar gingival changes, except for pregnancy tumors, are seen in adolescents as puberty gingivitis. These patients develop massive gingival enlargement that recurs even in the presence of little plaque.

After puberty, the enlargement regresses, but total disappearance only occurs after all local irritants are removed.

Drug-Influenced Gingival Enlargement

Clinically, drug-induced gingivitis is seen as a generalized overgrowth of the gingiva, especially of the interdental papillae on the facial gingiva, of the maxillary and mandibular teeth, particularly the anterior sextent, and does not often occur in edentulous areas (Figures 15–2 ■, 15–3 ■). Enlargement of the gingiva may result in malpositioning of teeth and interference with normal chewing, speech, and oral hygiene (Pihlstrom, 1990). The gingival tissue in cyclosporine-induced overgrowth tends to be more soft, red or bluish red, and fragile, and it bleeds more easily on probing than tissue undergoing phenytoin-induced overgrowth (Hallmon & Rossmann, 1999). Other medications that may cause gingival enlargement are the calcium channel blockers (e.g., nifedipine, amlodipine, diltiazem).

In most cases, maintaining strict plaque control can prevent this enlargement, but surgical intervention frequently is required to obtain physiologic gingival contours and aesthetics.

Rapid Dental Hint

Determine the cause when gingival inflammation and enlargement are recognized.

■ **FIGURE 15–2**   A 38-year-old woman taking phenytoin for seizures for the last three years. Note the generalized gingival enlargement, especially the interdental papillae.

■ **FIGURE 15–3**   A 56-year-old woman taking nifedipine for hypertension. Note the enlargement of the interdental papillae. The enlarged papillae take on a lobulated or nodular appearance.

Gingival Bleeding

The next step in the gingival examination is to determine the presence of marginal bleeding. This can be done by several methods, including stroking the lining of the sulcus or inserting a wooden or plastic wedge to assess proximal bleeding (Caton & Polson, 1985). If the stroke method is used, the probe is placed within the gingival crevice and is dragged from one interproximal space to the other interproximal space on the same tooth. Any bleeding seen within 30 seconds is labeled as a bleeding site. Bleeding measured at the gingival margin or crevice is often indicative of gingival inflammation. On the other hand, **bleeding on probing** (BOP) (bleeding coming from a pocket during periodontal probing) indicates a deeper inflammatory involvement. In private practice or a clinic setting, bleeding on probing usually is recorded as being either absent or present by placing a red dot over the site that bleeds. For research purposes, a bleeding index is used to standardize measurements. It is important to note that bleeding may be masked if the gingiva is fibrotic. Former heavy and current heavy smokers have been reported to show a significant suppression of high BOP compared to never smokers (Shimazaki et al., 2006). Many patients are taking low-dose aspirin for prevention of stroke and heart attack. It has been documented that aspirin intake of 325 mg/day for seven days moderately increased the appearance of bleeding on probing in a patient population that had ≥20% BOP sites.

Bleeding occurs when there is disruption of the sulcular and junctional epithelium allowing for passage

Rapid Dental Hint

Bleeding on probing indicates clinical inflammation. This is similar to getting a splinter in your finger. The same inflammatory process occurs.

of blood or exudate from the lamina propria into the sulcus. The epithelium is avascular and receives its blood supply and nutrients from the underlying vascular lamina propria. When the epithelium becomes inflamed, it reacts by forming microulcerations. Thus, sweeping the lining of the crevice or probing allows for blood to pass through from the engorged and newly formed blood vessels in the lamina propria subjacent to the epithelium.

Rapid Dental Hint

The easiest way to record bleeding is either the site bleeds (+) or it doesn't.

Bleeding traditionally is accepted as an objective clinical sign of inflammation; however, some visually inflamed gingival sites do not bleed. Therefore, it can be stated that bleeding is not always an early sign of gingival inflammation, and the actual mechanisms responsible for bleeding probably are not truly understood. In addition, the presence of bleeding from a periodontitis site is a poor predictor of future attachment loss (Armitage, 1996). On the other hand, the absence of bleeding is strongly indicative of low levels of inflammation (Lang et al., 1990) and high periodontal stability (Goodson, 1992). Thus, it can be stated that bleeding on probing is a poor positive predictor of periodontal disease, but conversely is a very strong negative predictor. The clinical interpretation of this research is that while BOP presence may not indicate periodontal disease, continued absence of BOP is a strong predictor (approximately 98%) of continued periodontal health. Gingival bleeding has been related to increased gingival crevicular fluid flow rate, which is associated with the presence of inflammation (Armitage, 1996). Another limitation of the use of bleeding as an inflammatory parameter is the possibility that healthy tissues may bleed on stimulation or probing (Lang et al., 1990) when excessive probing forces are used or improper toothbrushing methods or improper use of interdental cleaning aids has occurred. Also, healthy tissue may bleed if the patient is a smoker

or taking certain medications such as warfarin, aspirin, or clopidogrel (Schrodi et al., 2002). Thus, the dental hygienist must discriminate between bleeding sites that are inflamed and those that bleed for other reasons. In order to eliminate bleeding, the pathologic process must be changed. Traditionally, altering plaque levels by periodontal debridement and improved oral hygiene has been successful, especially in the reduction of gingivitis.

DENTAL HYGIENE NOTES

After the gingival assessment is completed, the findings are summarized according to location, distribution, and severity of the gingival changes. The findings can be either localized or generalized (localized to certain areas such as the mandibular lingual teeth or generalized throughout the entire mouth). Distribution is either marginal, papillary, or diffuse. If the marginal gingiva is affected, it is called marginal inflammation. If the interdental papillae are affected, it is called papillary inflammation. If the free, attached, and/or alveolar mucosa is affected, it is referred to as diffuse. Severity is classified as mild, moderate, or severe.

KEY POINTS

- The purpose of performing a gingival evaluation is to determine the status of the gingiva and the presence or absence of gingival inflammation and/or gingival enlargement.
- Gingival enlargement can be due to an inflammatory response to dental plaque or to certain drugs.
- The steps involved in a gingival evaluation include assessing for gingival color, contour, consistency, surface texture, size, and bleeding.
- The absence of bleeding indicates periodontal stability.

SELF-QUIZ

1. Which one of the following features describes the gingival appearance in a patient who is a 30 pack-years smoker? (p. 204)
   a. Red gingiva and cratered interdental papillae
   b. Red gingiva and bulbous gingival margins
   c. Whitish gingiva and absent interdental papillae
   d. Whitish gingiva and rolled, receded gingival margins

2. Which one of the following considerations must be addressed by the dental hygienist when performing a gingival assessment? (p. 199)
   a. Determine inflammatory changes.
   b. Evaluate periodontal disease activity.
   c. Assess destruction of supporting and alveolar bone.
   d. Evaluate probing depth changes.

3. Which one of the following statements is related to bleeding on probing or sulcular stimulation? (pp. 205–206)
   a. The absence of bleeding is strongly indicative of low levels of inflammation.
   b. The presence of bleeding from a periodontitis site is a good predictor for future attachment loss.
   c. All visually inflamed gingival sites bleed.
   d. Bleeding occurs when there is disruption of the oral epithelium.

4. All of the following factors are related to gingival enlargement except one. Which one is the exception? (p. 204)
   a. Gingival inflammation
   b. Hormonal changes
   c. Cigarette smoking
   d. Mouth breathing

5. Tissue redness should be used as the primary indicator of inflammation because it is strongly associated with future periodontal disease activity. (p. 199)
   a. Both the statement and the reason are correct and related.
   b. Both the statement and the reason are correct but not related.
   c. The statement is correct, but the reason is not.
   d. The statement is not correct, but the reason is correct.
   e. Neither the statement nor the reason is correct.

6. Which of the following statements regarding bleeding on probing and disease activity is correct? (pp. 205–206)
   a. Good positive indicator
   b. Poor negative indicator
   c. Strong negative indicator
   d. Is not correlated to disease activity

7. A patient is taking 325 mg/day of aspirin. Which of the following would be anticipated to occur while probing? (p. 206)
   a. Increased bleeding
   b. Decreased bleeding
   c. No affect on bleeding
   d. Should not probe a patient taking aspirin or other anticoagulants

8. Bleeding on probing is a clinical sign of (pp. 205–206)
   a. disease activity.
   b. inflammation.
   c. clinical attachment loss.
   d. bone loss.

9. All of the following are drugs that can cause gingival enlargement *except* one. Which one is the exception? (pp. 204–205)
   a. Aspirin
   b. Cyclosporine
   c. Nifedipine
   d. Diltiazem

10. Bleeding that occurs in the gingival crevice originates from the (p. 205)
    a. epithelium.
    b. lamina propria.
    c. alveolar bone.
    d. periodontal ligament.

REFERENCES

American Academy of Periodontology. 1996. Tobacco use and the periodontal patient. *J. Periodontol.* 67:51–56.

Armitage, G. C. 1996. Periodontal diseases: Diagnosis. *Ann. Periodontol.* 1:37–215.

Caton, J., and A. Polson. 1985. The interdental bleeding index: A simplified procedure for monitoring gingival health. *Compend. Contin. Educ. Dent.* 6:88–92.

Goodson, J. M. 1992. Diagnosis of periodontitis by physical measurement: Interpretation from episodic disease hypothesis. *J. Periodontol.* 63:373–382.

Haber, J. 1994. Cigarette smoking: A major risk factor for periodontitis. *Compend. Contin. Educ. Dent.* 15:1002, 1004–1008, 1014.

Halazonetis, T. D., A. D. Haffajee, and S. S. Socransky. 1989. Relationship of clinical parameters to attachment loss in subsets of subjects with destructive periodontal diseases. *J. Clin. Periodontol.* 16:563–568.

Hallmon, W. W., and J. A. Rossmann. 1999. The role of drugs in the pathogenesis of gingival overgrowth. *Periodontology 2000* 21:176–196.

Lang, N. P., R. Adler, A. Joss, and S. Nyman. 1990. Absence of bleeding on probing: An indicator of periodontal stability. *J. Clin. Periodontol.* 17:714–721.

Pihlstrom, B. L. 1990. Prevention and treatment of Dilantin®-associated gingival enlargement. *Compend. Contin. Educ. Dent. 11*(Suppl. 14):S506–S510.

Schrodi, J., L. Recio, J. Fiorellini, et al. 2002. The effect of aspirin on the periodontal parameter bleeding on probing. *J. Periodontol.* 73:871–876.

Shimazaki, Y., T. Saito, Y. Kiyohara, et al. 2006. The influence of current and former smoking on gingival bleeding: The Hisayama Study. *J. Periodontol.* 77:1430–1435.

Silness, J., and H. Löe. 1963. Periodontal disease in pregnancy. *Acta Odontol. Scand.* 21:533–551.

Stafne, E. E. 1997. Cigarette smoking and periodontal disease: The benefits of smoking cessation. *Northwest Dent.* (September–October): 25–29.

Chapter 16

Clinical Examination: Periodontal Assessment

Theodore L. West

OUTLINE

Introduction
Rationale for Periodontal Assessment
Periodontal Terminology
Examination Techniques
Dental Hygiene Notes
Key Points
Self-Quiz
References

EDUCATIONAL OBJECTIVES

Upon completion of this chapter, the reader should be able to:

- Describe the components of a periodontal assessment.
- Explain the clinical significance of each component of a periodontal assessment.
- Differentiate the significance of measuring clinical attachment level from probing depth.
- List several factors that can affect the accuracy of probe readings.
- Discuss the problems associated with a mucogingival defect.
- Describe the various causes of gingival recession.
- Discuss the concept of periodontal disease activity.

GOAL: To provide the basic elements for performing a periodontal examination.

KEY WORDS

attachment loss 212
clinical attachment
  level 211
gingival recession 219
monitoring 210
outcome measure 210

periodontal
  assessment 210
periodontal disease
  activity 210
periodontal disease
  severity 210
screening 210

INTRODUCTION

The periodontal examination performed by a dental hygienist has many purposes. First, large population groups in health fairs, schools, hospitals, clinics, and other institutions may need to be examined rapidly for periodontal diseases requiring further evaluation and subsequent treatment—the periodontal **screening.** For visual detection of periodontal diseases, rapid screening can be performed with as little instrumentation as two disposable wooden tongue blades and a flashlight to evaluate tooth loss, migration, and mobility; gingival recession, redness, suppuration, and swelling; and calculus and plaque levels. Essentially, screening is done in a single visit to differentiate between health and disease.

RATIONALE FOR PERIODONTAL ASSESSMENT

A more thorough examination requires a mouth mirror, a periodontal probe, and radiographs. The periodontal assessment includes complete medical and dental histories, and the recording of gingival findings, probing depths, clinical attachment levels, tooth mobility, tooth malposition, level of oral hygiene, occlusal relationships, and bone levels.

This **periodontal assessment** provides the baseline for the long-term monitoring of periodontal disease activity (Armitage, 2004). Such **monitoring** is often performed by the dental hygienist from one to four times a year at the periodontal maintenance visit. Such monitoring for increases in clinical attachment loss, gingival recession, swelling, bleeding, tooth mobility, and so on, because of the episodic and recurrent nature of periodontal diseases, is vitally necessary if the patient is to be maintained in a state of periodontal health. It often becomes the dental hygienist's responsibility to find and point out areas of recurrent periodontal disease activity in a patient's mouth.

Finally, the periodontal assessment examination should be used by the practitioner as an **outcome measure** to evaluate the success of periodontal treatment and the need for and frequency of periodontal maintenance visits (Douglas, 2006).

It seems likely that some general dental practices do not adequately assess periodontal diseases (McFall, Bader, Rozier, & Ramsey, 1988). In a study of almost 2,500 patient records from thirty-six general practices, radiographic bone loss was seen in over half the film sets.

However, in only one in five records was there a periodontal diagnostic entry or a notation about pocket formation. This random sample of adult patient records had very infrequent recordings of bleeding, recession, furcation invasions, pocketing, tooth mobility, and so on. These findings can be compared with an epidemiologic study in the same state of North Carolina (Bawden & DeFriese, 1981) that indicated that 55 to 75% of the adult population was affected by periodontal disease.

If periodontal disease assessment in the general dental practice is inadequate, then it certainly must follow that the monitoring of periodontal disease progression becomes an impossibility. It seems probable that the burden for assessing and monitoring periodontal diseases in a general practice may fall, to a greater or lesser extent, on the shoulders of the dental hygienist.

Although periodontal diseases occur primarily in the adult population, they also can occur in young people, occasionally in a very severe form. Therefore, a periodontal evaluation should be performed for all patients regardless of their age. A national survey of over 2,600 individuals 19 years of age and older, using a mouth mirror, explorer, and periodontal probe, showed 28% with periodontitis, 53.9% with gingivitis, and only 17.3% free of periodontal disease in the youngest group (19–44 years). In the 45- to 64-year age group, only 8.3% were free of periodontal disease, and 47.6% had pocket depths of 4 mm or more (Brown, Oliver, & Löe, 1989). Periodontal diseases have now been associated with increased risk for heart disease, stroke, diabetic complications, and premature, low-birth-weight babies. Since race, socioeconomic factors, nutrition, tobacco use, and various systemic diseases can further increase the prevalence of periodontal diseases at any age, the importance of the periodontal examination is obvious.

Periodontal disease severity represents the total destruction and healing that occur during the lifetime of a tooth (Jeffcoat, 1994). It is the status of the periodontium or extent of tissue damage at the time of the examination (Lamster, Celenti, Jans, Fine, & Grbic, 1993) and is determined by visual inspection, single measurements of probing depths, and evaluating radiographs for bone loss.

Periodontal disease activity, which is different from periodontal disease severity, is defined as the current or ongoing (at the time of the examination) loss of soft-tissue attachment, specifically destruction of the gingival fibers and apical migration of the junctional epithelium with subsequent alveolar bone loss. Periodontal disease activity is usually seen as episodic periods of exacerbation or active periodontal tissue destruction (loss of connective tissue attachment and alveolar bone) with intervening periods of quiescence or disease inactivity (Greenstein & Caton, 1990; Jeffcoat, 1994; Lamster et al., 1993). Periodontal disease activity is difficult to determine because it is a measurement of the continued breakdown of periodontal pockets between two points in time (separated by several weeks to months). Destruction must have occurred at some time between these two measurements.

While periodontal probing and radiographic assessment are retrospective views of disease activity and cannot identify an active disease site from an inactive one (nor accurately predict future destruction), they are still the foundation on which the classification of the disease and its treatment is made (Haffajee, Socransky, & Goodson, 1983). The clinical importance of distinguishing between a progressive or active periodontal lesion and a stable or inactive lesion is apparent. Therefore, more sophisticated techniques and assessments have been introduced recently that are designed to determine current periodontal disease activity and/or if a site will break down in the future (Williams, Beck, & Offenbacher, 1996). For a review of these adjunctive assessment tests, see Chapter 18.

PERIODONTAL TERMINOLOGY

Periodontal Probing Depths

Screening Method

Periodontal probing is the most commonly used physical screening method for measuring the depth of the gingival crevice and the **clinical attachment level.** Periodontal probing is a clinical approximation of the depth of a gingival sulcus or periodontal pocket (Armitage, 1995). Measurement of probing depths allows the practitioner to make certain presumptions about the state of health of the periodontium. Periodontal pockets are the result of the destruction of the coronal part of the junctional epithelium and the connective tissue attachment to the tooth surface at the apical aspect of the junctional epithelium (Figure 16–1 ■). The clinical significance of having pockets greater than 5 mm in depth is that such pockets may be difficult or impossible for the dental team to maintain in a state of health even with a patient's best oral hygiene self-care efforts and frequent professional cleanings.

Clinically, probing depth is defined as the distance from the gingival margin to the most apical extent of the probe or where physical resistance of the probe is met.

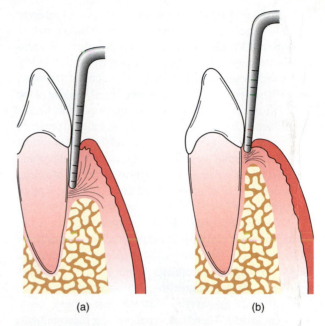

■ **FIGURE 16–1**   Probing depth measurement. (a) Deep pocket with apical migration of the junctional epithelium and bone loss. Probing depth is 6 mm. (b) Shallow probing depth (2 mm). There is no attachment loss or bone loss.

This approximates the level of soft tissue attachment (junctional epithelium) to the tooth. In healthy gingiva the free gingival margin is approximately 0.5 to 2 mm coronal to the cementoenamel junction (CEJ).

It should be noted that here we are using the term probing depth rather than pocket depth because what is being probed could be a pocket or a sulcus. This text will continue to use the term probing depth unless otherwise indicated.

Limitations of Probing   In health, the apical extent of the periodontal probe routinely penetrates the coronal to middle portion of the junctional epithelium (Listgarten, Mao, & Robinson, 1976; Robinson & Vitaek, 1979; Spray, Garnick, Doles, & Klawitter, 1978). When the gingiva is inflamed, the probe can transverse the junctional epithelium to deeper levels within the tissue. It can stop at, enter, or go through the lamina propria to the alveolar bone crest. Thus this measurement may be greater than the actual tissue destruction. Therefore, the clinical probing depth noted may be greater than the histologic probing depth due to probe penetration of inflamed tissue (Armitage, Svanberg, & Löe, 1977).

Probing depth measurements have several inherent limitations besides the degree of gingival inflammation (Robinson & Vitaek, 1979). The apical extent of probe penetration depends on the force used to probe (van der Velden, 1979), variations in placement and angulation of the probe, the site being probed, the type of probe used, the size of the probe (Keagle et al., 1989), and tooth anatomy. Other factors that influence the accuracy of probing include the presence of calculus, the visibility of the area, and the level of patient sensitivity. Despite these limitations, periodontal probing remains the most accurate and widely used method of assessing periodontal destruction. When done carefully, a probing difference of 2 mm or more can be clinically meaningful.

Disease Progression   Periodontal probing is important in determining past periodontal disease activity and is used to evaluate the results of periodontal treatment. Single probing measurements do not adequately reflect periodontal disease progression; they only signify past disease activity or the severity of attachment or bone loss at one point in time. Therefore, serial probing measurements must be done (e.g., at periodontal maintenance visits) and compared with previous measurements to determine whether the disease is progressing (Jeffcoat, 1994).

Probing depth measurements therefore are good for identifying areas that are potential therapeutic problems on a site-by-site basis (Armitage, 1995) and to determine the type of treatment needed. However, in longitudinal monitoring (e.g., at periodontal maintenance visits) for disease progression, probing depths are not reliable in determining the amount of detachment of the soft tissues from the root surface because the gingival margin may change its position over time due to gingival recession or gingival enlargement. This was first described in 1961 by Garguilo, Wentz, and Orban (Figure 16–2 ■).

Level of Attachment

Clinical attachment level (CAL) is the distance from the CEJ to the most apical extent of the periodontal probe or where resistance is met. Clinical attachment level is a clinical approximation of the loss of connective tissue attachment from the root surface (Armitage, 1996). Measuring the level of attachment of the base of the pocket on the tooth surface gives a better indication of the severity of periodontal disease.

Since the position of the gingival margin changes over time, probing depth measurements are not reliable for determining the extent of detachment of soft tissue from the root surfaces. Measurement of the clinical attachment level is the reference method used to establish

disease progression. The CEJ is a stable reference point that does not move over time. If the stationary point used is a part of the tooth other than the CEJ (e.g., cusp tip or restoration), the term used is relative attachment level. Although probing depth measurements are considered to be less valid for monitoring disease progression, they still should be considered as a clinical measure (Carlos, Brunelle, & Wolfe, 1987; Reddy, 1997).

When performing a periodontal charting, it is advisable to measure probing depths and to record the location of the free gingival margin. Future comparisons can then determine disease activity. In addition, the position of the gingival margin relative to the CEJ should be drawn on the chart.

Connective Tissue Attachment Loss   Attachment level measurements determine the amount of attachment loss if it has occurred on a tooth. **Attachment loss** is defined as the pathologic detachment of the gingival collagen fibers from the root surface with the concomitant apical migration of the junctional epithelium along the root surface. Supporting and alveolar bone resorption also occurs as a result of the inflammatory events, but is a consequence of the attachment loss.

A significant increase in CALs is the gold standard for measurement of periodontal disease activity or a site that is actively losing connective tissue attachment at a given site (Goodson, 1986). Currently, a change in clinical attachment level of between 2 and 3 mm, measured at different examination visits, must occur before a site can be labeled disease-active (with attachment loss). Clinical attachment level measurements are important because over time it will determine if a site has experienced further connective tissue attachment loss or gain.

Individuals who have extensive attachment loss also may have gingival recession, but if they have shallow probing depths and no bleeding, they are considered to have a healthy periodontium and not periodontitis at that point in time. Such patients could have been treated successfully and the disease progression stopped, or they may be in remission with no disease activity present.

Other Uses of the Periodontal Probe

The periodontal probe can be used not only to determine the level of the soft tissue attachment to a tooth but also to establish the presence of bleeding, the location of the mucogingival junction, the amount of gingival recession, the width of keratinized/attached gingiva, and the consistency of the gingiva.

A. Sulcus depth
B. Attached epithelium
C. Apical point of
   epithelial attachment
   below cementoenamel
   junction
D. Bottom of sulcus from
   cementoenamel
   junction
E. Cementoenamel
   junction to alveolar
   bone
F. Deepest point of
   epithelial attachment
   to alveolar bone

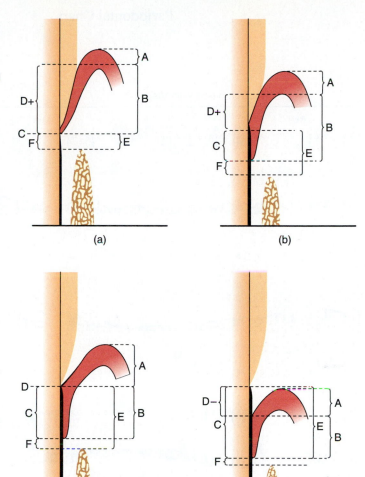

(a)   (b)   (c)   (d)

■ **FIGURE 16–2**   Schematic illustrations showing the different positions of the gingival margin. (a) Periodontal health. (b–d) The junctional epithelium has migrated onto the root surface.

─ **Did You Know?** ─────────

There are many types of periodontal probes with different calibration. For example, the Michigan O probe with William markings goes up to 10 mm; the North Carolina probe has markings up to 15 mm. Try different probes and choose the probe you like.

Controlled-Force Probes

Within the past decade, automated pressure-sensitive or controlled-force probes have been developed that provide a fixed 20 to 25g probing force in order to reduce examiner error and to make changes of less than 2 mm clinically meaningful. Examples of these probes include the Florida probe (Florida Probe® Corporation, Gainesville, FL) and the Interprobe™ (The Dental Probe Inc., Richmond, VA). Most such probes are connected to a computer for storage of data (see Figure 16–3 ■). Automated recording of the CEJ also has been developed.

With automated probing, the loss of tactile sense inherent in manual probing has been shown to increase rather than decrease probing errors. This is especially true in probing the patient with untreated periodontitis in whom subgingival calculus deposits are present. In the treated patient, controlled-force probing has been shown

■ **FIGURE 16–3**   (a) Example of a periodontal chart generated from a controlled-force probe. (Courtesy of Florida Probe Corporation, Gainesville, FL, www.floridaprobe.com)

Chart #:
Name:
Examiner:
Examination Date:

FLORIDA PROBE

Tests Performed: ☒Recession   ☒Probing,Bleeding,Suppuration
☒Furcation   ☒Plaque   ☒Mobility

Tooth #	DB	B	MB	ML	L	DL	
1	2.8 B	2.4 R=2 F=1 P	2.4	1.4 F=0	1.6 R=3	2 B F=0	M=1
2	2.2	1.6 R=1 F=0	1.6 P	3.8 F=0	2.2 B R=3 P	2.6 F=0	M=1
3	2 P	1.4 R=1 F=0	2.4 B P	2.4 BS F=0	2 R=2	2.4 F=0	M=0
4	2.8 P	2.6 R=0	1.4	1.8	2.6 R=1	2	M=0
5	2 B F=0 P	3 R=1	1.6 F=0	2.2	1.8 R=1	2.6	M=0
6	2.4	1.0 R=0	2	2.8	2.4 R=0 P	2.8 B	M=0
7	2.4	1.4 R=0	2.4	1	0.4 R=0.0	0.8	M=0
8	0.8	0.8 R=0	1.4	1.4	1.4 R=0.0	1	M=0

Tooth #	MB	B	DB	DL	L	ML	
9	1	2.2 R=0	2	0.8	0.8 R=0.0	1	M=0
10	1.4	1 R=0	1	0.6	0.4 R=1	0.6	M=0
11	2.6	2.4 B R=1 P	2.2 P	1.2	2.8 R=1	2.4	M=0
12	1 F=0 P	2.6 R=1	1.2 BS F=0 P	2.8	2.2 R=2 P	2.4	M=0
13							
14	1.2	2.6 R=1 F=0	2.4	3.2 B F=0	2.2 S R=1 P	1.4 S F=0	M=0
15	2.6	2 R=2 F=0	2 B P	2 BS F=0	1.6 S R=2 P	1.8 F=0	M=0
16	3	2.6 R=2 F=0	4.8 S P	2.2 B F=0	2.6 R=2 P	2.4 F=0	M=1
17	2.6	2.6 R=2 F=0 P	4 P	3.4	2.4 B R=2 F=0 P	2	M=1
18	1.2	0.6 F=0 P	1.6 BS P	1.6	0.6 R=2 F=0 P	1	M=0
19	1.4	1.2 R=2 F=1	2.0	2.8 S	3.2 R=2 F=0 P	2.2 B	M=0
20	0.6 P	1.6 R=2	1.4 B	1.8	2.4 R=1	2.2	M=0
21	1.0 P	1.2 R=2	1	2	2.4 R=1	2.0	M=0
22	2.2	1.4 B R=0	0.6	1	1.4 R=0	2	M=0
23	0.8	1.6 R=0	0.8	1	1 R=0.0	0.6	M=0
24	0.4	1.6 R=0	1.8	1	1 R=0.0	1.8	M=0

Tooth #	DB	B	MB	ML	L	DL	
25	1	0.8 R=0.0	0.8	2	2 R=0	2.6	M=0
26	1.6	1.2 R=0.0	0.6	0.8 B	2.2 R=1	1.4	M=0
27	1 P	1 R=2	0.8	2.2	1.2 R=2	1.8	M=0
28	4.6	2.6 S R=0	2	2.6	2.8 R=2 P	2.8	M=0
29	1.2	1.2 R=1	1.8	2	1.6 BS R=2	2.6	M=0
30							
31	2.0 P	3 S R=2 F=1 P	2.4 BS	2.6	2.6 R=1 F=0	2.4	M=1
32	1.6 B	2.0 R=2 F=0 P	2.6	1.6	0.4 R=1 F=0	2.2	M=1

Plaque Index Scores

All surfaces:	26%
Molar:	45%
Inter-proximal:	26%
Buccal Lingual:	26%
Buccal:	20%
Lingual:	33%

Probing Summary

30 Teeth   22 Bleeding sites   13 Suppurating
11 sites progressing deeper by at least 1mm.
5 moderate sites with 2 progressing deeper by at least 1mm.
0 severe sites with 0 progressing deeper by at least 1mm.
3 furcations were found.
6 teeth were found to have some degree of mobility.

■ **FIGURE 16–3**   (b) Example of a periodontal chart generated from a controlled-force probe. (Courtesy of Florida Probe Corporation, Gainesville, FL, www.floridaprobe.com)

to be more accurate in some studies but not in others (Armitage, 1996).

Although the Florida probe has been used in a number of research studies to reduce the interexaminer error, and the Interprobe was designed for routine clinical practice, their use has not been widely accepted. The automated probing examination may be more time consuming when compared with manual probing with no clear advantage of increased accuracy. It seems likely, however, that rapid, accurate, and easy-to-use automated probes will be available in the near future.

Periodontal Screening and Recording

The Periodontal Screening and Recording (PSR) system provides a rapid, 2- to 3-minute periodontal screening examination for detecting and monitoring of periodontal diseases. This system was developed by the American Dental Association and the American Academy of Periodontology with financial support from the Procter & Gamble Company. PSR indicates when a more comprehensive full-mouth periodontal examination should be performed.

The key component of the system is a thin, plastic or metal, ball-end periodontal probe. The ball tip enhances patient comfort and aids in detecting overhanging margins and subgingival calculus. The probe has a colored band extending from 3.5 to 5.5 mm for classifying pocket depth. The mouth is divided into six sextants or sections. Although six sites are probed on each tooth as in a conventional periodontal examination, only the deepest site in each sextant is scored and recorded in the patient's chart. The PSR code score is determined by how much of the colored band is visible when the PSR probe is placed in the gingival crevice.

The following are the codes used:

- Code 0: Colored probe area completely visible; no bleeding; no calculus or roughness
- Code 1: Colored probe area completely visible; bleeding; no calculus or roughness
- Code 2: Colored probe area completely visible; bleeding; calculus and/or roughness
- Code 3: Colored probe area partially visible (4–5 mm depth)
- Code 4: Colored probe area submerged completely (5.5 mm depth)

An asterisk is used to denote a furcation defect, tooth mobility, mucogingival involvement, or soft tissue recession.

The treatment of patients is based on their sextant scores. A code 3 or code 4 indicates that a more comprehensive periodontal examination and charting of the affected sextant is required to determine the treatment. When this system is used in the long-term monitoring of periodontal patients whose deep probing sites are being maintained nonsurgically, recording the tooth number and attachment level alongside the PSR coding box facilitates rapid monitoring of these sites at each periodontal maintenance visit.

EXAMINATION TECHNIQUES
Periodontal Probing Depths

To assess the probing depth, six measurements are recorded for each tooth: three on the facial surface (mesiofacial, facial, distofacial) and three on the lingual surface (mesiolingual, lingual, distolingual). It is best to develop a standardized sequence when probing. For instance, probing should start on the facial tooth surfaces of the maxillary right quadrant, proceeding to the maxillary left quadrant, then to the palatal surfaces of the maxillary right quadrant, then to the maxillary left quadrant, and finally to the mandibular quadrants in the same sequence. The probe is "walked" in approximately 1 mm increments to follow the level of attachment (Figure 16–4 ■). Spot probing is not adequate for a thorough periodontal examination. When a reading is between two millimeter marks on the probe, the higher reading is used.

Most errors occur in interproximal readings. When probing interproximal sites on posterior teeth, the probe is angled slightly so that the tip of the probe reaches the

■ **FIGURE 16–4** Walking the probe around the tooth allows exploration of the morphology of the gingival crevice. (Reprinted with permission of Procter & Gamble, Cincinnati, OH)

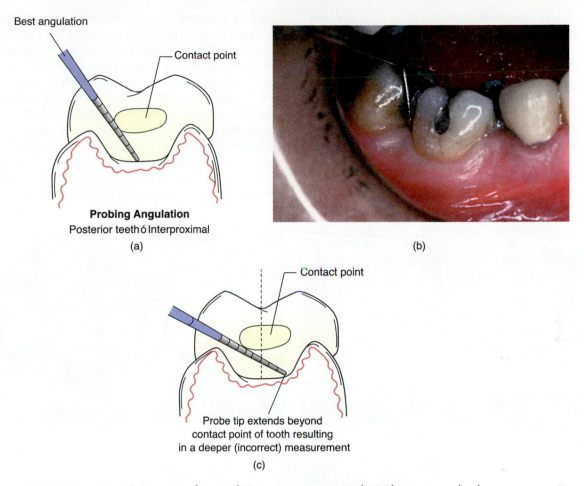

Probing Angulation
Posterior teeth ó Interproximal
(a)

(b)

(c)

■ **FIGURE 16–5**   (a) Correct probe angulation on a posterior tooth. Probe inserts under the contact area into the col. (b) Clinically, the probe is angled to reach the col. (c) Incorrect probe angulation.

col area, just under the contact area of the tooth (Figure 16–5 ■). When probing interproximal sites on anterior teeth, the probe needs to be parallel to the long axis of the tooth but at the same time should be as close to the interproximal area and not at the line angle (Figure 16–6 ■). The probe is parallel to the long axis of all teeth on the facial and lingual surfaces.

Bleeding Sites

In clinical practice, the primary value of bleeding on probing as a diagnostic sign is that its presence indicates that the tissues are inflamed and not healthy (Armitage, 1995). Bleeding points should be recorded on the chart with a small red dot over the probing depth measurement. Bleeding on probing indicates inflammation in the deeper tissues, whereas bleeding or stroking the gingival crevice indicates gingivitis. Sites that bleed with deep

■ **FIGURE 16–6**   Correct probe placement on an anterior tooth. Probe is not angled, but it must reach interproximally with the shank against the teeth.

pockets and clinical attachment loss are at greater risk for future tissue destruction and should be monitored (Lang, Joss, & Nyman, 1990; Lang & Löe, 1993). Sites that do not bleed on probing are likely not breaking down.

Clinical Attachment Level

The CAL must take into account the probing depth and location of the gingival margin. To assess the CALs, two measurements are needed: probing depth and the distance of the gingival margin from the CEJ at each of the six sites around the tooth. If gingival recession is present (Figure 16–7a ■), the CAL is determined by adding the gingival recession value and the probing depth. If there is gingival overgrowth or a pseudopocket (see Figure 16–7b), the CAL is determined by subtracting the amount of gingiva (in millimeters) coronal to the CEJ from the probing depth. If the free gingival margin is located at the CEJ (see Figure 16–7c), the CAL is equal to the probing depth. There is more tissue destruction or loss of attachment when gingival recession is present. When the attachment loss is 5 mm or greater with deep periodontal pockets, the patient should be referred to a specialist.

Another method to determine the CAL is to give a negative number to the amount of recession and then sub-

(a)

(b)

(c)

■ **FIGURE 16–7** Probing depth versus clinical attachment level. Probing depth is the distance from the free gingival margin to the attached gingival tissues. Clinical attachment level is the distance from the CEJ to the attached gingival tissues. When the free gingival margin is apical to the CEJ (a), add the amount of recession to the probing depth (3 mm + probing depth [2 mm] = 5 mm clinical attachment level). When the free gingival margin is coronal to the CEJ (b), the distance to the CEJ is measured and subtracted from the probing depth (5 mm probing depth – 2 mm gingival enlargement = 3 mm clinical attachment level). (c) When the free gingival margin is at the CEJ, the probing depth equals the clinical attachment level (2 mm probing depth = 2 mm clinical attachment level).

tract it from the probing depth. A positive number is given to the amount of gingival overgrowth and then subtracted from the probing depth.

Repeated measurements, when done in this manner, have been shown in numerous studies to be reproducible to within 61 mm 90% of the time and within 62 mm 99% of the time (Armitage, 1996). Attachment loss of more than 2 mm has become the gold standard for the assessment of periodontal disease progression (Armitage, 1996). This change is necessary to take into consideration the inherent errors, as mentioned earlier, in periodontal probing.

A patient has clinical attachment loss when there is periodontitis with apical migration of the junctional epithelium (Bouchard, Boutouyrie, Mattout, & Bourgeois, 2006; López, Fernández, Jara, & Baelum, 2001). Determination of attachment loss is part of the calculation of clinical attachment levels.

Rapid Dental Hint

When doing a periodontal charting, a good way to monitor CAL on your patient is to write the amount of gingival recession on the root of the tooth. You can easily read the probing depth and then calculate the CAL. This will then determine if there is any attachment loss.

Gingival Position

In health, the free gingival margin is located approximately 0.5 to 2 mm coronal to the CEJ. **Gingival recession** is defined as a shift in the gingival margin apical to the CEJ with exposure of the root surface to the oral environment. Actually, since the soft tissue margin may not always be composed of gingiva, the term soft tissue recession rather than gingival recession may be more appropriate. However, since this is currently not universally accepted, this text will continue to use gingival recession (Wennström, 1996). Gingival recession may be localized to one tooth or generalized throughout the mouth. Usually, the facial surface is involved, but all other tooth surfaces could be involved as well.

Measurement of Gingival Recession

Visible recession, which is seen clinically, is measured from the CEJ to the gingival margin and represents the apparent position of the gingiva. Hidden recession, which

is covered by the gingiva and therefore not visible, can only be measured by placing a periodontal probe at the level of attachment. This represents the actual position of the gingiva or the level of soft tissue attachment (junctional epithelium) to the tooth surface (Figure 16–8 ■). The visible recession added to the hidden recession equals the clinical attachment level. The clinical importance of measuring recession is often overlooked. There can be loss of attachment or gingival recession without a corresponding increase in probing depth. This often can be misleading, and it could be assumed that there is no tissue destruction occurring when actually there is.

Etiology of Gingival Recession

The principal predisposing factor that determines whether recession occurs is the anatomy of the area, specifically the thickness of the alveolar bone and overlying gingiva. The etiology of gingival recession is multifactoral. Etiologic factors include the following:

1. Mechanical trauma: soft tissue trauma from overzealous toothbrushing (Figure 16–9 ■).
2. Orthodontic movement.
3. Dental procedures.
4. Crown margins.
5. Clasps from partial dentures.
6. Destructive inflammatory periodontal disease, where there is loss of attachment (destruction of gingival fibers and apical migration of the junctional epithelium; Figure 16–10 ■).
7. Tooth malposition (rotated, lingually or facially displaced teeth), where the alveolar bone over a prominent root such as a maxillary canine is thin or absent.
8. Periodontal therapy (periodontal debridement or surgery), where tissue shrinkage has occurred.
9. Oral habits causing injury to the gingiva, such as fingernail biting.
10. Anatomic variations that may accelerate gingival recession include a high frenum attachment pulling the free gingival margin (Figure 16–11 ■).
11. Occlusal trauma (this has been suggested to cause gingival recession but has not been demonstrated).
12. Cigarette smoking and chewing tobacco (Figure 16–12 ■), but the exact mechanism has not been elucidated (Gunsolley et al., 1998).

It is imperative that the cause be determined in individual cases so that the progressive nature of the recession can be controlled and interceptive therapy initiated

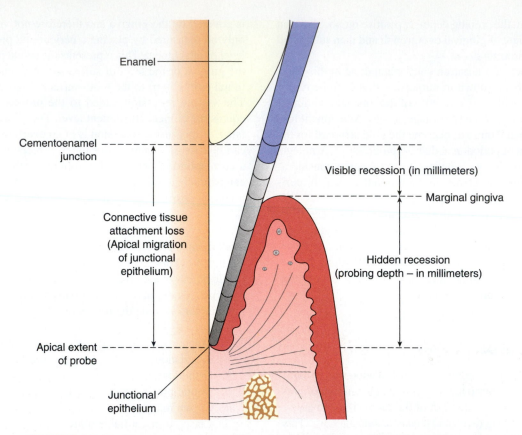

Enamel

Cementoenamel junction

Connective tissue attachment loss (Apical migration of junctional epithelium)

Visible recession (in millimeters)

Marginal gingiva

Hidden recession (probing depth – in millimeters)

Apical extent of probe

Junctional epithelium

■ **FIGURE 16–8** Diagram showing visible and hidden recession. Clinically, visible recession is determined by measuring with a periodontal probe from the CEJ to the free gingival margin. Hidden recession corresponds to the probing depth. The visible recession measurement added to the hidden recession measurement equals the clinical attachment level (CAL).

■ **FIGURE 16–9** Generalized gingival recession due to overzealous tooth brushing.

■ **FIGURE 16–10** Gingival recession in a refractory periodontitis patient. Note the presence of inflammation. Gingival recession is due to the disease process.

■ **FIGURE 16–11**   Recession on the mandibular incisors caused by the high frenum attachment pulling on the free gingival margin. Note the heavy accumulation of plaque and calculus.

■ **FIGURE 16–12**   A 55-year-old man who placed chewing tobacco in the facial vestibule of the anterior teeth. Note the gingival recession on the anterior teeth.

if necessary. Gingival recession can be seen in healthy gingiva; inflammation may or may not be present. The association with age does not necessarily suggest a physiologic effect of aging on recession. It may just reflect the fact that older people have been subject to the force of brushing for longer periods of time (Joshipura, Kent, & DePaola, 1994).

Rapid Dental Hint

Gingival recession should be documented on the periodontal chart. The cause of the recession must be determined to offer the appropriate treatment.

Clinical Significance of Gingival Recession

Identification of gingival recession has clinical significance. Root surfaces exposed to the oral environment are more vulnerable to the development of root caries. The thin layer of cementum on the exposed root surface may wear away easily, exposing the underlying dental tubules to the oral environment. Fluid in the exposed dentinal tubules contracts or expands when an external stimulus such as cold or touch is applied. This may stimulate nerves to produce pain. In addition, the col shape changes when gingival recession is present. If the interdental area is open so that no col exists, the facial and palatal gingiva become continuous and keratinized. Thus interproximal recession may create areas of food impaction.

Pathogenesis

The pathogenesis of gingival recession is debatable. As mentioned earlier, it has been considered perhaps to be a normal physiologic process that occurs with increasing age, but there is limited documentation to uphold this concept. Others consider it to be a pathologic condition. When the free gingiva is thin, the inflammatory lesion will occupy and degrade the entire connective tissue portion, resulting in collapse of the free gingiva (Wennström, 1994). If there is less than 1 mm or more of attached gingiva, the free gingival margin may be movable, which allows microorganisms to enter into the crevice, initiating an inflammatory response.

The amount of attached gingiva needed for gingival health is controversial. Experimental studies (Wennström & Lindhe, 1983a, 1983b) have failed to consistently support the concept of a minimal width of gingiva for maintenance of periodontal health.

Mucogingival Considerations

A mucogingival involvement or defect is defined as a discrepancy in the relationship between the free gingival margin and the mucogingival junction. Pathology or loss of attachment may not be involved. Common mucogingival conditions may be the result of

- Gingival recession, resulting in inadequate or diminished attached gingiva.
- Probing depths extending to or beyond the mucogingival junction into the alveolar mucosa (Figure 16–13 ■).
- Anatomical variations that may complicate the management of these conditions, including a high frenum attachment pulling the gingival margin away from the tooth surface (surgical intervention may be necessary to augment the amount of attached gingiva and correct the mucogingival problem).

Mucogingival Examination

A thorough mucogingival examination using appropriate screening techniques and recording the free gingival margin and mucogingival junction on the chart is necessary to detect these conditions. This also enables the practitioner to monitor the progressive nature at future periodontal maintenance visits so that appropriate treatment can be rendered. While radiographs are not used in the identification of mucogingival problems, appropriate radiographs may be used as part of a preoperative appraisal.

Recording the free gingival margin on the chart will identify the presence or absence of gingival recession or overgrowth. Recession on all six tooth surfaces should be recorded. It is important to measure the amount of recession (in millimeters) because it provides information for determining total attachment loss.

The next step in the mucogingival examination is to determine the total width or height of keratinized gingiva. The width of keratinized gingiva is determined by measuring with a periodontal probe the distance from the gingival margin to the mucogingival junction. The width of attached gingiva is determined by subtracting the probing depth (free gingiva) from the amount of keratinized gingiva (Figure 16–14 ■). Mucogingival involvement exists when no attached gingiva is present on a tooth. To establish the position of the mucogingival junction, move the side of the periodontal probe gently across the alveolar mucosa in an apical-coronal direction until the tissue stops moving (Figure 16–15 ■). At this point, elastic fibers are not present, and attached gingiva is coronal to the mucogingival junction. Other methods include the visual method. The problem with this technique is that with inflammation, the gingiva is red, and it will be difficult to differentiate between the red alveolar mucosa and the gingiva. Another method is to pull the lip outward, and the mucogingival junction is seen at the point of tension. This is sometimes misleading, and the actual location of the mucogingival junction is not always distinguished.

To determine if any frenal attachments are encroaching on the gingival margin, retract the cheeks and

■ **FIGURE 16–14** (*Left probe*) Determination of the amount of gingiva (free + attached) by measuring from the free gingival margin to the mucogingival junction. (*Right probe*) Determination of the amount of attached gingiva by subtracting the probing depth (right probe measurement) from the total width of gingiva (left probe measurement).

■ **FIGURE 16–13** There is no attached gingiva present on this tooth. This is a mucogingival defect.

■ **FIGURE 16–15**   The periodontal probe is gently placed on the alveolar mucosa and moved coronally until the tissue does not move. This is the mucogingival junction.

lips laterally by pulling with the thumb and index finger, and watch for movement of the gingival margin in the frenal attachment area.

> ┌─ **Did You Know?** ───────
>
> The alveolar mucosa is more movable than the attached/free gingiva because it contains loose connective tissue.

Delayed Passive Eruption

Delayed passive eruption occurs in adults when the free gingival margin failed to migrate apically toward the CEJ and still remains on or near the cervical bulge of the enamel, creating a "gummy smile" (Figure 16–16 ■). This condition is also seen in children up to the time of completed eruption of permanent teeth. This is a normal situation, and the process of passive eruption ultimately will move the free gingival margin apically.

RDH Rapid Dental Hint

Patients with "gummy smiles" should be evaluated for delayed passive eruption.

Suppuration

Suppuration, also referred to as purulent exudate or pus, is a clinical feature of inflammation. Pus is composed

■ **FIGURE 16–16**   A 40-year-old patient exhibiting delayed passive eruption. Note that the gingival margin is located on the cervical bulge of the enamel.

of dead cells, polymorphonuclear leukocytes (PMNs or neutrophils), and tissue fluids. The presence of suppuration indicates an ongoing infection in the periodontal pocket. Pus can be detected visually coming from the pocket by either probing the gingival crevice or using digital pressure from the base of the crevice on the outer surface of the gingiva moving in a coronal direction (Figure 16–17 ■).

Tooth Mobility

Tooth mobility is classified as either physiologic or pathologic. Physiologic movement of a tooth is limited to the width of the periodontal ligament space. All teeth have some degree of physiologic mobility that occurs

■ **FIGURE 16–17**   Suppuration detected from the maxillary central incisors. Deep probing depths were noted.

with normal function. The range of physiologic mobility varies according to the time of the day and the tooth. It is most evident on teeth with short roots, such as mandibular incisors, and early in the morning. Increased tooth mobility in the hours just after awakening is due to slight extrusion of the tooth as a result of limited occlusal contact during sleep.

Pathologic mobility of teeth results from bone loss, gingival inflammation, periapical pathology, hormonal imbalance (e.g., pregnancy gingivitis), or occlusal trauma, where excessive occlusal forces are placed on a tooth. Periodontal disease can be advanced without any evidence of increased tooth mobility. Therefore, the severity of tooth mobility is not always due to the amount of bone loss. Since tooth mobility may not result from periodontal problems, identification of the cause is important so that the appropriate treatment can be rendered.

Measurement of Tooth Mobility

The degree of mobility can be measured either manually or with electronic devices. Although the most common classification for measuring pathologic tooth mobility is the Miller classification, it remains very subjective. Mobility is assessed by using the handles of two hand instruments on the facial and lingual aspects of the crown and applying force. The Miller classification is summarized in Box 16–1 (Miller, 1950). Mobility requires treatment when the patient feels discomfort or when the mobility increases over time.

Box 16–1 Classification of Pathologic Mobility (Miller's Classification)

1 First distinguishable sign of tooth movement greater than normal in a facial/lingual direction
2 Movement of the tooth in a facial/lingual direction up to 1 mm
3 Movement of the tooth in a facial/lingual direction more than 1 mm and/or depressed in a vertical direction

The amount of fremitus is subjective, but the following guide can be used:
+ (slight vibrations can be felt);
++ (obvious, palpable vibrations can be felt, but movement of the tooth is barely visible); or
+++ (visible movement is seen).

Rapid Dental Hint

When you detect mobility on a tooth, the next step is to determine the cause. Without knowing the cause, you cannot effectively treat the patient.

Fremitus

Fremitus is the vibrational movement of a tooth under occlusal forces. Fremitus is determined by gently placing the index finger on the facial surfaces of the maxillary teeth while instructing the patient to tap the teeth together and grind them side to side. Only the maxillary teeth are checked for fremitus because the arch is fixed whereas the mandibular arch is moving.

Fremitus should be eliminated by occlusal adjustment by means of, say, selective grinding.

Did You Know?

You can only check for fremitus on the maxilla because it is a fixed structure. The mandible moves.

Pathologic Tooth Migration

Pathologic tooth migration is defined as the movement of teeth due to the disruption of forces that normally maintain physiologic tooth position. Tooth movement can occur in any direction. Clinically, this may be seen as increased spacing between teeth, dramatic overjet of anterior teeth (anterior flaring), rotation of teeth, or extrusion where tooth migration occurs in an occlusal or incisal direction (Figure 16–18 ■). Usually, tooth mobility is also present. Any of these symptoms is a common chief complaint of a patient that may prompt a professional evaluation. As part of the clinical examination, it is important to ask the patient if spaces between the teeth have increased over time or if they have always been present. It is important to recognize signs and symptoms of pathologic migration and determine the cause of the problem in order to render appropriate treatment.

Periodontal disease destruction of the attachment apparatus plays a major role in the etiology of pathologic migration (Towfighi et al., 1997). Other contributing factors include parafunctional habits such as tongue thrusting or bruxism, teeth adjacent to edentulous areas, and drug-induced gingival enlargement.

■ **FIGURE 16–18** Pathologic tooth migration in a 26-year-old woman with rapidly progressive periodontitis. The patient complained of flaring and increasing space between the maxillary central incisors.

Furcation Involvement

A furcation or furca is the area of root division on multirooted teeth, including the maxillary first and second molars, maxillary first premolar, and mandibular first and second molars. The third molars usually have fused conical roots. Since the maxillary molars have three roots (mesiobuccal, distofacial, palatal), they are trifurcated. There are three furcation entrances: mesial, distal, and buccal. The mandibular molars are bifurcated; that is, they have two roots (mesial and distal). There are two

■ **FIGURE 16–19** Surgical flap reflection shows a furcation defect on the maxillary first premolar. Fluting of the root is evident also.

furcation entrances: buccal and lingual. The maxillary first premolar is also bifurcated, having a buccal and lingual root (Figure 16–19 ■). There are two furcation entrances: mesial and distal.

Furcation involvement occurs when interradicular bone (bone between the root branches of the same tooth) destruction occurs. Furcation involvement is affected by factors such as the length of the root trunk and the presence of root concavities, which create a plaque trap. The root trunk is the area on the tooth from the CEJ to the roof or entrance of the furca (Figure 16–20 ■). As seen radiographically, high furcation with a short root trunk will have a greater chance of interradicular bone destruction early in the disease

Root trunk

Roof of furca

(a)

(b)

■ **FIGURE 16–20** (a) Dry-skull specimen of a furcation involvement on the mandibular molars. Root trunk length is the distance from the CEJ to the entrance (roof) of the furca. (b) Flap is reflected during surgery. There is bone loss around the molar but the furcation is intact without bone loss.

process than a low furcation with a long root trunk. The average root trunk length on a maxillary molar is about 4 mm at the mesial, 5 mm at the distal, and 4 mm at the buccal furcation. The root trunk length of the mandibular molar is 3 mm on the buccal aspect and 4 mm on the lingual aspect (Dunlap & Gher, 1985; Gher & Dunlap, 1985). This suggests that a minimum of 5 mm of attachment loss on a molar may result in early furcation involvement.

Rapid Dental Hint

Observe your patient as he or she talks to you. If you notice the maxillary incisors are spaced apart, and/or there is an extreme overjet (buck teeth), and/or the teeth are supraerupted, ask the patient if he or she noticed these signs previously. The patient who presents with these symptoms most likely has advanced bone loss.

Classification of Furcation Involvement

The clinical detection of furcation involvements is important because it is difficult for both the patient and the dental hygienist to effectively clean these areas. Radiographic interpretation does not allow sufficient detection of furcation involvement. The anatomy of the tooth and location of the furca are determined from both the radiograph and clinical examination. The pattern of interradicular bone loss is both horizontal and vertical. Although many classifications of horizontal furcation involvement have been suggested, Glickman's classification is described in Table 16–1 ■. Classification of vertical bone loss (Tarnow & Fletcher, 1984) is described in Figure 16–21 ■.

Table 16–1   Glickman's Classification of Furcation Involvement (Horizontal Pattern of Bone Destruction)

Source: From Carranza, F. A., and H. H. Takei. 1996. Treatment of furcation involvement and combined periodontal-endodontic therapy. In eds. F. A. Carranza and M. G. Newman, *Clinical periodontology,* 640. Philadelphia: W. B. Saunders. Illustrations courtesy of James A. Simonds, D.D.S., Copyright 1991 Practical Periodontics. Continental Education. Santa Rosa, CA.

Root trunk

Grade A 1–3 mm

Grade B 4–6 mm

Grade C 7 mm +

■ **FIGURE 16–21** Schematic drawing of a mandibular molar demonstrating the vertical classification of furcation involvement. The amount of vertical bone loss is determined from the roof of the furca apically.

Rapid Dental Hint

Do not forget that the maxillary first premolar has furcas. When there is furcation involvement, that tooth most likely does not have a good prognosis because it has a long root trunk.

Technique for Locating Furcation Involvements

A calibrated curved Nabers probe is used to clinically locate the furcation entrances and degree of horizontal pattern of bone destruction (Figure 16–22a ■). In the maxillary molar, the mesial furcation is not centered. The entrance is usually located about two-thirds of the buccal-lingual width toward the palatal aspect of the tooth (see Figure 16–22b). Thus, the mesial furcation is approached from the palatal side. The distal furcation is centered equally from the buccal and palatal aspects of the tooth (in the interproximal area), and thus the Nabers probe can be positioned from either the buccal or palatal side. The instrument handle is placed parallel to the long axis of the tooth. When a furcation defect is found, it is noted in the chart on the involved root. Furcations thus can be classified according to their horizontal and vertical component of bone loss, for example, IIA.

Did You Know?

The Nabers probe was named after a famous periodontist, Claude Nabers.

Cervical Enamel Projections

Cervical enamel projections (CEPs) are extensions of enamel toward and often into the furcation area. This area is thought to be a plaque trap, enhancing plaque accumulation. This area may be more prone to attachment loss because instead of a connective tissue attachment, the periodontal attachment on enamel will be via a junctional

(a)

(b)

■ **FIGURE 16–22** (a) Placement of the Nabers probe in determining the presence of a buccal furcation. Note that the handle is parallel to the occlusal plane. (b) Nabers probe placed to determine the presence of a mesial furcation of a maxillary molar. Note that the handle is parallel to the long axis of the tooth when probing interproximal furcations. (Reprinted with permission from the American Academy of Periodontology. Copyright 1984. Tarnow D., and P. Fletcher. Classification of the vertical componenent of furcation involvement. *J. Periodontol.* 1983;55:283–284.)

epithelium, which may not be as strong (Easly & Drennan, 1969). However, it has been demonstrated that an epithelial attachment may be just as resistant as a connective tissue attachment to inflammatory disease.

Palatogingival Groove

Palatogingival groove is a common developmental anomaly of maxillary incisors. A midpalatal groove usually extends apically into the root surface. Grooves allow for plaque accumulation and may contribute to the pathogenesis of periodontal and endodontic lesions (Figure 16–23 ■). Treatment involves periodontal and endodontic consultations to see the viability of keeping the tooth. (Ballal, Jothi, Bhat, & Bhat, 2007)

DENTAL HYGIENE NOTES

Documentation of clinical findings is done on a periodontal chart. Many types of charts are available. An example of a chart is given in Figure 16–24 ■. It is important to accurately date and record all clinical findings for legal reasons and to permit the comparison of pretreatment measurements with posttreatment values. Documentation includes the medical and dental histories, chief complaint, oral hygiene evaluation (plaque index), and gingival and periodontal evaluations.

Findings from the periodontal examination should be interpreted together with the medical, dental, oral hygiene, gingival, and radiographic assessments. Recording of clinical attachment level is important for long-term monitoring of patients for periodontal destruction.

KEY POINTS

• All new and maintaining patients should receive a periodontal examination.
• Probing depth is measured from the gingival margin to wherever the tip of the probe stops (in the junctional epithelium).
• Clinical attachment level is measured from the CEJ to the apical extent of the probe and is a more accurate long-term measurement for disease progression than probing depths.

SELF-QUIZ

1. Which one of the following reasons explains why measuring the clinical attachment levels (CALs) is a more reliable method for determing clinical attachment loss over time than probing depth measurements? (p. 211)
   a. Less penetration into the junctional epithelium occurs.
   b. Stable reference point is used (e.g., CEJ).
   c. More measuring points are used on the tooth.
   d. Less bleeding occurs at periodontal active sites.
2. Which one of the following instruments is best to measure the amount of horizontal bone loss in a furcation? (p. 227)
   a. Periodontal probe
   b. Nabers probe
   c. No. 11/12 explorer
   d. CH3 explorer

(a)

(b)

■ **FIGURE 16–23**   (a) Palatogingival groove on the maxillary lateral incisor. (b) Probing reveals a deep pocket that is difficult to maintain.

PERIODONTICS RECORD

FILE NO. ☐☐☐☐☐☐

NAME	BIRTHDATE	CLINICIAN	EXAM DATE

CHIEF PERIODONTAL COMPLAINT

ORAL HYGIENE METHODS
Current:

Rx:

HISTORY OF PERIODONTAL ILLNESS

PLAQUE INDEX (P.I.)

Date							
P.I.							

PREVIOUS PERIO (prophylaxis, other perio, inc. dates)

HABIT HISTORY

OCCLUSAL OBSERVATIONS

Arch Rel. (angle):   Overbite: Overjet:

Teeth in fremitus:

C.R. ⟶ C.O.:

C.O. ⟶ P.:

P.:

R.L. working:

    non-working:

L.L. working:

    non-working:

TMD:

RADIOGRAPHIC FINDINGS

B

SOFT TISSUE EXAM

ETIOLOGY

Local Factors:

GINGIVAL EXAM (color, form, density, bleeding on probing, etc.)

Microbiological Findings:

Occlusal Factors:

Systemic Factors:

DIAGNOSIS

TREATMENT PLAN

PRE-TREATMENT PROGNOSIS

SYSTEMIC FACTORS OF IMPORTANCE IN TREATMENT

(Courtesy Department of Oral Biology, School of
Dental Medicine, State University of New York at Buffalo, Buffalo, NY)

■ **FIGURE 16–24** A periodontal charting form that records initial and final probing depths, clinical attachment levels, tooth mobility, bleeding points, furcation involvement, and gingival recession.

PERIODONTAL EXAMINATION

PATIENT'S NAME: _____   DATE: _____

A

■ **FIGURE 16–24** (*cont.*)

3. Which one of the following techniques describes how visible recession is recorded? (p. 220)
   a. Use a periodontal probe to measure from the cementoenamel junction to the free gingival margin.
   b. Use a periodontal probe to measure from the free gingival margin to the base of the pocket.
   c. Use an explorer to determine the location of the cementoenamel junction.
   d. Use an explorer to determine the apical extent of the junctional epithelium.

4. Which one of the following conditions is related to gingival recession? (p. 219)
   a. Grinding and clenching of teeth
   b. Tongue thrusting
   c. Tooth malposition
   d. Mouth breathing

5. Which one of the following is a cause of a mucogingival involvement or defect? (p. 222)
   a. Mouthrinses with a high alcohol content
   b. Brushing with a hard-bristle toothbrush
   c. Inadequate amount or width of attached gingiva
   d. Inadequate amount or width of alveolar mucosa

6. Which of the following teeth with class II furca involvement has the worst prognosis? (pp. 225–226)
   a. Mandibular first molar
   b. Mandibular second molar
   c. Maxillary first premolar
   d. Maxillary first molar

7. Loss of attachment indicates that the (p. 212)
   a. gingival fibers have been detached from the enamel.
   b. periodontal ligament fibers have regenerated.
   c. junctional epithelium has migrated apically along the root.
   d. circular fibers have detached from the root.

8. A mucogingival involvement or defect is defined as a discrepancy in the relationship between the mucogingival junction and the (p. 222)
   a. cementoenamel junction.
   b. free gingival margin.
   c. nonkeratinized epithelium.
   d. junctional epithelium.

9. Which of the following terms describes the current or ongoing (at the time of the examination) loss of soft-tissue attachment? (p. 210)
   a. Periodontal disease activity
   b. Periodontal disease severity
   c. Clinical attachment loss
   d. Furcation involvement

10. Visible recession added to the hidden recession equals the (p. 220)
    a. Clinical attachment level
    b. Relative attachment level
    c. Probing depth
    d. Mucogingival defect

REFERENCES

Armitage, G. C. 1995. Clinical evaluation of periodontal diseases. *Periodontology 2000* 7:39–52.

Armitage, G. C. 1996. Periodontal diseases: Diagnosis. *Ann. Periodontol.* 1:37–215.

Armitage, G. C. 2004. The complete periodontal examination. *Periodontology 2000* 34(1):9–21.

Armitage, G. C., G. K. Svanberg, and H. Löe. 1977. Microscopic evaluation of clinical measurements of connective tissue attachment levels. *J. Clin. Periodontol.* 4:173–190.

Ballal, N.V., V. Jothi, K.S. Bhat, and K.M. Bhat. 2007. Salvaging a tooth with a deep palotogingival groove: An endo-perio treatment—a case report. *Int. Endod. J.* 40(10):808–817.

Bawden, J. W., and G. H. DeFriese. (eds.). 1981. *Planning for dental care on a statewide basis: The North Carolina Dental Manpower Project.* Chapel Hill: The Dental Foundation of North Carolina.

Bouchard, P., P. Boutouyrie, C. Mattout, and D. Bourgeois. 2006. Risk assessment for severe clinical attachment loss in an adult population. *J. Periodontol.* 77(3):479–489.

Brown, L. J., R. C. Oliver, and H. Löe. 1989. Periodontal diseases in the U.S. in 1981: Prevalence, severity, extent, and role in tooth mortality. *J. Periodontol.* 60:363–380.

Carlos, J. P., J. A. Brunelle, and M. D. Wolfe. 1987. Attachment loss versus pocket depth as indicators of periodontal disease: A methodologic note. *J. Periodont. Res.* 22:524–525.

Douglas, C.W. 2006. Risk assessment and management of periodontal disease. *JADA* 137 (suppl. 3):27S–32S.

Dunlap, R. M., and M. E. Gher. 1985. Root surface measurements of the mandibular first molar. *J. Periodontol.* 56:234–238.

Easly, J. R., and G. A. Drennan. 1969. Morphological classification of the furca. *J. Can. Dent. Assoc.* 35:105–107.

Garguilo, A. W., F. M. Wentz, and B. Orban. 1961. Dimensions and relations of the dentogingival junction in humans. *J. Periodontol.* 32:261–267.

Gher, M. E., and R. W. Dunlap. 1985. Linear variation of the root surface area of the maxillary first molar. *J. Periodontol.* 56:39–43.

Goodson, J. M. 1986. Clinical measurements of periodontitis. *J. Clin. Periodontol.* 13:446–455.

Greenstein, G., and J. Caton. 1990. Periodontal disease activity: A critical assessment. *J. Periodontol.* 61:543–552.

Gunsolley, J. C., S. M. Quinn, J. Tew, C. M. Gooss, C. M. Brooks, and H. A. Schenkein. 1998. The effect of smoking on individuals with minimal periodontal destruction. *J. Periodontol.* 69:165–170.

Haffajee, A. D., S. S. Socransky, and J. M. Goodson. 1983. Clinical parameters as predictors of destructive periodontal disease activity. *J. Clin. Periodontol.* 10:257–265.

Jeffcoat, M. K. 1994. Current concepts in periodontal disease testing. *J. Am. Dent. Assoc.* 125:1071–1078.

Joshipura, K. J., R. L. Kent, and P. F. DePaola. 1994. Gingival recession: Intra-oral distribution and associated factors. *J. Periodontol.* 65:864–871.

Keagle, J. G., J. J. Garnick, J. R. Searle, G. E. King, and P. K. Morse. 1989. Gingival resistance to probing forces: I. Determination of optimal probe diameter. *J. Periodontol.* 60:167–171.

Lamster, I. B., R. S. Celenti, H. H. Jans, J. B. Fine, and J. T. Grbic. 1993. Current status of tests for periodontal disease. *Adv. Dent. Res.* 7:182–190.

Lang, N. P., A. R. Joss, and S. Nyman. 1990. Absence of bleeding on probing: An indicator of periodontal stability. *J. Clin. Periodontol.* 17:714–721.

Lang, N. P., and H. Löe. 1993. Clinical management of periodontal diseases. *Periodontology 2000* 2:128–139.

Listgarten, M. A., R. Mao, and P. J. Robinson. 1976. Periodontal probing and the relationship of the probe tip to periodontal tissues. *J. Periodontol.* 47:511–513.

López, R., O. Fernández, G. Jara, and V. Baelum. 2001. Epidemiology of clinical attachment loss in adolescents. *J. Periodontol.* 72(12):1666–1674.

McFall, W. T., Jr., J. D. Bader, G. R. Rozier, and D. Ramsey. 1988. Presence of periodontal data in patient records of general practitioners. *J. Periodontol.* 59:445–449.

Miller, S. C. 1950. *Textbook of periodontia,* 3rd ed., 125. Philadelphia: Blakiston.

Reddy, M. S. 1997. The use of periodontal probes and radiographs in clinical trials of diagnostic tests. *Ann. Periodontol.* 2:113–122.

Robinson, P. J., and R. M. Vitaek. 1979. The relationship between gingival inflammation and resistance to probe penetration. *J. Periodont. Res.* 14:230–243.

Spray, J. R., J. J. Garnick, L. R. Doles, and J. J. Klawitter. 1978. Microscopic demonstration of the position of periodontal probes. *J. Periodontol.* 49:148–152.

Tarnow, D., and P. Fletcher. 1984. Classification of the vertical component of furcation involvement. *J. Periodontol.* 55:283–284.

Towfighi, P. P., M. A. Brunsvold, A. T. Storey, R. M. Arnold, D. E. Willman, and C. A. McMahan. 1997. Pathologic migration of anterior teeth in patients with moderate to severe periodontitis. *J. Periodontol.* 68:967–972.

van der Velden, U. 1979. Probing force and the relationship of the probe tip to the periodontal tissues. *J. Clin. Periodontol.* 6:106–114.

Wennström, J. L. 1994. Mucogingival surgery. In eds. N. P. Lang and T. Karring, *Proceedings of the 1st European Workshop on Periodontology,* 193–199. London: Quintessence.

Wennström, J. L. 1996. Mucogingival therapy. *Ann. Periodontol.* 1:671–701.

Wennström, J. L., and J. Lindhe. 1983a. Plaque-induced gingival inflammation in the absence of attached gingiva in dogs. *J. Clin. Periodontol.* 10:266–276.

Wennström, J. L., and J. Lindhe. 1983b. The role of attached gingiva for maintenance of periodontal health: Healing following excisional and grafting procedures in dogs. *J. Clin. Periodontol.* 10:206–221.

Williams, R. C., J. D. Beck, and S. N. Offenbacher. 1996. The impact of new technologies on the diagnosis and treatment of periodontal disease: A look to the future. *J. Clin. Periodontol.* 23:299–305.

Chapter 17

Radiographic Assessment

Herbert Frommer

OUTLINE
Introduction
Conventional Radiographs: Intraoral Technique
Conventional Radiographs Used in Periodontics
Periodontal Structures
Periodontal Interpretation
Radiographically Detectable Periodontal Changes
Frequency of Radiographs (Selection Criteria)
Digital Imaging
Digital Subtraction Radiology
Radiographs in Implantology
Dental Hygiene Notes
Key Points
Self-Quiz
References

EDUCATIONAL OBJECTIVES

Upon completion of this chapter, the reader should be able to:

- Identify and discuss the periodontal structures seen on a radiograph.
- Discuss the rationale for radiographs in periodontics.
- Explain the features of conventional and computer-based digital imaging.
- List and discuss the benefits and limitations of radiographs used in periodontics.
- Explain the radiographic improvements aimed at decreasing patient radiation exposure.
- Discuss the types of radiographs used in the treatment planning and evaluation of implants.

GOAL: To provide a radiology background that is used in conjunction with clinical data to recognize and classify periodontal diseases.

KEY WORDS

computed tomographic (CT) scans 244
conventional radiographs 234
direct digital radiography 243
full-mouth survey 234
paralleling technique 235

233

INTRODUCTION

The proper classification, evaluation, and treatment of the periodontal diseases can be accomplished only with a combination of radiographic and clinical examinations (Figure 17–1 ■). One must be aware of the diagnostic limitations of radiographs because periodontal diseases have both soft tissue and bony components. Soft-tissue changes such as inflammation, gingival enlargement, and recession cannot be seen on radiographs because such tissues are radiolucent and therefore appear black. Owing to the superimposition of the buccal and lingual alveolar bone plates, bone loss in some areas also may not be seen. Radiographs essentially portray a three-dimensional disease process in two planes. This point must be kept in mind when viewing radiographs because the appearance can be very misleading.

Despite these limitations, a proper periodontal classification cannot be made without a **full-mouth survey.** Radiographs serve to (1) identify predisposing factors, (2) detect early to moderate bone changes where treatment can preserve the dentition, (3) approximate the amount of bone loss and its location, (4) help in evaluating the prognosis of affected teeth and the restorative needs of these teeth, and (5) serve as baseline data and as a means to evaluate posttreatment results.

This chapter will discuss the role of **conventional radiographs** (i.e., radiographs taken on film with an X-ray machine) and computer-based image processing (i.e., the use of a computer to display and enhance images of teeth and bone).

■ **FIGURE 17–1** Radiographs are used to obtain a visual image of the bone and teeth or dental implants. (Courtesy of Procter & Gamble, Cincinnati, OH)

CONVENTIONAL RADIOGRAPHS: INTRAORAL TECHNIQUE

Parameters

The three parameters, or choices, that the dental professional selects at the control panel of an X-ray machine are kilovoltage, milliamperage, and exposure time. Understanding the effect of each of these parameters on the diagnostic X-ray beam is important and will help in making a correct classification of the disease process (i.e., dental hygiene diagnosis).

Kilovoltage

The amount of penetration of the X-ray beam is controlled by the kilovoltage. The suitable range for dental radiography is 65 to 100 kilovolt peak (kVp). This range is determined by the density of the objects to be radiographed (e.g., teeth, bone). Kilovoltage settings above 100 kVp result in overpenetration, and settings below 45 kVp would result in underpenetration. Kilovoltage settings in the range of 45 to 65 kVp, although producing a diagnostic beam, are never used because of the excess secondary radiation that results.

The question to be answered is: "Within the acceptable kilovoltage range, what kilovoltage is most appropriate for periodontal diagnosis?" The answer is determined by the degree of density and contrast that is most diagnostic for the clinician. Density is the degree of blackness on a film, and contrast is the difference in the degrees of blackness between adjacent areas.

Radiographs have a high degree of (short scale) contrast when low kilovolt-peak settings are used. The X-ray photons either penetrate the tissue or are absorbed—a sort of yes or no, black or white reaction. When higher kilovolt-peak settings are used, there is less contrast, and the overall tone of the radiograph is gray (Figure 17–2 ■). This occurs because there is much more partial penetration with the resulting long-scale contrast. Such low contrast is not as satisfying visually as high contrast, but early changes in object density such as early bone loss may be seen in the gradations of gray as a result of more selective penetration, which is not present in high-contrast films. Theoretically, therefore, higher kilovolt-peak settings with their resulting long-scale contrast produce better results in terms of periodontal diagnosis. A number of clinicians, however, feel that the human eye is not capable of seeing these very subtle gray changes and recommend using 75 kVp, where bony changes are distinguished more easily.

■ FIGURE 17–2 Selection of settings. (Courtesy of Procter & Gamble, Cincinnati, OH)

Milliamperage

The milliamperage setting controls the number of X-rays generated in a given exposure time. As noted above, the kilovoltage determines the quality (penetration) of the X-rays produced, but the milliamperage determines the quantity of X-rays produced.

It is more precise, however, to consider the concept of milliampere seconds (mAs) than milliamperage alone because the milliamperage setting and duration of exposure are interdependent values. In order to make a diagnostic exposure, different types of film need different milliamperage-second settings, and this is determined by the sensitivity of the film and the focal distance of the film. If the milliamperage setting is increased, then the exposure time can be reduced. For example, an exposure, at a given kilovolt-peak setting, of 1 s using 10 mA is 10 mAs. A 2 s exposure at the same kilovolt-peak setting using 5 mA would produce an identical film because the resulting exposure is again 10 mAs ($10 \times 1 = 10$ and $5 \times 2 = 10$). Both patients would receive the same amount of radiation. The only advantage of the higher milliamperage is the decrease in exposure time, which lessens the chance of patient movement. Common practice today is to use short exposure times at a magnitude of 6 impulses (1/10 s), so patient movement is less of a factor (see below). This reduction in exposure time to 1/10 s alone, however, will not prevent patient movement or gagging; it just facilitates obtaining the radiograph before such movement occurs. Thus, it is apparent that it makes no diagnostic and little technical difference if we work at 5, 6, 7, 10, or 15 mA. It should be pointed out that conventional dental X-ray machines do not have

milliamperage settings higher than 15 because of heat limitations within the tube.

Dental X-ray machines do not emit a continuous stream of radiation when an exposure is made; rather, they emit a series of radiation impulses. The number of impulses depends on the number of cycles per second in the electric current being used. With 60-cycle alternating current, which is standard, there are 60 X-ray pulses per second. Newer-generation X-ray machines have timer dials calibrated in impulses, not in seconds. On the timer dial, 15 would mean 15 impulses or 15/60 s exposure. These extremely short exposure times can only be controlled by an electric timer. The old mechanical timers are not this precise, and all X-ray machines should have electronic timers that are capable of delivering short, accurate exposure times.

Film Type

Even with the introduction of digital radiographs, film remains by far the most commonly used image receptor in dentistry. In periodontal diagnostic radiology, the most commonly used sizes are number 1 (narrow anterior), number 2 (adult size), and number 3 (long bitewing). Number 2 film with either loops or stick-on tabs can be converted into a bitewing film.

The film sensitivity, or speed, determines how much radiation for how long (e.g., milliampere seconds) is necessary to produce an image on the film. The speed of the film is determined mainly by the size of the silver halide crystals in the film emulsion.

Films are designated by American National Standards Institute (ANSI) categories, with category A film being the slowest and category F film being the fastest. The category E film speed is twice as fast as category D film and thus needs half the radiation exposure. Both films are equally diagnostic. The early objections to category E film based on decreased definition and lack of contrast have not been supported by studies in the literature. Thus, because it has the same diagnostic capability and results in 50% less radiation exposure than category D film, category E speed film generally should be used.

Paralleling versus the Bisecting Technique

In periodontal radiographic diagnosis, use of the **paralleling technique** with a 16-inch film focal distance for periapical radiographs is the method of choice. In this technique, the teeth and the film are parallel to each other, and the central ray of the X-ray beam is directed perpendicular (right angle) to both. With this technique, there will be no dimensional distortion or false and misleading indications of bone levels. The 16-inch focal distance, the so-called long cone, is used to compensate for the image enlargement caused by the increase in tooth-to-film distance necessary to achieve the parallelism between the teeth and the film.

In the bisecting technique, the film is placed as close to the tooth as possible, and the central ray of the X-ray beam is directed perpendicular to an imaginary line between the angle formed by the long axis of the tooth and the plane of the film. This technique is not recommended for periodontal diagnosis because it results in a distortion and exaggeration of the alveolar bone level. Excess vertical angulation (i.e., distortion of the length of the roots, either foreshortening or elongation) may lead to a perception of early furcation involvement when there is actually no interradicular bone loss (Figure 17–3 ■).

CONVENTIONAL RADIOGRAPHS USED IN PERIODONTICS

Table 17–1 ■ reviews the different types of conventional intraoral and extraoral radiographs used in conjunction with clinical data to recognize and classify periodontal diseases (Hodges, 1997). Many radiographs are available, but periapical, bitewing, and panoramic radiographs

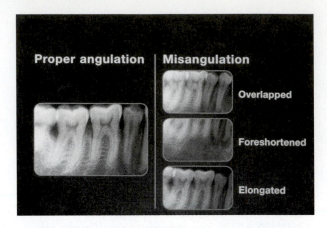

■ **FIGURE 17–3** Diagnostic quality. (Courtesy of Procter & Gamble, Cincinnati, OH)

are used most commonly in periodontics to evaluate periodontal structures.

Conventional radiographs give a history of past periodontal disease destruction but do not provide information on current periodontal disease status. As mentioned earlier, radiographs represent a two-dimensional view of three-dimensional objects, so it is difficult to recognize the slight changes in alveolar bone that would indicate early or mild periodontal disease. Other limitations and benefits of radiographs are discussed in Box 17–1. As a result, radiographs are used primarily in periodontics to

Table 17–1	Selection Criteria of Conventional Radiographs for Periodontics	
Type of Film	*Indications*	*Limitations*
Periapical	Viewing the apex of the root for any pathology (i.e., periapical radiolucency) Determining morphology (shape) of roots and root length Recognizing horizontal and vertical patterns of bone loss Evaluating implants Viewing interproximal dental caries	Technique errors may reduce the ability to detect crestal bone loss. Detection of incipient interproximal dental caries. Detection of pathologic lesions in the mandible and maxilla. Evaluation of other structures such as sinuses and the mandibular canal.
Bitewing	Viewing the alveolar crest bone height (use vertical bitewings) Evaluation of defective restorations (i.e., overhang)	Cannot view the apical area of a tooth. Evaluation of the morphology and length of roots.
Panoramic	Viewing the area of the maxilla and mandibular arches (i.e., impacted teeth, sinuses, and pathologic lesions)	Not used for recognizing periodontal diseases or dental caries.

Box 17–1 Benefits and Limitations of Conventional Radiographs

Radiographs *do* show:

- crestal alveolar bone levels
- clinical crown-to-root ratio
- calculus on proximal tooth surfaces
- metallic restorations
- morphology of roots (i.e., root length, root shape)

Radiographs *do not* show:

- periodontal pockets
- buccal and lingual plates of bone
- hard-to-soft-tissue relationship
- a successfully treated patient
- bone loss until about 30 to 50% of loss of mineralization occurs

determine the severity and pattern of bone loss, the morphology (i.e., length and shape) of roots, root proximity, pathologic lesions such as a cyst or an abscess, and the effects of occlusion.

Just as a single periodontal probing recording only provides information on past disease activity, it is important to compare several sets of full-mouth radiographs over a period of time to evaluate for periodontal disease progression (Hollender, 1992; Jeffcoat & Reddy, 1991). In addition, radiographic findings always should be correlated with the corresponding probing depth measurements.

Periapical Radiographs

A periapical radiograph shows the entire area around a tooth, including the apex of the root. Periapical radiographs are part of the full-mouth survey and are taken of anterior and posterior teeth. The number of periapical films taken for a full-mouth survey varies from fourteen to twenty.

Film technique errors occur quite often with periapical radiographs as a result of improper alignment of the film with the tooth and the X-ray beam with the film. Excessive vertical angulation causes foreshortening (roots appear shorter and the alveolar crest appears to be closer to the cementoenamel junction than it truly is) and occlusal surfaces to be cut off. This can result in inaccurate recording of the crestal alveolar bone level. Insufficient vertical angulation causes elongation and roots to

be cut off from the X-ray. Overlapping of proximal tooth surfaces is caused by improper horizontal angulation of the radiographic beam.

Bitewing Radiographs

The bitewing radiograph is by far the best radiograph to interpret posterior alveolar bone levels and bone loss with the least amount of distortion or technique error. Bitewing radiographs show the crowns of the maxillary and mandibular teeth and the alveolar crest. Identification of carious lesions is best with bitewing radiographs. Posterior bitewing radiographs are part of the full-mouth survey and can include up to four views. Bitewing films can be placed either horizontally or vertically (Figure 17–4 ■). Vertical bitewing radiographs are especially useful in periodontal patients with moderate to severe bone loss (this is determined by periodontal probing and previous radiographs, if available) in order to evaluate crestal bone. Horizontal bitewing radiographs do not show the entire bone height. Two posterior vertical bitewing radiographs may be sufficient, however, for visualization of both maxillary and mandibular teeth. The radiographs are taken perpendicular to the alveolar crest so that the crestal bone is depicted accurately. Anterior vertical bitewing radiographs also can be taken.

RDH Rapid Dental Hint

It is best to take vertical bitewings on a patient with bone loss. The crest of bone may not be seen on horizontal bitewings.

■ **FIGURE 17–4** View selection—bitewing. (Courtesy of Procter & Gamble, Cincinnati, OH)

Panoramic Radiology

The image on a panoramic film shows the entire dentition and supporting bone structure from condyle to condyle on one film (Figure 17–5 ■). The resulting image, however, does not have the same degree of definition seen on an intraoral periapical or bitewing radiograph. This shortcoming is inherent to the pantomographic process and is also caused by the use of intensifying screens.

Many diagnostic problems in dentistry require a high degree of radiographic definition. Early detection of such conditions as disruption of the periodontal ligament, loss of crestal alveolar bone, a thickened periodontal ligament, and ongoing caries requires the maximum amount of radiographic definition. Because of this, panoramic films have very limited value in the diagnosis of periodontal disease. If a panoramic film is used instead of a full-mouth survey, it must be augmented with both anterior and posterior bitewing radiographs and selected periapical films where indicated. Many technique errors can occur with panoramic radiographs, including improper patient positioning and operator errors.

Rapid Dental Hint

Remember, panoramic X-rays are not used to recognize periodontal disease.

PERIODONTAL STRUCTURES

In order to recognize disease, the normal anatomy must be understood. Periodontal anatomy identified on radiographs includes the supporting structures such as the alveolar bone, periodontal ligament space, and cementum (Figure 17–6 ■). Since gingiva is a noncalcified soft tissue structure, the X-rays go completely through it and are not absorbed, thus the gingiva is not seen as a radiopaque structure.

Interdental Septum

The normal crest of interproximal bone runs parallel to a line drawn between the cementoenamel junctions on adjoining teeth at a level approximately 2.0 mm apical to the cementoenamel junction (Figure 17–7 ■). The shape of the alveolar crest is determined primarily by the contact area of adjacent teeth and the shape of the cementoenamel junction. The alveolar crest is flatter in posterior areas and more convex and pointed anteriorly. The width of the interdental septum can be determined by viewing a radiograph. The interdental septum can be narrow in cases of close root proximity. In some instances, the roots of adjacent teeth are so close that there may be little to no cancellous bone. Teeth that frequently show close root proximity include the distobuccal root of the maxillary first molar and the mesiobuccal root of the maxillary second molar and the mandibular anteriors.

■ **FIGURE 17–5** View selection—panoramic. (Courtesy of Procter & Gamble, Cincinnati, OH)

■ **FIGURE 17–6** Radiograph of the periodontal structures (1 = lamina dura; 2 = periodontal ligament space; 3 = interproximal bone; 4 = alveolar bone crest; 5 = trabecular bone; 6 = interradicular bone; 7 = pulp).

■ **FIGURE 17–7** Radiograph showing the normal relationship of the crestal bone level being parallel with the cementoenamel junctions of adjacent teeth. No bone loss is depicted in this radiograph.

■ **FIGURE 17–8** The maxillary second premolar shows a widened periodontal ligament space due to an excessive occlusal load placed on it.

Radiographically, a thin radiopaque line surrounds the entire tooth and is continuous with the alveolar crest (see Figure 17–6). This is referred to as the lamina dura. Clinically, it represents the alveolar bone that lines the tooth socket.

> **Did You Know?**
>
> Approximately 50% of bone must be demineralized before it is evident on an X-ray.

Periodontal Ligament Space

The periodontal ligament fibers (or principal fibers) transverse from the cementum to the alveolar bone. Since these fibers are soft tissue, they are not evident on radiographs. Instead, the space where the fibers are located appears as a radiolucent area surrounding the entire tooth (see Figure 17–6). On one side of the space is the cementum, and the other border is the lamina dura. Evaluating the width of the periodontal ligament (space) is important during the occlusal examination. If a tooth has excessive occlusal loads placed on it, the periodontal ligament compensates for the resulting tooth mobility by becoming thicker. This shows up on a radiograph as a widened periodontal ligament (Figure 17–8 ■).

> **Did You Know?**
>
> Fibroblasts from the periodontal ligament are responsible for regeneration of lost periodontal structures. This concept is called guided tissue regeneration.

PERIODONTAL INTERPRETATION

Using radiographs as an evaluation tool in the recognition of periodontitis has several limitations that are listed in Box 17–1. It is difficult to determine changes in bone simply by viewing radiographs. For this reason, clinical data must be incorporated with radiographic findings in an assessment of periodontal status. For example, a patient's radiographs may show moderate bone loss, but previously the patient may have had periodontal surgery for pocket reduction. Thus, the radiographs still show bone loss, but the periodontal charting shows probing depths from 1 to 3 mm without bleeding on probing. At this time the patient does not have periodontitis. The radiographs show past disease activity, not what is occurring presently.

Bone Loss

Conventional radiographs represent an insensitive technique in detecting early, small bony defects (bone loss). Before bone loss is identified on a radiograph, approximately 30 to 50% loss of mineralization must occur (Jeffcoat, 1992; Jeffcoat & Reddy, 1991). In addition, radiographically, the cortical bone plates may hide slight bone loss.

Radiographic evaluation of alveolar bone loss associated with periodontitis is based on the status of the interdental septum (Kasaj, Vasiliu, & Willerhausen, 2008). Fuzziness or breaks in the continuity of the lamina dura have been described as the earliest radiographic signs of bone loss. However, the radiographic observation that the loss of crestal lamina dura is a sign of periodontitis is not totally accurate (Armitage, 1996). Clinical studies have shown that sites did not break down, even though there was a break in the lamina dura. Moreover, absence of crestal lamina dura is a common radiographic finding in normal, nondiseased interproximal sites (Rams, Listgarten, & Slots, 1994). Thus, it is more accurate to state that the presence of an intact crestal lamina dura represents a stable site than that the absence of a crestal lamina dura indicates a disease site (Armitage, 1996; Rams et al., 1994).

Patterns of Bone Loss

The severity, distribution, and pattern of bone loss can be determined from radiographs. Clinically, as measured with a periodontal probe, two types of bony pockets exist: suprabony and infrabony. A gingival pocket or pseudopocket is not associated with bone loss. These bony pockets are associated with two patterns of bone loss: horizontal and vertical. In horizontal bone loss, interdental bone is destroyed equally along the surfaces of adjacent teeth (Figure 17–9a ■). Suprabony pockets, where the base of the pocket is coronal to the alveolar bone crest, are characterized by horizontal bone loss. In vertical (angular) bone loss, the resorption on one tooth sharing the septum is greater than on the other tooth (Figure 17–9b). Infrabony pockets, where the base of the pocket is apical to the alveolar crest, are associated with vertical bone loss.

Severity of Bone Loss

The severity, or amount, of bone loss is classified as mild, moderate, or severe. One way to determine the amount of bone loss is to determine the percentage of bone loss. This is done by measuring the length from the cementoenamel junction to the tip of the root and the distance from the cementoenamel junction to the alveolar crest. The percentage of bone loss is calculated by dividing this number by the root length and multiplying by 100 (Hodges, 1997). Bone loss of less than 20% is usually classified as mild; bone loss between 20 and 50% is moderate; and bone loss of more than 50% is severe. It also

(a)

(b)

■ **FIGURE 17–9** (a) A periapical radiograph showing a horizontal pattern of bone loss. (b) Vertical or angular bone loss on the mesial surface of the first molar with furcation involvement.

should be remembered that 30 to 50% bone loss must be present before it is evident radiographically.

Determination of Bone Loss

The first step in determining if there is radiographic bone loss is to draw an imaginary line connecting the cementoenamel junction of adjacent teeth and then a line on the alveolar crest. If the alveolar crest is more than approximately 2 mm apical to the cementoenamel junction, there is bone loss. The next step is to determine if the pattern of bone loss is horizontal or vertical. In vertical bone loss, the bone level is not parallel to the cementoenamel junctions of adjacent teeth. In horizontal bone loss, the bone level is parallel to the cementoenamel junctions of adjacent teeth. If a tooth is not in the normal occlusal plane (e.g., extruded, intruded, or tipped), the bone level will not be in a straight line, but neither will the cementoenamel junctions, so the lines will still be parallel to each other (Figure 17–10 ■).

Despite these limitations, conventional radiographs are still mandatory in the recognition and treatment of periodontal diseases. They provide an excellent measurement of the history of periodontal disease in a patient and provide important information about the interproximal bone changes that occur over time (Douglass, Levine, Otomo-Corgel, Sims, & Taggart, 1991). The detection of predisposing factors is one of the most important roles of radiography in periodontal diseases, and the detection and elimination of local irritants are essential steps in prevention or actual periodontal therapy.

Calculus

Early deposits, small and not fully calcified, are not seen radiographically. Even calcified supragingival calculus, which is seen most often on the lingual surfaces of lower anterior teeth and the buccal surfaces of upper molars, is not seen clearly in its early stage because of superimposition of tooth structure (e.g., roots) and cortical plates. Subgingival calculus on the proximal surfaces is more easily detected in the early calcified stages. Calculus appears as an irregularly pointed radiographic projection from the proximal root surface (Figure 17–11 ■).

Anatomic Configurations

Only through radiographic examination can information about the size, shape, and positions of the roots of periodontally involved teeth be obtained. It is important to document the lengths of the root trunks of multirooted teeth to ensure tooth survival. A tooth with a short root trunk has "higher" furcation entrances and longer roots. A tooth with a long root trunk has shorter roots, but the furcation entrance is more apical. Therefore, more bone has to be destroyed in the development of a furcation involvement.

■ **FIGURE 17–10**   *The area between the premolar and molar shows uneven crestal alveolar bone that parallels the uneven cementoenamel junctions. There is horizontal bone loss but not angular bone loss.*

■ **FIGURE 17–11**   Calculus spurs evident on all tooth surfaces.

Another important factor in the overall periodontal prognosis is the shape of the roots. The space between the roots is important. Roots of multirooted teeth can be diverging, converging, or conical. Diverging roots have a larger surface area for periodontal attachment including bone. Teeth with thicker, diverging, longer roots have a better prognosis than conical or converging roots. Roots also can be long and tapered or short, bulbous, and conical. These factors are important in evaluating the present condition and planning periodontal and restorative therapy.

In restorative case planning, the crown-to-root ratio is an important factor. This ratio is the relationship of the length of the root embedded in bone compared with the length of the rest of the tooth. The greater the length of the tooth embedded in bone, the better is the prognosis for support of a fixed or removable prosthesis. A 2:1 crown-to-root ratio is desirable. Teeth with bulbous roots have more area for attachment than those with fine tapered roots.

RADIOGRAPHICALLY DETECTABLE PERIODONTAL CHANGES

Gingivitis

Because gingivitis is a soft-tissue change, there are no radiographic findings other than the presence of predisposing or contributing factors (e.g., condition of restorations).

Slight (Mild) Periodontitis

This stage of periodontal disease is characterized radiographically by changes in the crest of the interproximal bone septum and triangulation of the periodontal ligament space (Figure 17–12 ■). Triangulation is widening of the periodontal ligament space at the crest of the interproximal septum that gives the appearance of a radiolucent triangle to what is normally a radiolucent band. Fading of the density of the crest with cup-shaped defects appears in the early stages of periodontitis.

Moderate Periodontitis

In this stage, bone loss may be apparent in both horizontal and vertical planes. Radiolucencies appear in the furcations of multirooted teeth, indicating interradicular bone loss. This is a furcation involvement and is confirmed clinically using a Nabers probe. In this stage, horizontal bone loss on the buccal or lingual surface may

■ **FIGURE 17–12**   Slight (mild) chronic periodontitis. Generalized slight horizontal bone loss of less than 20%.

go undetected because of superimposition. Careful examination of the radiograph in most cases reveals a difference in density indicating different levels of bone on the buccal and lingual surfaces (Figure 17–13 ■).

Severe Periodontitis

This stage of periodontal disease is easily identified radiographically by the advanced vertical and horizontal patterns of bone loss, furcation involvement, thickened periodontal ligament, and indications of changes in tooth position (Figure 17–14 ■).

■ **FIGURE 17–13**   Moderate chronic periodontitis. Localized furcation involvement on the mandibular molar.

■ **FIGURE 17–14**   Severe chronic periodontitis. Generalized extensive horizontal and vertical bone loss of more than 50% and furcation involvement.

Periodontal Abscess

The radiographic signs of a periodontal abscess may vary greatly. Such a diagnosis is dictated by an acute clinical manifestation. Clinically, a deep periodontal pocket is usually found. The periodontal abscess is caused by the occlusion of an existing pocket; therefore, the radiograph of the acute episode may not vary greatly from previous radiographs of the existing condition that produced the pocket. In other instances, there may be signs of rapid and extensive bone destruction.

FREQUENCY OF RADIOGRAPHS (SELECTION CRITERIA)

Among the many methods of reducing a patient's radiation exposure (e.g., collimation, filtration, and fast film), selection criteria also are very important and are the responsibility of the dentist. Selection criteria are descriptions of clinical conditions and historical data that identify patients who are most likely to benefit from a particular radiographic examination. These guidelines help the practitioner select which patient needs radiographs and determine which radiographs are needed. The final decision rests with the individual dentist and is determined by professional judgment.

The practice of taking radiographs based on a time interval rather than patient needs, as determined by clinical examination and dental history, is not considered the appropriate way to practice dental radiology. In relation to periodontal care, there should never be a policy, for

example, that mandates a new full-mouth survey every two years or bitewing radiographs every six months. The radiographic needs of each patient are different and should not be based on the calendar but rather on a complete clinical examination and the history of previous periodontal therapy or signs and symptoms of the disease.

An expert panel of dentists under the auspices of the Public Health Service (U.S. Department of Health and Human Services, 1987) has developed guidelines for the prescription of dental radiographs. One of the patient categories is "Periodontal disease or a history of periodontal treatment." The recommendations call for a full-mouth survey for every new patient, comprised of periapical and bitewing films. For the recall examination, radiographs should be taken for evaluation of previous periodontal therapy (e.g., surgery, bone grafting, implants, or when there is a dramatic change in the probing depth measurement). In any patient, radiographs should never be taken before there is a complete clinical examination. Based on this examination, a radiographic prescription is formulated, the films are taken, and a final classification and treatment plan are determined.

DIGITAL IMAGING

Radiographic improvements are designed to reduce patient radiation exposure and to simplify identification and measurement of changes in alveolar bone height. The most recent addition to dental radiology is **direct digital radiography.** Presently, about fifteen systems are available on the market, each with its own variations. Many clinicians are converting from film to digital imaging. With digital imaging, there is an up to 90% reduction in radiation exposure compared with conventional radiographs (Jeffcoat, 1998). Direct digital radiography replaces the film used in a conventional intraoral radiograph with an electronic sensor. This sensor, the approximate size of intraoral film, is placed in the patient's mouth in the same manner as one would place film. The exposure is made, and the sensor sends impulses based on the penetration of the object by the X-ray photons to a computer. These impulses are then digitized and formed into an image by the computer. The image can be stored, printed in hard copy, darkened or lightened, reversed, colorized, magnified, measured, or transmitted to a remote site.

A computer monitor creates an image using pixels or tiny dots that become a recognizable form when projected on the screen. Viewing the digital radiograph allows the clinician to determine bone loss through the percentage of lightness and darkness of pixels. White, the

■ **FIGURE 17–15** An example of a direct digital radiograph. This radiograph was taken during implant surgery to guide in the placement of the implant. Digital images can be changed electronically to improve contrast and density and can magnify the image. The mandibular canal (arrows) is well visualized. (Courtesy of Procter & Gamble, Cincinnati, OH)

lightest shade, indicates the maximum amount of bone mineral, whereas black, the darkest shade, indicates absence of bone mineral (Figure 17–15 ■).

From a periodontal standpoint, all the diagnostic criteria mentioned previously in terms of conventional radiographs stay the same. The instant imaging is a time advantage and the substantial reduction in patient exposure is desirable, and the periodontal diagnostic capabilities, when compared with film, are about equal. There may be some advantage in determining bone levels by image reversal or colorization, but this varies among practitioners. These systems are available for commercial in-office use.

DIGITAL SUBTRACTION RADIOLOGY

Digital subtraction radiology (DSR) magnifies images, allowing detection of osseous changes (bone loss) that are too small to be seen in a visual examination of conventional film. As mentioned earlier, comparing radiographs from different time periods is important in detecting progressive bone loss. Because of the superimposition of cortical plates and roots of teeth, it is almost impossible to detect changes in the bone level unless there was a dramatic loss of bone (Jeffcoat, 1994). In digital subtraction radiology, two images taken at two different visits are compared, and all structures that do not change, such as cortical plates and roots of teeth, are not shown on (subtracted from) the image. Any changes in bone level are indicated by a color-shaded area; red is for bone loss, and green is for bone gain (Figure 17–16 ■). DSR has not been used much in clinical practice because it is a difficult technique to master, but it is used frequently in clinical research.

RADIOGRAPHS IN IMPLANTOLOGY

At the present time, the basic diagnostic radiographs used in screening implant patients are conventional radiographs such as periapical, occlusal, and panoramic films. In addition, **computed tomographic (CT) scans** are used for a three-dimensional view of the bone. It is most important to realize that to diagnose and plan for implant placement, one must be able to view the implant site in three dimensions or planes. As dental professionals, we are used to seeing objects in two planes, mesiodistal and incisoapically. We do not see objects in a three-dimensional view except with occlusal films in the buccolingual plane, and this information is critical in implant planning. Of the techniques used, only CT images can supply this information.

Periapical/Occlusal Films

If the film can be placed parallel to the ridge and the field size allows for visualization of the entire proposed alveolar area, then periapical films can be used. Unfortunately, there are very few patients who fit this criterion, and thus periapical views are of limited value. Occlusal films, if they can be positioned, can augment the periapical film to view the third dimension.

Pantomograms (Panoramic Films)

The panoramic film is currently the most commonly used radiograph in treatment planning for an implant patient. Pantomograms are ideal for showing the structures of the mandible and maxilla, including the locations of nerves. Although the field size is large enough in panoramic films, there is still no cross-sectional visualization. There is also an uneven amount of magnification (27%) in different areas of the mouth, and this can be very misleading in interpreting the radiograph. The exact location of

FIGURE 17–16   Computerized digital radiography is used to quantify the change in bone mineral. A baseline radiograph was taken (*left*). The shaded area indicates 0.84 mm of bone loss between examinations taken over a six-month period (*right*). This shading allows the area of change to be readily seen. (Courtesy of Procter & Gamble, Cincinnati, OH)

the mandibular canal is difficult to determine on a pantomogram. Thus, pantomograms should not be used as the only method for evaluating osseous structures.

Conventional Tomograms

Cross-sectional tomograms are an excellent way to obtain the necessary field visualization. Tomograms are cross-sectional images perpendicular to the edentulous ridge. Images are often blurry or indistinct, and this procedure is time consuming. Since very few offices have tomographic units, referral to medical radiologists or hospitals is necessary. If one is to refer a patient to this type of facility, it is probably better to refer for CT imaging.

Computed Tomography (CT Scanning)

Traditional CT: Three-dimensional computed tomography (CT) imaging is essentially digitized tomography that results in an enhanced image in all three dimensions or planes that is much easier to read than a conventional tomogram. The CT scanner makes a 1.0 to 1.5 mm thick slice or cut of the edentulous area (Figures 17–17 ■, 17–18 ■). The tomogram measures the amount of energy transmitted through the object. The information is transmitted to a computer, which displays the image on a monitor.

CT scans are ideal for locating the amount and quality of bone available for implant placement above

the mandibular canal (this is where the mandibular nerve is located) in the posterior area of the mandible. When maxillary areas are being used as implant sites, CT scans should be used to locate the sinuses and determine the amount and quality of available bone.

Cone Beam CT: Limitations of CT include radiation, machine size, and cost. Recently, cone beam computed tomography (CBCT) has been introduced (Misch, Yi, & Sarment, 2006). It uses smaller, cheaper machines with high-quality results. Cone beam CT imaging system also allows pinpointing the exact location and dimensions of a tumor in the jaw. CBCT can take

FIGURE 17–17   CT scan showing cross sections or "slices" of the mandible.

■ **FIGURE 17–18** Axial CT at the level of the maxillary sinus.

images of both the maxilla and mandible at the same time and emits less radiation than a panoramic radiograph. Typical CT scans require separate scans for the maxilla and mandible. There is much less radiation with cone beam CT; each scan subjects the patient to 200 to 300 times the radiation required for a panoramic radiography. When both jaws need to be scanned, the patient is collectively receiving 400 to 600 times the radiation dose for a panoramic radiograph. These machines not only are used for implant placement but can also measure periodontal defects and image the temporomandibular joint. CBCT scanners utilize a narrow, columninated cone beam of radiation that requires only two to eight times the amount of radiation used in a panoramic radiograph. Additionally, CBCT is accurate to one-tenth of a millimeter (0.1 mm), while traditional CT scanners are off by 0.5 mm or more.

Postoperative Implant Evaluation

Baseline radiographs are taken to verify the fit of the abutment to the fixture head and document bone levels around an implant. After placement of implants, clinical and radiographic evaluations are necessary at continuing care or supportive periodontal therapy visits (Degidi, Nardi, & Piatelli, 2008; Joly et al., 2003; Pontes et al., 2007). Periapical and panoramic films are used for post-treatment evaluation. The primary reason for taking radiographs postoperatively is to help monitor the bone level around the implant. Periapical films are best for this

purpose. For the edentulous patient, followup radiographs should be taken annually for three years and then once every other year. Pantomograms are also used to determine bone changes and the status of the abutment and fixture. Alveolar bone loss of less than 0.2 mm per year after the first year of placement is considered acceptable for a successful implant (Albrektsson, Zarb, Worthington, & Eriksson, 1986). CT scans cannot be used because the metallic implants produce image "noise" that interferes with proper interpretation.

DENTAL HYGIENE NOTES

Adequate radiographs and imaging systems are necessary for a complete periodontal and implant examination. Many techniques and systems are available. Conventional radiographs are adequate for visualizing the tooth and surrounding tissues. Conventional radiographs are also used to determine the amount and quality of bone available for implant placement in the anterior sextant of the mandible and maxilla. However, CT scans are necessary to evaluate the implant site in the maxilla and posterior areas of the mandible for its osseous status and proximity to vital structures (e.g., sinuses and mandibular canal).

KEY POINTS

• Radiographic interpretation is used to supplement clinical findings from the periodontal assessment (e.g., probing depths, clinical attachment levels).
• Posterior vertical bitewing radiographs are ideal for visualizing the level of the alveolar bone crest.
• Radiographs do not show gingival and periodontal pockets or mobile teeth.
• The CT and cone beam CT scan is the most commonly used imaging system for visualizing implant sites in the maxilla and posterior areas of the mandible.

SELF-QUIZ

1. The radiographic evaluation of alveolar bone loss associated with periodontitis is based on the status of which one of the following structures? (p. 238)
   a. Interdental septum
   b. Cementoenamel junction
   c. Periapical bone
   d. Periodontal ligament fibers

2. Which one of the following radiographic structures is described as a thin radiopaque line surrounding the entire tooth and is continuous with the alveolar crest? (pp. 238–239)
   a. Dentin
   b. Cementum
   c. Lamina dura
   d. Periodontal ligament fibers
   e. Gingival fibers
3. Which one of the following types of images uses less radiation and is used before implant placement? (p. 245)
   a. Panoramic
   b. Periapical
   c. Cone beam CT
   d. Vertical bitewing
4. Which one of the following types of radiographs is best to evaluate the alveolar bone crest for moderate to severe bone loss? (p. 237)
   a. Periapical
   b. Horizontal bitewing
   c. Vertical bitewing
   d. Panoramic
   e. Computed tomography
5. Which one of the following predisposing factors of periodontal diseases can be seen on radiographs? (pp. 239–241)
   a. Gingival recession
   b. Periodontal pockets
   c. Furcation involvement
   d. Tooth mobility
6. All the following types of radiographs are currently used in the treatment planning of implants except one. Which one is the exception? (pp. 244–245)
   a. Periapicals
   b. Bitewings
   c. Panoramic
   d. CT scan
7. Which one of the following features does the computed tomographic (CT) process provide? (p. 245)
   a. A three-dimensional view of the area of interest
   b. A two-dimensional view of the area of interest
   c. A global view of all oral structures
   d. A closeup view of the periapical structures

8. All the following are reasons for using radiographs in periodontics except one. Which one is the exception? (pp. 238–240)
   a. Identify predisposing factors.
   b. Detect early to moderate bone changes.
   c. Determine the shape and depth of periodontal pockets.
   d. Serve as baseline data and as a means of evaluating posttreatment results.
9. The normal crest of interproximal bone is located at a level (p. 238)
   a. 2.0 mm apical to the cementoenamel junction.
   b. 3.0 mm coronal to the cementoenamel junction.
   c. 2.0 to 3.0 mm coronal to the cusp tip of the crown.
   d. 3.5 mm apical to the cusp tip of the crown.
10. Which one of the following types of radiographs is used primarily in clinical research rather than clinical practice? (p. 244)
    a. Panoramic films
    b. Direct digital radiography
    c. Digital subtraction radiography
    d. Computed tomography

REFERENCES

Albrektsson, T. G., Zarb, P. Worthington, and A. R. Eriksson. 1986. The long-term efficacy of currently used dental implants: A review and proposed criteria of success. *Int. J. Oral Maxillofac. Implants* 1:11–25.

Armitage, G. C. 1996. Periodontal diseases: *Diagnosis. Ann. Periodontol.* 1:37–215.

Degidi, M., D. Nardi, and A. Piattelli. 2008. Peri-implant tissue and radiographic bone levels in the immediately restored single-tooth implant: A retrospective analysis. *J. Periodontol.* 79(2): 252–259.

Douglass, G. L., S. M. Levine, J. Otomo-Corgel, T. N. Sims, and E. J. Taggart. 1991. Periodontal examination, diagnosis and treatment. *Can. Dent. Assoc. J.* 19:16–30.

Hodges, K. O. 1997. Recommendations for radiographs. In ed. K. O. Hodges, *Concepts in nonsurgical periodontal therapy,* 118–149. Albany, NY: Delmar.

Hollender, L. 1992. Decision making in radiographic imaging. *J. Dent. Educ.* 56:834–843.

Jeffcoat, M. K. 1992. Imaging techniques for the periodontium. In eds. T. J. Wilson, K. S. Kornnan, and M. G. Newman, *Advances in periodontics,* 47–57. Chicago: Quintessence.

Jeffcoat, M. K. 1998. Periodontal diseases: Epidemiology and diagnosis. Consensus reports from the 1996 World Workshop in Periodontics. *J. Am. Dent. Assoc.* 129:9S–14S.

Jeffcoat, M., and M. S. Reddy. 1991. A comparison of probing and radiographic methods for detection of periodontal disease progression. *Curr. Opin. Dentistry* 1:45–51.

Joly, J. C., A. F. Martorelli de Lima, and R. Carvalho da Silva. 2003. Clinical and radiographic evaluation of soft and hard tissue changes around implants: A pilot study. *J. Periodontol.* 74(8): 1097–1103.

Kasaj, A., C. H. Vasiliu, and B. Willershausen. 2008. Assessment of alveolar bone loss and angular bony defects on panoramic radiographs. *Eur J Med Res.* (January 23) 13(1):26–30.

Misch, K. A., E. S. Yi, and D. P. Sarment. 2006. Accuracy of cone beam computed tomography for periodontal defect measurements. *J. Periodontol.* 77(7): 1261–1266.

Pontes, A. E. F., F. S. Ribeiro, V. C. da Silva, R. Margonar, et al. 2008. Clinical and radiographic changes around dental implants inserted in different levels in relation to the crestal bone, under different restoration protocols, in the dog model. *J. Periodontol.* 79(3): 486–494.

Rams, T. E., M. A. Listgarten, and J. Slots. 1994. Utility of radiographic crestal lamina dura for predicting periodontitis disease activity. *J. Clin. Periodontol.* 21:571–576.

U.S. Department of Health and Human Services. 1987. *The selection of patients for x-ray examinations* (HHS Publication FDA 88-8273). Washington, DC: U.S. Government Printing Office.

Chapter 18

Advances in Detecting and Monitoring Periodontal Diseases

Denise Estafan

OUTLINE
Introduction
Gingival Crevicular Fluid Assays
Microbial Tests
Immunologic Assays
Enzyme-Based Assays
Genetic Assays
Clinical Applications
Dental Hygiene Notes
Key Points
Self-Quiz
References

GOAL: To introduce diagnostic methods that can be used as a supplement to conventional periodontal assessments for recognizing and monitoring periodontal diseases.

EDUCATIONAL OBJECTIVES

Upon completion of this chapter, the reader should be able to:

- Evaluate the role of using adjunctive diagnostic aids as a predictor for periodontal breakdown.
- Explain the advantages and disadvantages of the various adjunctive diagnostic methods for detecting periodontal disease activity.
- Distinguish the type of patient who may benefit from adjunctive diagnostic testing.

KEY WORDS

genetics 254
gingival crevicular fluid 250
host-derived enzymes 252

periodontal disease activity 250
periodontal pathogens 252

INTRODUCTION

Currently, identifying inflammatory periodontal diseases involves recognizing disease severity. Such traditional tests as visual inspection, probing depths, clinical attachment levels, and radiographs have not changed in the last forty years and are considered the foundation for a periodontal examination. However, newer examination techniques may provide additional information beyond that which can be obtained from a clinical examination. Such information may offer predictions about the future of periodontal disease progression and patient evaluation. Approximately 30% of periodontal diseases are recurrent, so it is necessary to monitor the patient to identify problem sites before further tissue damage occurs. Research is ongoing to determine the overall plausibility and effectiveness of these tests. Ultimately, the screening of at-risk patients may allow for improved treatment and prevention of periodontal diseases.

The past decade has seen the evolution of several diagnostic methods designed to be used as an adjunct or in combination with the clinical examination (Estafan et al., 1999). These methods help in identifying **periodontal disease activity** or patients at risk for an episode of active disease and are designed to help determine the most appropriate mode of treatment. The present standard for periodontal disease activity is a change in clinical attachment level of 2 to 3 mm. Various methods are used to analyze the products of the host response to dental plaque and to identify specific microbial (bacterial) species. The greatest value of diagnostic testing may lie in the ability to monitor patients after treatment, as well as those in the supportive periodontal therapy phase. Hopefully, appropriate testing will allow the practitioner to make therapeutic decisions before the onset of disease activity or at an early stage in its development. The initial determination of the need for active periodontal therapy still depends on use of a periodontal probe, gingival inspection, and radiographs (Bader, 1995). Therefore, these new assessment methods shift the focus from determining disease severity to evaluating disease progression or the risk of future periodontal breakdown—in essence, quantifying ongoing disease activity.

Adjunctive tests for the evaluation of periodontal diseases are divided into three main groups: gingival crevicular fluid assays, microbial tests, and genetic assays (Estafan, Weinberg, Estafan, 1999) (Box 18–1). Only a

---

Box 18–1   Supplemental Diagnostic Tests in Periodontics

Methods of detecting bacteria:
- Culture and sensitivity techniques
- DNA probes (DMDx®; MicroDenteX, Fort Myers, FL; Micro-IDent®plus, Advanced Dental Diagnostics, Franklin, TN)
- Dark-field or phase-contrast microscopy (available commercially)
- Immunologic assays (not available commercially)
- Enzyme-based assays (not available commercially)

Methods of detecting sites actively breaking down or at risk for future destruction:
- Gingival crevicular fluid assays (not commercially available)
  - Collagenase
  - Aspartate aminotransferase
- Genetic susceptibility test:
  - Interleukin-1 genotype (PST™ Genetic Test; Advanced Dental Diagnostics, Franklin TN)

---

few of the tests are available in the United States for in-office use. Table 18–1 ■ reviews the advantages and disadvantages of various tests.

GINGIVAL CREVICULAR FLUID ASSAYS

Of the three most common fluids found within the oral cavity (**gingival crevicular fluid** [GCF], serum, and saliva), GCF has been the focus of most research in recent years. GCF is a fluid that originates from the gingival connective tissue (lamina propria) and flows into the gingival crevice. As a result of inflammation, GCF is formed when fluids leak from dilated blood vessels within the lamina propria. As this fluid flows through the inflamed connective tissue, it picks up tissue breakdown products, enzymes, and other substances involved in the immune response. In this regard, it is an "inflammatory soup" containing subgingival bacteria, inflammatory cells, and a vast array of other substances (mediators) produced by bacteria and host cells. GCF is relatively easy to collect by placing paper strips into selected pockets (Figure 18–1 ■). It is these features that make GCF a

Table 18–1	Advantages and Limitations of Selective Adjunctive Tests	
Test	**Advantages**	**Limitations**
Culture	• Identifies specific microorganisms • Only test available that determines antibiotic sensitivity	• Expensive and time-consuming • Technique sensitive; diverse data from different labs (use of different media, sampling, transport) • Cell vitality must be preserved during transportation to lab • Some organisms may be lost through sampling
DNA probe assays	• Highly sensitive and specific for targeted periodontal pathogens • Viable organisms not needed • Samples sent by mail after collection chairside • Rapid identification (18 hours)	• Need special disposal procedures for radioactive waste • Certain bacterial species may not be detected due to highly sensitive nature of the test • Performed in a lab
Microscopic test (phase-contrast microscopy)	• Good for chairside patient awareness of the importance of bacteria in periodontal disease • Not suitable to monitor disease activity • Motivational tool for patient's plaque-control habits	• Does not specifically identify bacterial species, only shape, size, and mobility
GCF enzyme assays	• Rapid and inexpensive • Technique insensitive, so easy to perform chairside • Good for screening purposes • In-office use	• Cannot identify specific bacteria, but allows for rapid assessment of bacterial enzymatic activity • Need sufficient amount of enzymes

■ **FIGURE 18–1**   Collection of gingival crevicular fluid (GCF). Placement of filter paper strips into the gingival crevice. (Courtesy of Zila Pharmaceuticals)

good source of potential markers of periodontal destruction (Pradeep et al., 2007).

In areas affected by periodontal disease, GCF is an abundant source of substances (e.g., inflammatory mediators) that appear to play a central role in the tissue breakdown processes associated with periodontitis. This idea has led to the investigation of certain inflammatory mediators and their possible role as markers for active periodontitis (Armitage, 1992). Although these investigations have, over the past twenty years, resulted in the evolution of many techniques for assessing various aspects of disease, currently none are commercially available. Among the mediators that have been looked at most closely are host-derived enzymes (enzymes produced by host cells), inflammatory mediators, and tissue breakdown products.

Host-Derived Enzymes

During the disease process, certain host cells found in the body, such as polymorphonuclear leukocytes (neutrophils), release certain enzymes, including β-glucuronidase and elastase. These **host-derived enzymes** are components of GCF and have been reported to be associated with an increased risk of clinical attachment loss and bone loss (Lamster, Holmes, et al., 1995; Lamster, Oshrain, et al., 1988). Elevated levels of these enzymes in the GCF, which can be used as markers for periodontitis, are most evident six months before the occurrence of disease (Palcanis et al., 1992).

Aspartate aminotransferase (AST) is an intracellular enzyme (e.g., it stays inside the cell) that indicates cell death when it is present extracelluary (e.g., outside the cell). Cell death leads to the release of the contents of the cell into the extracellular fluid. When AST is present at elevated levels in GCF, it has been shown to predict clinical attachment loss (Persson, DeRouen, & Page 1990), but over a shorter period than β-glucuronidase and elastase. Evidence from studies on AST in the GCF of patients at risk for periodontal disease indicates that elevated levels of the enzyme can predict clinical attachment loss an average of three months in advance (Chambers et al., 1991). Currently, however, no test is available commercially.

Collagenase is an enzyme that breaks down collagen and is responsible for normal collagen remodeling. In the presence of inflammation, however, excessive amounts of collagenase are produced that cause periodontal tissue destruction during periodontal inflammation. Collagenase is produced by and released from host cells such as neutrophils (Overall, Sodek, McCulloch, & Birek, 1991). Fibroblasts also produce and release collagen and collagenase, but this occurs during normal tissue remodeling. Currently, however, no test is available commercially to detect "high" collagenase levels in the GCF.

Prostaglandin E₂

Prostaglandin E_2 (PGE_2) is a metabolite of arachidonic acid that is associated with many inflammatory effects, including bone loss. PGE_2 concentrations in the GCF of patients with clinical attachment loss of 3 mm or more have been shown to be significantly higher than in patients without this level of attachment loss (Offenbacher, Odler, & van Dyke, 1986). Identification of high levels of PGE_2 in GCF can indicate an increased risk of periodontal disease up to six months prior to its appearance clinically. Currently, however, no test is available commercially in the United States.

MICROBIAL TESTS

Bacterial plaque is the primary cause of the initiation and progression of inflammatory periodontal diseases. Suggested **periodontal pathogens** include *Actinobacillus actinomycetemcomitans, Porphyromonas gingivalis, Tannerella forsythensis, Prevotella intermedia, Campylobacter rectus, Eikinella corrodens, Fusobacterium nucleatum, Capnocytophaga sputigena, Peptostreptococcus mitis, Selenomonas* spp., *Eubacterium* spp., and *Haemophilus* spp. (Loomer, 2004; Socransky & Haffajee, 1991; Tanner, 1992).

Over the past few decades, the understanding of periodontal diseases has changed dramatically. Since specific bacterial types have been well documented to cause periodontal diseases, including localized and generalized aggressive periodontitis, and refractory cases, treatment of periodontal diseases is best aimed at identification of the periodontal pathogens responsible. While no single one of these pathogens has been indicated as the organism responsible for disease progression, all the preceding bacteria are considered potential periodontal pathogens when identified in subgingival plaque samples. Identification of these pathogens allows for faster and better treatment aimed at eliminating or reducing bacterial levels.

Since gingivitis and chronic periodontitis are not commonly associated with specific bacteria, identification of these diseases probably would not benefit from the use of microbial testing.

Many methods for bacterial testing are available for research and clinical use. These include culturing, microscopic DNA and probe, and immunologic techniques.

Culture Techniques

Culturing allows for the growth of certain microorganisms found in periodontal pockets. Specific in-office procedures must be followed. After removal of supragingival plaque, samples of subgingival bacteria are taken from the plaque with a curet and are placed in a transport fluid and sent to a licensed clinical laboratory within a day or two to maintain bacterial viability (bacteria must be alive on reaching the laboratory). The laboratory then disperses the sample, dilutes it, and plates it on selective and non-selective media. The most common pathogens are identified, and antibiotic susceptibility is determined. A detailed report of the findings is then sent back to the dental office, including the systemic antibiotics to which the cultured bacteria are sensitive. Knowing the susceptibility or resistance of specific microorganisms to these antibiotics provides important guidelines for antibiotic use in conjunction with periodontal therapy.

Cost and time constraints limit the use of such a process, so it is not appropriate for all patients. However, culture analysis may be useful for patients who do not respond to conventional therapy, especially if they have taken antibiotics previously (Armitage, 1993). In addition, culturing is limited in that it can only detect living bacteria; some bacteria may not survive transportation to the laboratory.

Microscopic Techniques

Identification of subgingival biota also may be accomplished through various microscopic techniques such as phase-contrast and dark-field microscopy. Rather than identifying specific bacteria, phase-contrast microscopy categorizes bacteria by motility (motile), and dark-field microscopy identifies the morphology or shape (e.g., cocci, rods) (Sixou, 2003). Bacterial shifts from non-motile to motile species often indicate a change from health to disease (Listgarten & Levin, 1981). Genus and species determination, as well as antibiotic susceptibility, is not possible using these techniques. Many dental offices use microscopic techniques solely for patient education. Clinically, a digital camera and monitor are attached to the microscope.

Nucleic Acid (DNA) Probe Analysis

All living organisms contain DNA (deoxyribonucleic acid), which carries all genetic information needed for the coding for proteins, the basic building blocks of life (Papapanou, Engelbretson, & Lamster, 1999). The DNA of each species consists of a specific sequence that is unique to that organism. Nucleic acid probe analysis identifies DNA sequences specific for certain subgingival periodontal pathogens. In the dental office, plaque samples are collected by inserting a special sterile paper point into the base of a pocket. This paper point is then placed in an air-filled vial and mailed to a testing service. Bacterial DNA is so stable that no special transport fluid is required before mailing the sample, and the bacteria do not have to be living. This is a key advantage to using DNA as a biochemical marker in the identification of periodontal pathogens. The microorganism's DNA is cut into single-strand fragments. The DNA probe is made in the laboratory and labeled with either a radioactive or enzyme marker. If binding of the labeled DNA probe strands occurs, the test organism is thus identified. DNA probe reports are rapid, relatively inexpensive, and can detect nonviable species (Loesche, 1992; Sonnier, 1996). This test (DMDx® Test) is available through a few laboratories, including MicroDenteX in Fort Myers, FL. Another test, Micro-IDent® Plus (Advanced Dental Diagnostics, Franklin, TN) identifies eleven pathogens including *Actinobacillus actinomycetemcomitans* (Aa), *Prevotella intermedia* (Pi), *Porphyromonas gingivalis* (Pg), *Eikenella corrodens* (Ec), *Campylobacter rectus* (Cr), *Tannerella forsythensis*, *Treponema denticola* (Td), and *Fusobacterium nucleatum* (Fn). *P. gingivalis*, *T. forsythensis* and *A. a.* are very strongly considered to be pathogenic for periodontal disease. A sterile paper point is inserted into the pocket for 10 seconds. After removal it is placed in a vial and shipped to the lab. This test also gives a list of antibiotics that the bacteria are susceptible to.

Currently, there is no reason to use DNA probes routinely in every patient. DNA probes should be reserved for difficult refractory cases where previous treatments have failed to control disease progression. It can also be used to monitor therapy outcome after the disease is controlled and to evaluate implant sites. Susceptibility testing should only be done when usual antibiotic regimens have failed or when unusual pathogens are present. Since certain antibiotics are almost always effective against anaerobic pathogens (infections), these infections are usually treated empirically or hypothetically.

IMMUNOLOGIC ASSAYS

The enzyme-linked immunosorbent assay (ELIZA) is based on the specific binding of an antibody to an antigen on the surface of a microorganism. The primary antibody is detected by labeling with a fluorescent secondary antibody. ELIZA is able to identify specific bacteria. It is an expensive test and currently used only in research.

ENZYME-BASED ASSAYS

The enzymatic approach is based on the ability to screen for the presence of an enzyme unique to one or more bacterial species. In this assay, a plaque sample is exposed to a substance that is degraded by the specific enzyme in question. For example, *Treponema denticola, Porphyromonas gingivalis,* and *Tannerella forsythensis* produce a trypsin-like enzyme that degrades a substance called BANA (benzoyldi-arginine-2-naphthylamide). A positive test indirectly indicates the presence of one or more of the three bacteria (Papapanou et al., 1999).

GENETIC ASSAYS

Numerous established and potential risk factors are associated with periodontal diseases, including smoking, smokeless tobacco, systemic diseases, age, medications, stress, and genetics (heredity). All these factors, except for genetics and age, are acquired or environmental and can be controlled or eliminated. **Genetics** is an innate risk factor that one is born with and cannot be altered or modified. Kornman and colleagues (1997) addressed the first association between genetics and periodontal diseases. Interleukin-1 (IL-1) is a cytokine produced and secreted by inflammatory cells such as macrophages as a result of accumulation of bacterial plaque. IL-1 is responsible for inflammation and bone loss. Some individuals produce too much IL-1 in response to bacterial challenge. These individuals are more susceptible to the onset and rapid progression of periodontal diseases than individuals who do not show an IL-1 genotype (gene). IL-1 does not cause periodontal disease directly, but it predisposes the patient to the disease process by increasing inflammation when bacteria are present (Newman, 1998). This information allows the patient to be monitored more closely and helps dental practitioners recommend optimal preventive therapy and supportive care programs (Newman, 1998).

A saliva-based genetic test is available that determines if a patient has an IL-1 genotype. This test is called Genotype PST™ Plus (Periodontal Susceptibility Testing; Advanced Dental Diagnostics, Franklin, TN). The test is performed by collecting saliva from the patient. The sample is analyzed in a licensed medical laboratory to determine if the patient is positive or negative for the IL-1 genotype. An IL-1 gene-positive patient is about seven times more likely to develop or have advanced periodontal disease than a gene-negative patient,

and this genotype occurs in approximately 30% of the population.

CLINICAL APPLICATIONS

Although at present a good clinical judgment as to the presence of periodontal disease can be made using existing diagnostic procedures, this decision may be very subjective and sometimes unreliable. Therefore, there is a need for more precise decision making, and care should be taken in evaluating and using these new systems. However, presently, there are no completely validated assessment procedures that can identify progressing or active periodontitis.

Since the etiology of and risk factors for periodontal diseases are multifaceted, the most important steps for patient evaluation include a comprehensive clinical and radiographic analysis and identification of modifying systemic risk factors, including cigarette smoking and diabetes mellitus. Additionally, the host response contributes to the development and progression of the disease. Therefore, no microbial or host response test will definitively determine the initiation or progression of disease.

It is without foundation to use these tests on all periodontal patients. A critical factor that needs to be considered when a practitioner chooses to introduce diagnostic testing as part of patient care is when to use the tests. At a time when there is great pressure to reduce healthcare costs, judicious application is critical (Lamster, 1996).

Culture and sensitivity testing can provide guidelines for antibiotic selection in certain cases, including periodontitis patients who are refractory to previous treatment. Such patients probably have been treated previously with numerous antibiotics, and bacterial resistance could have developed. DNA probe analysis can be helpful in these patients, providing rapid results within 24 hours. Assessment of the genetic susceptibility of a patient or of children of parents with advanced periodontal disease may soon prove to be an important tool in the initiation of preventive measures.

DENTAL HYGIENE NOTES

Traditional clinical assessments usually will detect inflammatory lesions and direct practitioners to areas requiring therapy and possible additional testing (Greenstein & Rethman, 1998). Presently, microbial assays and host-response diagnostic tests appear to have meager use and limited applicability in routine diagnosis in periodontics. These adjunctive diagnostic tests may improve clinical decision making but require further confirmation followed by controlled clinical studies. Additional testing may be beneficial at specific sites or for individual patients when there is diagnostic uncertainty regarding the absence or presence of diseases or when the medical or dental history suggests that a patient is at risk of developing periodontitis (Greenstein & Rethman, 1998). Currently, however, few of these tests are available commercially, and no test is available that will definitively determine if a site is actively losing attachment and bone or will lose attachment in the future. There are no specific guidelines to follow, but some factors to consider include cost of testing, age of the patient, patient motivation, and systemic health of the patient.

KEY POINTS

- No clinical test is available that will currently determine if a site is actively breaking down or predict periodontal breakdown; more research is needed.
- A combination of traditional and new diagnostic testing can, in some cases, provide more complete information for treatment planning.
- Additional bacterial tests are used for site-specific treatment, additional information to assist treatment, and to rule out other causes of disease.

SELF-QUIZ

1. Which one of the following tests is used to determine the susceptibility of certain bacteria to antibiotics? (pp. 253)
   a. Phase-contrast microscopy
   b. DNA probe
   c. Dark-field microscopy
   d. Temperature
2. All the following types of patients may require adjunctive periodontal diagnostic testing except one. Which one is the exception? (p. 254)
   a. New patients who have not received therapy previously
   b. Treated patients who initially present with advanced periodontal disease
   c. Patients not responding to periodontal treatment
   d. Patients with previously treated gingivitis

3. Which one of the following is the role of genetics as a risk factor for periodontal diseases? (p. 254)
   a. Destruction of bone early in life
   b. Production of excessive amounts of interleukin-1
   c. Demonstration of high levels of bacteria in childhood
   d. Presentation with highly inflamed soft tissues
4. Which one of the following is a goal for using host-based diagnostic periodontal tests? (p. 252)
   a. Determine the need for future maintenance care
   b. Identify periodontal sites that are bleeding
   c. Evaluate the need for more aggressive periodontal treatment
   d. Distinguish between active and inactive disease sites
5. Which one of the following tests is highly sensitive for specific periodontal pathogens present in a subgingival sample of plaque? (p. 253)
   a. Culture
   b. DNA probe
   c. GCF enzyme assay
   d. Microscopic technique
6. In which one of the following secretions are high levels of host-derived enzymes found? (pp. 250–251)
   a. Whole saliva
   b. Crevicular fluid
   c. Sweat
   d. Serum
7. Which one of the following statements is related to adjunctive periodontal tests? (p. 254)
   a. Eventually they will replace conventional periodontal assessment techniques.
   b. They are used on all periodontal patients presenting in the office.
   c. Established guidelines need to be determined.
   d. They are cost-effective and easy to perform.
8. Which one of the following tests identifies the motility of bacteria? (p. 253)
   a. Enzyme-linked immunosorbent assay (ELIZA)
   b. Phase-contrast microscopy
   c. DNA probe
   d. GCF enzyme
   e. Temperature

9. Which one of the following host cells synthe-sizes and releases beta-glucuronidase and elas-tase? (p. 252)
   a. Mast cells
   b. Lymphocytes
   c. Neutrophils
   d. Eosinophils
   e. Fibroblasts
10. All of the following statements are correct con-cerning the use of DNA probe assays except one. Which one is the exception? (p. 251)
    a. They are highly sensitive and specific for tar-geted periodontal pathogens.
    b. Samples are sent to an outside laboratory.
    c. They require viable microorganisms.
    d. They provide rapid identification.

REFERENCES

Armitage, G. C. 1992. Diagnostic tests for periodontal diseases. *Curr. Opin. Dent.* 21(1): 53–62.

Armitage, G. C. 1993. Periodontal diagnostic aids. *Calif. Dent. Assoc. J.* 21(11):35–46.

Bader, H. I. 1995. Contemporary periodontics and a vision for the future: Diagnostics and monitoring the treated case. *Dentistry Today* 1:42–45.

Chambers, D. A., P. B. Imrey, R. L. Cohen, J. M. Crawford, M. E. Alves, and T. A. McSwiggin. 1991. A longitudinal study of aspartate aminotransferase in human gingival cervicular fluid. *J. Periodont. Res.* 26:65–74.

Estafan, D., M. A. Weinberg, and A. Estafan. 1999. Adjunctive diagnostic methods for monitoring progressive periodontal diseases. *Gen. Dent.* (Jul-Aug) 47(4):374–80.

Greenstein, G. S., and M. P. Rethman. 1998. Diagnosing de-structive periodontal diseases. In eds. M. Nevins and J. T. Mellonig, *Periodontal therapy: Clinical approaches and ev-idence of success,* Vol. 1. Chicago: Quintessence.

Kornman, K. S., A. Crane, H.-Y. Wang, et al. 1997. The inter-leukin-1 genotype as a severity factor in adult periodontal disease. *J. Clin. Periodontol.* 24:72–77.

Lamster, I. B. 1996. In-office diagnostic tests and their role in sup-portive periodontal treatment. *Periodontology 2000* 12:49–55.

Lamster, I. B., L. G. Holmes, K. B. Gross, R. L. Oshrain, D. W. Cohen, et al. 1995. The relationship of β-glucuronidase ac-tivity in crevicular fluid to probing attachment loss in pa-tients with adult periodontitis: Findings from a multicenter study. *J. Clin. Periodontol.* 22:36–44.

Lamster, I. B., R. L. Oshrain, D. S. Harper, R. S. Celenti, C. A. Hovliaras, and J. M. Gordon. 1988. Enzyme activity in crevicular fluid for detection and prediction of clinical at-tachment loss in patients with chronic adult periodontitis: Six-month results. *J. Periodontol.* 59:516–523.

Listgarten, M. A., and S. Levin. 1981. Positive correlation be-tween the proportions of subgingival spirochetes and motile bacteria and susceptibility of human subjects to periodontal deterioration. *J. Clin. Periodontol.* 8:122–138.

Loesche, W. J. 1992. DNA probe and enzyme analysis in peri-odontal diagnostics. *J. Periodontol.* 63:1102–1109.

Loomer, P.M. 2004. Microbiological diagnostic testing in the treat-ment of periodontal diseases. *Periodontology 2000* 34(1):49–56.

Newman, M. 1998. Genetic, environmental, and behavioral in-fluences on periodontal infections. *Compend. Contin. Educ.* (special issue) 19(1):25–31.

Offenbacher, S., B. M. Odler, and T. E. van Dyke. 1986. The use of crevicular fluid prostaglandin E_2 as a predictor of peri-odontol attachment loss. *J. Periodont. Res.* 21:101–112.

Overall, C. M., J. Sodek, C. A. G. McCulloch, and P. Birek. 1991. Evidence for polymophonuclear leukocyte collage-nase and 92-kilodalton gelatinase in gingival crevicular fluid. *Infect. Immun.* 59:4687–4692.

Palcanis, K. G., I. K. Larjara, B. R. Wells, K. A. Suggs, J. P. Landis, et al. 1992. Elastase as an indicator of periodontal disease progression. *J. Periodontol.* 63:237–242.

Papapanou, P. N., S. P. Engelbretson, and I. B. Lamster. 1999. Current and future approaches for diagnosis of periodontal diseases. *N. Y. State Dent. J.* (April):32–38.

Persson, G. R., T. A. DeRouen, and R. C. Page. 1990. Rela-tionship between gingival crevicular fluid levels of aspar-tate aminotransferase and active tissue destruction in treated chronic periodontitis patients. *J. Periodont. Res.* 25:81–87.

Pradeep, A. R., S. G. Manjunath, P. P. Swati, C. Shikha, and P. B. Sujatha. 2007. Gingival crevicular fluid levels of leukotriene B_4 in periodontal health and disease. *J Periodon-tol.* 78:2325–2330.

Sixou, M. 2003. Diagnostic testing as a supportive measure of treatment strategy. *Oral Dis.* 9 (Suppl 1):54–62.

Socransky, S. S., and A. D. Haffajee. 1991. Microbial mecha-nisms in the pathogenesis of destructive periodontal dis-eases: A critical assessment. *J. Periodont. Res.* 26:195–212.

Sonnier, K. E. 1996. Microbial testing: Present and future. *Clin. Update* 18(4):7.

Tanner, A. 1992. Microbial etiology of periodontal diseases: Where are we? Where are we going? *Curr. Opin. Dent.* 2(1):12–24.

INTRODUCTION

Controlling inflammation is the initial treatment objective of therapies for the periodontal diseases. The key to controlling inflammation is to eliminate, reduce, or change the makeup of microbes residing in the mouth. Of course, once inflammation is brought under control, the prevention of recurrent periodontitis is essential (Hancock, 1996; Van Dyke, 2007).

Research findings have shown that plaque microbes and their by-products are responsible for the initiation and progression of the periodontal diseases (Haffajje & Socransky, 2006; Ismail, Morrison, Burt, Caffesse, & Kavanagh, 1990; Kolenbrander et al., 2006). Additional research has found that the host's immune response to infection plays an important role in determining how periodontal destruction manifests itself by producing chemical modulators that actually may accelerate periodontal destruction (Grossi et al., 1994, 1995; Van Dyke & Serhan, 2003). Therefore, comprehensive periodontal therapy may include tactics to modulate the host's immune response in addition to traditional efforts to suppress periodontal pathogens.

This chapter explores current concepts of periodontal treatment planning with a focus on **problem-based** learning.

PROBLEM-BASED LEARNING (PBL) APPROACH TO TREATMENT

A problem-based recording system is designed to introduce the student to a technique for developing an individualized treatment plan for each patient. Problem-based learning (PBL) initially identifies significant problems from the patient's medical/dental history from which a differential dental hygiene diagnosis (or interpretation) will be made for each sign and/or symptom on the problem list. The problem list will be used as a guide to develop a treatment plan and a co-management or a referral system. A decision-making tree can be also be used to help decide on the proper treatment in each case. Therapeutic decision making refers to the process of the use of the decision theory, which is the study of the best possible outcomes for decisions made under varying conditions, in making decisions about treatment of individual cases.

Tables 19–1 ■ through 19–3 ■ provide an overall concept of therapeutic decision making when treatment planning a periodontal case.

The American Academy of Periodontology has developed practice parameters on the diagnosis and treatment of periodontal diseases. The *Parameters of Care* (American Academy of Periodontology, 2000a) are strategies to assist oral healthcare practitioners in making clinical decisions from a range of treatment options to achieve a desired outcome.

For many years, periodontitis was thought to be the inevitable result of poor oral hygiene along with uncontrolled dental plaque biofilm and calculus accumulation. This was termed the nonspecific plaque hypothesis (Loesche, 1976). In recent decades, research has suggested instead that there are microbial species whose presence tends to signal a greater likelihood of progressive periodontal destruction (Haffajee et al., 1991). Furthermore, for most patients, evidence suggests that procedures aimed at suppressing these species will improve clinical outcomes. (American Academy of Periodontology, 2000b; Haffajje & Socransky, 2006). However, for adults, front-line periodontal therapy remains largely nonspecific in design—because conventional clinical and self-care procedures often succeed among this predominating group of patients with periodontal diseases. For periodontal diseases in young people, for refractory disease in adults, and in special situations, periodontal therapy may include procedures aimed at specific putative periodontal pathogens.

Goals of Periodontal Therapy

The ideal goal of periodontal therapy is to restore the periodontium to a comfortable and functional state of health for the balance of the patient's life. Therefore, most periodontal therapy aims to prevent the initiation, progression, or recurrence of periodontal diseases, termed arrestive periodontal therapy. The first step in developing a treatment plan should be to determine individual treatment goals for each patient.

Periodontal Therapy: Ongoing Care

The management of most patients with periodontal diseases demands continued reassessments and adjustments to ongoing care. Reassessment and adjustments are necessary because periodontal care is not permanent in the sense that many other highly successful dental therapies are considered permanent (e.g. the permanent crown on a decayed tooth). For most cases of chronic periodontitis, the only permanent periodontal end point is tooth (or

Table 19–1	Consensus Findings: Diagnosis of Periodontitis			
Test	*Application*	*Strengths*	*Weaknesses*	*Type of Evidence*
Periodontal screening and recording	All patients in every practice.	Cost-effective, quick, easy, detects patients with periodontal disease.	Does not provide a tooth-by-tooth assessment for later comparison during maintenance therapy; a full periodontal examination recording is needed for this purpose.	Epidemiologic studies. Only the deepest pockets are recorder per sextant.
Probing pocket depths	All patients.	Shallow probing depths associated with a lack of future disease progression.	Moderate to deep pockets in a single probing depth examination will not distinguish with certainty which teeth will undergo progressive periodontal destruction.	Longitudinal studies.
Gingival inflammation assessment	All patients.	Absence of inflammation is associated with a lack of future disease progression; in treated patients, bleeding on probing is associated with an increased risk of progressive loss of attachment.	Presence of inflammation will not distinguish with certainty which teeth will undergo progressive periodontal destruction.	Longitudinal studies.
Radiographic evidence of bone loss	At-risk patients as determined by PSR screening or periodontal examination.	Absence of bone loss is associated with a lower risk of future disease progression.	Presence of bone loss on a single radiograph will not distinguish with certainty which teeth will undergo progressive periodontal destruction.	Longitudinal studies.
Microbial plaque biofilm tests	High-risk or refractory patients.	Absence of supragingival plaque is associated with a lack of disease progression. In compromised or refractory patients, may be useful in determining the presence of pathogens.	Routine testing offers limited benefit in chronic periodontitis.	Cross-sectional and longitudinal studies. Case reports.

Biochemical profiles in gingival crevicular fluid	Not yet determined.	A number of biochemical markers may identify individuals at risk.	At present, there are no specific biochemical profiles that characterize specific periodontal diseases.	Cross-sectional and longitudinal studies.

Source: From M. K. Jeffcoat, M. McGuire, and M. G. Newman. 1997. Evidence-based periodontal treatment: Highlights from the 1996 World Workshop in Periodontics. *J. Am. Dent. Assoc.* 128:713–724. Copyright 1997 by the American Dental Association. Reprinted by permission of ADA Publishing Co., Inc.

Table 19–2 Consensus Findings: Nonsurgical Treatment of Gingivitis and Periodontitis

Treatment Category	Treatment	Strengths	Weaknesses	Type of Evidence
Professional mechanical therapy— used in the treatment of gingival diseases and periodontitis	Scaling and root planing with manual instruments.	Decreases gingival inflammation by 40% to 60%; decreases probing depth; facilitates gain in clinical attachment level.	Requires attention to detail and meticulous technique.	Longitudinal, cohort, and randomized clinical trials.
	Ultrasonic and sonic scaling and root planing.	Results are similar to those for manual scaling and root planing.	Requires attention to detail and meticulous technique.	Longitudinal, cohort, and randomized clinical trials.
Chemical plaque biofilm control with mouthrinses and toothpastes	Chlorhexidine; triclosan with copolymer or triclosan with zinc citrate; essential oils; stannous fluoride.	Significant reduction in gingival inflammation.	No clear evidence that there is a substantial long-term benefit in periodontitis except to control coexisting inflammation.	Randomized, double-blind clinical trials.
Irrigation	Supragingival and subgingival irrigation used as an adjunct to brushing.	Aids in the reduction of gingivitis.	Some evidence that there is a substantial long-term benefit for periodontitis.	Randomized, double-blind clinical trials.
Sustained-release antimicrobials	Intrapocket resorbable or nonresorbable delivery systems containing an antimicrobial.	When used as an adjunct to scaling and root planing, gains in clinical attachment level and decreases in probing depth and bleeding.	A few reported side effects include transient discomfort, erythema, recession, allergy and, rarely, *Candida* infection.	Randomized, double-blind clinical trials.
Systemic antibiotics	Tetracyclines, metronidazole, spiramycin, clindamycin, and combinations such as metronidazole and amoxicillin.	May be useful to treat aggressive, destructive periodontitis.	Not indicated for gingivitis; not indicated for most patients with chronic periodontitis.	Assessment of risk-benefit ratio; randomized, double-blind clinical trials; longitudinal assessment of patients' conditions.

Source: From M. K. Jeffcoat, M. McGuire, and M. G. Newman. 1997. Evidence-based periodontal treatment: Highlights from the 1996 World Workshop in Periodontics. *J. Am. Dent. Assoc.* 128:713–724. Copyright 1997 by the American Dental Association. Reprinted by permission of ADA Publishing Co., Inc.

Table 19–3 **Consensus Findings: Surgical Periodontal Therapy—Selected Procedures**

Category and Goal	Treatment	Strengths	Weaknesses	Type of Evidence
Pocket therapy for access to root surfaces and bony defects, reduces probing depths, facilitates plaque control, and enhances restorative and cosmetic dentistry.	Modified Widman flap to provide access to roots and bony defects for debridement; apically repositioned flap with or without bony recontouring; gingivectomy.	All procedures decrease pocket depth; with the exception of gingivectomy, all increase clinical attachment level (junctional epithelium attachment); after five years, greatest reduction in probing depth with osseous recontouring; apically repositioned flap with or without bony recontouring used in crown lengthening procedures to provide biologic width.	Procedures designed to reduce probing depths may increase recession; lack of professional maintenance and patient compliance can be detrimental to the long-term success.	Randomized clinical trials; longitudinal studies.
Regenerative procedures to facilitate growth of new periodontal ligament, cementum and bone over previously diseased root surfaces.	Extraoral autogenous bone grafts.	High potential for bone growth.	Second surgical site (such as iliac crest); root resorption may be associated with fresh grafts.	Limited case report data.
	Intraoral autogenous grafts (such as maxillary tuberosity, healing extraction sites, osseous coagulum).	Case reports indicate bone gain of more than 50%; controlled studies comparing grafts with nongrafted bone show improved clinical attachment levels and bone, but not as great as those in case reports.		Case reports; comparative controlled clinical studies.
	Allografts—tissues transferred from one person to another; freeze-dried bone allograft.	Bone fill has been reported in a high proportion of defects involving freeze-dried bone allograft.	Osteogenic potential may vary from vial to vial; patient differences; clinician variability.	Field test; controlled clinical trials.
	Alloplasts—synthetic grafts: • Absorbable: plaster, calcium carbonates, ceramics such as tricalcium phosphate and absorbable hydroxyapatite (HA).	Improved probing depth and attachment level. Some evidence of histologic regeneration in calcium calcium-coated polymer polymethylmethacrylate and hydroxy methylmethacrylate.	Histologic findings indicate that synthetic grafts primarily act as fillers, with little if any regeneration.	Controlled clinical trials.

	• Nonabsorbable: dense HA, porous HA, bioglass. • Calcium-coated polymer polymethylmetha crylate and hydroxymethyl methacrylate.			
Guided tissue regeneration—physical barriers are used to facilitate selective cell population of the root surface after periodontal surgery to promote regeneration.	Nonresorbable membranes.	Significant improvement in clinical attachment level compared with debridement alone; most favorable results are in Class II furcations in the mandible and infrabony defects; no need for second-stage surgery (resorbable only).	Less favorable results in maxillary molar and Class III defects; nonresorbable membrane requires a second surgery to remove the membrane.	Randomized, controlled clinical trials; uncontrolled studies; and case reports.
	Resorbable materials.		Clinical results similar to those for nonresorbable membranes but less evidence available to allow a comparison of predictability with respect to nonresorbable membranes.	
Gingival augmentation to promote root coverage.	Pedicle grafts. Free soft tissue grafts (epithelialized or connective-tissue graft). Combination grafts • Connective tissue or biodegradable membrane barrier plus pedicle graft. • Coronally positioned, previously placed soft tissue graft. • Nonbiodegradable membrane barrier plus pedicle graft.	Improve aesthetics/cosmetic results; decrease root sensitivity; manage defects resulting from root caries removal or cervical abrasion; manage mucogingival defects.	Not as predictable in smokers.	Case reports; comparison studies.

Table 19–3	Consensus Findings: Surgical Periodontal Therapy—Selected Procedures (*cont.*)			
Endosseous dental implants.	Two-stage and one-stage implants; titanium; titanium alloy; hydroxyapatite-coated implants.	Dental implants are predictable replacements for missing teeth in fully and partially edentulous patients.	While there are few studies in the literature, the clinician should use caution in the following cases: smoking, untreated periodontitis, poor oral hygiene, uncontrolled systemic disease, history of radiation therapy, active skeletal growth.	Longitudinal studies.

Source: From M. K. Jeffcoat, M. McGuire, and M. G. Newman. 1997. Evidence-based periodontal treatment: Highlights from the 1996 World Workshop in Periodontics. *J. Am. Dent. Assoc.* 128:713–724. Copyright 1997 by the American Dental Association. Reprinted by permission of ADA Publishing Co., Inc.

Did You Know?

The most frequently performed periodontal surgical procedure by periodontists is flap surgery to provide access for root debridement.

---

implant) loss. Furthermore, no single periodontal treatment produces ideal outcomes for all patients.

Once a patient is practicing thorough daily oral hygiene, the ideal interval between patient appointments—even for patients in periodontal maintenance programs—may be as brief as every two to three months (American Academy of Periodontology, 2000b; Axelsson & Lindhe, 1981). Frequent reexaminations, reevaluations, and adjustments to therapy often are necessary for many years. Given this context, practitioners need to comply with their ethical and medical/legal responsibilities to refer periodontitis patients to specialists, provide comparable periodontal care in the general practice, or partner with a specialist to share responsibilities for periodontal patients. Suggestions governing what, when, and why to refer are made where appropriate throughout this chapter.

PROBLEM LIST

A problem list should be set up for individual periodontal patients (Table 19–4 ■). The problem list will identify the patient's problems by reviewing the chief complaint and medical, social (habit), and dental histories. For each problem identified, a solution should be written and expected outcomes (the result of taking care of the problem), prognosis (predication of recovery), and any major concerns must be addressed. Identified problems may have multiple solutions.

Risk Assessment for Periodontal Diseases

An important aspect of treatment planning is to perform **risk assessment** to determine either predisposition for developing periodontal conditions or for susceptibility for further breakdown. Numerous risk factors have been identified that predispose an individual to periodontitis. Risk factors that cannot be modified—known as risk indicators or determinants—include increased age, male gender, lower socioeconomic status, and genetics. Modifiable risk factors include the presence of plaque biofilm and

Rapid Dental Hint

Developing the problem list, solutions, and expected outcomes addresses not only the clinical concerns of the patient but helps identify the patient's subjective concerns as well.

Table 19–4   Periodontal Problem List

Problems	Solutions (Plan)	Expected Outcome/Prognosis/ Major Concerns
Chief Complaint	Address chief complaint	Treat the chief complaint first
Risk Factors		
Medical History (e.g., diabetes, HIV)	• Detailed assessment • Consultations required • Advise patient of relationship between systemic diseases and periodontal disease	Concern with possible delayed healing
Dental History (e.g., previous periodontal care)	• Detailed assessment • Previous periodontal surgery • Frequency of maintenance care	Compliance is a deciding factor in prognosis
Genetics	Blood test determines possible susceptibility to periodontal diseases	If determined to be susceptible, patient must be compliant with periodontal care
Smoking	Smoking cessation program	• Concerned with periodontal and systemic diseases • Good prognosis if patient is willing to quit
Iatrogenic dentistry	Look for open margins, overhangs, open contacts, and replace or modify exisiting restorations	Concerned with food impaction and plaque biofilm traps
Poor oral hygiene	Patient education	Non-adherence may increase incidence or progression of periodontitis
Soft Tissues		
Gingival inflammation	Eliminate/reduce gingival inflammation with mechanical debridement and oral hygiene	Concerned with development/progression of gingivitis
Soft tissue recession	Determine etiology; may need periodontal surgery (mucogingival)	Future attachment loss
Abnormal tissue architecture: Gingival overgrowth	Determine etiology; drug-induced or hereditary or plaque-induced inflammation; may need periodontal surgery to correct	Difficulty with oral hygiene
Lack of attached gingiva	Determine etiology; determine if prosthetics will be done; may need gingival plastic surgery to correct	Increased incidence of inflammation
Probing depths	Deep probing depths: mechanical debridement followed by reevaluation and if needed periodontal surgery	Deep probing depths difficult to perform oral hygiene and mechanical debridement; future attachment loss likely

Table 19–4   Periodontal Problem List (cont.)

Problems	Solutions (Plan)	Expected Outcome/Prognosis/ Major Concerns
Hard Tissue		
Ridge defects	Surgical intervention; planning for implants	Implant placement/esthetics
Teeth		
Missing teeth	Replacement of missing teeth	Concerned with movement of teeth, function, and comfort
Mobility	Determine etiology: bone loss, occlusal trauma, inflammation, and treat accordingly	Concerned with increasing mobility and patient comfort
Fremitus	Determine etiology: bone loss, occlusal interferences and treat accordingly to eliminate fremitus	Concern with patient comfort and continued occlusal trauma
Parafunctional habits	Eliminate parafunctional habits; counseling or appliances	Concerned with occlusal trauma/good prognosis if eliminated
Radiographic Findings		
Horizontal bone loss	With deep probing depths surgery is needed	Prognosis depends on several factors including amount of bone remaining, mobility, furcation involvement
Vertical bone loss	Surgical intervention	Prognosis depends on several factors including amount of bone remaining, mobility, furcation involvement
Root proximity	Identify teeth and monitor for periodontal breakdown	Concerned with amount of interproximal bone remaining
Pathology		
Mucosal lesions	Determine size, shape, color, and location; refer to specialist; brush biopsy; excisional biopsy	Concerned with oral cancer
TMD/pain	Excercises/appliances/referral to specialist	Reduced function

Source: Adapted from New York University College of Dentistry Problem List. (This list is filled out to show an example.)

microbiota and poor oral hygiene. The primary risk factor for developing periodontitis is tobacco smoking, while certain systemic conditions—most notably diabetes—are also factors (American Academy of Periodontology, 2008). Risk assessment for periodontal diseases is typically performed by the patient filling out a form indicating specific habits or conditions. The clinician then subjectively interprets the findings to determine disease susceptibility. Research has shown that such methods are not accurate and can lead to inappropriate treatment (Pers-

son, Mancl, Martin, & Page, 2003). An objective, computer-based tool could result in more uniform and accurate periodontal clinical decision making, improved oral health, reduction in the need for complex therapy, and reduction in healthcare costs. One such tool is the Oral Health Information Suite® (PreViser Corporation, Mount Vernon, WA). Risk scores calculated using the periodontal risk calculator (PCR) and information gathered during a standard periodontal examination predict future periodontal status with a high level of accuracy and validity (Page, Martin, Krall, Mancl, & Garcia, 2003). Clinically validated periodontal disease risk and severity analysis as well as suggested treatment options for a patient are calculated by entering 23 data points. Risk is reported on a clinically validated 1 (very low) to 5 (very high) numeric scale, while disease severity is described on a validated 1 (health) to 100 (severe periodontitis) numeric scale. Reports are generated while the patient is still in the chair. Patients are given this analysis as simple-to-understand numeric scores that demonstrate improvement or deterioration in their periodontal health status.

Frequent and regular patient education in self-diagnosis and self-care techniques (Axelsson, Nystrom, & Lindhe, 2004; Douglass 2006) can also be used as a risk assessment tool for periodontal diseases.

Did You Know?

Risk assessment is commonplace for medical conditions, yet its potential for oral conditions remains largely untapped.

Treatment Planning

Once the examination and risk assessment are completed, the data must be analyzed. Data include the patient's medical and dental history, complete radiographs, detailed periodontal data, tooth conditions (including vitality, caries, and morphologic abnormalities), and dental awareness.

PATIENT CO-MANAGEMENT AND REFERRAL TO A PERIODONTIST

While patients experiencing periodontal problems may be referred to a periodontist at any time, preliminary phases of periodontal therapy often are performed in the general practice. Sometimes, especially for mild cases, this is all that is necessary to achieve the goal of periodontal therapy (Dockter et al., 2006). However, even for patients who are ultimately referred, the benefits of self-care training, motivation, and emphasis on team building in the general practice increase the likelihood of treatment success by the periodontist. Hygienists, general practitioners, and periodontists who function as a team maximize the likelihood of optimal outcomes.

Although a licensed general practitioner legally may provide comprehensive periodontal therapy to any informed and consenting patient, he or she is ethically and legally required to meet the same standard of care for such therapy as a specialist. Therefore, with the wel-

fare of periodontal patients in mind, the following co-management and referral guidelines are proposed—with the knowledge that exceptions occur.

Did You Know?

One survey showed that about 80% of general dentists treat periodontal disease.

Guidelines for Referral and Co-management

Any patient who has one or more periodontal sites that show persistent signs of inflammation should be considered for referral. Often these patients fit in one or more of the following categories:

1. Chronic periodontitis with deeper probing depths, furcation involvement, and/or problematic gingival recession
2. Aggressive (localized, generalized) periodontitis
3. Periodontitis associated with systemic diseases (such as diabetes mellitus)
4. Periodontitis with significant or increasing tooth mobility
5. Periodontal lesions adjacent to necrotic (or endodontically treated) teeth
6. Refractory (considered nonresponsive to treatment) or recurrent periodontitis (responsive, but still headed downhill)
7. Patients who have aesthetic concerns about the interplay between teeth, restorations, and the gingiva or alveolar arches
8. Patients with mucocutaneous disorders affecting the oral soft tissues (e.g., pemphigus, lichen planus)

In 2006, the American Academy of Periodontology released the *Guidelines for the Management of Patients with Periodontal Diseases.* (American Academy of Periodontology, 2006) This document was developed to assist clinicians in identifying individuals most at risk for developing periodontal diseases. Along with the practitioner's skill and judgment, the *Guidelines* can help identify patients at risk as early as possible, thus hopefully preventing more severe conditions. The *Guidelines* are not mandates, nor do they specify treatment modalities. When used as a framework for patient management, they can enhance communication among all members of the oral healthcare team and determine those patients most appropriate for specialty care. Box 19–1 contains the *Guidelines* document.

Box 19–1   **Guidelines for the Management of Patients with Periodontal Diseases**

LEVEL 3: PATIENTS WHO SHOULD BE TREATED BY A PERIODONTIST

Any patient with:

Severe chronic periodontitis

Furcation involvement

Vertical/angular bony defect(s)

Aggressive periodontitis (formerly known as juvenile, early-onset, or rapidly progressive periodontitis)

Periodontal abscess and other acute periodontal conditions

Significant root surface exposure and/or progressive gingival recession

Peri-implant disease

Any patient with periodontal diseases, regardless of severity, whom the referring dentist prefers not to treat.

LEVEL 2: PATIENTS WHO WOULD LIKELY BENEFIT FROM CO-MANAGEMENT BY THE REFERRING DENTIST AND THE PERIODONTIST

Any patient with periodontitis who demonstrates at reevaluation or any dental examination one or more of the following risk factors/indicators* known to contribute to the progression of periodontal diseases:

Periodontal Risk Factors/Indicators

Early onset of periodontal diseases (prior to the age of 35 years)

Unresolved inflammation at any site (e.g., bleeding upon probing, pus, and/or redness)

Pocket depths > 5 mm

Vertical bone defects

Radiographic evidence of progressive bone loss

Progressive tooth mobility

Progressive attachment loss

Anatomic gingival deformities

Exposed root surfaces

A deteriorating risk profile

*It should be noted that a combination of two or more of these risk factors/indicators may make even slight to moderate periodontitis particularly difficult to manage (e.g., a patient under 35 years of age who smokes).

Medical or Behavioral Risk Factors/Indicators

Smoking/tobacco use

Diabetes

Osteoporosis/osteopenia

Drug-induced gingival conditions (e.g., phenytoins, calcium channel blockers, immunosuppressants, and long-term systemic steroids)

Compromised immune system, either acquired or drug induced

A deteriorating risk profile

LEVEL 1: PATIENTS WHO MAY BENEFIT FROM CO-MANAGEMENT BY THE REFERRING DENTIST AND THE PERIODONTIST

Any patient with periodontal inflammation/infection and the following systemic conditions:

Diabetes

Pregnancy

Cardiovascular disease

Chronic respiratory disease

Any patient who is a candidate for the following therapies who might be exposed to risk from periodontal infection, including but not limited to the following treatments:

Cancer therapy

Cardiovascular surgery

Joint-replacement surgery

Organ transplantation

FREQUENTLY ASKED QUESTIONS (FAQS)

The American Academy of Periodontology's Guidelines for the Management of Patients with Periodontal Diseases

1. What are the *Guidelines?*
    *   The *Guidelines* provide information to assist in the timely identification of patients who would benefit from co-management by the referring dentist and the periodontist.

2. Why did the Academy develop the *Guidelines?*
    *   The Academy's objective is to encourage referring dentists and periodontists to work together to optimize the health of patients. Determining if and when a patient should be referred to a periodontist are sometimes difficult issues. These *Guidelines* are intended to help the general practitioner in the rapid identification of those patients at greater risk for the consequences of periodontal inflammation and infection and, therefore, those patients most appropriate for specialty referral.

- Despite recent advancements in periodontal therapy, periodontal diseases continue to present significant challenges for the public and dental profession. Periodontal diseases remain a major cause of tooth loss in adults. In addition, periodontal diseases are associated with systemic conditions, such as cardiovascular disease, diabetes, adverse pregnancy outcomes, and respiratory disease. Periodontists are experts in assessing and treating periodontal diseases.
- Accumulating evidence, including recent literature, suggests that an increasing number of patients would benefit from periodontal specialty care. This evidence also suggests that these patients are being referred later in the disease process than in the past.

3. Who needs/benefits from the *Guidelines?*
   - All dental teams and their patients need and will benefit from the *Guidelines.*
4. How were the *Guidelines* developed, and who developed them? Did the Academy collaborate with organized dentistry or any other groups or individuals on these *Guidelines?*
   - A Board of Trustees–appointed task force consisting of periodontal practitioners, academicians, and researchers developed the *Guidelines.*
   - The Academy distributed a draft version of the *Guidelines* to all members, the American Dental Association, Academy of General Dentistry, and American Dental Hygienists' Association for commentary.
   - All organizations and more than 375 members provided commentary.
   - The task force revised the *Guidelines* based on the comments received.
5. What are the benefits of using the *Guidelines?* The *Guidelines* will:
   - Help the practitioner in triaging patients who currently have or who are at risk for the development of periodontal diseases.
   - Help the general practitioner more effectively address the association of periodontal diseases and systemic diseases/conditions.
   - Assist the general dentist and hygienist in the management of periodontal diseases.
   - Result in appropriate and timely treatment of periodontal diseases.

In addition, the *Guidelines:*
- Should enhance the restorative outcome of dental treatment by establishing and maintaining a healthy periodontal foundation.
- Are clear, concise, and should be easy to incorporate into daily practice and will enhance the partnership between periodontists and referring dentists.

6. Where do the *Guidelines* fit in the process of care?
   - The *Guidelines* will become an integral part of patient management.
   - The *Guidelines* do not replace the knowledge, skills, and abilities of the dental team.
7. The *Guidelines* mention the concept of risk assessment. What is risk assessment, and why is it so important?
   - Risk assessment is the process of determining the qualitative or quantitative estimation of the likelihood of adverse events that may result from exposure to specified health hazards or from the absence of beneficial influences. Upon dental examination, many practitioners incorrectly assume that a patient in a state of periodontal health is not at risk for developing periodontitis. Indeed, the patient may have risk factors/indicators (e.g., a smoking habit, diabetes, and young age) that could increase the probability of the occurrence of periodontitis in the future. Therefore, risk assessment helps predict a patient's disease state at some future point in time or the rate of progression of current disease.
8. Why are patients with furcation involvement considered among those patients who "should be treated by a periodontist"?
   - Periodontists are specialists trained to assess and treat the more advanced forms of periodontal diseases and associated lesions. Furcation involvements are among the most problematic periodontal lesions. Therefore, it is often appropriate that earlier manifestations of these lesions be evaluated and managed by a periodontist.
9. The *Guidelines* suggest that certain patients can only be treated by a periodontist. Is this true?
   - No. Some patients can be well managed within the general dental practice, whereas others would benefit from co-management with a periodontist.

Box 19–1 **Guidelines for the Management of Patients with Periodontal Diseases** (*cont.*)

The Academy understands that the education, experience, and interests of individual general practitioner dentists vary, and, therefore, specialty referral may occur at different stages of a patient's disease state and risk level. Referral is not only associated with treatment but also includes consultation.

10. Do all patients who are referred to periodontists require surgery?
    • No. Comprehensive care by a periodontist includes nonsurgical and/or surgical therapies depending on the needs of the individual patient.

11. Dental implants, oral reconstructive and corrective procedures, and tissue engineering are not included in the *Guidelines*. Why aren't these procedures included?
    • These *Guidelines* are focused on the management of patients with periodontitis. They do not include all areas of periodontal specialty care or specific treatment modalities. Dental implants, periodontal plastic surgery, oral reconstructive surgery, and tissue-engineering procedures are currently performed by periodontists. The development of clinical guidelines for these other areas of periodontics is being considered by the Board of Trustees.

12. Where is the research to support statements made in the *Guidelines?*
    • The Academy's Web site includes many resources that support the *Guidelines for the Management of Patients with Periodontal Diseases*. These resources are located at www.perio.org/resources-products/posppr2.html.

13. Is the Academy implying a medicolegal standard with the dissemination of these *Guidelines?*
    • This document is intended to serve as a guide for the dental team in managing patients with periodontal diseases.
    • The Academy believes that all dentists have the right to practice according to their education, training, and experience. Clearly, each dentist has an obligation to render treatment in the best interests of the patient. It is hoped that this document will help dentists identify patients at greatest risk for periodontal diseases so that these patients receive appropriate and timely periodontal care.

EXPLANATION OF TERMS
• May: A choice to act or not; indicates freedom or liberty to follow a suggested alternative.
• Should: A highly desirable direction but does not mean mandatory.
• Must: Used to express a command; indicates an imperative or duty. This term does not appear in the document and is provided as a comparison to the terms "may" and "should."
• Co-management: A shared responsibility for patient care between a periodontist and referring dentist. This patient management may consist of consultation and/or treatment.
• Reevaluation: Assessment of a patient's periodontal status and risk profile after therapy to be used as a basis for subsequent patient management.
• Deteriorating risk profile: Adverse changes in risk factors/indicators suggestive of disease onset or progression.
• Disease definitions: For disease definitions such as severe chronic periodontitis, aggressive periodontitis, and acute periodontal conditions, please refer to volume 4 of the *Annals of Periodontology* at www.perio.org/resources-products/classification.htm.
• Peri-implant disease: Chronic inflammation and/or bone loss around dental implants that may influence implant status.
• Periodontal inflammation: Most periodontal diseases including chronic and aggressive periodontitis are inflammatory diseases. Chronic periodontitis has an infectious etiology from the endogenous plaque biofilm. This type of opportunistic infection results in a chronic release of inflammatory cytokines, prostaglandins, and destructive enzymes from neutrophils and mononuclear cells in the periodontium. The ensuing chronic inflammation in the tissue is what leads to the pathologic anatomic changes clinically detectable as periodontal pockets and alveolar bone loss. Furthermore, some

microorganisms of the biofilm and inflammatory mediators from the affected tissue may adversely affect systemic chronic inflammatory diseases and pregnancy outcomes.

- Significant root surface exposure: Gingival recession of sufficient magnitude that results in the loss of tooth structure, sensitivity, esthetic concerns, or attachment loss.

Source: Reprinted with permission from the American Academy of Periodontology. The *Guidelines* were approved by the Board of Trustees of the American Academy of Periodontology in August 2006. Any citation of this document must be to the *Journal of Periodontology* as: American Academy of Periodontology. Guidelines for the management of patients with periodontal diseases. *J Periodontol* 2006;77:1607-1611. The *Guidelines* will be updated periodically. The most current version of the *Guidelines* is available online at www.perio.org/resources-products/posppr3-1.html.

Did You Know?

Younger dentists (< 31 years) are more likely to treat periodontal disease in their practice, while dentists between 31 and 45 are more likely to refer patients to a periodontist. Sixty percent of dentists ≥ 46 referred fewer patients and were more likely to treat themselves.

Phases of Treatment

Ideal **treatment planning** incorporates a logical interplay between periodontal and nonperiodontal procedures. This is because successful management of the periodontal diseases is a multifaceted discipline that can be affected by other dental conditions and treatments. Box 19–2 depicts four sequential phases that are guidelines for overall case management. In addition to developing a "best case" treatment plan, reasonable alternatives should be considered and presented to the patient. Flowcharts may help delineate the general route a patient takes during treatment (Boxes 19–3 through 19–8).

Phase I: Nonsurgical/Initial Preparation The goal of Phase I therapy is to reduce all etiologic and risk factors to the maximum extent possible—short of surgical intervention. Conditions associated with pain, such as a periodontal abscess, necrotizing ulcerative gingivitis, or traumatic injury, should be treated at this time. Nonrestorable teeth should be identified and extracted. Teeth needing endodontic therapy should be treated.

Oral hygiene instruction and patient education are performed. Patients need to learn that diligent self-care is the critical foundation for successful periodontal treatment. Boxes 19–5 through 19–10 emphasize self-care training, professional analyses, and technique refinement to a degree some may consider excessive. However, failure to provide compulsive clinical emphasis on patient motivation and self-care techniques invites many treatment failures that could be avoided.

Oral prophylaxis and periodontal debridement may be performed. The tissue responses to in-office and improved self-care may be assessed as soon as a week later.

Multiple appointments during this phase help the patient better understand his or her role as cotherapist. They also help build the key concept of a patient–hygienist–dentist team—organized to fight together against periodontitis on a site-by-site basis.

As this phase draws to a close, if signs of inflammation persist at deeper probing sites—especially those the patient is keeping free of supragingival plaque—the need for periodontal surgery is often obvious to everyone.

Phase II: Periodontal Surgery Although evidence exists suggesting an approximate equivalence between arrestive outcomes of closed debridement procedures and open (surgical) procedures in many types of periodontal defects, practitioners need to know that the design of these nonsurgical studies (e.g., 20 minutes of root planing per tooth) is clinically unrealistic (Froum, Weinberg, Tarnow, 1998; Lindhe et al., 1984; Pihlstrom, McHugh, Oliphant, & Ortiz-Campos, 1983; Ramfjord et al., 1987). In addition, root anatomy (such as concavities), furcations, and deep probing depths can compromise the ability to effectively instrument areas via root planing (American Academy of Periodontology, 2001).

Many periodontal surgical procedures are performed to provide the practitioner with better and faster access to deep periodontal pockets. These surgeries may

 Rapid Dental Hint

Tailor the appointment to the needs of the patient. Certain procedures may or may not be provided based on the individual's presentation at the time.

Box 19–2 **Phases of Periodontal Treatment**

Phase I or initial therapy: Disease control
- Emergency care; relief of acute symptoms*
- Oral hygiene instruction*
- Nutritional counseling*
- Correction of inadequate restorations (e.g., over-hang or poorly contoured restorations,* open proximal contacts)
- Periodontal debridement*
- Antimicrobial therapy (oral rinses, oral irrigation for patient self-care, controlled-release products)*
- Systemic antibiotics, if indicated, in aggressive cases
- Fluoride application (varnish or other) for caries control or desensitization, if indicated*
- Smoking cessation*
- Minor orthodontic movement
- Occlusal therapy (including night guards)*
- Extraction of hopeless teeth
- Reevaluation of initial therapy*

Phase II therapy: Surgical correction

Phase III therapy: Restorative/prosthetic care
- Final restorations fabricated

Phase IV therapy: Maintenance care
- Evaluation of patient's oral hygiene*
- Smoking cessation*
- Treatment depends on the condition of the peri-odontium

*Procedures that may be performed by dental hygienists in some jurisdictions. Check with individual state practice regulations.

Box 19–3 **Periodontal Health**

Gingival tissues are healthy and there is no bleeding after gentle probing.

First appointment: 45 minutes to 1 hour
- Comprehensive oral evaluation (new patients) or periodic oral evaluation (existing patients)—consisting of a medical and dental history update, vital signs, head and neck examination, and oral cancer screening.
- Complete X-ray series, including vertical bitewings (new patients) or indicated radiographs (existing patients).
- Oral hygiene instruction.
- Oral prophylaxis.
- Selective polishing, if needed.
- Nutritional counseling for the control of dental caries.
- Fluoride application (varnish or other) for moderate or high caries risk individuals.
- Tobacco counseling for the control and prevention of oral disease, if indicated.
- Suitable maintenance interval established (3, 6, or more months).

---

be arrestive or regenerative. A single surgical procedure may incorporate both elements. For example, an osseous (bone) graft may be placed in a deep infrabony defect on one tooth, whereas bone in adjacent areas may be reduced to facilitate the placement of a pocket-eliminating apically positioned surgical flap that establishes a maintainable gingival form.

Other periodontal surgical procedures may be performed to address gingival recession. The indications for such surgery include dentinal sensitivity, aesthetic complaints, or continuing recession. Many times these procedures are both arrestive and regenerative in character.

Additional periodontal surgical procedures may be performed to maximize the aesthetic results associated with new restorative dentistry. Examples include ridge augmentation and crown lengthening. Procedures per-formed for aesthetics alone are usually termed periodontal plastic surgery.

Phase III: Restorative Care Restorative dentistry is performed in this phase. Ideally, periodontal and prosthetic dentists work together to design restorations that satisfy aesthetic, comfort, and functional needs without compromising future periodontal health.

Phase IV: Maintenance Care Phase IV consists of periodontal maintenance (also termed recall or continuing care). The goal of periodontal maintenance is to prevent continued periodontal destruction. Maintenance care includes reexamination and assessment of the periodontal condition and patient self-care. It often includes an oral prophylaxis and may include periodontal debridement and other local therapies that target persistently inflamed sites.

The frequency of periodontal maintenance visits is individualized and depends on the patient's periodontal status, medical condition, and self-care motivation and effectiveness. Regular periodontal maintenance care is especially important following surgical procedures to ensure success of treatment (DeVore et al., 1986).

Box 19–4   Gingivitis

Probing depths of less than 4 mm; plaque and calculus present; no bone loss or mobility.

First appointment: 1 hour
- Comprehensive oral evaluation (new patients) or periodic oral evaluation (existing patients)—consisting of a medical and dental history update, head and neck examination, and oral cancer screening. Make referrals to appropriate physicians if necessary.
- Periodontal examination.
- Complete X-ray series, including vertical bitewings (new patients) or indicated radiographs (existing patients).
- Note and record sites that bleed on gentle probing.
- Oral hygiene instruction after staining for plaque and relating stained areas to bleeding sites.
- Full-mouth instrumentation.
- Nutritional counseling for the control of dental caries.
- Tobacco counseling for the control and prevention of oral disease, if indicated.

Second appointment: At least 45 minutes, scheduled seven to ten days after first appointment.
- Review medical and dental history.
- Stain for plaque.
- Note and record sites that bleed on gentle probing.
- Evaluate tissue response to previous treatment on a site-by-site basis. If inflammation persists, determine the cause. If plaque or calculus are present, debride the area(s) and reinforce oral hygiene. Adjunctive antimicrobial mouthrinses may be recommended.
- Reinforce plaque control instruction.
- Selective polishing, if indicated.
- Nutritional counseling for the control of dental caries, if needed.
- Fluoride application (varnish or other) for moderate or high caries risk individuals.
- Tobacco counseling for the control of oral disease, if needed.
- If gingival health has been achieved, a suitable maintenance interval is established (three to six months), or after seven to ten days, a third appointment is scheduled if needed.
- Referral to periodontist, if necessary, with alternating maintenance visits planned.

INFORMED CONSENT

Before examination and treatment, the patient must give consent. For medicolegal reasons, **informed consent** is usually recorded using a document signed by the patient and the practitioner, because any treatment provided without consent legally may constitute a battery. Furthermore, a valid consent requires that the patient be made reasonably knowledgeable about the risks and benefits associated with the proposed treatments, alternative treatments, and no treatment. Some individuals cannot execute a valid consent, including minor children.

For periodontal patients, the informed consent form should clearly reflect that the patient understands and accepts the need for periodontal maintenance and oral hygiene self-care.

TREATMENT GUIDELINES

The following treatment guidelines were written for new patients but can be adapted for existing patients. Although treatment-planning guidelines are helpful, it is important to remember that treatment must be tailored to each patient. Experience and the scientific literature have demonstrated that responses to therapy can vary from one patient to another or even in the same patient at different sites and at different times. Therefore, each patient may respond uniquely to the therapy provided.

This section contains guidelines for treating typical periodontal patients and patients with other periodontal conditions, including medication- and hormone-influenced gingivitis, gingivitis and periodontitis related to systemic conditions, aggressive periodontitis, and acute periodontal conditions.

As discussed previously, these guidelines include intensive and continual emphasis on self-care, self-care assessment (by the practitioner), and professional reassessments (of tissue status) on a site-by-site basis. For many patients, these are essential for long-term treatment success. Furthermore, the suggested time allowance for each appointment is subject to change based on the patient's response to care. Of course, these are only guidelines. The ultimate decision and responsibility for how to treat a patient rests with the individual practitioner.

Periodontal Health

Patients presenting with no bleeding on gentle probing and light to no supragingival plaque biofilm and calculus only require an oral prophylaxis (see Box 19–2).

Box 19–5 Slight (Mild) Chronic Periodontitis

Probing depths of 4 to 5 mm; clinical attachment loss (CAL) of 1 to 2 mm; slight horizontal bone loss (up to 20%); no mobility or furcation involvement; supra- and subgingival deposits; bleeding on probing.

First appointment: 1 hour

- Comprehensive oral evaluation (new patients) or periodic oral evaluation (existing patients)—consisting of a medical and a dental history update, head and neck examination, and oral cancer screening. Make referrals to appropriate physicians if necessary.
- Supragingival debridement, if needed, to facilitate a periodontal examination.
- Periodontal examination. Sites that bleed on probing should be recorded.
- Complete X-ray series, including vertical bitewings (new patients) or indicated radiographs (existing patients).
- Stain for plaque and relate stained areas to bleeding sites as part of oral hygiene instruction (patient learns cause and effect).
- Periodontal debridement by quadrant (use of local anesthesia is determined by the practitioner; local anesthesia is a big part of successful treatment).
- Adjunctive antimicrobial irrigation or mouthrinse, if indicated.
- Nutritional counseling for the control of dental caries.
- Tobacco counseling for the control and prevention of oral disease, if indicated.
- Application of desensitizing medicaments, if needed.

Second, third, and fourth appointments: At least 45 minutes (each scheduled seven to ten days after previous appointment)

- Review medical and dental history.
- Evaluate tissue response from previous treatment.
- Stain for plaque.
- Relate stained areas to any bleeding sites as part of oral hygiene instruction (patient learns cause and effect).
- Reinforce plaque biofilm-control instruction.
- Continue debridement procedures by quadrant.
- Nutritional counseling for the control of dental caries.
- Tobacco counseling for the control and prevention of oral disease, if indicated.

- Sustained, slow-release, local-delivery antimicrobials may be used at sites not fully responsive to self-care and debridement (as long as clinical parameters are promptly reassessed and nonresponders are referred, this tactic should offer little or no risk).
- Application of desensitizing medicaments, if needed.

Fifth appointment (reevaluation of therapy): At least 45 minutes (scheduled four to eight weeks after previous appointment (Segelnick & Weinberg, 2006).

- Review medical and dental history.
- Evaluate tissue response from previous treatment.
- Oral and dental examination.
- Periodontal examination; record sites that bleed on probing.
- Stain for plaque and relate stained areas to any bleeding sites as part of oral hygiene instruction (patient learns cause and effect).
- Selective polishing, if indicated.
- Nutritional counseling, if needed.
- Fluoride application (varnish or other) for moderate or high caries risk individuals.
- Tobacco counseling, if indicated.
- Application of desensitizing medicaments, if needed.

At this time, the patient may be put on a suitable maintenance interval of every two to four months if inflammation appears arrested (e.g., no bleeding on probing from deep pockets at sites that patient is maintaining plaque-free) and there is no other reason to refer to a specialist (e.g., unresolved dentinal hypersensitivity, gingival recession, desire or need for periodontal plastic surgery). Over time, this interval can be increased in patients who remain inflammation-free.

If there are nonresponsive sites characterized by deep (4 mm or more) probing depths that bleed on probing or at sites of previous attachment loss, referral to or co-management with the periodontist is appropriate. Given the potential for rapid loss of attachment at any susceptible site, a decision to engage in "watchful waiting" is ethically and legally problematic.

If bleeding on probing persists at shallower sites (gingivitis), the practitioner should reevaluate the patient's self-care techniques and remove any subgingival calculus from suspect sites. Referral to the periodontist is an option for these patients as well.

Box 19–6 Moderate Chronic Periodontitis

Probing depths of 6 to 7 mm; clinical attachment loss (CAL) of 3 to 4 mm; moderate horizontal/vertical bone loss (20 to 50%); mobility and early furcation involvement; supra- and subgingival deposits; bleeding on probing.

First appointment: 1 hour
- Comprehensive oral evaluation (new patients) or periodic oral evaluation (existing patients)—consisting of a medical and dental history update, head and neck examination, and oral cancer screening. Make referrals to appropriate physicians if necessary.
- Complete X-ray series, including vertical bitewings (new patients) or indicated radiographs (existing patients). Referral to the periodontist depends on the type and amount of bone loss.
- Supragingival debridement, if needed, to facilitate a periodontal examination.
- Periodontal examination. Sites that bleed on probing should be recorded.
- Stain for plaque and relate stained areas to bleeding sites as part of oral hygiene instruction (patient learns cause and effect).
- Nutritional counseling for the control of dental caries.
- Tobacco counseling for the control and prevention of oral disease, if indicated.
- Application of desensitizing medicaments, if needed.

Second, third, and fourth appointments: 1 hour (each scheduled seven to ten days after previous appointment)
- Review medical and dental history.
- Evaluate tissue response from previous treatment.
- Stain for plaque and relate stained areas to any bleeding sites as part of oral hygiene instruction (patient learns cause and effect).
- Reinforce plaque biofilm-control instruction.
- Periodontal debridement by quadrant (local anesthesia may be indicated).
- Recommend home adjunctive antimicrobial irrigation or mouthrinse, if indicated.
- Nutritional counseling for the control of dental caries.
- Tobacco counseling for the control and prevention of oral disease, if indicated.
- Application of desensitizing medicaments, if needed.

Fifth appointment (reevaluation of therapy): 1 hour (scheduled four to eight weeks after previous appointment (Segelnick & Weinberg, 2006):
- Review medical and dental history.
- Evaluate tissue response from previous treatment.
- Oral and dental examination.
- Periodontal examination; record sites that bleed on probing.
- Stain for plaque and relate stained areas to any bleeding sites as part of oral hygiene instruction (patient learns cause and effect).
- Periodontal debridement by quadrant (local anesthesia may be indicated).
- Recommend home adjunctive antimicrobial irrigation or mouthrinse, if indicated.
- Sustained, slow-release, local-delivery antimicrobials may be used at nonresponsive sites. (if clinical parameters are promptly reassessed and nonresponders are referred, this tactic should offer little or no risk.)
- Selective polishing, if indicated.
- Nutritional counseling, if needed.
- Fluoride application (varnish or other) for moderate or high caries risk individuals.
- Tobacco counseling, if indicated.
- Application of desensitizing medicaments, if needed.

At this time, the patient may be put on a suitable maintenance interval of two to four months if inflammation appears arrested (e.g., no bleeding on probing from deep pockets at sites that patient is maintaining plaque-free) and there is no other reason to refer to a specialist (e.g., unresolved dentinal hypersensitivity, gingival recession, desire or need for periodontal plastic surgery).

However, if bleeding on probing persists at sites with deeper (4 mm or more) probing depths or at sites of previous attachment loss, referral to the periodontist is indicated—probably for periodontal surgery at those sites.

If no bleeding on probing is present but deep pockets persist, referral to the periodontist may be considered. Research suggests that deep pockets will not break down further if they repeatedly fail over time to demonstrate bleeding on probing (Lang, Adler, Joss, & Nyman, 1990). However, this should be viewed in light of other research showing that deeper pockets are more likely than shallower pockets to experience additional attachment loss due to periodontitis (Grbic & Lamster, 1992; Haffajee et al, 1991).

Box 19–7   Severe Chronic Periodontitis

Probing depths of more than 8 mm; clinical attachment loss (CAL) of > 5 mm; horizontal and vertical bone loss (> 50%); mobility and furcation involvement.

First appointment: 1 hour

- Comprehensive oral evaluation (new patients) or periodic oral evaluation (existing patients)—consisting of a medical and dental history update, head and neck examination, and oral cancer screening. Make referrals to appropriate physicians if necessary. If the patient does not want to be referred to the periodontist, document the refusal in the patient's chart.
- Complete X-ray series, including vertical bitewings (new patients) or indicated radiographs (existing patients). If severe bone loss and heavy deposits exist, consider immediate referral to the periodontist for legal ramifications. If it is decided that initial therapy is to be done in the general practitioner's office, the following steps should be performed.
- Supragingival debridement, if needed, to facilitate a periodontal examination.
- Periodontal examination. Sites that bleed on probing should be recorded.
- Stain for plaque and relate stained areas to bleeding sites as part of oral hygiene instruction (patient learns cause and effect).
- Nutritional counseling for the control of dental caries.
- Tobacco counseling for the control and prevention of oral disease.
- Application of desensitizing medicaments, if needed.

Second appointment: 1 hour (scheduled as soon as possible after initial visit)

- Review medical and dental history.
- Stain for plaque and relate stained areas to bleeding sites as part of oral hygiene instruction (patient learns cause and effect).
- Reinforce plaque biofilm-control instruction.
- Periodontal debridement by quadrant (use of local anesthesia may be indicated).
- Recommend home adjunctive antimicrobial irrigation or mouthrinse, if indicated.
- Nutritional counseling for the control of dental caries.

- Tobacco counseling for the control and prevention of oral disease, if indicated.
- Application of desensitizing medicaments, if needed.

Third, fourth, and fifth appointments: 1 hour (scheduled every 7 to 10 days)

- Review medical and dental history.
- Evaluate tissue response from previous treatment.
- Stain for plaque and relate stained areas to bleeding sites as part of oral hygiene instruction (patient learns cause and effect).
- Reinforce plaque-control instruction.
- Continue debridement procedures by quadrant.
- Recommend home adjunctive antimicrobial irrigation or mouthrinse, if indicated.
- Sustained, slow-release, local-delivery antimicrobials may be used at nonresponsive sites (if clinical parameters are promptly reassessed and nonresponders are referred, this tactic should offer little or no risk).
- Nutritional counseling for the control of dental caries.
- Tobacco counseling for the control and prevention of oral disease, if indicated.
- Application of desensitizing medicaments, if needed.

Sixth appointment (reevaluation of therapy): 1 hour (scheduled four to eight weeks after previous appointment (Segelnick & Weinberg, 2006).

- Review medical and dental history.
- Evaluate tissue response from previous treatment.
- Periodontal examination; record sites that bleed on probing.
- Stain for plaque and relate stained areas to bleeding sites as part of oral hygiene instruction (patient learns cause and effect).
- Reinforce plaque-control instruction.
- Selective polishing, if indicated.
- Sustained, slow-release, local-delivery antimicrobials may be used at nonresponsive sites (if clinical parameters are promptly reassessed and nonresponders are referred, this tactic should offer little or no risk).
- Nutritional counseling for the control of dental caries.

- Fluoride application (varnish or other) for moderate or high caries risk individuals.
- Tobacco counseling for the control and prevention of oral disease, if indicated.
- Application of desensitizing medicaments, if needed.
- At this time, referral to the periodontist is necessary for legal ramifications.

Only rarely will the procedures outlined above result in resolution of inflammation in pockets of more than 8 mm. (If this occurs, treat as for moderate chronic periodontitis.) Therefore, these patients are often referred early on to a periodontist.

Box 19–8   Refractory Periodontitis (Nonresponsive Cases)

The patient does not respond to conventional therapy.
First appointment: 1 hour
- Comprehensive oral evaluation (new patients) or periodic oral evaluation (existing patients)—consisting of a medical and dental history update, head and neck examination, and oral cancer screening. If this is an existing patient and previous treatment in the office has been ineffective, immediate referral to the periodontist is appropriate.
- If the patient does not want to be referred to the periodontist and wants treatment in the general practitioner's office, document the patient's informed refusal in the chart.
- Complete X-ray series, including vertical bitewings (new patients) or indicated radiographs (existing patients). If severe bone loss and heavy deposits, consider immediate referral to a periodontist for legal ramifications. Even though referral is indicated, if it is decided that therapy is to be done in the general practitioner's office, the following steps should be performed.
- Supragingival debridement, if needed, to facilitate periodontal examination.
- Periodontal examination. Sites that bleed on probing should be recorded.
- Stain for plaque and relate stained areas to bleeding sites as part of oral hygiene instruction (patient learns cause and effect).
- Periodontal debridement by quadrant (use of local anesthesia is determined by the practitioner)

in conjunction with systemic antibiotics (four to five appointments).
- Consider adjunctive diagnostic/bacteriologic tests (e.g., genetic test, culture, DNA probe).
- Nutritional counseling for the control of dental caries.
- Tobacco counseling for the control and prevention of oral disease, if indicated.
- Application of desensitizing medicaments, if needed.
- Referral to a periodontist.

Third, fourth, and fifth appointments: 1 hour (scheduled every seven to ten days)
- Review medical and dental history.
- Evaluate tissue response from previous treatment.
- Chart sites that bleed on gentle probing.
- Stain for plaque and relate stained areas to bleeding sites as part of oral hygiene instruction (patient learns cause and effect).
- Reinforce plaque-control instruction.
- Continue debridement procedures by quadrant.
- Nutritional counseling for the control of dental caries.
- Fluoride application (varnish or other) for moderate or high caries risk individuals.
- Tobacco counseling for the control and prevention of oral disease, if indicated.
- Application of desensitizing medicaments, if needed.

These patients are best treated by a periodontist.

Subgingival root debridement is contraindicated. Once oral hygiene efficacy is assured, a suitable periodontal maintenance schedule is determined, usually every six to twelve months.

The motivated and periodontally healthy patient is often "dentally aware." Indeed, past dental therapy may be responsible for the healthy state the patient now enjoys. Such patients generally like discussing new advancements in dentistry. They usually welcome improvements in professional care and self-care and may question the practitioner about new treatment concepts. Oral hygiene instruction time may be used to discuss new oral hygiene products and their applications. The patient must be reminded of the need for future examinations (since problems may occur even though the patient currently appears healthy).

Gingival Diseases

Dental Plaque-Induced Gingivitis

Most cases of gingivitis are plaque-related and are best treated by instrumentation and oral hygiene instructions (see Box 19–4). Dental plaque-induced gingival diseases can be related to dental plaque only, or can be modified by systemic factors, medications or malnutrition. (Armitage, 1999). An example of a dental-plaque-induced gingival disease modified by systemic factors is hormone-associated gingivitis. Pregnancy, oral contraceptives, and puberty can contribute to gingival inflammation. Treatment of hormone-influenced gingivitis is aimed at lowering dental biofilm levels by maintaining meticulous oral hygiene. Frequent periodontal maintenance also may help.

With all cases of gingivitis, the therapeutic goal is to establish gingival health by eliminating the etiologic factors. The ultimate objective is to prevent sites from progressing to periodontitis, and initial periodontal debridement and oral hygiene instructions are the key to minimizing microbial plaque accumulation.

Since we are unable to predict which sites will progress, the entire mouth must be treated. Patients need to be aware of the need for adequate toothbrushing and the use of interdental cleaning aids. Supplemental use of antimicrobial agents (e.g., as mouthrinses or used as home irrigation agents) is recommended in certain patients, such as those with severe bleeding that interferes with debridement procedures or those with poor manual dexterity. Following initial therapy, the patient is placed on a well-monitored periodontal maintenance program.

For all types of gingival diseases, sulcular sites that bleed on gentle probing should be noted and recorded and pointed out to the patient. Plaque staining will reveal areas of dental biofilm accumulation. These should be recorded as well. Bleeding often occurs at these sites. The patient needs to understand this relationship. The patient also needs to appreciate that if a site bleeds as a result of self-care, that site usually needs more self-care attention, not less. This runs counter to the intuition of most patients, whose common response to bleeding is to "leave the area alone."

If the patient is taught to understand that the destructive process is at an early stage and that proper professional care and self-care likely will return the tissues to health, treatment is more likely to succeed. Involve the patient as a co-therapist.

Non-Plaque-Induced Gingival Diseases

This category of gingival diseases was included in the latest classification of periodontal diseases and conditions. (Armitage, 1999). It includes gingival conditions where the primary etiologic agent is not dental plaque biofilm, yet plaque biofilm is a modifying factor. They include diseases of bacterial, viral, fungal, and genetic origin. Also included are manifestations of systemic conditions, traumatic lesions, and foreign body reactions. One of the more commonly encountered non-plaque-induced gingival diseases is drug-induced gingival disease.

Drug-Induced Gingival Disease

Gingival enlargement is sometimes seen in patients taking certain medications. Removal of dental plaque biofilm and calculus by meticulous oral hygiene and regular professional mechanical debridement may help to prevent or slow gingival overgrowth. Therefore, initial treatment should focus on improved self-care and professional plaque and calculus removal. Unfortunately, gingival enlargement still may occur, making it difficult to perform effective self-care and may even interfere with chewing, speech, and appearance. For patients with drug-induced gingival enlargement, overgrowth usually requires surgical intervention. Recurrence is common if the drug is continued. Therefore, it is important to inform the patient's physician about the oral condition and inquire if an alternative drug could be prescribed.

Gingival overgrowth may also be seen in patients with orthodontic appliances. For orthodontic patients, surgical removal of fibrotic pseudopockets can be performed at any time, but recurrence is likely if orthodontic appliances remain.

Periodontitis

The current list of periodontitis classifications includes chronic, aggressive, periodontitis as a manifestation of systemic conditions; necrotizing periodontal diseases; abscesses of the periodontium; periodontitis associated with endodontic lesions; and developmental or acquired deformities and conditions (Armitage, 1999). Chronic periodontitis (formerly termed adult periodontitis) is the most common form of periodontitis seen in otherwise healthy patients. Aggressive periodontitis (formerly termed early-onset periodontitis) is less common but more difficult to treat and should be referred. A brief overview of chronic, aggressive, and necrotizing diseases follows below as well as peri-implantitis. Other chapters cover these conditions in greater detail.

Chronic Periodontitis

In general, the treatment of patients with chronic periodontitis begins with oral hygiene instructions and periodontal debridement, followed by surgical therapy if needed. Patients are then monitored, and treatment is modified as necessary as part of an ongoing periodontal maintenance program. Repeated surgeries sometimes are necessary.

Periodontal patients who demonstrate attachment loss and probing pocket depths of 4 to 5 mm (slight periodontitis) often respond adequately (e.g., elimination of bleeding on probing) to periodontal debridement and effective oral self-care (see Box 19–5). In moderate periodontitis (attachment loss with probing depths of 6 to 7 mm; see Box 19–6) and severe periodontitis (attachment loss with probing depths of more than 8 mm; see Box 19–7), periodontal debridement is less predictable (Stambaugh, Dragoo, Smith, & Carasali, 1981). Following oral hygiene instruction and periodontal debridement, such patients are usually referred to the periodontist—often for periodontal surgery at nonresponsive sites.

Patients with gingival recession should be evaluated. If the recession causes tooth pain, is progressing, or interferes with aesthetics, gingival grafting may be indicated.

It should be noted that chronic periodontitis is site-specific. Some patients demonstrate clinical attachment loss and/or probing depths that are normal at some sites, suggestive of slight periodontitis at other sites, and indicative of moderate or severe periodontitis at others. Therefore, periodontal debridement and improved self-

care may be adequate at some sites but inadequate at others in the same patient. The most problematic sites guide ideal patient management. In other words, the persistence of even one diseased site is sufficient to justify referral for more aggressive therapy.

Refractory periodontal patients who do not respond to proper periodontal treatment (see Box 19–8) despite quality self-care and participation in a well-monitored periodontal maintenance program should be referred to a periodontist.

Aggressive Periodontitis

Apparently healthy young people (younger than 30 years of age) can have underlying immune system irregularities that may manifest as periodontitis with rapid attachment loss and bone destruction (American Academy of Periodontology, 2003; Tonetti & Mombelli, 1999). Treatment of this type of periodontitis is similar to that for chronic forms of periodontitis except that surgical intervention and/or antibiotic therapy often are used immediately. Therefore, these patients should be referred promptly to a periodontist.

Necrotizing Periodontal Diseases

Necrotizing ulcerative gingivitis (NUG) and necrotizing ulcerative periodontitis (NUP) are collectively referred to as necrotizing periodontal diseases. Necrotizing ulcerative gingivitis (NUG) is an infection localized to the gingiva. Contributory risk factors include emotional stress, poor oral hygiene, cigarette smoking, and HIV infections (Rowland, 1999). NUP involves the attachment apparatus and is seen primarily in individuals with systemic conditions including, but not limited to, HIV infection, severe malnutrition, and immunosuppression (Novak, 1999). Treatment includes prescribing analgesics and systemic antibiotics, periodontal debridement and referral to a periodontist for periodontal surgery, if indicated.

Peri-Implantitis

Treatment of peri-implant diseases may include periodontal debridement, oral hygiene instructions, mouthrinses, systemic antibiotics, arrestive and regenerative periodontal surgery, and/or implant removal. Referral to a periodontist is recommended.

Prognosis

Prognosis is a prediction of the future course of a malady with or without treatment. All aspects of the patient's history, data from the clinical examination, and the patient's healing capacity are factors.

Common clinical factors used in assigning a prognosis are reviewed in Box 19–9 (McGuire & Nunn, 1996). This checklist can be reviewed as part of developing a prognosis for each patient. The more unfavorable factors noted, the worse the prognosis. Furthermore, prognosis determination and risk assessment help develop a more appropriate treatment plan both before and after active therapy.

Prognosis is usually reported using a graded scale. This may be a simple scale such as good, guarded, or poor or a scale with more intervals such as good, fair, poor, questionable, or hopeless (Box 19–10; McGuire & Nunn, 1996).

Determination of prognosis is important in treatment planning so that the practitioner and patient can agree on a plan that best satisfies the patient's overall goals while minimizing disappointments if setbacks occur. Realistic prognoses are of amplified importance in complex cases that combine periodontal and restorative therapies. This is because in these patients, the unexpected loss of a key

---

Box 19–10 Prognostic Classification for Individual Teeth

- Good prognosis: Adequate periodontal support around the tooth and can be easily maintained by the practitioner and the patient.
- Fair prognosis: About 25% bone loss. Class I furcation involvement present and can be properly maintained.
- Poor prognosis: About 50% bone loss. Class II furcation involvement present and can be maintained but with difficulty.
- Questionable prognosis: Greater than 50% bone loss around the tooth. Class II and III furcation involvements present that cannot be maintained.
- Hopeless prognosis: Not enough bony support around the tooth to maintain it in its socket. Extraction of tooth recommended.

Source: McGuire and Nunn, 1996.

Box 19–9 Common Clinical Factors Used in Determining a Prognosis

Factors affecting prognosis of individual teeth:
- Amount of bone remaining
- Depth of pockets
- Pattern of bone loss, horizontal or vertical
- Tooth mobility
- Type of infrabony defect: one, two, or three walls
- Root anatomy, favorable or unfavorable
- Furcation involvement
- Crown-to-root ratio, favorable or unfavorable
- Caries or pulpal involvement, yes or no
- Missing teeth and restorative dentistry

Factors affecting overall prognosis:
- Age
- Significant medical history (e.g., diabetes)
- Smoker, yes or no, past smoker
- Family history of periodontal diseases, yes or no
- Oral hygiene: good, fair, or poor
- Compliant with treatment and home care, yes or no

Source: Adapted from McGuire and Nunn, 1996.

---

abutment tooth may necessitate replacement of complicated and expensive crown and bridge prosthetics.

ADJUNCTIVE TREATMENT

Antimicrobials

Systemic antibiotics often are prescribed as part of the treatment of aggressive periodontitis or of periodontitis patients with systemic maladies. For example, administration of a systemic antibiotic, debridement, and surgery constitute an appropriate course of therapy for a patient with a localized aggressive periodontitis. Systemic antibiotics are not used in patients with chronic periodontitis or gingivitis. In the case of refractory periodontal diseases, specific antibiotics are selected based on identification of the suspected pathogens.

The regimens governing the use of systemic antibiotics in patients with periodontitis are frequently changing. Therefore, clinicians who consider using systemic antimicrobials to treat aggressive and refractory periodontitis must remain very up-to-date with the appropriate biomedical literature.

Controlled-release antimicrobial drug systems as supplements to periodontal debridement may be indicated when clinical signs of inflammation (bleeding upon probing) persist in pockets of 5 mm or greater at localized sites. However, continuing reassessment is needed to determine if other therapies are indicated.

Chlorhexidine gluconate rinses are prescribed frequently for specified periods when mechanical plaque control is not feasible (e.g., after surgery, after acute infection). Antimicrobial rinses are not indicated in patients with periodontitis, since rinses are only delivered supragingivally. Use of mouthrinses is as an adjunct to oral self-care and should not be as a substitute.

GERIATRIC PATIENTS

Although the same general guidelines already provided for chronic periodontitis patients apply to the elderly, geriatric patients often have special needs. They may present with uncontrolled dental plaque biofilm and/or xerostomia. Other oral pathologies, including oral cancers, are more common among members of this age group.

Plaque Control

Age-related factors may limit the ability of a patient to perform adequate oral self-care. Using a toothbrush or dental floss may be impossible for patients with arthritis or stroke-related impairments. Dementia may affect an individual's ability or motivation to perform daily oral hygiene procedures. Virtually any debilitating systemic illness may predispose patients to periodontitis—and many of these maladies are seen more commonly in aged populations. Most important, periodontal treatment may be complicated by multiple medical conditions.

Xerostomia

Decreased saliva production occurs with advancing age (Ghezzi & Ship, 2003). Furthermore, many of the hundreds of medications known to decrease salivary flow are used by older people. Antidepressants, antihistamines, antihypertensives, antipsychotics, diuretics, antiparkinsonians, and antianxiety agents all may contribute to xerostomia (Brangan, 1994). Older patients, with decreased protective properties of saliva, are at increased risk for dental caries and periodontal diseases (Rees, 1998).

If a patient complains of xerostomia, or if dryness seems to be contributing to oral problems, relevant systemic medications should be identified and alternatives considered. Saliva substitutes may be recommended, but these have limited effectiveness and can be expensive.

Treatment Considerations

When treating geriatric patients, the practitioner must consider systemic concerns that may complicate the management of periodontal conditions. It may be important for the dentist and hygienist to consult with a patient's physician to review pertinent details of the patient's medical conditions.

Treatment goals for the elderly are the same as for the young, that is, the preservation (or restoration) of an aesthetic, comfortable, and functional dentition. This is not to suggest that age should not be a factor in planning how best to achieve these goals; indeed, conservative therapy may be more appropriate in older patients for a number of reasons. Whatever treatment is planned, it should be flexible and adapted to each patient's particular needs. As these needs change, so should the therapy.

Successful treatment of the elderly often requires a high degree of cooperation between the practitioner, patient, and other supporting caregivers. Modified self-care routines may be necessary, such as use of a toothpick or interdental brush instead of floss, a toothbrush with a modified handle such as a tennis ball, and the frequent use of antimicrobial agents (such as fluorides or chlorhexidine) along with mechanical plaque control. Automated oral hygiene devices may facilitate more effective plaque control.

DENTAL HYGIENE NOTES

Research supports the majority of procedures routinely performed by the dental hygienist to prevent or arrest the progression of the common periodontal maladies. Science, combined with clinical experience and inferential skills, has produced the periodontal parameters of care for today. As time passes, continued scientific testing of new and old therapeutic tactics along with clinical experience will continue to underpin future parameters for periodontal care.

Periodontal treatment planning remains complicated. For now, ongoing periodontal care should be modulated based on the response of the patient to self-care and treatment rendered previously. If a desired and optimal response is not achieved, some other reasonable approach must be used and assessed. Critical analyses of outcomes will sometimes suggest that referral to a specialist is in the best interest of the patient.

Quality assessment has been defined as "a measure of care provided in a particular setting" (Burt & Eklund,

1992). Quality assurance is a broader concept that encompasses assessment of care along with the "implementation of any necessary changes to either maintain or improve the quality of care rendered" (Burt & Eklund, 1992).

Dental hygienists have the professional responsibility to promote the oral health of the public in the most effective ways possible. As excerpted from the American Dental Hygienists Association's (2007-2008) Code of Ethics, "We acknowledge the following responsibilities to patients or clients:

- Provide oral health care utilizing high levels of professional knowledge, judgment, and skill.
- Maintain a work environment that minimizes the risk of harm.
- Serve all clients without discrimination and avoid action toward any individual or group that may be interpreted as discriminatory.
- Hold professional client relationships confidential.
- Communicate with clients in a respectful manner.
- Promote ethical behavior and high standards of care by all dental hygienists.
- Serve as an advocate for the welfare of clients.
- Provide clients with the information necessary to make informed decisions about their oral health and encourage their full participation in treatment decisions and goals.
- Refer clients to other healthcare providers when their needs are beyond our ability or scope of practice.
- Educate clients about high-quality oral heath care."

KEY POINTS

- Evidence-based periodontal treatment based on dental literature focuses on the recognition of risk, prognosis, and treatment factors.
- The evidence-based approach is a good model for evaluating the results of periodontal therapy.
- Problem-based learning identifies patient's dental problems.
- The ideal goal of periodontal therapy is to restore the periodontium destroyed by disease to a comfortable and functional state of health.
- Periodontal treatment involves ongoing care and demands continued reassessments.

SELF-QUIZ

1. Which one of the following factors improves the treatment decisions made by dental/medical practitioners? (p. 259)
   a. Clinical experience of the practitioner and use of scientific literature
   b. Following the advice of fellow dental practitioners
   c. Following the advice of fellow medical practitioners
   d. Consulting with the dental companies
2. Which one of the following statements is the ideal goal of periodontal therapy? (p. 259)
   a. Control or eliminate and prevent the initiation, progression, or recurrence of periodontal diseases.
   b. Promote tissue healing by regeneration or replacement of the lost tissue with new bone, cementum, and periodontal ligament.
   c. Restore the periodontium to an attractive, comfortable, and functional state of health for the balance of the patient's life.
   d. Allow the attachment apparatus to relax.
   e. Remove all microbial plaque every day.
3. Which one of the following steps should be first in developing a plan to treat a patient? (p. 264)
   a. Teach proper use of oral hygiene aids.
   b. Perform risk assessment.
   c. Discuss the case with the patient.
   d. Decide on the proper maintenance interval.
   e. Obtain informed consent for periodontal maintenance.
4. All the following are phases of treatment except one. Which one is the exception? (p. 272)
   a. Phase I: disease control
   b. Phase II: surgical correction
   c. Phase III: restorative/prosthetic care
   d. Phase IV: maintenance care
   e. Phase V: implant care
5. In which one of the following phases of treatment is reevaluation of initial therapy completed? (p. 272)
   a. I
   b. II
   c. III
   d. IV
   e. V

6. Which one of the following treatment steps is most appropriate in controlling pregnancy-associated gingivitis? (p. 278)
   a. Surgical intervention
   b. Oral irrigation with chlorhexidine
   c. Plaque control with toothbrushing and flossing
   d. Systemic antibiotics
   e. Estrogen supplements

7. Which one of the following treatments is most appropriate for patients with localized aggressive periodontitis? (p. 279)
   a. Periodontal debridement, systemic antibiotics, and surgery
   b. Periodontal debridement and surgery
   c. Oral rinsing and periodontal debridement
   d. Oral irrigation and periodontal debridement
   e. Improved oral hygiene and watchful waiting

8. Which one of the following sequences is the best initial treatment for a patient with gingival enlargement caused by phenytoin? (p. 278)
   a. Oral hygiene instructions, periodontal debridement, systemic antibiotics, and surgery
   b. Oral hygiene instructions and periodontal debridement
   c. Periodontal debridement and systemic antibiotics
   d. Periodontal debridement and surgery
   e. Discontinuation of phenytoin

9. Which one of the following definitions best describes the term *prognosis*? (p. 279)
   a. Prediction of the future course of a condition with or without treatment
   b. Prediction of the future course of a condition without treatment
   c. Identification and naming of the type of condition present
   d. Patient's healing capacity

10. Which one of the following is the most important consideration when treating geriatric patients? (p. 281)
    a. Therapy may be complicated by multiple medical conditions.
    b. The ability to properly understand oral hygiene instructions may be impaired.
    c. Anxiety level is higher in this age group.
    d. Severe frailty inhibits normal maneuvering in the dental office.
    e. Physical impairments are possible.

REFERENCES

American Academy of Periodontology. 2000a Parameters of Care. *J. Periodontol.* 71 (Suppl.):847–883.

American Academy of Periodontology. 2000b. Parameter on Periodontal Maintenance. *J. Periodontol.* 71:849–850.

American Academy of Periodontology. 2001. Academy Report: Treatment of plaque induced gingivitis, chronic periodontitis, and other clinical conditions. *J. Periodontol.* 72:1790–1800.

American Academy of Periodontology. 2003. Position paper: Periodontal diseases of children and adolescents. *J. Periodontol.* 74:1696–1704.

American Academy of Periodontology. 2006. Guidelines for the management of patients with periodontal diseases. *J. Periodontol.* 77:1607–1611.

American Academy of Periodontology. 2008. Position paper: Risk assessment. *J. Periodontol* 79:202.

American Dental Hygienists' Association. 2007. *2007–2008 Bylaws and code of ethics.* Chicago: Author.

Armitage, G. 1999. Development of a classification system for periodontal diseases and conditions. *Ann. Periodontol.* 4: 1–6.

Axelsson, P., B. Nystrom, and J. Lindhe. 2004. The long-term effect of a plaque control program on tooth mortality, caries, and periodontal disease in adults: Results after 30 years of maintenance. *J. Clin. Periodontol.* 31(9):749–57.

Axelsson, P., and J. Lindhe. 1981. The significance of maintenance care in the treatment of periodontal disease. *J. Clin. Periodontol.* 8:281–294.

Burt, B., and S. Eklund. 1992. *Dentistry, dental practice and the community.* Philadelphia: W. B. Saunders.

Brangan, P. 1994. Dental hygiene care for the older adult. In eds. M. L. Darby and M. Walsh, *Dental hygiene theory and practice,* 873–912. Philadelphia: W. B. Saunders.

DeVore, C. H., D. M. Duckworth, F. M. Beck, M. J. Hicks, F. W. Brumfield, and J.E. Horton. 1986. Bone loss following periodontal therapy in subjects without frequent periodontal maintenance. *J. Periodontol.* 57:354–359.

Dockter, K. M., K. B. Williams, K. S. Bray, et al. 2006. Relationship between prereferral periodontal care and periodontal status at time of referral. *J. Periodontol.* 77:1708–1716.

Douglass, C. W. 2006. Risk assessment and management of periodontal disease. *JADA* 137(3):27S–32S.

Froum, S. J., M. A. Weinberg, and D. Tarnow. 1998. Comparison of bioactive glass and open debridement. *J. Periodontol.* 68:698–709.

Ghezzi, E. M., and J. A. Ship. 2003. Aging and secretory reserve capacity of major salivary glands. *J Dent Res.* (October) 82(10):844–8.

Grossi, S. G., R. J. Genco, E. E. Machtei, A. W. Ho, G. Koch, et al. 1995. Assessment of risk for periodontal disease: II. Risk indicators for alveolar bone loss. *J. Periodontol.* 66:23–29.

Grossi, S. G., J. J. Zambon, A. W. Ho, G. Koch, R. G. Dunford, et al. 1994. Assessment of risk for periodontal disease: I. Risk indicators for attachment loss. *J. Periodontol.* 65:260–267.

Haffajee, A. D., and S. S. Socransky. 2006. Introduction to microbial aspects of periodontal biofilm communities, development and treatment. *Periodontology 2000* 42(1):7–12.

Haffajee, A. D., S. S. Socransky, J. Lindhe, R. L. Kent, H. Okamoto, and T. Yoneyama. 1991. Clinical risk indicators for periodontal attachment loss. *J. Clin. Periodontol.* 18:117–125.

Hancock, E. B. 1996. Prevention. *Ann. Periodontol.* 1:223–249.

Ismail, A. I., E. C. Morrison, B. A. Burt, R. G. Caffesse, and M. T. Kavanagh. 1990. Natural history of periodontal disease in adults: Findings from the Tecumseh Periodontal Disease Study, 1959–1987. *J. Dent. Res.* 69:430–435.

Kolenbrander, P. E., R. J. Palmer, A. H. Rickard, et al. 2006. Bacterial interactions and successions during plaque development. *Periodontology 2000* 52(1):47–79.

Lindhe, J., E. Westfelt, S. Nyman, S. S. Socransky, I. L. Heij, G. Bratthall. 1984. Long-term effect of surgical/nonsurgical treatment of periodontal disease. *J. Clin. Periodontol.* 11:448–458.

Loesche, W. 1976. Chemotherapy of dental plaque infections. *Oral Sci. Rev.* 9:65–107.

McGuire, K. M., and M. E. Nunn. 1996. Prognosis versus actual outcome: II. The effectiveness of clinical parameters in developing an accurate prognosis. *J. Periodontol.* 67:658–665.

Novak, M. J. 1999. Necrotizing ulcerative periodontitis. *Ann. Periodontol.* 4:74–77.

Page, R. C., J. Martin, E. A. Krall, L. Mancl, and R. Garcia. 2003. Longitudinal validation of a risk calculator for periodontal disease. *J. Clin. Periodontol* 30(9):819–27.

Persson, G. R., L. A. Mancl, J. Martin, and R. C. Page. 2003. Assessing periodontal disease risk: A comparison of clinicians' assessment versus a computerized tool. *J Am Dent Assoc.* (May) 134(5):575–82.

Pihlstrom, B., R. McHugh, T. Oliphant, and C. Ortiz-Campos. 1983. Comparison of surgical and nonsurgical treatment of periodontal disease: A review of current studies and additional results after 6 1/2 years. *J. Clin. Periodontol.* 10:524–541.

Ramfjord, S. P., R. G. Caffesse, E. C. Morrison, R. W. Hill, G. J. Kerry, et al. 1987. Four modalities of periodontal treatment compared over 5 years. *J. Clin. Periodontol.* 14:445–452.

Rees, T. D. 1998. Drugs and oral disorders. *Periodontol 2000* 18:21–36.

Rowland, R. W. 1999. Necrotizing ulcerative gingivitis. *Ann. Periodontol.* 4:65–73.

Segelnick, S., and M. A. Weinberg. 2006. Reevaluation after initial therapy. When is the appropriate time? *J. Periodontol.* (September) 77(9):1598–601.

Stambaugh, R. V., M. Dragoo, D. M. Smith, and L. Carasali. 1981. The limits of subgingival scaling. *Int. J. Periodont. Restor. Dent.* 1(5):31–41.

Tonetti, M. S., and A. Mombelli. 1999. Early-onset periodontitis. *Ann. Periodontol.* 4:39–52.

Van Dyke, T. 2007. Control of inflammation and periodontitis. *Periodontology 2000* 45(1):158–166.

Van Dyke, T. E., and C. N. Serhan, 2003. Resolution of inflammation: A new paradigm for the pathogenesis of periodontal diseases. *J. Dent Res* 82(2): 82–90.

Chapter 20

Oral Hygiene for the Periodontal Patient: Beyond the Basics

Judith Kreismann

Khalid Almas

OUTLINE

Introduction
Definition of Oral Hygiene Self-Care
Periodontal Disease Control
Preventive Measures
Oral Hygiene Self-Care Methods
Oral Home Care for Patients with Periodontal
 Disease
Advice to the Patient
Effects of Improper Use of Oral Hygiene Devices
Dentinal Hypersensitivity
Dental Hygiene Notes
Key Points
Self-Quiz
References

EDUCATIONAL OBJECTIVES

Upon completion of this chapter, the reader should be able to:

• Describe measures to prevent and control the progression of periodontal diseases.
• Introduce protocols for different types of hygiene care recommended to the patient with periodontal diseases.
• Discuss the consideration of the patients' goals for their oral and systemic health.
• Discuss the importance of interdental cleaning in maintaining periodontal health.
• Discuss the significance of halitosis; how to control, cure, and the role of the dental hygienist in patient care.
• Describe the standards for plaque-control regimen following periodontal and implant surgery.

GOAL: To provide information about the fundamentals of counseling patients with periodontal disease on oral hygiene self-care.

KEY WORDS

dentifrice **300**
halitosis **287**
oral biofilms **292**
oral hygiene self-care **286**
patient education **286**
primary prevention **287**
secondary prevention **287**

INTRODUCTION

There is no alternative to well-performed oral hygiene self-care as a preventive measure. The willingness and ability of patients to keep dental plaque below the threshold for disease is essential. Preventive measures are important for a healthy periodontium as well as to achieve a successful outcome of periodontal therapy. Preventive measures in periodontics depend on the removal of supra- and subgingival dental plaque biofilms. The most common preventive methods involve both personal and professional mechanical plaque control. Preventive measures should control or eliminate etiologic factors as well as eliminate risk factors for inflammatory periodontal diseases (Hancock, 1996). The control of supragingival plaque in conjunction with professional tooth cleaning subgingivally forms the basis for the management of progressive periodontal diseases (Corbet & Davies, 1993). Supragingival plaque control contributes to preventing or moderating subgingival microbial recolonization. This chapter focuses on fundamental information related to oral hygiene self-care for the periodontal patient.

DEFINITION OF ORAL HYGIENE SELF-CARE

Oral hygiene self-care, also known as oral physiotherapy or oral home care, is defined as physical therapy for the mouth or oral cavity. It refers to daily oral healthcare practices employed by the patient to prevent dental and gingival diseases and maintain optimal oral health. The rationale for oral hygiene self-care as well as professional periodontal debridement is to eliminate or suppress harmful microorganisms found in supragingival biofilms. Consequently, plaque control prevents the potential detrimental effects of pathogenic microorganisms on the teeth and periodontium. The primary method of oral hygiene self-care is the use of such mechanical oral hygiene measures as a toothbrush and interdental cleaning devices. Since not all bacteria in biofilms are pathogenic (disease-producing), the objective of treatment is not total elimination of all bacteria but rather control of the bacteria.

Did You Know?

In 200 CE, the Romans used a mixture of bones, eggshells, oyster shells, and honey to clean their teeth.

Periodontal Health: Motivation and Behavior

Since dental and periodontal health is taking on increasing importance for both patients and family members, evaluation of a patient's motivation and behavior in terms of oral self-care is important in the overall treatment plan.

In the process of evaluating a patient's oral hygiene, it is necessary to assess the clinical aspects of oral hygiene as well as relate the patient's attitude toward oral hygiene and his or her commitment to oral hygiene practices.

PERIODONTAL DISEASE CONTROL

It is well known that the accumulation of supragingival dental plaque on tooth surfaces near the free gingival margin is associated with the development of gingivitis. Thus, removal of dental plaque from tooth surfaces is a basic step in the prevention and treatment of gingivitis. Subgingival bacteria are derived from the supragingival dental plaque. If supragingival plaque is not removed, subgingival plaque develops. Subgingival bacteria play an important role in the progression of periodontal diseases. Therefore, meticulous mechanical supragingival plaque control can reduce the risk for the development of periodontitis or for disease recurrence after periodontal therapy or prevent further loss of attachment if periodontitis is already present (Addy & Adriaens, 1998; Westfelt, 1996). Clinical trials have shown that professionally delivered and frequently repeated supragingival tooth cleaning, combined with optimal self-performed plaque control, has a marked effect in controlling subgingival microbiota in moderate to deep periodontal pockets (Hellström, Romberg, Krok, & Lindhe, 1996).

Patient Education

Informing the periodontal patient about oral hygiene self-care is one of the most important roles of the dental hygienist. **Patient education** provides the patient with the necessary information and skills for the prevention of dental caries and periodontal diseases. A thorough knowledge of oral hygiene self-care is essential for dental hygienists to help plan successful preventive strategies related to a patient's individual plaque-control needs.

One way to highlight the presence of dental plaque is by using disclosing agents. The purpose of using disclosing tablets or liquid is for supragingival plaque detection. The most commonly used disclosing agent is erythrosin, which is FD & C Red No. 28. Erythrosin stains newly formed dental plaque, making it visible to the naked eye.

Studies have shown that the method used to educate patients about oral hygiene self-care techniques is not critical (Glavid, Christensen, Pedersen, Rosendahl, & Attström, 1985). Therefore, instructions can be given personally by the dental hygienist, and/or the patient may be provided with a self-instruction manual, pamphlet, or videotape.

PREVENTIVE MEASURES

The primary goal of prevention is to achieve the lowest plaque level possible. Total elimination of bacteria is neither possible nor desirable, because a number of beneficial bacteria exist in the oral cavity that are necessary for a balanced oral environment.

Preventive measures are classified into two main groups depending on when mechanical plaque control is instituted during the disease process. **Primary prevention** describes preventive measures taken to prevent disease from occurring. It aims at reducing plaque in all individuals regardless of their susceptibility to disease. On the other hand, if periodontal disease is already present in an individual, the goal of treatment changes from preventing the occurrence of disease to preventing the disease from progressing further or preventing the recurrence of the disease after treatment. This is **secondary prevention** (Garmyn, van Steenberghe, & Quirynen, 1998).

Halitosis

Halitosis is the general term used to describe unpleasant breath, regardless of its sources, oral or nonoral (e.g., expired air). *Oral malodor* is the term especially used to describe the odor from the oral cavity.

Oral malodor, bad breath, or halitosis is a common complaint encountered by dental practitioners. It may be due to poor oral hygiene, local factors, or systemic involvement. Oral malodor affects a large proportion of population and may cause a significant social or psychological handicap to those suffering from it.

It has been estimated that 10 to 30% of the U.S. population suffers from bad breath on a regular basis (Meskin, 1996). In other studies, 20 to 60% of the population suffers from chronic oral malodor, and in approximately half of these individuals, the problem becomes serious enough to create personal discomfort and social embarrassment (Bosy, 1997; Brunete, Proskin, & Nelson, 1998). There is potential impact of oral malodor on personal life, so sufferers often make desperate attempts to mask their oral malodor with mints and chewing gum, compulsive brushing, and repeated use of mouthrinses.

In most cases, the problem of oral malodor has been shown to originate in the oral cavity, where conditions that favor the retention of anaerobic, mainly Gram-negative bacteria, lead to the development of bad breath (Ratcliff & Johnson, 1999). In addition to the periodontal pockets, the most important retention site is the dorsum of the tongue with its numerous papillae (Delanghe et al., 1999; Scully, El-Maaytah, Porter, & Greenman, 1997). There are various compounds that produce unpleasant smells in the human oral environment, such as hydrogen sulfide, methanethiol, dimethylsulfide, n-dodecanol, n-tetradecanol, phenol, indole, diphenylamine, pyridine, and others (Kostelc, Preti, Zelson, et al., 1980). Especially volatile sulfur compounds (VSC; hydrogen sulfide, methylmercaptan, and dimethyl sulfide), which arise from bacterial metabolism of amino acids, mainly contribute to oral malodor. It has been demonstrated that the intensity of clinical bad breath is significantly associated with amount of intraoral VSC level (Replogle & Beebe, 1996). The periodontal pocket is an ideal environment for VSC production with respect to the bacterial profile and sulfur source. In addition, VSC also accelerate periodontal tissue destruction. This may explain why patients with periodontal diseases often complain of oral malodor (Morita & Wang, 2001). Many people still believe that bad breath originates in the stomach. Halitosis is rarely a gastrointestinal condition (Page, 1997). Research reports now agree that, in the vast majority of cases, halitosis (80 to 90%) originates within the oral cavity, where anaerobic bacteria degrade sulfur-containing amino acids to the foul-smelling volatile sulfur compounds (Rosenberg, 1996; Tonzetich, 1997). The oral and systemic factors predisposing toward bad breath are given in Boxes 20–1 and 20–2.

Classification of Patients with Halitosis

Although halitosis involves oral, systemic, and psychological pathologies, a clear classification has not been established, and mismanagement of psychological or systemic cases of halitosis can occur. The classification system reported by Miyazaki and colleagues (1999) has three categories: genuine halitosis, pseudo-halitosis, and

Box 20–1   Oral Conditions That May Cause Bad Breath

- Periodontal pockets
- Xerostomia (dryness of mouth)
- Carious lesions
- Bacterial biofilms
- Interdental areas debris
- Spaces between the papillae of the tongue
- Poor restorations
- Calculus
- Erupting wisdom teeth (pericoronitis)
- Remaining roots
- Gangrenous pulps (necrosed pulp tissue)
- NUG (necrotizing ulcerative gingivitis)

Box 20–2   Causes to Consider in a Patient with Halitosis

Non-pathologic causes
Oral: morning breath, xerostomia due to mouth breathing and medications
Hunger
Tobacco
Foods: onion, garlic, pastrami, other meats
Alcohol
Pathologic causes
Periodontal disease, xerostomia (underlying illness), gingivitis, stomatitis, glossitis, cancer, candidiasis, parotitis
Gastrointestinal disorders
Gastroesophageal reflux, hiatal hernia, cancer
Nasal
Rhinitis, sinusitis, tumors, foreign bodies
Pulmonary
Bronchitis, pneumonia, tuberculosis, cancer
Systemic
Diabetes, uremia, hepatic disease, blood dyscrasias, rheumatologic disease, dehydration, fever
Psychiatric
Delusions

halitophobia. Genuine halitosis is subclassified as physiologic halitosis and pathologic halitosis. Pathologic halitosis is categorized as oral pathologic halitosis and extraoral pathologic halitosis (Table 20–1 ■).

Pseudo-halitosis and halitophobia both involve a psychosomatic condition. Patients complain of the presence of bad breath, but offensive malodor is not perceived by others. Improvement of the condition of pseudohalitosis is expected by the explanation of examination results, counseling, and simple treatment measures, such as tongue cleaning. Thus, pseudohalitosis is treatable by dental practitioners. In contrast, patients who are halitophobic believed that there are definite physical or social factors that contribute to their belief in having halitosis, and they cannot be convinced that they do not have malodor. Because of the difficulty in treating halitophobia, it is not considered within the realm of dentistry (Yaegaki & Coil, 2000b). Treatment needs for breath odor are described in detail in Table 20–2 ■.

Diagnosis and Assessment of Oral Malodor

There are many methods available for examination, diagnosis, and assessment of oral malodor.

1. Self-Assessment

Patients have been found to be incapable of scoring their own malodor in an objective fashion. Inability to smell one's own oral malodor has been attributed to adaptation or dulling of sensation resulting from continued exposure. Patients should follow the instructions in Box 20–3 before receiving a breath examination.

2. Gas Chromatography

A few halitosis clinics use a gas chromatography (GC) equipped with a flame photometric detector for diagnosing halitosis (Yaegaki & Coil, 2000a). GC is the gold standard for oral malodor measurement (Miyazaki et al., 1999; Yaegaki & Coil, 2000a). It is an objective means to obtain exact values for the various odorous volatiles. It is a very sensitive method. A flame photometer detector is usually employed for the detection of VSC. Gas chromatography may also be combined with mass spectrometry (an instrument used to identify chemicals in a substance by their mass and charge) enlarging the scope of the method (Preti et al., 1992).

3. Halimeter

The Halimeter (Interscan, CA), using an electrochemical gas sensor cell, has become the primary tool in chronic halitosis research and diagnosis. The Halimeter is twice as sensitive to hydrogen sulfides as it is to methylmercaptan. Halimeter measurements are significantly influenced by other oral gases such as from chewing gum, strong mouthrinse odors, alcohol, shampoo, body lotion, smoking, and even water vapor.

Table 20–1 **Classification of Halitosis with Corresponding Treatment Needs (TN) (Yaegaki & Coil, 2000a; Miyazaki et al., 1999)**

Classification	Subdivision and Treatment Needs	Description
I. Genuine Halitosis A. Physiologic Halitosis	TN – 1	• Obvious malodor intensity beyond socially acceptable level. • Malodor arises through putrefactive process within the oral cavity. • Neither specific disease nor pathologic condition that could cause halitosis is found. • Origin is mainly the dorsoposterior region of the tongue. (Temporary halitosis as a result of dietary factors [e.g., garlic bread] should be excluded)
B. Pathologic Halitosis	1. Oral Pathologic TN-1 and TN-2	• Halitosis caused by disease, pathologic condition, or malfunction of oral tissues. • Halitosis derived from tongue coating modified by pathological condition (e.g. periodontal disease, xerostomia, etc.) is included in this subdivision.
	2. Extraoral Pathologic TN-1 and TN-3	• Malodor originates from nasal, paranasal, and laryngeal regions. • Malodor originates from pulmonary tracts. • Malodor originates from upper digestive tracts. • Malodor originates from disorders anywhere in the body whereby the odor is blood-borne and emitted via lungs (diabetes mellitus, hepatic cirrhosis, uremia, internal bleeding, etc).
II. Pseudo-Halitosis	TN-1 and TN-4	• Obvious malodor is not perceived by others, although a patient stubbornly complains of the existence of his or her halitosis. • Improvement of this condition is highly promising by explanation of examination results, counseling, and simple treatment measures.
III. Halitophobia	TN-1 and TN-5	• After treatment for genuine halitosis or pseudo-halitosis, a patient persists in believing that he or she has halitosis, although no physical or social evidence exists.

Source: Yaegaki and Coil, 2000a; Miyazaki et al., 1999.

Table 20–2 Treatment Needs (TN) for Breath Odor

Category	Description
TN-1*	Explanation of halitosis and instruction for oral hygiene. Support and reinforcement of the patient's self-care for further improvement of his or her oral hygiene.
TN-2	Oral prophylaxis, professional cleaning, and treatment for oral diseases, especially periodontal diseases.
TN-3	Referral to a physician or medical specialist.
TN-4	Explanation of examination data, further professional instruction, education, and reassurance for improvement.
TN-5	Referral to a clinical psychologist, psychiatrist, or other psychological specialist.

*TN-1 is applicable to all cases requiring TN-2 through TN-5.

4. **Organoleptic Measurement**

Organoleptic (the taste and aroma properties of a food or chemical) scoring (Miyazaki et al., 1999) is simply done by smelling the patient's breath and assigning a score of oral malodor (Yaegaki, 2000). (Box 20–4). A translucent tube is inserted into the patient's mouth. The patient exhales as the clinician smells the breath. When the recognition threshold (score 2 or over) is identified, a diagnosis of genuine halitosis is made.

The patient is required to refrain from drinking coffee, tea, juice; smoking; eating garlic; and using scented cosmetics before the assessment. The clinician must have a normal sense of smell. The clinician can regularly check

Box 20–3 Instructions to Patients before Receiving Examination (Miyazaki et al., 1999)

Before the day of assessment, patients are instructed to abstain from:
1. Taking antibiotics for three weeks before the assessment.
2. Garlic, onions, and spicy foods for 48 hours before assessment.
3. Scented cosmetics for 24 hours before assessment.
On the day of the assessment, patients are instructed to abstain from:
1. Food and drink.
2. Oral hygiene practices.
3. Use of oral rinse or breath fresheners.
4. Smoking for twelve hours before assessment.
Source: Miyazaki et al. (1999)

his or her specific sense of smell by sniffing VSC from a freshly boiled egg or nori (seaweed that can be purchased in an Oriental food store) (Yaegaki, 2000).

5. **Simple Determination of Oral Malodor**

When a simple determination of oral malodor is required, the spoon test is preferred. In the spoon test, the posterior area of the dorsal surface of the tongue is assessed by thorough scraping, using a disposable plastic spoon. Afterwards, the spoon can be smelled; it has a very repulsive odor in patients with severe oral malodor (Yaegaki & Coil, 2000b).

6. **Psychological Assessment**

Halitophobia patients and many pseudo-halitosis patients have a psychosomatic condition (Miyazaki et al., 1999; Yaegaki, 2000). Because halitophobia is easily diagnosed using the halitosis classification of Miyazaki and colleagues (1999), corresponding patient management is improved. Psychological assessment is facilitated by specified, tested, and established questionnaires used to acquire medical history as a routine practice.

7. **Tongue Sulfide Probe**

Recently, a tongue sulfide probe for detecting oral malodor has been developed (Morita, Musinski, & Wang, 2001). The tongue sulfide level on the tongue dorsum (VSC level) is determined by using the tongue sulfide probe (Diamond General Development Corporation, Ann Arbor, MI). The probe is applied on the anterior, the middle, or the posterior part of the tongue along the median groove of the tongue dorsum with a light pressure for 30 seconds. The probe is composed of an active sulfide-sensing element and a stable reference element. The sulfide-sensing element generates an electrochemical voltage proportional to the concentration of sulfide ions present. This voltage is measured relative to the operating point of the reference element.

Box 20–4   Organoleptic Scoring Scale (Miyazaki et al., 1999)

0 Absence of Odor	Detectable odor is completely absent.
1 *Questionable*	Odor is detectable, although a judge could not recognize it as a malodor. This is defined as the detection threshold.
2 *Slight Malodor*	Odor is deemed to exceed the threshold of malodor recognition. This is defined as the recognition threshold.
3 *Moderate Malodor*	Malodor is definitely detected.
4 *Strong Malodor*	Strong malodor, but examiner can tolerate.
5 *Severe Malodor*	Overwhelming malodor. Examiner cannot tolerate malodor at this level (the examiner instinctively averts the nose).

Source: Miyazaki et al; 1999.

Treatment of Oral Malodor

The first step in treating oral malodor is to assess and treat all oral diseases and conditions that may contribute to oral malodor. The following treatment methods have proven their effectiveness to a variable level (Roldán et al., 2005) for treating oral malodor.

1. **Tongue Cleaning**

   Treatment needs (TN) corresponding to the classification of halitosis in dental practice has been categorized into five levels (see Table 20–2) (Miyazaki et al., 1999). Practical management of physiologic halitosis requires TN-1 with cleaning the tongue being more essential than mouth rinsing, because the origin of physiological halitosis is mainly the dorsoposterior region of the tongue. Tongue coating is comprised of desquamated epithelial cells, blood cells, and bacteria. Cleaning the tongue reduces VSC. Tongue brushing is preferred over tongue scraping (Yaegaki & Coil, 2000a). It is postulated that brush bristles sweep between papillae and remove microorganisms (Kleinberg & Codipilly, 2001). Tongue cleaning should be carried out before toothbrushing, because mint flavor in toothpaste sensitizes the oropharyx to an elevated gag reflex (Yaegaki & Coil, 2000b). The middle and posterior parts of the tongue dorsum should be focused for a cleaning as high proportional sulfide (pS) levels are found there (Morita et al., 2001).

Did You Know?

Like fingerprints, everyone's tongue print is different.

---

2. **Oral Hygiene and Mouthrinses**

   Mechanical reduction of microorganisms through improved oral hygiene procedures has been associated with reductions in oral malodor.

   Additional treatments in TN-1 include routine oral hygiene procedures and mouthrinsing. Some clinical trials of mouthrinses claim to reduce VSC determined by gas chromatography or Halimeter (Yaegaki & Coil, 2000a). Mouthrinses containing cetylpyridinium chloride (CPC), chlorhexidine, or hydrogen peroxide have very limited role in controlling VSC. Currently, it has been recommended that patients use a zinc-containing mouthwash (Yaegaki & Coil, 2000b) such as BreathRx, because zinc strongly inhibits bacterial cysteine proteinase and inhibits the destruction of shed epithelial cells and blood cells (Yaegaki & Suetaka, 1989).

3. **Toothpastes**

   Toothpastes containing triclosan and a copolymer or sodium bicarbonate were reported to reduce certain amounts of VSC, and these toothpastes also may be recommended (Niles et al., 1999). Such toothpastes include Colgate Total®, and Arm and Hammer® Toothpaste.

4. **Chewing Gums**

   When people are concerned with oral malodor, approximately 70% use chewing gum (Yaegaki et al. 2000a). Chewing gum containing sugar was shown to reduce VSC in mouth air through an active pH change in the oral cavity (Kleinberg & Westbay, 1992). However, sugarless gum only masks halitosis with its flavors, producing a short-term effect (Reingewirtz, Girault, Reingewirtz, Senger, & Tenenbaum, 1999).

5. **Periodontal/Restorative Dental Treatment and Xerostomia**

Periodontal treatment is frequently required as TN-2 because periodontal diseases contribute to oral pathologic halitosis. The reduction of salivary secretion may cause oral pathologic halitosis; the treatment of xerostomia may reduce oral malodor. Increased salivary flow may contribute to decreased oral malodor. Although dental caries may not be a significant cause of oral malodor, caries treatment may be recommended (Yaegaki & Coil, 2000b).

Management of Patients with Pseudo-Halitosis (Patient with Extraoral Halitophobia)

Because extraoral pathologic halitosis treatments are out of the realm of dental clinicians, patients with extraoral halitophobia should be referred to medical practitioners (TN-3) (Yaegaki & Coil, 2000b). Patients with pseudo-halitosis are able to accept the clinician's diagnosis that oral malodor does not exist after receiving literature support, education, and explanation of examination results (TN-4). If a patient is not able to accept the diagnosis of pseudo-halitosis or if a patient with halitosis believes that halitosis exists after the halitosis was treated, the patient should be diagnosed as halitophobic by the dentist. The dentist should be referred to a psychological specialist (TN-5) (Yaegaki & Coil, 2000b).

Over-the-Counter (OTC) Products

Over-the-counter oral health products are numerous in the market. The products include tongue brushes, tongue scrapers, mouthrinses, chewing gums, chewable aromatic tablets, mouth fresheners, oral sprays, and gels. Some OTC products may be genuinely effective as a result of actually reducing the number of bacteria, while others may mask the odors, though their masking effect may only last for a brief period (Loesche & Kazor, 2002).

Did You Know?

Upper-class Romans added expensive imported urine to their teeth whitening mix (unaware that it was the ammonia molecules that were brightening their teeth).

Mechanical Plaque Control

Plaque control involves the regular removal of **oral or dental biofilms** from the teeth and adjacent oral tissues and the prevention of its accumulation. Since dental plaque is not always visible to the naked eye, patients may be unaware of it until it is disclosed. For this reason, a disclosing agent is recommended for patient education and prior to the patient's daily oral hygiene self-care regimen.

Evaluation

Exposure of plaque is a necessary first step in evaluation and can be accomplished with either disclosing tablets or liquid. Disclosing solutions show only gross changes and the quantity of stainable plaque. Disclosing agents do not differentiate between food and plaque, nor do they reveal the presence of microorganisms. The disclosing dye in the form of a solution or tablet absorbs into the dental plaque. The red solution does not contain FD&C red #3 or saccharin. The dental hygienist can use this visual resource to demonstrate the appropriate techniques of oral hygiene self-care to the patient. It is important to show the patient areas where plaque accumulates in proximity to the gingiva. Patients can self-disclose dental biofilms periodically to determine the effectiveness of their oral hygiene self-care techniques. However, merely teaching patients about the use of disclosing agents in their dental health education instruction frequently is not sufficient to motivate them to clean their teeth more effectively. Visual feedback may play an important part in health education. Photographs can be taken before treatment and after treatment to show the patient results.

ORAL HYGIENE SELF-CARE METHODS

Proper oral hygiene self-care accomplishes plaque control, improves appearance, refreshes the breath, and provides a sense of oral cleanliness. The oral hygiene plan designed for the patient should be based on the patient's specific oral hygiene needs. Numerous mechanical cleansing devices, including toothbrushes and interdental aids, are available commercially in today's highly competitive product market. The dental hygienist should be familiar with the particular characteristics of each product in order to make an appropriate selection for each patient. Oral health promotions can improve oral hygiene and gingival health (Watt & Marinho, 2005).

Toothbrushes

Manual Toothbrushes: Design

Clinical evaluation of the efficiency of toothbrushes and other oral hygiene devices is constrained by such factors

Did You Know?

Early forms of the toothbrush have been in existence since 3000 BCE. Ancient civilizations used a "chew stick," which was a thin twig with a frayed end. These "chew sticks" were rubbed against the teeth.

■ **FIGURE 20–1**   Improper use of a toothbrush caused gingival recession and tooth abrasion, identified by a notching in the cervical area of the maxillary lateral incisors and canines.

as the time devoted to the method, the patient's hand pressure and dexterity, patient motivation, and the criteria used for measuring plaque (Yankell & Saxer, 1999). Therefore, toothbrush recommendations should be based on the toothbrushing method prescribed, the patient's intraoral characteristics, patient motivation, the patient's manual dexterity, and product cost.

The standard manual toothbrush consists of a handle and head with bristles and/or filaments. Toothbrush designs vary greatly depending on the desired characteristics. The handle may be straight (conventional) or angled, have a double angulation of the neck, come with or without thumb rests, and/or have a wavelike contour. The shank may be conventional (straight), offset, twisted, or curved. The head may have any of the following features: diamond shaped, squared, rounded, and of variable sizes for infants, children, young adults, and adults. The bristles/filaments (bristles are made of individual filaments) are most often made from nylon. Compared with natural bristles, nylon bristles have shown certain superior qualities, such as bristle durability, cleanliness, and resistance to the accumulation of bacteria and fungi. Bristle stiffness is classified as soft, medium, and hard. Soft bristles are the most highly recommended. Hard bristles have been shown to cause gingival recession and excessive tooth wear, resulting in cervical abrasion (Figure 20–1 ■). Toothbrush bristle planes vary greatly. The flat (conventional), dome, bilevel, rippled, and tuft profiles are unique to each toothbrush. Frandsen (1986) reported that daily brushing with a conventional flat-bristle brush removes only 50% of plaque from tooth surfaces, with removal of plaque from interproximal surfaces especially lacking. Newer brushes using more tapered and narrow bristles have been designed to more effectively reach interproximal areas, but more research and data evaluation must be done. Research on toothbrush bristles has focused much attention on end rounding of the bristles. End-rounded bristles aid in reducing damage to the gingival tissue. Despite manufacturers' attempts to fabricate toothbrushes with a high percentage of acceptable end-rounded bristles, studies have shown that poorly rounded, sharp and pointed, or flat bristle tips may be present in significant numbers even among brushes making claims of superior end rounding (Dellerman, Hughes, & Burkett, 1994).

Alternatives to conventional toothbrushes have been studied. One example is a disposable polyester foam sponge on a stick impregnated with a nonfoaming dentifrice. These spongelike brushes have been used frequently in hospitals and nursing homes and are shown to possess plaque-preventive capabilities. The spongelike brush was found to be effective in retarding accumulation of plaque from a plaque-free baseline on both facial and lingual tooth surfaces (Lefkoff, Beck, & Horton, 1995). It is especially useful after periodontal surgery.

Frequency of Toothbrushing

Toothbrushing must be carried out on a regular basis. It is difficult to determine the number of times a day an individual must brush, since the frequency of brushing is tailored to meet individual needs (Savolainen et al., 2005). An individual should brush as many times a day as it takes to effectively remove dental plaque. Factors that affect the recommendations for frequency of toothbrushing include rate of dental plaque formation, plaque visibility, state and susceptibility of oral disease, diet, and presence of contributory factors. Low-risk patients should be directed to brush at least twice a day. High-risk patients should brush more frequently, especially after meals. The use of disclosing agents is highly recommended because it allows meticulous removal of visible plaque from the teeth. The patient should individualize his or her own brushing technique to optimize plaque control. Current data on toothbrushing time suggests that people think they brush longer than they actually do. The average time spent brushing is between 24 and 60 seconds, but the recommended brushing time actually is about 3 minutes (Cancro & Fischman, 1995).

Powered Toothbrushes

Alternatives to manual toothbrushes include powered toothbrushes. A new generation of sonic and ultrasonic toothbrushes has become available. Powered toothbrushes were designed originally to simulate the action produced using a manual brush. However, effectiveness still depends on brush and bristle placement. Powered toothbrushes originally were recommended for patients lacking fine motor skills or patients with physical or mental impairments, but recent innovations in technology have increased their use for patients with periodontal disease, as well as patients with dental implants.

Mechanism of Action

There are many types of powered sonic and ultrasonic toothbrushes on the market today. Variations in brush head, bristle design, and brush movement exist. The various mechanical motions occur in rapid, short strokes in one or a combination of the following directions: reciprocating (in and out or up and down), rotational, counterrotational, oscillating (vibrational). A newer generation of powered toothbrushes work by sonic waves and ultrasonic action.

Effectiveness

Various studies with conflicting results have examined the effectiveness of powered toothbrushes compared with conventional brushes in plaque removal. Since most studies in the 1960s and 1970s failed to show that powered toothbrushes removed plaque better than manual toothbrushes, they were not so popular. In the 1996 World Workshop in Periodontics it was concluded that limited evidence supports the fact that powered toothbrushes offer additional benefits compared with manual toothbrushes (Hancock, 1996).

A few powered toothbrushes may be superior in removing plaque from interproximal areas than conventional manual toothbrushes (Bader, 1992; Saxer & Yankell, 1997). One study suggests that the sonic tooth-

brush (Sonicare®, Phillips Electronics) is more beneficial in resolving inflammation and reducing pocket depths in patients with moderate periodontal disease (O'Beirne, Johnson, Rutger Persson, & Spektor, 1996). However, other randomized, controlled clinical studies have not proven conclusively any differences in the efficacy of plaque removal between manual and powered toothbrushes (Preber, Ylipaa, Bergström, & Ryden, 1991; Van der Weijden, Danser, Nijboer, Timmerman, & Van der Velden, 1993). A recent clinical study using 62 adult patients with significant amounts of plaque, calculus, and inflammation demonstrated that brushing with either a manual or ultrasonic toothbrush significantly reduced bleeding and gingival inflammation. Neither toothbrush showed superiority over the other in removing plaque (Forgas-Brockmann, Carter-Hanson, & Killoy, 1998). The novelty of using a new device may in part increase self-care efforts, thus improving oral hygiene.

Powered toothbrushes have been found to be superior in removing tooth stains (Grossman, Cronin, Dembling, & Proskin, 1996). The Braun Oral-B® Plaque Remover (Braun, Oral-B, MA) and Sonicare® have been shown to be superior to a manual toothbrush in removal of chlorhexidine stains (Moran & Addy, 1995).

Recommending a Powered Toothbrush

Factors to consider when recommending a powered toothbrush include the toothbrush design, brushing motion, patient's interest and motivation, and the costs and benefits. Placement of bristles and the head of the toothbrush are important to avoid tissue trauma. The powered toothbrush should be moved slowly in sequence around the mouth using less pressure than with a manual toothbrush, thus producing less cervical abrasion and tissue trauma. Evaluation of a patient's ability to improve his or her plaque and gingival indices over time is the best method for determining the success of a specific powered toothbrush. Use of powered toothbrushes is safe on titanium dental implants.

The use of powered toothbrushes by patients with poor self-care compliance has shown some advantages (Hellstadius, Asman, & Gustafsson, 1993). Use of a powered toothbrush (counterrotational) in periodontal patients in a periodontal maintenance program has proved to be helpful in reducing plaque levels and enhancing gingival conditions (Yukna & Shaklee, 1993). Other patients that may benefit from the use of powered toothbrushes include those with limited manual dexterity, orthodontic patients, and children (parental brushing of children's teeth).

Interdental Care

Interdental cleaning is a primary area of neglect. A major factor in disease initiation and control is the anatomy of the interdental area. Cleansing of these interproximal areas depends on tooth alignment and tissue configuration. Supplemental aids are necessary because, despite new toothbrush designs, brushing alone is ineffective in the removal of interproximal plaque.

Various considerations are appropriate when recommending interdental cleaning devices. These factors are as follows:

- The presence or absence of interdental papillae
- Alignment of teeth
- Shape of teeth
- Tissue contour
- Condition of restorations
- Tightness of contact area
- Presence of bridges, dental implants, and orthodontic appliances
- Patient motivation and interest in interproximal cleaning
- Effectiveness of patient's self-care
- Size of gingival embrasure

Types of Gingival Embrasures

There are three types of gingival embrasures (Figure 20–2 ■): Type I, in which the embrasure is completely filled with gingiva; Type II, in which there is slight to moderate recession of the interdental papillae; and Type III, in which there is extensive or complete loss of interdental papillae.

(a)

(b)

(c)

■ **FIGURE 20–2**   Three types of gingival embrasures. Interdental cleaning devices are specific for each type of embrasure. (a) Type I embrasure is completely filled with interdental gingiva. (b) Type II embrasure has partial loss of interdental gingiva (mandibular anterior teeth). (c) Type III embrasure has complete loss of interdental gingiva.

┌───┐
Did You Know?

Boar bristles were used until 1938, when nylon bristles were introduced by Dupont de Nemours. The first nylon toothbrush was called Doctor West's Miracle Toothbrush. Later, Americans were influenced by the disciplined hygiene habits of soldiers from World War II. They became increasingly concerned with the practice of good oral hygiene and quickly adopted the nylon toothbrush.
└───┘

Available interdental cleaning devices include dental floss, dental tape, interdental brushes, interdental stimulators, and oral irrigators (Table 20–3 ■). Determination of which interdental aid is to be used depends on the type of gingival embrasure.

Dental Floss and Dental Tape   Numerous types of nylon dental floss are available: waxed, unwaxed, flat, round, colored, flavored, shred resistant, and impregnated with substances such as fluoride, baking soda, and tetrasodium pyrophosphate. Floss is indicated for use in Type I gingival embrasures, where the embrasures are completely filled with interdental papillae. It is also ef-

Table 20–3	**Clinical Features of Interdental Cleaning Devices**	
Type of Dental Device	*Use*	*Limitations*
Dental floss	Type I gingival embrasures.	Use caution not to cause tissue trauma. Not recommended for diastemas and Types II and III gingival embrasures.
Dental tape	Broad and flat for wider spaces and assists in polishing proximal surfaces.	Difficult to use for tight contact areas and Types II and III embrasures.
Dental floss threader	Floss is threaded through a plastic needle-like device. Best to use under pontics, around orthodontic wires, and where teeth are splinted or soldered.	Use caution not to injure the gingiva with the point of the threader.
Dental floss holder	Patients with limited manual dexterity or who do not want to place fingers in the mouth. For Type I embrasures.	Sometimes it is difficult to get the floss through the contact area; floss must be taut. Do not use in Types II or III embrasures.
Tufted floss	To clean beneath pontics, around orthodontic wires, and between splinted teeth. The yarn portion of the floss is used for actual cleaning where space permits (e.g., Superfloss).	Not intended for Type I gingival embrasures. Use caution with the tip of the floss.
Rubber-tip stimulator	Used for the removal of dental plaque along the gingival margin. Also can be used in an open embrasure.	To avoid tissue trauma, do not place tip subgingivally.
Wooden wedge	Use in Type II and III embrasures with shallow pockets.	Use caution not to cause tissue trauma. Difficult to adapt lingually.
Interdental brushes	Use in Type II and III embrasures and furcation involvement areas. Post-periodontal surgery.	Do not use in Type I embrasures.
Implant floss	Use around implant posts or abutments.	Avoid forcing floss into the gingiva.
Electric interdental cleaner	Good for patients with limited manual dexterity. Good for all types of embrasures, including around bridges and implants. Available with a filament and FlexiTip stimulator.	Follow manufacturer's instructions.

fective around implants. Dental floss is 80% effective in removing interproximal dental plaque (Lewis et al., 2004). Waxed dental floss may be more resistant to tearing or shredding but may be too bulky for tight contacts. Teflon-coated floss is made of polytetrafluoroethylene and is inserted easily into difficult access areas and resists fraying (Ciancio, Shilby, & Farber, 1992). Unwaxed floss is thin and easily manipulated through tight contact areas. Even though patients prefer to use waxed floss rather than unwaxed floss (Beaumont, 1990), there is actually no difference between the two flosses in efficacy in removing interproximal plaque (Hill, Levi, & Glickman, 1973). Floss may fray and tear where teeth are crowded or in areas where restorations are defective. Dental tape is broad and flat and should be used in open interdental spaces or between teeth without tight contacts and for polishing proximal tooth surfaces. The major advantage of colored floss is patient appeal and the patient's ability to see what is removed by flossing. This factor may help motivate the patient to floss regularly (Hague & Carr, 2007). A recent study found that four different floss products (unwaxed, woven, and shred-resistant floss and a powered flosser) in combination with a manual toothbrush removed plaque significantly better than the toothbrush alone. The powered flosser was superior to the traditional floss products but there were no significant treatment differences between the three traditional floss products (Terézhalmy, Bartizek, & Biesbrock, 2008).

A floss modification called tufted dental floss, made by many manufacturers, has a stiff straight end with a section of unwaxed floss and an area of thicker nylon meshwork. The stiff end allows the floss to be passed easily under bridges, around implant abutments, through exposed furcations, or between orthodontic appliances.

The floss holder is a yoke-like device with a space between the two prongs of the yoke. The floss is secured tightly between the two prongs designed to facilitate movement of the floss interproximally, as shown in

■ **FIGURE 20–3**   Floss holder. The floss is held tightly between two prongs.

Figure 20–3 ■. It is recommended for patients with limited manual dexterity.

The floss threader is a needle-like device (Figure 20–4 ■) to facilitate floss use under pontics and splinted crowns, between orthodontic appliances, through a gingival embrasure, or between teeth with tight contacts. It is used by threading approximately 12 inches of floss through the loop and then drawing it through the interproximal space. The floss is then engaged against the tooth surface.

■ **FIGURE 20–4**   The floss threader is a needle-like device. Floss is placed through the loop for access underneath pontics, exposed furcations, orthodontic appliances, and splinted crowns.

An article (Segelnick, 2004) reported that daily flossing was practiced 2.4 times more often in patients seen in a private periodontal practice (19.3%) than in a hospital dental clinic (7.9%). It was concluded that patients who do floss most likely are not using the proper technique. Looking at the flossing technique, the average number of times patients reported to floss with an up-and-down motion was 2.6 times. There is a statistically significantly higher floss frequency among middle-aged patients as compared to older and younger patients. Women flossed significantly more frequently than men, which was seen only at the hospital clinic. Almost 40% of the individuals who reported flossing are not practicing the proper technique of flossing around the tooth.

Caution is necessary in flossing to avoid injury to the gingiva. The floss may cut the gingiva if it is pulled too quickly past the contact and/or if it is positioned too forcefully beneath the gingiva. Damage to the junctional epithelium may occur, especially in healthy gingiva. The patient should be instructed to perform flossing procedures in a systematic fashion (hence all mandibular and maxillary teeth are included). Mastering the flossing technique requires time and patience. Patients are discouraged and less motivated to incorporate the flossing regimen into their oral hygiene program when they have difficulties with manual dexterity or when they do not have the patience to do the job well (Lewis et al., 2004).

Floss also has been designed specifically for cleaning implant supported dentures. The denture has to be removed before cleaning the abutments. The floss is looped from facial to lingual around the abutment and gently placed subgingivally until resistance is met. It is then crisscrossed and used in a sliding back-and-forth, up-and-down motion. Implant floss is made of braided nylon filaments and can be washed off after each use.

Interdental and Single-Tuft Brushes   Exposed furcations, root concavities (e.g., mesial concavity on the maxillary first premolar), and Type II and III gingival embrasures usually are best cleaned with an interdental or single-tuft brush (also called end-tuft brush) (Figure 20–5 ■). Other uses for such brushes include the distal surface of the terminal molar, around pontics and maligned teeth, and around orthodontic appliances or dental implant abutments. The premoistened brush is inserted interproximally and used in an in-and-out direction. However, such brushes should not be forced to fit into gingival embrasures.

Interdental brushes consist of nylon filaments twisted onto a metal wire or a nylon-coated plastic wire that does not scratch or cause tissue trauma. This special

■ **FIGURE 20–5**   Floss is not as effective as an interdental brush in removing interdental plaque from tooth concavities.

brush is recommended for titanium surfaces. Interchangeable bristles come in a variety of sizes, such as cylindrical, tapered, and large cylindrical (Figure 20–6 ■). A unique wireless soft foam insert is available for postoperative periodontal care, implant maintenance, and medicament applications.

The single-tuft brush, also called an end-tuft brush, consists of a group of small bristles or tufts that are flat or tapered on a straight or angled handle (Figure 20–7 ■).

Rubber-Tip Stimulator   The rubber-tip stimulator consists of a flexible rubber tip attached to a handle or at the end of a toothbrush. It is not recommended for healthy gingiva that completely fills the gingival embrasure, but it can be useful in Type II or Type III embrasures. Generally, it is used for removing plaque at the gingival margin, exposed furcation areas, concave surfaces, and open interdental areas. The tip is inserted gently into the interdental area and inclined approximately 45° away from the occlusal surface following the contour of the gingiva. It also can be placed interproximally at a 90° angle. A back-and-forth or rolling motion is used. It was thought originally that use of the rubber tip increased keratinization and vascular function through gingival stimulation, but there is no clinical evidence to support this (Rounds & Tilliss, 1999).

Wooden Toothpicks   Wooden toothpicks are available as either a toothpick-in-holder or a triangular balsa wood stimulator. These devices should be used where interdental papillae are missing (Type II and Type III embrasures). Since wooden toothpicks are difficult to

(a)

(b)

(c)

■ **FIGURE 20–6**   (a) Variations in types of interdental brushes. Uses of an interdental brush (b) in a Type II embrasure and (c) around implant abutments.

use on lingual surfaces and they do not reach subgingivally, they are not as effective as dental floss.

The triangular stimulator should be moistened with saliva and then inserted interproximally, flat side toward the papilla, moving in an in-and-out burnishing stroke. Discard the wedge if it becomes splayed.

The toothpick-in-holder is a plastic-handled instrument with a tapered, conical opening at one end where the toothpick is inserted; the excess portion is broken off. It is used for plaque removal along the gingival margin, within the sulcus, in root concavities, in furcation areas, and around orthodontic appliances; it also can be used for the application of medicaments (e.g., fluoride or a desensitizing agent). The blunt point and sides of the toothpick are placed in the sulcus to engage, debride, and dislodge adherent plaque.

Electric Interdental Cleaning Devices   One of the more recent advances in interdental cleaning is the Braun Oral-B Interclean®, an electric interdental cleaning device that consists of a thin, flexible cleaning filament (Figure 20–8 ■). This device has been shown to reduce plaque, gingivitis, and bleeding equal to or better than floss (Gordon, Frascella, & Reardon, 1996). Other automated interdental cleaners are available and include sonic devices, filament tips, brush tips, and flossers.

Tongue Cleansing

A number of tongue cleansing devices are available. These are used in a pull or forward motion. A soft-bristle toothbrush also may be used for tongue cleansing. When using a toothbrush, a brushing stroke starting on

■ **FIGURE 20–7**   (a) Variations in single-tufted brushes (tapered and nontapered). Use of a single-tufted brush (b) around orthodontic appliances, (c) dental implants, and (d) the distal surface of the terminal tooth. (Figure 20–7a courtesy of Oral-B Labs, MA)

the posterior-most aspect of the dorsum of the tongue is performed with a roll to the tip of the tongue. Tongue brushing will improve tongue appearance and halitosis by removing coatings associated with bacteria, food, and smoking.

 Rapid Dental Hint

Remind patients to brush their tongue.

Dentifrices

A **dentifrice** is a toothpowder, toothpaste, or gel used in conjunction with a toothbrush to help remove plaque,

materia alba, and stain from teeth. The word is derived from the Latin words dens ("teeth") and fricare ("to rub"). Although the mechanical action of brushing and flossing is the primary means of plaque removal, a dentifrice facilitates the oral hygiene process.

Dentifrices are considered to be either cosmetic or therapeutic. Cosmetically, they function in cleaning and polishing teeth, removing extrinsic stains, and freshening the oral cavity. There is a continuing effort by manufacturers to obtain additional dental benefits from dentifrices through the inclusion of agents designed to have a therapeutic action. Therapeutic agents are included in dentifrices to reduce caries; control of gingivitis, plaque, and calculus formation; and reduce of dentinal hypersensitivity (Tables 20–4 ■).

(a)   (b)

■ **FIGURE 20–8**   (a) Braun Oral-B Interclean®. (b) Interproximal use of the device. (Courtesy of Oral-B Labs, MA)

The main limitation of dentifrices as a therapeutic agent is the issue of patient compliance. Dental hygienists cannot control the frequency of use or amount or type of dentifrice used by a patient. Dentifrice selection is based most often on cosmetic qualities such as flavor, texture, appearance, and dispensability rather than on its therapeutic value. The public looks to dental professionals for specific recommendations. The dental hygienist must be up to date with product information and be able to recommend a dentifrice that will provide oral health benefits yet appeal to the patient for continued use. Dentifrices should be chemically stable, effective, and nontoxic. Products with the ADA seal of acceptance have sustained scrutiny and testing and can be safely recommended by dental hygienists.

Dentifrice Components

Dentifrices contain basic components along with an active ingredient for its intended use. The active agent provides the therapeutic benefit and can include fluoride for anticaries effect, potassium nitrate or strontium chloride for desensitization (reducing or eliminating dentin sensitivity), sodium pyrophosphate for calculus inhibition, or triclosan for plaque and gingivitis control. Recent formulations have incorporated a combination of these active ingredients for maximal patient benefits.

A typical dentifrice contains, besides water (15 to 50%), an abrasive (20 to 60%). Abrasives clean or polish tooth surfaces, allowing them to resist bacterial reaccumulation. The powders and pastes contain abrasives such as silicon oxides, chalk, hydrated aluminum oxide, and sodium bicarbonate. Generally speaking, commercial dentifrice powders are more abrasive than pastes. Abrasives usually do not damage the enamel, but they may dull tooth luster. Therefore, a polishing agent is incorporated into most dentifrices, forming an abrasive system (Fischman & Yankell, 1999). Although abrasives can result in tooth wear, other factors such as brushing habits, including technique, pressure, direction, and frequency of brushing, and toothbrush bristle stiffness can influence the incidence of tooth abrasion. The more abrasive the dentifrice, the more likely it is to cause tooth wear in the cervical area. This area is more prone to abrasion because enamel is approximately 20 times harder than dentin or cementum (Fischman & Yankell, 1999). There is no valid reason to use a dentifrice with a greater abrasiveness or polishing effect than necessary to prevent deposits, including stains on the teeth.

Table 20–4	Dentifrices with Therapeutic Benefits (ADA Seal of Acceptance)
Product Name	**Active Ingredients**
Anticavity/antiplaque/antigingivitis:	
Colgate® Total™ Toothpaste (Colgate-Palmolive Co., New York, NY)	0.30% triclosan 0.24% sodium fluoride
Anticavity/antigingivitis/sensitive teeth:	
Crest® ProHealth Toothpaste (anticavity, antigingivitis and sensitive teeth)	Stannous fluoride 0.454%, 0.16% sodium fluoride
Prevention of calculus	
Colgate® Tarter Control Gel/Toothpaste (Colgate-Palmolive Co., New York, NY)	Tetrasodium pyrophosphate, 0.15% sodium fluoride
Aquafresh® Tartar Control Toothpaste (GlaxoSmithKline, PA)	Tetrapotassium pyrophosphate, tetrasodium pyrophosphate, 0.221% sodium fluoride
Crest® Tartar Protection Fluoride Gel/Toothpaste (Procter & Gamble, Cincinnati, OH)	Tetrapotassium pyrophosphate, disodium pyrophosphate, tetrasodium pyrophosphate, 0.15% sodium fluoride

Humectants (20 to 40%) are a vehicle into which agents are incorporated to prevent hardening of the dentifrice when exposed to air. Common humectants are glycerin, sorbitol, mannitol, and polyethylene glycol. Surfactants (1 to 2%) act as detergents by contributing to the foaming action, lowering surface tension, and loosening deposits from the teeth. Sodium lauryl sulfate is the most commonly used detergent. Binders (1 to 2%; cellulose products, gums, alginates) prevent the separation of the solids and liquids in the dentifrice, maintain firmness and thickness, and ensure stability. Gels contain more binders to give the product a thicker quality. Flavoring and sweetening agents mask the poor-tasting ingredients and provide a pleasant flavor to the dentifrice. Flavorings include essential oils (peppermint, cinnamon, and wintergreen) and sodium saccharin. Colorants (1%) are dyes added to the dentifrice to enhance its attractiveness without staining or discoloring teeth or oral tissues or causing harm on ingestion.

Fluoride Dentifrices

Dentifrices are the most widely used form of self-applied fluoride. Recommended for both children and adults, fluoride dentifrices can reduce caries by 20 to 30% when used twice daily on a regular basis. First introduced in the 1950s, fluoride dentifrices contained stannous fluoride as the anticaries agent. Current fluoride dentifrices contain sodium fluoride (0.24%) or sodium monofluorophosphate (0.76%). The anticaries efficacy of these two fluoride agents continues to be evaluated (Proskin & Volpe, 1995). Although some analyses indicate that there is no statistically or clinically significant difference between the two fluoride agents (Volpe, Pretrone, Davies, & Proskin, 1995), it has been shown that the therapeutic benefit of fluoride depends on a dose-response relationship (Stephen, 1994); a decrease in caries with increasing dose of fluoride. Sodium fluoride dentifrices appear to be retained longer, however, when compared with dentifrices containing sodium monofluorophosphate (Shellis & Duckworth, 1994) and thus may be more effective clinically (Duckworth, Jones, Nicholson, Jacobson, & Chestnutt, 1994).

Indications for fluoride gels include rampant caries, patients susceptible to caries, root caries, orthodontic appliances, dentinal hypersensitivity, and patients undergoing radiation therapy. Since over 95% of dentifrices contain fluoride and the benefits have been shown clinically for decades, issues of safety are of minor concern. Numerous studies have evaluated fluoride therapies for their impact on dental fluorosis (Stookey, 1994). Dentifrices have been identified as a causative factor in the increased prevalence of mild enamel fluorosis. For this reason, young children must be monitored for inadvertent dentifrice ingestion.

The mechanism of fluoride's anticaries effect in root caries is not well understood. Fluoride gels may have a beneficial effect in the prevention of caries on exposed root surfaces. An example of a home-applied gel prescription product is 1.1% sodium fluoride (Prevident® 5000 Plus Gel, Colgate Oral Pharmaceuticals; Neutracare®, Oral-B). These gels should be applied daily after home-care procedures. The gel is applied either by brushing it on the root surface for 1 minute or using a custom-made or disposable tray for 4 minutes.

Stannous Fluoride Dentifrices

Before the introduction of sodium fluoride and sodium monofluorophosphate, stannous fluoride was incorporated into dentifrices. Stannous fluoride, in concentrations of greater than 0.3%, has been the most widely studied fluoride in controlling plaque and gingivitis. Clinical studies of caries and plaque prevention showed mixed results, therefore stannous fluoride does not have the ADA seal of acceptance.

Commonly reported adverse side effects include extrinsic tooth staining caused by the tin molecule and a metallic, bitter taste (Wilkins 2009). Recent dentifrice formulations contain flavoring agents that mask the taste. Removal of stains caused by stannous fluoride is no more difficult than stain removal resulting from other product use (Beiswanger et al., 1995). Stannous fluoride is available as a brush-on gel, a mouthrinse, and a dentifrice.

Triclosan-Containing Dentifrices

Triclosan is another type of therapeutic dentifrice. Triclosan is a phenolic compound with antiplaque/antigingivitis properties. It is a broad-spectrum antibacterial agent effective against Gram-positive and Gram-negative bacteria. Used as an antibacterial agent in soaps, deodorants, and cosmetics, triclosan recently has become available in the United States in a dentifrice formulation (Total™, Colgate Oral Pharmaceuticals, New York, NY).

Total contains 0.3% triclosan and 2.0% polyvinylmethylether maleic acid (PVM/MA), which enhances its retention (substantivity) on hard and soft oral surfaces and adds anticalculus properties (Ciancio, 1997). Triclosan binds to plaque, resulting in a sustained impact on bacteria for over 12 hours after brushing (Volpe, Petrone, DeVizio, & Davies, 1996). Triclosan affects the quality of existing plaque (Lindhe, Rosling, Socransky, & Volpe, 1993) and plaque regrowth (Binney, Addy, McKeowns, & Everatt, 1996). When compared with other dentifrices, triclosan is as effective as stannous fluoride (Binney, Addy, Owens, & Faulkner, 1997) and sodium fluoride dentifrices (Binney, Addy, McKeowns, & Everatt, 1995) in inhibiting plaque. In addition, this product is also claimed to prevent caries. No adverse effects have been reported, and it is safe for oral use. Triclosan has the ADA Seal of Acceptance for antiplaque/antigingivitis properties.

Sodium Bicarbonate/Hydrogen Peroxide Dentifrices

Sodium bicarbonate (baking soda) has been used as a cleansing agent for many years and has been the primary abrasive agent in dentifrices. The therapeutic benefit of sodium bicarbonate dentifrices results from reduction of plaque and gingivitis and stain removal (Koertge, 1996; Zambon, Mather, & Gonzales, 1996). The mechanism of action is disruption of the bacterial cell membrane (Drake, Vargas, Cardenzana, & Srikantha, 1995). Even though baking soda disintegrates quickly during brushing (so that its abrasive action is not sustained), it still removes stains (Koertge, 1996). An additional benefit of baking soda dentifrices is their control of oral malodor (Brunette, 1996).

Hydrogen peroxide is added to dentifrices for its antigingivitis properties. Some manufacturers claim that hydrogen peroxide–containing dentifrices were developed to whiten teeth by decolorizing stains. Others claim that hydrogen peroxide freshens the mouth because of its bubbling action. Consumers often view these agents as more "natural." The concept of combining sodium bicarbonate with hydrogen peroxide is based on the regimen supported by the Keyes technique. Most dentifrices contain a low level of hydrogen peroxide (<1%) that causes no harm to tissues (Marshall, Cancro, & Fischman, 1995).

The Keyes technique has received much attention in the lay press for the treatment of periodontal disease without surgical intervention. The Keyes technique, originally developed by Dr. Paul Keyes in the late 1970s, is based on monitoring of the disease with phase-contrast microscopy and treatment. The first phase of treatment involves mechanical therapy, and this is followed by local antimicrobial therapy, in which the patient uses a toothpaste composed of 3% hydrogen peroxide, salt, and sodium bicarbonate. Oral irrigation at home and in the office is also done. In the last phase of treatment, patients are prescribed systemic antibiotics such as tetracycline.

The Keyes technique was found not to be any more effective than conventional periodontal therapy (Pihlstrom et al., 1987). In addition, oral ulcerations have been reported to result from short-term use of 3% hydrogen peroxide in combination with a salt solution (Levine, 1987).

Research findings on the efficacy of sodium bicarbonate/peroxide are mixed. One study concluded that after 3 months of using a sodium bicarbonate/peroxide dentifrice there was a 52% reduction in bleeding sites (Fischman, Kugel, Truelove, Nelson, & Cancro, 1992). Dentifrices containing hydrogen peroxide may decrease plaque and gingivitis, but mechanical access to submarginal sites is required for them to deliver a therapeutic effect (Marshall et al., 1995). When applied with a sulcular brush and an interproximal toothpick, sodium bicarbonate/hydrogen peroxide had no benefit in reducing the microbiota in 4 to 7 mm pockets (Cerra & Killoy, 1982). No antimicrobial benefits were exhibited when compared with conventional dentifrices (sodium fluoride, stannous fluoride) and mouthrinses (essential oils) (Bacca et al., 1997). Arm and Hammer Dental Care Advanced Cleaning Mint toothpaste has the ADA Seal of Acceptance for anticaries properties.

Tartar-Control Dentifrices

Calculus, although not a primary causative factor for periodontal disease, does play a contributing role in dental plaque retention due to its porous surface. The introduction of soluble pyrophosphates into dentifrices provides a chemical means of reducing supragingival calculus formation. Calcium and phosphorus from saliva are prevented from incorporating into the plaque matrix to form calculus.

Pyrophosphates act as crystal growth inhibitors, especially large, organized crystals that may delay mineralization of the plaque and make it more susceptible to mechanical removal. Once calculus has formed into an organized matrix, pyrophosphates are ineffective. Their effectiveness is limited to new supragingival calculus. For this reason, recommendations for use are appropriate after prophylaxis or scaling/root planing.

> **Did You Know?**
>
> Ninety-four percent of Americans say they brush nightly; 81 percent say they brush their teeth first thing in the morning.

Many studies have evaluated the effectiveness of pyrophosphates on calculus formation (Addy & Koltai, 1994; Gaengler, Kurbad, & Weinert, 1993). Not only is there a reduction in new calculus formation, but also the number of sites in the mouth that are calculus-free is increased (Lobene, 1989). Results after three and six months indicated significant reductions in supragingival deposits (Schiff, 1987) by 35.5 and 45.9%, respectively. Calculus inhibitors cause the newly formed deposits to be softer and easier for the clinician to remove. The amount of force and number of strokes by the dental hygienist are reduced (White et al., 1996). The addition of a copolymer (methoxyethylene and maleic acid) to a pyrophosphate dentifrice enhances the anticalculus effect (Singh, Petrone, Volpe, Rustogi, & Norfleet, 1990).

Besides the effect on hard deposits, anticalculus dentifrices also may exhibit antimicrobial activity by killing or inhibiting bacterial growth (Drake, Grigsby, & Drotz-Dieleman, 1994). Pyrophosphates have been found to reduce chlorhexidine-induced extrinsic stain (Bollmer, Sturzenberger, Vick, & Grossman, 1995).

Tissue irritation has been reported in the form of tissue sloughing (peeling) and tooth surface sensitivity. Pyrophosphates in dentifrices also have been thought to interact with the fluoride compounds and interfere with the remineralization process. Fluoride uptake is not altered by pyrophosphates, however. The anticaries benefits are similar for regular-formula and tartar-control dentifrices. The ADA seal of acceptance has been given to tartar control dentifrices based on their anticaries properties.

Zinc Citrate–Containing Dentifrices

Viadent™ Advanced Care (Colgate Oral Pharmaceuticals, Canton, MA) has as its active ingredients 2% zinc citrate trihydrate, which is an antibacterial agent, and 0.8% sodium monofluorophosphate, which has anticaries properties. This formulation is also available as an oral rinse.

Other Dentifrice Categories

Herbal-based and "natural" dentifrices are attractive alternatives to some patients interested in maintaining oral hygiene. Although these products have been documented to perhaps be as effective as conventional dentifrices in their ability to control plaque and gingivitis (Mullaby, James, Coulter, & Linden, 1995), their efficacy remains questionable. As long as these "natural" toothpastes contain fluoride, patients receive anticaries benefit. Patients must be informed of the limitations of their choice of dentifrice. The primary benefit of some of these alternatives is motivational, in that patients may be encouraged to brush more regularly with their chosen dentifrice.

Dentifrices containing a lactoperoxidase system (Biotene®, Laclede Professional Products, Rancho Dominguez, CA) may be beneficial for special patient groups. Patients with xerostomia were relieved of their symptoms after a four-week daily use of a lactoperoxidase dentifrice and mouthrinse (Kirstila, Lenander-Lumikari, Soderling, & Tenovuo, 1996). Biotene does not have the ADA Seal of Acceptance.

ORAL HOME CARE FOR PATIENTS WITH PERIODONTAL DISEASE

Since not every patient has the same type and severity of periodontal disease, the hygienist must customize a oral hygiene self-care plan for every patient. Patients who have gingivitis with intact interdental papillae are going to have a different hygiene strategy than a patient with generalized chronic periodontitis with blunted and absent papillae (Table 20–5 ■).

Post-Periodontal Surgical Home Care

The important role of oral hygiene in controlling dental plaque growth and recolonization immediately after periodontal surgery cannot be overestimated (Sanz & Herrera, 1998). The degree of oral hygiene maintained by the patient also influences the healing response after periodontal surgery (Flores-de-Jacoby & Mengel, 1995; Palcanis, 1996). Presently, it is unknown if the healing response results from the improvement in and maintenance of low plaque levels by the patient (Westfelt, 1996) or is related to the increased frequency of periodontal maintenance visits after surgery (Ramfjord, 1987).

If a periodontal dressing was used, the patient should be informed not to dislodge it. It is likely that the patient will be inclined to avoid brushing the area, but he or she should be instructed to lightly brush the exposed tooth surfaces and all other areas of the dentition with a soft or ultrasoft toothbrush. The Bass method should be avoided; other methods that do not place the bristles directly into the gingival crevice are recommended to prevent trauma to the healing tissue. Chlorhexidine is usually recommended after periodontal surgery.

Patients with periodontal disease frequently have localized or generalized blunted papillae due to the disease process or as a consequence of periodontal surgery. Because of the open embrasures, the use of interdental brushes and single-tuft brushes is recommended. A fluoride dentifrice should be used. Assess the need for an antimicrobial rinse.

The patient's plaque control must be closely monitored postsurgery.

Implant Home Care

Diligent home care around tissue-integrated implant prostheses is imperative for long-term success. Plaque-control procedures must start immediately after uncovering the implants. It is important that the dental hygienist customize a home-care regimen based on the patient's awareness and ability and the type of prosthesis present (Orton, Steele, & Wolinsky, 1989).

A multitude of home-care devices exist to assist in mechanical oral hygiene regimes. These devices include various manual (Figure 20–9 ■) or powered toothbrushes (Figure 20–10 ■) and specific interdental aids (Balshi, 1986). Soft or ultrasoft manual toothbrushes are the traditional means of plaque removal. However, toothbrush heads come in many different shapes and sizes, and brushes should be prescribed individually depending on the implant type and the patient's abilities. An excellent area-specific soft nylon brush is the single-tufted brush for use with individual implants, one implant at a time; the shaft can be bent for better access.

Various interdental devices are available, including interdental brushes, rubber-tip stimulators, wooden cleaners, numerous types of dental floss, and a plastic toothpick (Ultradent, Oral B). The brush attachment for interdental brushes is available as a plastic or nylon-coated wire rather than a metal wire to prevent scratching of implant surfaces. Interdental brushes are used only if the interdental papilla is blunted or absent. Various floss types, such as tufted floss or floss cords (Post-Care™, Sunstar Americas Inc., Chicago), along with folded gauze or traditional floss, are effective and safe interproximal plaque-removal aids (Figure 20–11 ■).

Clinical use of antimicrobials (chemotherapeutic agents) can help to inhibit plaque and gingivitis around implants. These agents may be delivered by rinsing or applied topically (via toothbrush, floss, or cotton-tipped

---

Did You Know?

Americans spend $2 billion a year on dental products such as toothpaste, mouthwash, and dental floss.

Table 20–5   Oral Home Care for the Patient with Periodontal Disease

Type of Disease	Clinical Features	Toothbrush	Interdental Care and Adjunctive Care	Reasoning
Periodontal health	No clinical attachment loss or gingival recession. Intact interdental papillae. No bleeding.	Soft-bristled toothbrush; modified Bass technique.	Floss. If crowns are present, waxed floss may be easier for patient.	Since no disease is present, no modifications to home care are necessary. Observe proper technique and frequency of practice.
Gingivitis	Red and slight bleeding gingiva. No clinical attachment loss. Moderate to heavy plaque. Light/medium/heavy calculus. Most likely will Has type I gingival embrasures.	Soft-bristled toothbrush; modified Bass technique. If gingival recession is present, use the Charter's technique. For areas of edema use the Stillman's technique. *Antimicrobial toothpaste and rinses.*	Floss for type I gingival embrasures. Chemotherapeutics for rinsing or oral irrigation.	Emphasize brushing and flossing technique. Modify technique and frequency of practice. May include a mouth-rinse as an adjunct to help reduce bacterial load.
Chronic periodontitis	Numerous sites with blunted or absent papillae. Plaque and calculus accumulations. Bleeding may be evident except if the patient is a smoker.	A soft-bristled toothbrush with a modified Bass technique. Stillman's technique for gingival recession or blunted papillae. *Antimicrobial and fluoride toothpaste, desensitizing toothpaste for recession.*	Floss for type I gingival embrasures and interdental brush for type II and III. Oral irrigators and mouthrinses for reduction of microbial load in pockets. Local delivery of antibiotics (Arestin, Atridox).	Adjunctive use of mouthrinse or other chemotherapeutics and oral irrigators.
Aggressive periodontitis	Lack of clinical inflammation with normal appearance. Deep pockets in affected areas, absence of heavy plaque or calculus formation. Rapid bone destruction.	A soft-bristled toothbrush with a modified Bass technique. *Antimicrobial and fluoride toothpaste.*	Floss for type I gingival embrasures, interdental brushes for open embrasures. Adjunctive use of systemic antibiotics, chemotherapeutic agents and mouth-rinses.	Goal to slow progress of disease. Individualized instruction for plaque control and positive reinforcement for client. Antimicrobial therapy.
Periodontitis associated with immune dysfunction	Severe bone loss and tooth loss resulting from body's lack of resistance to bacterial infections.	A soft-bristled toothbrush with modified Bass technique. For gingival recession use Stillman's technique. *Antimicrobial and fluoride toothpaste.*	Floss for type I gingival embrasures. Interdental brushes for type II and III embrasures. Adjunctive use of chemotherapeutic agents and mouth-rinses.	Goal is to slow progress of periodontal disease exacerbated by the immune dysfunction.

Necrotizing ulcerative gingivitis (NUG)	Marginal gingiva is bright red, inflamed spontaneous bleeding, cratered punched out necrotic papillae, grayish-white pseudomembrane covering the gingiva, may include burning sensation, fetid odor, fever, enlarged lymph nodes.	Soft-bristled toothbrush with simple self-care, Gentle rolling strokes with minimal tissue movement. After inflammation begins to subside, more sulcular cleansing, gentle oral irrigation and microbials.	Careful slow addition of any products that could cause additional gingival irritation such as anti calculus toothpaste, rinses with high alcohol content. Gentle flossing after tissue healing begins appropriate to embrasures. Chemotherapeutics to complement antibiotic therapy.	Goal to allow for healing while adding in plaque removal techniques.
Necrotizing ulcerative periodontitis (NUP)	Extensive necrosis of gingiva, red band around marginal gingiva, severe pain, spontaneous bleeding, extensive clinical attachment loss with deep periodontal pockets.	Soft-bristled toothbrush with gentle rolling strokes with minimal tissue movement. After inflammation begins to subside, more sulcular cleansing, gentle oral irrigation and microbials	Interdental brush for type II and III gingival embrasures. Oral irrigators and mouth-rinses for microbial load in pockets.	Emphasize gentle brushing while healing, then add auxiliary plaque removal aides appropriate for embrasures.
Hormonal pregnancy gingivitis	Inflamed papillae, bright red, edematous tissue with a shiny smooth surface, Pregnancy tumors (pyogenic) in more severe cases.	Soft-bristled toothbrush; modified Bass technique after symptoms recede.	Floss for type I gingival embrasure and interdental brush for type II and III gingival embrasures. Adjunctive use of chemotherapeutic mouthrinses.	Since inflammation will usually regress postpartum plaque removal and meticulous home care must be stressed

applicator). Rinsing with chlorhexidine gluconate (Peridex®, Omni or PerioGard®, Colgate Oral Pharmaceuticals) and Listerine® (McNeil-PPC) has been shown to be advantageous in the inhibition of bacterial plaque with patients with implants (Ciancio et al., 1995). Irrigation can be used if pathologic changes are present (Meffert, Langer, & Frutz, 1992). A study conducted by Felo, Shibly, Ciancio, Lauciello, and Ho (1997) investigated the effects of subgingival irrigation with chlorhexidine gluconate diluted with water on peri-implant gingival health compared with rinsing with chlorhexidine when used as an adjunct to routine peri-implant maintenance. Results suggested that powered subgingival irrigation with chlorhexidine may be better than rinsing in implant maintenance. However, even though the results of this study were favorable toward the use of irrigation at home,

patients should not irrigate around implants until more controlled clinical studies can support its use.

While rinsing with antimicrobials has been proven to be beneficial, some rinses do have unwanted side effects, such as staining, altered taste, and increased calculus formation. Because of the potential side effects, patients may prefer alternative delivery by applying the solution in a site-specific fashion so as to avoid undesirable effects.

Orthodontic Home Care

Orthodontic appliances tend to increase the accumulation of supragingival plaque on the teeth leading to the development of gingival inflammation and bleeding. Meticulous oral hygiene is important to control the development of gingival inflammation. During orthodontic

■ **FIGURE 20–9**   Types of toothbrushes used on implants. (a) Single-tuft brush (also referred to as an end-tuft brush). (b) Powered brush used with fixed partial denture superstructure. (c) Powered brush used with overdenture abutments and retention bar.

■ **FIGURE 20–10**   Various types of powered brush heads. Many clinicians recommend powered brushes for use around dental implants.

treatment, the patient should be evaluated regularly. A soft-bristled toothbrush designed specifically for orthodontic appliances should be recommended to the patient, including an oral rinse if needed to supplement brushing. The Charters method of brushing is used to clean the brackets of cervical areas of the teeth. For interdental home care, use of a floss threader with floss or tufted floss is recommended.

ADVICE TO THE PATIENT

Noncompliance with oral hygiene self-care is a major factor in the recurrence of periodontal diseases. One role of the dental hygienist is to determine the patient's enthusiasm and manual dexterity in performing plaque control (Baker, 1995), which entails having good professional

■ FIGURE 20–11 Oral hygiene aids for interproximal tooth surfaces. (a) Tufted floss used under a fixed denture. (b) Tufted floss used under a fixed bridge. (c) Folded gauze strip can be efficient when access is good. (d) Interdental brush used under a fixed partial denture.

communication skills and patience, since it is not easy for patients to change their habits. Besides lack of motivation, other reasons for plaque control failure include poor technique, lack of knowledge, and inconsistent performance (Van Dyke, Offenbacher, Pihlstrom, Putt, & Trummel, 1999).

Oral hygiene self-care programs are based on a patient's individual needs. Keeping the program simple will increase patient compliance. Try to adapt the oral hygiene program to the patient's lifestyle. Establishing good oral hygiene habits involves having patients clean their teeth in a systematic pattern (e.g., starting on the maxillary right and ending on the mandibular right). However, strict adherence to one approach may not always be in the best interests of thorough plaque removal and improved gingival health.

Oral physiotherapeutic products have limitations. Brushing and flossing are effective in the mechanical removal of most supragingival plaque but are limited in removing subgingival plaque due to the design of the devices and the contour of the gingiva. A periodontal patient may be able to access the subgingiva only slightly. The techniques described in this chapter can be modified to permit cleansing of all accessible areas of the dentition. A different regimen is applied after periodontal surgery, and the patient must be familiar with the various cleaning aids needed. The dental hygienist must introduce these new aids to the patient.

The iatrogenic effects of dentistry need to be eliminated prior to setting expectations for plaque removal. For example, unpolished amalgam restorations retain more plaque than polished ones. Composite materials may accumulate plaque greater than amalgam. Ill-fitting margins, overhangs, and rough surfaces on restorations should be evaluated for replacement or finishing because of plaque-retentive possibilities.

EFFECTS OF IMPROPER USE OF ORAL HYGIENE DEVICES

Once the importance of oral hygiene is explained to the patient and he or she begins to use numerous oral hygiene devices, the next step is to ensure that the patient is using each device correctly.

Toothbrushing

Factors that can cause acute or chronic tissue problems include incorrect bristle angulation or placement, heavy or long brushing strokes, a toothbrush with hard bristles, extremely abrasive toothpaste, and loss of concentration. Acute soft tissue lesions appear as small ulcers, red areas, or denuded gingiva. Chronic, long-standing gingival lesions present as gingival recession, rolled marginal gingiva, or gingival clefting. Gingival recession was found to occur mostly on the buccal surfaces of maxillary first molars, premolars, and canines (Björn, Andersson, & Olsson, 1981). Hard tissue lesions present as toothbrush abrasions occurring at the cervical area of teeth (see Figure 20–11). Tooth abrasion in most cases is due to the combined effect of toothbrushing and the use of dentifrices containing abrasives (Sangnes, 1976). Cervical abrasion

may occur once the root surface has been exposed by gingival recession. Thus, in order for cervical abrasions to occur, they must be preceded by gingival recession.

Interdental Devices

Dental floss, interdental brushes, and single-tufted brushes can cause injury to the gingiva if improper techniques are used. Each device is indicated in different types of gingival embrasures. Gingival ulcers, cuts, and clefts can result from improper technique.

Floss should not be forced too deeply into the gingival crevices (Figure 20–12 ■). When floss is used as part of the daily plaque-control routine, the junctional epithelial cells adhering to the enamel are in a continuous state of disruption and healing (Waerhaug, 1981). Interdental brushes and single-tufted brushes should not be forced into gingival with intact papilla.

Interdental cleaning is easy to master if the dental hygienist provides proper teaching and supervision to the patient.

DENTINAL HYPERSENSITIVITY

Maintaining plaque control is of utmost importance in reducing the sensitivity of exposed root surfaces. Often patients have difficulty complying with oral hygiene procedures because of the discomfort experienced during toothbrushing. Identification of hypersensitive areas is difficult, and frequently, toothbrushing is a major factor in localizing the sensitivity. Accordingly, root surfaces must be desensitized and an adequate oral hygiene self-care

(a)

(b)

■ **FIGURE 20–12**   (a) Soft tissue trauma cause by improper flossing. (b) Soft tissue trauma caused by improper tooth-brushing.

program maintained. In patients with good oral hygiene but with dentinal hypersensitivity, use of a desensitizing agent is recommended (Orchardson & Gillam, 2006).

Gingival recession as a result of the disease process (attachment loss), tooth malposition, faulty toothbrushing, or periodontal surgery can result in exposed dentin, which can result in hypersensitivity near the cervical area of the tooth. Usually, movement of fluid within the dentinal tubules causes discomfort in the exposed areas.

Root sensitivity occurs in approximately half of the patients following subgingival scaling and root planing (von Troil, Needleman, & Sanz, 2002). The intensity of root sensitivity increases for a few weeks after therapy, after which it decreases. In clinical practice, it may be recommended that patients should be made aware of the potential for root sensitivity prior to treatment (von Troil, Needleman, & Sanz, 2002). A clinical study reported that scaling and root planing procedures in periodontal therapy resulted in an increase of teeth that respond to painful stimuli. However, pain experiences in general appeared minor, and only a few teeth in a few patients developed highly sensitive root surfaces following instrumentation (Tammaro, Wennström, & Bergenholtz, 2000).

Assessing The Patients' Need for Desensitization

The following steps are recommended to assess the type of desensitization needed:

1. Use the air syringe to assess whether there is sensitivity. Write on the tooth being evaluated a "+" if the tooth has a positive response to the stimulus.
2. Recommend use of a desensitizing dentifrice for about four to six weeks. The patient is instructed to brush two times a day for 1 minute.
3. Instruct the patient on proper brushing so that the situation does not get worse. The patient's brushing technique must be corrected if treatment is to be successful.
4. Discuss the role of diet with the patient. Acidic and citrus foods should be limited in the patient's diet. If the patient frequently consumes acidic foods or juices, he or she should be instructed to rinse the mouth with sodium bicarbonate to help neutralize the acidity.
5. At the next examination, do the air syringe test again, and if the sensitivity is gone, the patient can

go back to his or her regular dentifrice. If the sensitivity reappears later, the patient can use the desensitizing dentifrice again. If the sensitivity is still present, an in-office treatment should be tried.

Treatment

A number of treatments are available for sensitive teeth. The type of treatment depends on the severity of the problem and the history of prior intervention. Treatment of dentin hypersensitivity focuses on blocking the opened dentinal tubules to prevent transmission of the noxious external stimuli and decreasing the intradental nerve excitability. Therapeutic products can be applied either professionally or by the patient. Most of the patient-applied over-the-counter (OTC) products must be used for a prolonged period of time (up to several months) for greatest effect. Manufacturers have added fluoride to the formula for its anticaries effect. It must be stressed to patients that optimal plaque control will help to reduce the sensitivity.

Table 20–6 ■ lists the more commonly used dentifrices for dentinal hypersensitivity. Potassium nitrate is effective in reducing cold and tactile sensitivity as compared with regular toothpaste (Silverman et al., 1996). Potassium nitrate acts quickly and directly on the pulpal nerves. Potassium nitrate containing dentifrices are ADA approved for the relief of dentin sensitivity. Application of fluoride to the dentinal surface is a treatment option for dentinal hypersensitivity (Bartold, 2006; Jacobsen & Bruce, 2001).

Patient-Applied Treatment

Basically, potassium nitrate and stannous fluoride products are available for patient-applied treatments (Table 20–6).

Dentifrices

Patient-applied medicaments are available as dentifrices, gels, and rinses. Dentifrices are helpful when many tooth surfaces are sensitive. For patients with mild sensitivity without loss of substantial tooth structure, a densensitizing dentifrice is recommended. Because it can take several weeks to see results, fluoride has been added to most dentifrices. It appears that a potassium nitrate–containing dentifrice works the fastest.

The longer the dentifrice is in contact with the dentin surface, the greater is its success. Thus, more frequent applications are advised. Instead of using a dentifrice in the usual manner, it may be more effective if the

Table 20–6	Patient-Applied Desensitizing Agents	
Product	*Active Ingredient*	*Method of Use*
Crest Sensitivity Protection® (Procter & Gamble, Cincinnati, OH)	5% potassium nitrate, 0.15% sodium fluoride	Apply to toothbrush
Crest Pro-Health Toothpaste	Stannous fluoride 0.454%, 0.16% sodium fluoride	Apply to toothbrush
Gel-Kam® gel (Colgate Oral Pharm.,)	0.4% stannous fluoride	Apply to toothbrush and brush teeth. This product is available over-the-counter without a prescription. Available in 4.3 oz tubes or a pack with 2 to 3.5 oz tubes.
Gel-Kam® Oral Care Rinse (Colgate Oral Pharm.)	0.63% stannous fluoride	Patient places 1/8 fluid oz of concentrate in marked mixing vial (included in box) and adds water as directed to prepare a 0.1% stannous fluoride rinse. Rinse over a 3-week period.
STANIMAX™ Perio Rinse (SDI Labs, Glenview, IL)	0.63% stannous fluoride	1/8 fluid oz is diluted with warm water to make 1 oz of the rinse in a measuring cup that is provided.
STANIMAX™ Brush-on Gel (SDI Labs, Glenview, IL)	0.4% stannous fluoride	Apply gel to toothbrush and brush teeth.
Sensodyne® Toothpaste (GlaxoSmithKline)	5% potassium nitrate, sodium fluoride	Apply to toothbrush and brush teeth
Soothe Rx (Omni)	calcium, sodium, phosphorus, and silica	Prescription toothpaste. Tube-Stage 1: Use twice daily for 2 weeks. Packets-Stage 2: Use once weekly for 24 weeks. Apply a ribbon on toothrush. Brush for 2 minutes. Do not eat or drink for 30 minutes.

undiluted dentifrice is applied with a cotton applicator directly on the tooth surface.

Fluorides

Of all the fluorides, stannous fluoride shows the most promise for topical application in periodontal therapy as an antibacterial and desensitizing agent. Application of stannous fluoride (gel: 0.4%, rinse: 0.63%, toothpaste: 0.454%) on a daily basis, after some time, can be therapeutic in reducing dentinal hypersensitivity. However, it often stings the gingiva, and patients may not comply with treatment. In addition, stannous fluoride can cause a yellowish or light brown stain on dentin (Ellingsen, Eriksen, & Rölla, 1982) more than enamel because of its porous nature, making it unaesthetic (Terézhalmy et al., 2007).

In-Office Treatment

If therapeutic dentifrices are not successful, in-office application of medicaments is recommended. Several products are available, including ferric oxalate, fluoride (with or without iontophoresis), bonding agents, varnishes, and glass ionomers (Table 20–7 ■).

Oxalate Salts

Most oxalates (ferric oxalate and potassium oxalate) are available as acidic solutions. Oxalates are capable of blocking the dentinal tubules when they are placed on an area of exposed dentin. Often the patient brushes the oxalate off. Thus the patient must be instructed not to brush too vigorously so that the dentin will not be re-

Table 20–7   Chairside Desensitizing Products

Product	Active Ingredient	Method of Use
Seal & Protect® (Dentsply, PA)	methacrylate resins, PENTA, nanofillers, triclosan (a broad spectrum antibacterial agent), and acetone	Isolate area, rinse and dry. Apply product and keep wet for 20 seconds. A gentle stream of compressed air is used to volatilize the acetone solvent and the material is light cured for 10 seconds. A second coat is then applied, dried, and light activated. Dentsply/Caulk claims the product provides symptomatic relief for up to six months.
Gel-Kam Dentinbloc® (Colgate Oral Pharm.)	1.09% sodium fluoride, 0.40% stannous fluoride, 0.14% hydrogen fluoride	Saturate a cotton pellet and apply to dry exposed dentin. Do not burnish; use light pressure.
Sensodyne® Sealant	6% ferric oxalate	Saturate a cotton pellet and apply to dry exposed dentin. Do not burnish; use light pressure.
STANIMAX-PRO™ (SDI Labs, Glenview, IL)	3.28% stannous fluoride	Can be used as a gel or diluted one-to-one with water to form a 1.64% stannous fluoride rinse.
Duraflor® (Pharmascience Inc., Montréal, Canada) Duraphat® (Colgate Oral Pharm., NY)	50 mg sodium fluoride varnish 5% sodium fluoride varnish	Apply to affected area with a cotton pellet. Apply to affected area with a brush that comes with kit or with a cotton pellet.
Denclude™ Dental Cream (Ortek-Therapeutics, NY)	calcium carbonate, hydrated silica, arginine bicarbonate	Apply a thick ribbon to a soft toothbrush. Brush twice daily and expectorate. Don't eat of drink for 30 minutes afterwards.
Proclude™ Prophylaxis Paste (Ortek-Therapeutics, NY)	hydrated silica, calcium carbonate, arginine bicarcarbonate	Use as a polishing paste post-scaling and root planning to reduce sensitivity especially at cervical areas. Rinse after application.
NuCare™ Root Conditioner with NovaMin (SunStar-Butler)	calcium, sodium, phosphorus, and silica	Tooth remineralization.
NuCare™ Prophylaxis Paste with NovaMin (SunStar-Butler)	calcium, sodium, phosphorus, and silica	Tooth remineralization. Can apply after periodontal surgery.

moved. It is best to evaluate the patient's brushing technique in the office.

Fluorides

Stannous fluoride is applied topically on the exposed dentin, forming a sort of granular layer over the dentin surface that does not come off with brushing, so it seals or decreases dentin permeability.

Sodium fluoride is available as a paste (33% sodium fluoride, 33% kaolin, 33% glycerin). Sodium fluoride works best for about seven to fourteen days, and then its effects dissipate.

Various sodium fluoride solutions have been tried with limited success. When iontophoresis is used to allow the fluoride ion to penetrate into the dentinal tubules, longer-lasting effects, up to three to four months, are seen. A second application usually is necessary.

Restorative Materials/Restorations

Methacrylate resins, such as Seal and Protect, are used to seal the affected area but may provide relief for up to six months and then need to be reapplied. If all treatments discussed above have failed to resolve the hypersensitivity, a restoration can be placed, but the restoration is usually finished with a diamond bur, which may open up new tubules below the restoration, recreating sensitive dentin. Since the restoration is located at the cervical third of the tooth, overhangs or rough surfaces may create more problems.

If the sensitivity can be narrowed down to just one or two teeth, a glass ionomer can be used.

DENTAL HYGIENE NOTES

The primary reference standard for detection of oral malodor is the human nose (organoleptic assessment), because it provides an overall evaluation of the existing malodor condition. For the treatment of bad breath, improved oral hygiene, especially tongue cleaning, has been shown to reduce VSC significantly.

The incorporation of diagnosis and management of oral malodor should be considered part of comprehensive dental care. Although most oral malodor have a simple cause, no single therapy is always effective. A team approach to diagnosis and treatment may involve the dentist, periodontist, an ear, nose, and throat specialist, dietition, pharmacist, internal medicine specialist, and psychologist.

Supragingival and subgingival dental plaque biofilms play a major role in the initiation of periodontal diseases. Since the subgingival microbiota is derived originally from supragingival plaque, it is necessary to disrupt both groups of bacteria. This is accomplished through mechanical supragingival plaque removal by the patient using toothbrushes and interdental devices and by the dental hygienist by removing subgingival plaque.

It would seem that gingivitis should be treated easily with plaque removal. Unfortunately, many obstacles prevent the timely removal of plaque. Besides lack of motivation to learn and perform toothbrushing and flossing skills, many patients also perform inconsistently, lack knowledge, and employ poor technique.

Fluorides have successfully decreased the rate of dental caries. Thereafter, few advances in chemical plaque control (dentifrices) have been achieved in recent years, except for the introduction of triclosan. Tartar-control dentifrices offer a cosmetic benefit. Desensitizing toothpastes may aid in the alleviation of dentinal hypersensitivity. Baking soda/hydrogen peroxide dentifrices have not been shown to consistently elicit antiplaque/antigingivitis effects. Triclosan is the first chemical agent used in dentifrices that can claim benefits to periodontal health.

KEY POINTS

- Plaque removal prevents gingivitis.
- The removal of plaque through daily plaque-control practices and professional cleanings is important in controlling subgingival plaque formation.
- There are numerous periodontal, dental, and medical causes of bad breath that need to be explored to effectively treat halitosis.
- The main goal of prevention is to achieve the lowest plaque level possible.
- Plaque-control measures by the patient and professional maintenance appointments are both important in maintaining gingival health and are essential parts of primary and secondary prevention of periodontitis.
- Dental floss is indicated for interproximal plaque removal in Type I gingival embrasures.
- There is no difference in efficacy of plaque removal with waxed or unwaxed dental floss.

SELF-QUIZ

1. Which one of the following statements describes the rationale for periodontal oral hygiene self-care? (p. 286)
   a. Reduction in the risk for development of dental caries
   b. Augmentation of the immune reaction to a bacterial insult
   c. Elimination or suppression of harmful microorganisms found in supragingival plaque biofilms
   d. Disruption of the number of subgingival microbial biota with a delay in the repopulation of pathogens

2. Which one of the following oral hygiene regimens is best for a patient after periodontal surgery? (p. 305)
   a. Resume regular brushing and flossing regimens.
   b. Use a soft-bristle toothbrush and an antimicrobial mouthrinse.
   c. Use powered toothbrush and floss.
   d. Use oral irrigation with chlorhexidine.
3. A patient says that he is doing the best he can with his home care, but he still has moderate to heavy supragingival deposits. Which of the following recommendations should the dental hygienist give to this patient? (pp. 308–310)
   a. Don't worry because everyone gets some accumulations.
   b. Use an antimicrobial mouthrinse.
   c. Improve or change method of home care.
   d. Refer to a specialist.
4. Waxed dental floss has proven to be more effective in interdental cleaning than unwaxed dental floss because it is easier for the patient to handle. (pp. 296–297)
   a. Both the statement and the reason are correct and related.
   b. Both the statement and the reason are correct but not related.
   c. The statement is correct, but the reason is not.
   d. The statement is not correct, but the reason is correct.
   e. Neither the statement nor the reason is correct.
5. All of the following tests can be used for the assessment of halitosis except one. Which one is the exception? (pp. 288–290)
   a. Self-assessment
   b. Tongue sulfide probe
   c. Chew gum test
   d. Psychological assessment
   e. Simple determination of oral malodor
6. All the following factors need to be considered when recommending interdental cleansing devices except one. Which one is the exception? (pp. 295–298)
   a. Amount of plaque
   b. Manual dexterity
   c. Presence of a bridge
   d. Type of embrasure

7. Which one of the following methods best evaluates for effectiveness of a patient's oral hygiene? (pp. 286–287)
   a. Show and tell
   b. Feedback
   c. Disclosing agents
   d. Self-documentation
8. Which one of the following oral hygiene aids is best to remove dental plaque on the proximal surface of a tooth that has a Type I gingival embrasure? (p. 296)
   a. Toothbrush
   b. Interdental brush
   c. Rubber-tip stimulator
   d. Wooden wedge
   e. Dental floss
9. Which one of the following steps should be done first when treating a patient for dentinal hypersensitivity? (pp. 310–314)
   a. Recommend a desensitizing dentifrice for four to six weeks.
   b. Instruct the patient on the proper toothbrushing method.
   c. Identify the tooth/teeth that is (are) painful.
   d. Apply sodium fluoride.
10. Which of the following oral hygiene aids is best used for interdental removal of plaque from implants? (p. 305)
   a. Toothbrush
   b. Powered toothbrush
   c. Interproximal brush with plastic core
   d. Interproximal brush with metal core

REFERENCES

Addy, M., and P. Adriaens. 1998. Epidemiology and etiology of periodontal diseases and the role of plaque control in dental caries: Consensus report of group A. In eds. N. P. Lang, R. Attström, and H. Löe, *Proceedings of the European Workshop on Mechanical Plaque Control,* 99–101. Chicago: Quintessence.

Addy, M., and R. Koltai. 1994. Control of supragingival calculus. Scaling and polishing and anticalculus toothpastes: An opinion. *J. Clin. Periodontol.* 21:342–346.

Bacca, L. A., M. Leusch, A. C. Lanzalaco, D. Macksood, and O. J. Bouwsma, et al. 1997. A comparison of intraoral antimicrobial effects of stabilized fluoride dentifrice, baking soda/hydrogen peroxide dentifrice, conventional NaF dentifrice and essential oil mouthrinse. *J. Clin. Dent.* 8:54–61.

Bader, H. J. 1992. Review of currently available battery operated toothbrushes. *Compend. Contin. Educ. Dent.* 13:1163–1169.

Baker, K. 1995. The role of dental professionals and the patient in plaque control. *Periodontology 2000* 8:108–113.

Balshi, T. J. 1986. Hygiene maintenance procedures for patients treated with the tissue integrated prosthesis (osseointegration). *Quintessence Int.* 17:95–102.

Beis Wanger, B. B., P. M. Doyle, R. D. Jackson. The clinical effect of dentifrices containing stabilized stannous fluoride on plaque founa and gingivitis. A six-month study with adlibtum brushing. *J. Clin. Dent* 1995; 6; 46–53.

Bartold, P. M. 2006. Dentinal hypersensitivity: A review. *Australian Dental Journal* 51(3):212–218.

Beaumont, R. H. 1990. Patient preference for waxed or unwaxed dental floss. *J. Periodontol.* 61:123–125.

Binney, A., M. Addy, S. McKeowns, and L. Everatt. 1995. The effect of commercially available triclosan-containing toothpaste compared to a sodium-fluoride containing toothpaste and a chlorhexidine rinse on 4-day plaque regrowth. *J. Clin. Periodontol.* 22(1):830–834.

Binney, A., M. Addy, S. McKeowns, and L. Everatt. 1996. The choice of controls in toothpaste studies: The effect of a number of commercially available toothpastes compared to water on a 4-day plaque regrowth. *J. Clin. Periodontol.* 23(5):456–459.

Björn, A. L., U. Andersson, and A. Olsson. 1981. Gingival recession in 15-year-old pupils. *Swed. Dent. J.* 5:141–146.

Bollmer, B. L. V., O. P. Sturzenberger, V. Vick, and E. Grossman. 1995. Reduction of calculus and Peridex stain with Tarter Control Crest. *J. Clin. Dent.* 6(4):185–187.

Borden, L. C., E. S. Chaves, J. P. Bowman, B. M. Faith, and G. L. Hollar. 2002. The effect of four mouthrinses on oral malodor. *Compendium* 23:531–546.

Bosy, A. 1997. Oral malodor: Philosophical and practical aspects. *J. Can. Dent. Assoc.* 63:196–201.

Brunette, D. M. 1996. Effects of baking soda–containing dentifrices on oral malodor. *Compend. Contin. Educ. Dent. 17* (Suppl. 19):22–31.

Brunette D. M., H. M. Proskin, and B. J. Nelson. 1998. The effects of dentifrice systems on oral malodor. *J. Clin. Dent.* 9:76–82.

Cancro, L. P., and S. L. Fischman. 1995. The expected effect on oral health of dental plaque control through mechanical removal. *Periodontology 2000.* 8: 60–74.

Cerra, M. B., and W. J. Killoy. 1982. The effect of sodium bicarbonate and hydrogen peroxide on the microbial flora of periodontal pockets: A preliminary report. *J. Periodontol.* 53:599–603.

Ciancio, S. G., C. Lauciello, O. Shibley, et al. The effect of an antiseptic mouth rinse on implant maintenance plaque & peri-implant gingival tissues. *J Periodentol* 1995; 66(11): 962–965.

Ciancio, S. G. 1997. Triclosan: A new antigingivitis agent. *Biol. Ther. Dent.* 13:23–26.

Ciancio, S. G., O. Shilby, and G. A. Farber. 1992. Clinical evaluation of the effect of two types of dental floss on plaque and gingival health. *Clin. Prevent. Dent.* 14:14–18.

Corbet, E. F., and W. I. R. Davies. 1993. The flow of supragingival plaque in the control of progressive periodontal disease: A review. *J. Clin. Periodontol.* 20:307–313.

Delanghe, G., J. Ghyselen, C. Bollen, D. van Steenberghe, B. Vanderkerckhove, and L. Feenstra. 1999. An inventory of patients' response to treatment at a multidisciplinary breath odor clinic. *Quintessence Int.* 30:307–310.

Dellerman, P. A., T. J. Hughes, and T. A. Burkett. 1994. A comparative evaluation of the percent acceptable end-round bristles in the Crest Complete, the Improved Crest Complete and the Oral-B Advantage toothbrushes. *J. Clin. Dent.* 5:74–81.

Drake, D. R., B. Grigsby, and D. Drotz-Dieleman. 1994. Growth-inhibitory effect of pyrophosphate on oral bacteria. *Oral Micro. Immunol.* 9(1):25–28.

Drake, D., K. Vargas, A. Cardenzana, and R. Srikantha. 1995. Enhanced bacterial activity of Arm and Hammer Dental Care. *Am. J. Dent.* 8(6):308–312.

Duckworth, R. M., Y. Jones, J. Nicholson, A. P. Jacobson, and I. G. Chestnutt. 1994. Studies on plaque fluoride after use of F-containing dentifrices. *Adv. Dent. Res.* 8(2):202–207.

Ellingsen, J. E., H. M. Eriksen, and G. Rölla. 1982. Extrinsic dental stain caused by stannous fluoride. *Scand. J. Dent. Res.* (Feb) 90(1):9–13.

Felo, A., O. Shibly, S. G. Ciancio, F. R. Lauciello, and A. Ho. 1997. Effects of subgingival chlorhexidine irrigation of peri-implant maintenance. *Am. J. Dent.* 10:107–110.

Fischman, S. L., G. Kugel, R. B. Truelove, B. J. Nelson, and L. P. Cancro. 1992. Motivational benefits of a dentifrice containing baking soda and hydrogen peroxide. *J. Clin. Dent.* 3:88–94.

Fishman, S. L., and S. Yankell. 1999. Dentifrices, mouth rinses, and tooth whiteners. In eds. N. O. Harris and F. García-Godoy, *Primary preventive dentistry,* 5th ed., 103–125. Stamford, CT: Appleton and Lange.

Flores-de-Jacoby, L., and R. Mengel. 1995. Conventional surgical procedures. *Periodontology 2000.* 9:38–54.

Forgas-Brockmann, L. B., C. Carter-Hanson, and W. J. Killoy. 1998. The effects of an ultrasonic toothbrush on plaque accumulation and gingival inflammation. *J. Clin. Periodontol.* 25:375–379.

Frandsen, A. 1986. Mechanical oral hygiene practices. In eds. H. Löe and D. V. Kleinman, *Dental plaque control measures and oral hygiene practices,* 93–116. Oxford: IRL Press.

Gaengler, P., A. Kurbad, and W. Weinert. 1993. Evaluation of anti-calculus efficacy: An SEM method of evaluating the effectiveness of pyrophosphate dentifrice on calculus formation. *J. Clin. Periodontol.* 20:144–146.

Garmyn, P., D. van Steenberghe, and M. Quirynen. 1998. Efficacy of plaque control in the maintenance of gingival health: Plaque control in primary and secondary prevention. In eds. N. P. Lang, R. Attström, and H. Löe, *Proceedings of the European Workshop on Mechanical Plaque Control*, 107–120. Chicago: Quintessence.

Glavid, L., H. Christensen, E. Pedersen, H. Rosendahl, and R. Attström. 1985. Oral hygiene instruction in general dental practice by means of self-teaching manuals. *J. Clin. Periodontol.* 12:27–34.

Gordon, J. M., J. A. Frascella, and R. C. Reardon. 1996. A clinical study of the safety and efficacy of a novel electric interdental cleaning device. *J. Clin. Dent.* 7:70–73.

Grossman, E., M. Cronin, W. Dembling, and H. Proskin. 1996. A comparative study of extrinsic tooth stain removal with two electric toothbrushes and a manual brush. *Am. J. Dent.* 9:25–29.

Hague, A. L., and M. P. Carr. 2007. Efficacy of an automated flossing device in different regions of the mouth. *J. Periodontol.* 78(8):1529–1537.

Hancock, E. B. 1996. Prevention. *Ann. Periodontol.* 1:223–249.

Hellstadius, K., B. Asman, and A. Gustafsson. 1993. Improved maintenance of plaque control by electric tooth brushing in periodontitis patients with low compliance. *J. Clin. Periodontol.* 20:235–237.

Hellström, M. K., P. Romberg, L. Krok, and J. Lindhe. 1996. The effect of supragingival plaque control on the microflora in human periodontitis. *J. Clin. Periodontol.* 23:934–940.

Hill, H. C., P. A. Levi, and I. Glickman. 1973. The effects of waxed and unwaxed dental floss on interdental plaque accumulation and interdental gingival health. *J. Periodontol.* 53:411–414.

Jacobsen, P. L., and G. Bruce 2001. Clinical dentin hypersensitivity: Understanding the causes and prescribing a treatment. *J. Contemporary Practice* 2(1):1–8.

Jepsen, S. 1998. The role of manual toothbrushes in effective plaque control: Advantages and limitations. In eds. N. P. Lang, R. Attström, and H. Löe, *Proceedings of the European Workshop on Mechanical Plaque Control*, 121–137. Chicago: Quintessence.

Kirstila, V., M. Lenander-Lumikari, E. Soderling, and J. Tenovuo. 1996. Effects of oral hygiene products containing lactoperoxidase, lysozyme, and lactoferrin on the composition of whole saliva and on subjective oral symptoms in patients with xerostomia. *Acta Odontol. Scand.* 54:391–397.

Kleinberg, I., and M. Codipilly. 2001. Cysteine challenge testing as a method of determining the effectiveness of oral hygiene procedures for reducing oral malodor. *J. Dent. Rest.* 79 (special issue):425.

Kleinberg, I., and G. Westbay. 1992. Salivary and metabolic factors involved in oral malodor formation. *J Periodontol.* 63:768–775.

Koertge, T. E. 1996. Management of dental staining: Can low-abrasive dentifrices play a role? *Compend. Contin. Educ. Dent.* 17(Suppl 19):33–38.

Kostelc, J. G., G. Preti, P. R. Zelson, et al. 1980. Salivary volatiles as indicators of periodontitis. *J. Periodont. Res.* 15:185–192.

Lefkoff, M. H., F. M. Beck, and J. E. Horton. 1995. The effectiveness of a disposable tooth cleansing device on plaque. *J. Periodontol.* 66:218–221.

Levine, R. A. 1987. The Keyes technique as a cofactor in self-inflicted gingival lesions: A case report. *Compend. Contin. Educ. Dent.* 8:266–269.

Lewis, M. W., C. Holder-Ballard, R. J. Selders, Jr., M. Scarbecz, H. G. Johnson, and E. W. Turner. 2004. Comparison of the use of a toothpick holder to dental floss in improvement of gingival health in humans. *J. Periodontol.* 75(4): 551–556.

Lindhe, J., B. Rosling, S. S. Socransky, and A.R. Volpe. 1993. The effect of a triclosan containing dentifrice on established plaque and gingivitis. *J. Clin. Periodontol.* 20:327–334.

Lobene, R. R. 1989. A study to compare the effects of two dentifrices on adult dental calculus formation. *Clin. Dent.* 1:67–69.

Loesche, W. J. and C. Kazor. 2002. Microbiology and treatment of halitosis. *J. Periodontol.* 28:256–79.

Mariotti, A. J. 1998. Mouthrinses and dentifrices. In *ADA Guide to Dental Therapeutics*, 210–212. Chicago: ADA Publishing Co.

Meffert, R., B. Langer, and M. Frutz. 1992. Dental implants: A review. *J. Periodontol.* 63:859–870.

Meskin, L. H. 1996. A breath of fresh air. *J. Am. Dent. Assoc.* 127:1282–86.

Miyazaki, H., M. Arao, K. Okamura, K. Yaegaki, and T. Matsuo. 1999. Tentative classification of halitosis and its treatment needs. *Niigata Dent. J.* 32: 7–11.

Moran, J. M., and M. Addy. 1995. A comparative study of stain removal with two electric toothbrushes and a manual brush. *J. Clin. Dent.* 6:188–193.

Morita M., D.L. Musinski, and H.L. Wang. 2001. Assessment of newly developed tongue sulfide probe for detecting oral malodor. *J. Clin. Periodontol.* 28: 494–496.

Morita, M., and H.L. Wang. 2001. Association between oral malodor and adult periodontitis: A review. *J. Clin. Periodontol.* 28:813–819.

Mullaby, B. H., J. A. James, W. A. Coulter, and G. H. Linden. 1995. The efficacy of a herbal-based toothpaste on the control of plaque and gingivitis. *J. Clin. Periodontol.* 22:686–689.

Niles, H.P., K. Rustogi, M. Pestrone, et al. 1999. Long lasting breath freshening effects of a trichlosan/coplymer/NaF toothpaste. *Proceedings of the 4th International Conference on Breath Odor,* 13. Los Angeles: Wiley.

O'Beirne, G. O., R. H. Johnson, G. Rutger Persson, and M. D. Spektor. 1996. Efficacy of a sonic toothbrush on inflammation and probing depth in adult periodontitis. *J. Periodontol.* 67:900–908.

Orchardson, R., and D. G. Gillam. 2006. Managing dentin hypersensitivity. *JADA* 137(7):990–998.

Orton, G. S., D. L. Steele, and L. T. Wolinsky. 1989. The dental professional's role in monitoring and maintenance of tissue-integrated prosthesis. Int J Oral Maxillofac implants. 4(4): 305–310.

Page, R. C. 1997. Causes of halitosis. *Oral Care Rep.* 7(4):7–8.

Palcanis, K. G. 1996. Surgical pocket therapy. *Ann. Periodontol.* 1:589–617.

Pihlstrom, B. L., L. F. Wolff, M. B. Bakdash, E. M. Schaffer, J. R. Jensen, et al. 1987. Salt and peroxide compared with conventional oral hygiene: I. Clinical results. *J. Periodontol.* 58:291–300.

Preber, H., V. Ylipaa, J. Bergström, and H. Ryden. 1991. A comparative study of plaque removing efficiency using rotary electric and manual toothbrushes. *Swed. Dent. J.* 15:229–234.

Preti, G., L. Clark, B. J. Cowart, R. S. Feldman, L. D. Lowry, et al. 1992. Non-oral etiologies of oral malodor and altered chemosensation. *J. Periodontol.* 63:790–796.

Proskin, H. M., and A. R. Volpe. 1995. Comparison of the anticaries efficacy of dentifrices containing fluoride as sodium fluoride or sodium monofluorophosphate. *Am. J. Dent.* 8:51–58.

Ramfjord, S. P. 1987. Maintenance care for treated patients. *J. Clin. Periodontol.* 14:433–437.

Ratcliff, P. A., and P. W. Johnson. 1999. The relationship between oral malodor, gingivitis, and periodontists. A review. *J. Periodontol.* 70:485–489.

Reingewirtz, Y., O. Girault, N. Reingewirtz, B. Senger, and H. Tenenbaum. 1999. Mechanical effects and volatile sulfur compounds reducing effects of chewing gums and a control group. *Quintessence Int.* 30:319–323.

Replogle, W. H., and D. E. Beebe. 1996. Halitosis. *American Family Physician.* 53:1215–1223.

Roldán, S., D. Herrera, A. O'Connor, et al. 2005. A combined therapeutic approach to manage oral halitosis: A 3-month prospective case series. *J. Periodontol.* 76(6):1025–1033.

Rosenberg, M. J. 1996. Clinical assessment of bad breath: Current concepts. *J. Am. Dent. Assoc.* 127:475–482.

Rounds, M. C., and T. S. I. Tilliss. 1999. Personal oral hygiene: Auxiliary measures to complement toothbrushing. In eds. N. O. Harris, and F. Garcia-Godoy, *Primary preventive dentistry,* 125–154. Norwalk, CT: Appleton & Lange.

Sangnes, G. 1976. Traumatization of teeth and gingiva related to habitual tooth cleaning procedures. *J. Clin. Periodontol.* 3:94–103.

Sanz, M., and D. Herrera. 1998. Role of oral hygiene during the healing phase of periodontal therapy. In eds. N. P. Lang, R. Attström, and H. Löe, *Proceedings of the European Workshop on Mechanical Plaque Control,* 248–267. Chicago: Quintessence.

Savolainen, J. J., A. L. Suominen-Taipale, A. K. Uutela, T. P. Martelin, M. C. Niskanen, and M. L. E. Knuuttila. 2005. Sense of coherence as a determinant of toothbrushing fre-

quency and level of oral hygiene. *J. Periodontol.* 76(6):1006–1012.

Saxer, U. P., and S. L. Yankell. 1997. Impact of improved toothbrushes on dental diseases: II. *Quintessence Int.* 28:573–593.

Schiff, T. G. 1987. The effect of a dentifrice containing soluble pyrophosphate and sodium fluoride on calculus deposits. *Clin. Prev. Dent.* 9:13–16.

Scully, C., M. El-Maaytah, S. R. Porter, and J. Greenman. 1997. Breath odor: Etiopathogenesis, assessment and management. *Eur. J. Oral Sci.* 105:287–293.

Segelnick, S. 2004. A survey of floss frequency, habit and technique in a hospital dental clinic and private periodontal practice. *NYSDJ* (May/June):28–33.

Shellis, R. P., and R. M. Duckworth. 1994. Studies on the cariostatic mechanisms of fluoride. *Int. Dent. J.* 44(3 Suppl. 1):263–273.

Silverman, G., E. Berman, C. B. Hanna, A. Salvato, P. Fratarcangelo, et al. 1996. Assessing the efficacy of three dentifrices in the treatment of dentinal hypersensitivity. *J. Am. Dent. Assoc.* 127:191–201.

Singh, S. M., M. E. Petrone, A. R. Volpe, K. N. Rustogi, and J. Norfleet. 1990. Comparison of the anticalculus effect of two soluble pyrophosphate dentifrices with and without a copolymer. *J. Clin. Dent.* 2:53–55.

Stephen, K. W. 1994. Fluoride toothpastes, rinses and tablets. *Adv. Dent. Res.* 8:185–189.

Stookey, O. K. 1994. Review of fluorosis risk of self-applied topical fluorides, dentifrices, mouthrinses and gels. *Comm. Dent. Oral Epidemiol.* 22(3):181–186.

Tammaro, S., J. L. Wennström, and G. Bergenholtz. 2000. Root-dentin sensitivity following nonsurgical periodontal treatment. *J. Clin. Periodontol.* 27:690–69.

Terèzhalmy, G. T., R. D. Bartizek, and A. R. Biesbrock. 2008. Plaque-removal efficacy of four types of dental floss. *J. Periodontol.* 79(2):245–251.

Terèzhalmy, G., E. Chaves, S. Bsoul, R. Baker, and T. He. 2007. Clinical evaluation of the stain removal efficacy of a novel stannous fluoride and sodium hexametaphosphate dentifrice. *Am J Dent.* (Feb) 20(1):53–8.

Tonzetich, J. 1997. Production and origin of oral malodor: A review of mechanisms and methods of analysis. *J. Periodontal.* 48:13–20.

Van der Weijden, G. A., M. M. Danser, A. Nijboer, M. F. Timmerman, and U. Van der Velden. 1993. The plaque-removing efficacy of an oscillating/rotation toothbrush: A short-term study. *J. Clin. Periodontol.* 20:273–278.

Van Dyke, T., S. Offenbacher, B. Pihlstrom, M. Putt, and C. Trummel. 1999. What is gingivitis? Current understanding of prevention, treatment, measurement, pathogenesis and relation to periodontitis. *J. Int. Acad. Periodontol.* 1:3–10.

Volpe, A. R., M. E. Petrone, R. Davies, and H. M. Proskin. 1995. Clinical anticaries efficacy of NaF and SMFP dentifrices: Overview and resolution of the scientific controversy. *J. Clin. Dent.* 6:1–28.

Volpe, A. R., M. E. Petrone, W. DeVizio, and R. M. Davies. 1996. A review of plaque, gingivitis, calculus and caries clinical efficacy studies with a fluoride dentifrice containing triclosan and PVM/MA copolymer. *J. Clin. Dent.* 7(Suppl):1–14.

von Troil, B., I. Needleman, and M. Sanz. 2002. A systematic review of the prevalence of root sensitivity following periodontal therapy. *J. Clin. Periodontol.* 29(Suppl. 3):173–177.

Waerhaug, J. 1981. Healing of the dentoepithelial junction following the use of dental floss. *J. Clin. Periodontol.* 8:144–150.

Watt, R. G., and V. C. Marinho. 2005. Does oral health promotion improve oral hygiene and gingival health? *Periodontology 2000* 37(1):35–47.

Westfelt, E. 1996. Rationale of mechanical plaque control. *J. Clin. Periodontol.* 23:263–267.

White, D. J., B. W. Bollmer, R. A. Baker, E. R. Cox, M. A. Perlich, et al. 1996. Quantical assessment of the clinical scaling benefits provided by phyrophosphate dentifrices with and without triclosan. *J. Clin. Dent.* 7(special issue):46–49.

Wilkins, E. M. 2009. *Clinical practice of the dental hygienist,* 320. Baltimore, MD. Wolters Kluwer, Lippinoctt, Williams & Wilkins.

Yaegaki, K. 2000. Organoleptic measurement of oral malodor. In ed. K. Yaegaki, *Clinical guideline for halitosis,* 35–44. Tokyo: Quintessence.

Yaegaki, K., and J. M. Coil. 2000a. Examination, classification, and treatment of halitosis, clinical perspectives. *J. Can. Dent. Assoc.* 66:257–261.

Yaegaki, K., and J. M. Coil. 2000b. Genuine halitosis, pseudo-halitosis, and halitophobia: Classification, diagnosis and treatment. *Compendium.* 21:880–890.

Yaegaki, K., and T. Suetaka, 1989. The effect of zinc chloride mouthwash on the production of oral malodor, the degradation of salivary cellular elements and proteins. *J. Dent. Health.* 9:377–386.

Yankell, S. L., and U. P. Saxer. 1999. Toothbrushing and toothbrushing techniques. In eds. N. O. Harris and F. Garcia-Godoy, *Primary preventive dentistry,* 77–102. Norwalk, CT: Appleton and Lange.

Yukna, R. A., and R. L. Shaklee. 1993. Evaluation of a counterrotational powered brush in patients in supportive periodontal therapy. *J. Periodontol.* 64:859–864.

Zambon, J. J., M. L. Mather, and Y. Gonzales. 1996. A microbiological and clinical study of the safety and efficacy of baking-soda dentifrices. *Compend. Contin. Educ. Dent. Suppl.* 17:39–44.

Chapter 21

Topical Drug Delivery Systems: Oral Rinses and Irrigation

Mea A. Weinberg

OUTLINE

Introduction
Oral Rinses
Antiplaque/Antigingivitis Agents
Oral Irrigation
Dental Hygiene Notes
Key Points
Self-Quiz
References

EDUCATIONAL OBJECTIVES

Upon completion of this chapter, the reader should be able to:

- Describe measures, using chemical agents, taken to prevent and control the progression of periodontal diseases.
- List the different oral rinses available for the periodontal patient.
- Describe the indications for oral irrigation.

GOAL: To provide an understanding of the fundamentals of counseling periodontal patients on the adjunctive use of chemotherapeutic agents for supragingival plaque control.

KEY WORDS

chemotherapeutic agents 321
periodontal pathogens 327
substantivity 321
topical delivery 321

320

INTRODUCTION

Topically applied **chemotherapeutic agents** have been developed based on a need for treatment of gingival bleeding and inflammation in association with gingivitis. Mouth rinsing and oral irrigation are two approaches used for supragingival application of antiseptic solutions. Oral rinses are the most common form of **topical delivery.** Oral rinses are ideal vehicles for the delivery of topical antimicrobials because of their relative simplicity of formulation and ease of use for patients.

ORAL RINSES

Mouthrinses generally are divided into two classifications: therapeutic rinses, used to treat diseases such as gingival diseases, and cosmetic rinses, used to freshen the breath. Indications for using oral rinses are as follows:

- As an addition to home care regimens that have failed to achieve plaque-control goals by other means.
- As an addition to periodontal instrumentation.
- Where oral hygiene may be inadequate or difficult to accomplish for many people, as in the physically or mentally compromised.
- Following surgical procedures, when brushing and flossing are generally not practical.
- As a preprocedural rinse to reduce aerosolized bacteria in the dental office (when masked, the clinician is protected; however, after the mask is removed, aerosols remain in the dental operatory);
- For maintenance of dental implants.

Topical antimicrobial agents delivered by a rinse are effective only against supragingival bacteria. Antimicrobial rinses when used in conjunction with brushing and flossing have been reported to be an important method of reducing plaque and gingivitis (Barnett, 2006; Silverman & Wilder, 2006). No antimicrobial rinse has been shown to be effective against periodontitis because oral rinses do not reach the subgingival area. Mouthrinses may be discontinued if oral health conditions can be maintained without their use.

ANTIPLAQUE/ANTIGINGIVITIS AGENTS

Antimicrobial agents ideally should inhibit microbial colonization on tooth surfaces and prevent the subsequent formation of plaque. They also should eliminate or suppress the pathogenicity of existing plaque. Antiseptics have a greater potential to prevent the formation of plaque than to resolve established plaque and gingivitis.

An antimicrobial agent relies on two factors for efficacy. Success depends on the amount of time the agent stays in contact with the target site and how well the agent gains access to the target site. A major requirement for the success of antimicrobial therapy is **substantivity,** which is the ability of the drug to adsorb or bind to intraoral surfaces such as teeth and soft tissues with subsequent release of the drug in its active form (Stabholz et al., 1993). Substantivity involves the ability of the drug to stay at the target site for longer periods of time, thus maintaining therapeutic levels. It is ideal to have a drug with high substantivity that will be bound in the oral cavity and released over a period of hours in order to prolong the effects. Lack of substantivity can be overcome by more frequent use of the agent, but this would likely result in noncompliance and undesirable side effects.

> **Did You Know?**
> The total annual consumer spending on oral antiseptics/rinses is $885 million.

Classification of Oral Rinses

Topical antimicrobial oral rinses can be classified as either first- or second-generation agents. First-generation agents have antibacterial properties with low substantivity and limited therapeutic value in reducing plaque and gingivitis. Examples include phenolic compounds, quaternary ammonium compounds, peroxide, and sanguinarine. Second-generation agents have antibacterial properties in addition to substantivity. Chlorhexidine gluconate is an example of a second-generation agent and is currently the only second-generation agent proven to prevent and control gingivitis. It is available in the United States only by prescription. All first-generation mouthrinses are available over the counter (OTC) without a prescription.

In 1986, the American Dental Association (ADA) established guidelines for evaluation of the therapeutic effectiveness of products against gingivitis. For example, studies should be conducted over a minimum of six months, two studies with independent investigators should be conducted, and the active product should be used as part of a normal regimen and compared with a placebo or control product.

Most mouthrinses contain alcohol as a flavor enhancer and as a vehicle for the active ingredients. There has been some concern about the association of alcohol in mouthrinses with oral cancer. Various studies have shown inconsistent findings. Some studies document that there is no reason for patients to refrain from use of alcohol-containing mouthrinses (Ciancio, 1993), while research from the National Cancer Institute has drawn an association between alcoholic mouthrinses to mouth and throat cancers (Winn et al., 1991). Additionally, a vitro (laboratory) studied the effect of acetaldehyde, a toxic compound produced by alcohol metabolism (breakdown) in the body. It was reported that acetaldehyde caused changes in gingival fibroblasts (cells involved in oral connective tissue maintenance) (Poggi, Rodriguez y Baena, Rizzo, & Rota, 2003).

Bisbiguanides

Description and Mechanism of Action Chlorhexidine gluconate (Peridex® Omni 3M, St. Paul, MN; PerioGard®, Colgate Oral Pharmaceuticals, New York, NY) is a cationic (positively charged) molecule. Originally, chlorhexidine was used in medicine as an antiseptic cream for wounds, as a preoperative skin cleanser, and as a surgical scrub. In 1970, the first study on the ability of chlorhexidine to inhibit the formation of plaque and maintain soft tissue health was released (Löe & Schiott, 1970). It was not until 1986 that chlorhexidine became available in the United States by prescription at a 0.12% concentration with an alcohol concentration of 11.6%. It has the ADA seal of acceptance for the treatment of gingivitis (Cheng, Leung, & Corbet, 2008).

After rinsing, chlorhexidine (positively charged) is attracted to and attaches onto the negatively charged bacterial cell walls, causing lysis or breakage of the cell wall and the contents of the cells leak. Chlorhexidine enters the cell through the opening, resulting in death of the bacteria. By binding to the pellicle on the tooth surface, chlorhexidine inhibits plaque attachment. Chlorhexidine exhibits substantivity, with approximately 30% of the drug binding to oral tissues and the plaque on the teeth (Rölla, Löe, & Schiott, 1971) and showing antimicrobial activity for 8 to 12 hours afterwards (Addy & Wright, 1978; Schiott et al., 1970).

In 2006 the FDA approved a nonalcoholic chlorhexidine oral rinse 0.12%. Alcohol is an inactive ingredient so the effectiveness is the same as chlorhexidine with alcohol. This product is ideal for patients susceptible to dry mouth, those who experience irritation of soft tissues (mucositis), and patients who are sensitive to alcohol.

Indications Rinsing with chlorhexidine is indicated before, during, and after periodontal debridement to reduce plaque levels and gingival inflammation. Chlorhexidine rinses can improve wound healing and provide better plaque control after periodontal surgery when brushing and flossing is not feasible (Sanz, Newman, Anderson, & Motaska, 1987). A clinical study showed that even intermittent rinsing with chlorhexidine may provide a preventive benefit in reducing levels of bacteria but only in subjects without alveolar bone loss (Persson et al., 2007). In the office, before using dental devices that produce an aerosol, such as power-assisted instruments or air polishing, it has been shown that a preoperative rinse with chlorhexidine markedly reduces contamination of the dental office (Warrall, Knibbs, & Glenwright, 1987). Rinsing with chlorhexidine has been shown to decrease the severity of mucositis in patients receiving chemotherapy. Since peri-implantitis is similar to gingivitis, rinsing with chlorhexidine may be effective in implant plaque control (Kozlovsky et al., 2006).

Usage It is recommended to rinse twice a day for 30 seconds. The positive charge of chlorhexidine causes it to bind to the negatively charged molecules in toothpastes such as fluorides and sodium lauryl sulfate (a detergent) and thus inactivates them. Therefore, it is best to rinse either 30 minutes before or after toothbrushing or rinse very well with water after toothbrushing. Because of this inactivation by anionic compounds, chlorhexidine is not available in toothpaste form. Chlorhexidine can be used as an irrigant, but it is usually diluted with water to reduce the incidence of staining. A recent clinical study compared the effectiveness of scaling and root planing alone or in combination with chlorhexidine in 29 patients with chronic periodontitis (Faveri et al., 2006). Results showed that scaling and root planing in combination with chlorhexidine was more effective in reducing plaque than scaling and root planing alone.

Adverse Effects Chlorhexidine is a relatively safe drug because it is poorly absorbed from the oral membranes and systemic circulation if swallowed. The

> **Did You Know?**
>
> Chlorhexidine 0.12% is used as an oral rinse but chlorhexidine surgical 4.0% is used as a surgical scrub.

most common adverse effect is a yellow, brownish extrinsic staining of the teeth, tongue, and restorations (McCoy et al., 2008). Staining is more frequent with chlorhexidine than with other agents because of its affinity for oral surfaces. The staining may be associated with food dyes found within certain foods and beverages. This staining is not permanent and can be removed mechanically during professional prophylaxis. If the patient is compliant with oral home care, the staining is more likely on proximal tooth surfaces than facial or lingual surfaces. Other adverse effects include a temporarily impaired taste perception and increased supragingival calculus formation.

 Rapid Dental Hint

Remind patients using chlorhexidine to brush well to help prevent calculus buildup.

Phenolic Compounds

Listerine® (McNeil, Titusville, NJ) is a combination of phenolic compounds or essential oils, including thymol, eucalyptol, menthol, and methyl salicylate, in an alcohol vehicle. The mechanism of action is cell wall disruption, resulting in leakage of intracellular components and lysis of the cell (Fine et al., 2007; Stoeken, Paraskevas, & van der Weijden, 2007). The original-formula Listerine contains 26.9% alcohol, whereas Cool Mint and Fresh Burst Listerine contain 21.6% alcohol. The newest product, Natural Citrus, also contains 21.6% alcohol.

Because of low substantivity, effectiveness is strongly related to the duration of tooth contact. Clinical studies have shown it to significantly reduce plaque development in patients with minimal plaque levels (Gordon, Lamster, & Sieger, 1985). A six-month study comparing Listerine with a control product found that Listerine reduced plaque and gingivitis from 20 to 34%. The subjects had preexisting plaque and gingivitis, and no prophylaxis was performed at the beginning of the study (Lamster, Alfano, Seiger, & Gordon, 1983). In-office preprocedure rinsing with Listerine reduced the level of bacteria in the aerosol generated during ultrasonic scaling (Fine et al., 1992).

Recommendations are to rinse for 30 seconds with 2/3 oz once in the morning and once at night. Possible adverse effects include a burning sensation and bitter taste.

Quaternary Ammonium Compounds

Quaternary ammonium compounds are positively charged (cationic) compounds similar to chlorhexidine, except that after rinsing they readily bind to oral surfaces and are released more rapidly or lose their activity upon binding to the surface (Moran & Addy, 1984). Substantivity is only approximately three hours (Roberts & Addy, 1981). An increase in bacterial cell wall permeability leads to cell lysis and decreased attachment of bacteria to tooth surfaces. Cetylpyridinium chloride is the active ingredient in Scope® Original (Procter & Gamble, Cincinnati, OH), Cepacol® (J. B. Williams, Glen Rock, NJ), and Viadent™ Advanced Care (Colgate Oral Pharmaceuticals, New York, NY). The alcohol concentration is 14% for Cepacol, 18.9% for Scope Original, and 5.5% for Viadent™ Advanced Care.

Clinical data on plaque reduction and gingivitis control have been relatively inconclusive because of the variability in results between studies. Following an initial professional prophylaxis and suspension of all oral hygiene, chlorhexidine was found to be superior to cetylpyridinium in the reduction of plaque (Renton-Harper, Addy, Moran, Doherty, & Newcombe, 1996). Cetylpyridinium chloride may have some antiplaque action but less effect on gingivitis when used as an adjunct to conventional oral home care. Lack of substantivity limits clinical efficacy. As with chlorhexidine, to obtain the maximum effect, the patient should rinse very well or wait 30 minutes after brushing with a dentifrice before using the rinse. Adverse effects are similar to those of chlorhexidine, including some staining, calculus formation, and mucosal ulceration.

 Rapid Dental Hint

Remember, not every patient needs to use a mouthrinse. Follow your treatment plan.

A clinical study reported that in combination with toothbrushing, a mouthrinse containing 0.1% cetylpyridinium chloride or 0.06% chlorhexidine may be more effective than flossing in reducing interproximal plaque (Zimmer et al., 2006).

> ### Did You Know?
>
> Hippocrates also offered advice for bad breath. He suggested a mouthwash containing oil of anise seed, myrrh, and white wine.

Oxygenating Agents

Oxygenating agents such as peroxides and perborates have been used in mouthrinse formulations primarily for acute necrotizing ulcerative gingivitis and pericoronitis. Since hydrogen peroxide liberates gaseous oxygen, it provides a cleansing action and gentle effervescence for oral wounds. Its antimicrobial effect is directed at anaerobic microorganisms that cannot live in the presence of oxygen, and it has a physical effect on plaque through the bubbling of oxygen as it is released from the peroxide (Marshall, Cancro, & Fischman, 1995). The Food and Drug Administration has approved its use as a temporary debriding agent in the oral cavity. However, antiplaque/antigingivitis claims are not well supported.

The safety of hydrogen peroxide has been disputed. Long-term use of 3% hydrogen peroxide has resulted in gingival irritation (Marshall et al., 1995; Rees & Orth, 1986) and delayed tissue healing, and it may serve as a cocarcinogen in animals (Weitzman, Weitberg, Stossel, Schwartz, & Shklar, 1986). A cocarcinogen is a compound that when administered with a low dose of a known carcinogen results in increased incidence of tumors. On the other hand, other studies found that adverse effects from exposure to 3% or less hydrogen peroxide were rare. It was concluded that exposure to less than 3% hydrogen peroxide was safe (Marshall et al., 1995). Long-term studies do not demonstrate any additional benefit over regular home care, however. Since many patients use hydrogen peroxide on a regular basis, the dental hygienist should question patients about their oral home-care practices.

Povidone-Iodine

Povidone-iodine is antibacterial and antiseptic. Its primary use is in the prevention and treatment of surface infections. Often povidone-iodine is combined with hydrogen peroxide as a subgingival irrigant for the reduction of gram-negative microorganisms. Most studies confirm that iodine may be a beneficial adjunctive treatment for the prevention and control of gingivitis when used with optimal oral hygiene self-care procedures (Clark, Magnusson, Walker, & Marks, 1989). Iodine can stain teeth, clothing, skin, and restorations, however.

Fluorides

Fluorides have been used in dentistry primarily for dental caries prevention by reducing demineralization and enhancing remineralization. Fluoride rinses have not been proven clinically to prevent root caries (Paine, Slots, & Rich, 1998). Its role as an antiplaque/antigingivitis agent is less well documented and shows controversial results.

Stannous fluoride (SnF_2) has been documented to exhibit antimicrobial properties in the control of gingival inflammation and bacterial repopulation. The tin molecule supposedly prevents bacterial adhesion to the tooth surface. Another indication for stannous fluoride is for dentinal hypersensitivity. Stannous fluoride is available as a dentifrice, a gel, and a concentrated oral rinse that is diluted with water. For home rinsing, available products include Gel-Kam® (available over-the-counter; Colgate Oral Pharmaceuticals, New York, NY) and Stanimax (0.63% SnF_2). Extrinsic tooth staining occurs with extended use. Sodium fluoride is indicated for caries prevention and has not been documented to have any antiplaque/antigingivitis action.

Prebrushing Rinses

A prebrushing rinse (Plax®, Pfizer, New York, NY) that contains surfactants such as sodium lauryl sulfate (which functions as a detergent to help loosen and remove plaque), sodium benzoate (a preservative), and tetrasodium pyrophosphate (an anticalculus agent) is intended to be used before brushing. Studies have shown limited beneficial effects of this agent over rinsing with water alone (Grossman, 1988).

Alcohol-Free Mouthrinses

Most mouthrinses contain alcohol as a vehicle to carry other ingredients and as a flavor enhancer. The form of alcohol in the rinse is either ethanol (ethyl alcohol) or a specially denatured (SD) alcohol that is made synthetically. Alcohol can cause drying of the oral mucosal tissues, especially when the agent is used for extended periods of time. These rinses are primarily used as cosmetic rinses rather than therapeutic rinses. Indications for a nonalcoholic mouthrinse include pregnant women, former alcoholics, patients who are taking medications that would additionally dry the mouth, patients taking metronidazole (an antibiotic), and patients who prefer to avoid alcohol. Box 21–1 lists some nonalcoholic antimicrobial mouthrinses.

> **Box 21–1 Selective Alcohol-Free Antimicrobial Mouthrinses**
>
> - Rembrandt® (DenMat, Santa Maria, CA)
> - Oral B® Antibacterial Rinse (Oral-B, Redwood City, CA)
> - Listermint® (Warner-Lambert, Morris Plains, NJ)
> - BreathRX® (Discus Dental, Culver City, CA)
> - Biotène (Laclede, Rancho Dominguez, CA)

ORAL IRRIGATION

Oral irrigation emerged in the late 1960s as an adjunct to brushing and flossing. Early studies indicated that mechanical water-pressure devices did not remove significant amounts of supragingival plaque but only loosened food debris and less adherent materials (Lobene, 1969). However, regardless of the plaque index, reductions in gingivitis and calculus formation were evident as early as 1969 (Lobene, 1969; Lobene & Soparkar, 1970). Today, there is a preponderance of clinical studies that address the use of oral irrigation on gingivitis and periodontitis maintenance patients and show significant reductions in clinical parameters (e.g., bleeding on probing and gingival inflammation).

According to the American Academy of Periodontology (2005), supragingival and marginal irrigation play an important role in the treatment of gingivitis and maintenance of periodontal patients. However, there is not much data to support a single episode of subgingival irrigation will increase the immediate impact or duration of root planing effectiveness.

Home Oral Irrigation

The primary use of oral irrigation is to nonspecifically reduce bacteria and their by-products that lead to the initiation or progression of periodontal diseases. The target area of irrigation is unattached or loosely attached microorganisms at the subgingival level, regardless of where the tip of the device is placed. It is a misconception that if the tip is placed at the gingival margin, it is only effective on supragingival plaque; it is effective against both supragingival and subgingival bacteria. Cobb, Rodgers, and Killoy (1988) found that supra-

gingival irrigation had an effect on subgingival microorganisms at probing depths of up to 6 mm. Irrigation attempts to reduce the potential of developing gingivitis or decreases existing gingivitis and directly reduces pocket microbiota in an attempt to control or prevent the initiation of periodontitis.

With our current understanding of the pathogenesis of periodontal infections and the role endotoxins play in the immune response, irrigation may have a more significant place in self-care routines, especially since the highest concentrations of endotoxins have been found within the loosely adherent subgingival plaque. Supragingival irrigation dilutes (Ciancio, 1990) and flushes away bacteria coronal to the gingiva, which helps to prevent or treat gingivitis and also reduces subgingival bacteria. Subgingival irrigation attempts to directly reduce the pocket microbiota in an effort to prevent initiation of periodontitis or to help its reduction. However, irrigation does not remove adherent dental plaque, calculus, or stains.

Home irrigation has been proven to reach farther into the pocket than rinsing (Braun & Ciancio, 1992; Eakle, Ford, & Boyd, 1986; Flotra, Gjermo, Rölla, & Waerhaug, 1972; Mashimo, Umemoto, Slots, Genco, & Ellison, 1980). The addition of an antimicrobial agent has reduced clinical parameters in some studies. Flemming and colleagues (1990) demonstrated an enhanced effect on reducing gingivitis when a 0.06% solution of chlorhexidine was used as the irrigant compared with rinsing and water irrigation. Conversely, the addition of Listerine® (Warner-Lambert, Morris Plains, NJ) as an irrigant was as effective as placebo in reducing gingivitis and improving gingival health (Ciancio, Mather, Zambon, & Reynolds, 1989). However, the addition of Listerine® resulted in greater reductions in plaque and gingival bleeding and a moderate decrease in total bacteria counts, although it was not statistically significant. Subgingival irrigation with chlorhexidine has been shown to decrease subgingival microbiota and inflammation around implants (Lavigne, Drust-Bay, Williams, Killoy, & Theisen, 1994).

Devices

Oral irrigation devices generally are power-driven pulsating devices that deliver water or a medicament to the site. The pulsations create two zones of hydrokinetic activity. The impact zone is the area where the irrigant comes in contact with the tooth surface, and the flushing zone is the deflection of the irrigant subgingivally (Cobb et al., 1988). A pulsating stream of water provides better flushing than a continuous stream because it incorporates a compression and decompression phase, which allows debris and bacteria to be displaced more efficiently. Products are available that are nonpulsating and non-power-driven, but to date, there is no evidence that they are clinically effective.

Water Pik (Teledyne Water Pik, Fort Collins, CO; Figure 21–1a ■) is one such home irrigation device (Table 21–1 ■). Water or a medicament is delivered to the gingival margin with a standard jet tip (Figure 21–1b) placed at a 90° angle to the long axis of the tooth. The jet tip is positioned directly interproximally so that the stream of water or medicament reaches the target slightly subgingivally. The tip is passed along the gingival margin to the next proximal area and held in place for 5 to 6 seconds. The procedure is usually performed over a bathroom sink beginning with a low-pressure setting. Pressure may be increased as needed or according to patient comfort and gingival health. Eakle and colleagues (1986) found that a standard jet tip delivered an irrigant 44 to 71% into the depth of pockets. In addition, use of a standard jet tip with a Water Pik® oral irrigator placed on medium pressure was found to have a positive effect on subgingival microorganisms at probing depths of up to 6 mm (Cobb et al., 1988). Some home irrigation devices have accessory delivery tips designed for targeted direct subgingival delivery. A Water Pik® oral irrigator using a Pik Pocket® subgingival irrigation tip (Figure 21–2 ■) delivers an irrigant to approximately 90% of the depth of pockets ranging from 0 to 6 mm (Braun & Ciancio, 1992). The Pik Pocket® tip is designed for controlled, targeted low-pressure delivery of a medicament or water. Water Pik® dental water jets come in many models including a cordless unit.

In-Office Irrigation

Efficacy An alternate route of topical drug delivery is through patient or professionally applied oral irrigation. An antimicrobial agent also can be applied professionally in-office. This can be accomplished by using an air- or power-driven device (e.g., Perio Pik Subgingival Irrigation Handpiece, Teledyne Water Pik®, Fort Collins, CO; Figure 21–3 ■), ultrasonic unit (piezoelectric) scaler (Piezon Master 400, EMS, Richardson, TX; Figure 21–4 ■), or handheld syringe. Caution must be taken when using a handheld syringe because the delivery pressure cannot be controlled and may exceed a safe pressure for delivery into a periodontal pocket. Control is also compromised because of the inability to fulcrum and may affect the delivery to the apical aspect of the pocket. Penetration of an irrigant with an ultrasonic unit may be limited due to little lateral dispersion of agents and inaccessibility of the tip to certain areas (Nosel, Scheidt, O'Neal, & Van Dyke, 1991).

At present, a single episode of in-office irrigation has been shown only to have limited or no beneficial effects by itself, but it may be of some advantage if patients perform subgingival irrigation at home between continuing-care appointments (Jolkovsky et al., 1990). Repeated irrigations over a period of time or longer exposure to an antibiotic has shown efficacy in some patients (Christersson, Norderyd, & Puchalsky, 1993; Clark et al., 1989). The use of 2% chlorhexidine alone over a

(a)

(b)

■ **FIGURE 21–1** (a) Water Pik® dental systems. (b) Placement of standard jet tip. (© Courtesy of Teledyne Water Pik, Fort Collins, CO)

Table 21–1	Home Oral Irrigators
Product	**Description**
Water Pik® dental systems (various) (Teledyne Water Pik, Fort Collins, CO)	Two tips are available; standard jet tip for supragingival irrigation and the Pik Pocket™ tip for subgingival irrigation.
Braun Oral-B™ Oxy Jet (Oral-B, Belmont, CA)	Mixes air and water, then pressurizes it to form micro bubbles that attack bacteria. Use in conjunction with toothbrush.
Viajet™ (Oratec Corporation, Herndon, VA)	Two standard tips for supragingival irrigation and two sulcus tips for marginal application are available. For office use: A cannula (stainless steel tube) adapter for subgingival application is also available.
Braun Oral-B™ Plaque Removal System (Oral-B, Belmont, CA)	This device is only available with the powered brush (sold as one unit). Plastic tips are available for supragingival use only, and the tips cannot be removed.

fifteen-week period was nearly as effective in reducing clinical parameters as periodontal debridement alone (Southard, Drisko, Killoy, Cobb, & Tira, 1989).

Many different chemical agents have been used as irrigants (Box 21–2). Owing to differences in protocol, type of agent used, concentrations, and levels of disease, oral irrigation is inconclusive in terms of efficacy, and research is ongoing.

Studies repeatedly show statistically significant reductions in gingivitis, bleeding on probing, probing depth, and **periodontal pathogens** in gingivitis and periodontal maintenance patients with the use of oral irrigation over normal oral hygiene (Cobb et al., 1988; Flemming et al., 1990; Newman et al., 1994). Subgingival calculus must be removed before irrigation because

it interferes with penetration of the agent (Pitcher, Newman, & Strahan, 1980).

It appears that using a standard jet tip or a specialized delivery tip is effective with specific home irrigation devices. Caution must be taken when evaluating the research because not all products have been studied in

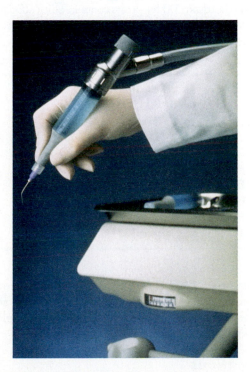

■ **FIGURE 21–3** Perio Pik™ subgingival irrigation handpiece for in-office subgingival irrigation fits into a standard handpiece holder. (Courtesy of Teledyne Water Pik®, Fort Collins, CO)

■ **FIGURE 21–2** Pik Pocket® subgingival delivery tip placement in furcation of mandibular first molar. (Courtesy of Teledyne Water Pik®, Fort Collins, CO)

■ FIGURE 21–4 Ultrasonic scaler (Piezon Master 400, EMS, Richardson, TX) for professional in-office subgingival irrigation of solutions during ultrasonic scaling. There is a built-in reservoir for the irrigant.

Box 21–2 Chemical Agents Used as Irrigants

- Water
- Chlorhexidine
- Povidone-iodine
- Essential oils
- Hydrogen peroxide
- Fluoride
- Tetracycline

clinical trials. Therefore, established efficacy with one product may not be true for another. It is always advisable to contact the manufacturer and request copies of the clinical trials that support product claims.

Indications

Adjunctive oral irrigation may not be necessary for all patients. However, Chaves and colleagues (1994) found an added benefit for patients with good oral hygiene. Oral irrigation is an ideal adjunct when supragingival mechanical aids (e.g., toothbrushes, floss, and interproximal brushes and devices) are not sufficient to keep the bacterial load below the threshold of disease. It is also ideal for delivering antimicrobial agents deeper into pockets. Patients with physical challenges, orthodontic appliances, or prosthodontic replacements such as implants and crowns or those who need an adjunctive method to reduce repopulation of bacteria between periodontal maintenance appointments are also ideal candidates for supplemental home oral irrigation. Subgingival irrigation may be better than rinsing in the maintenance of gingival health around dental implants (Felo, Shibly, Ciancio, Lauciello, & Ho, 1997).

Patients with plaque-induced gingivitis can benefit most from oral irrigation because the disease is in its early stage. Patients with slight and moderate chronic periodontitis also may benefit from oral irrigation. However, patients with severe chronic periodontitis and refractory periodontitis require more aggressive treatment and referral to a periodontist.

Cautions

Controlled powered-driven home irrigation devices are safe for patients to use on a daily basis. Thorough patient evaluation is always necessary prior to recommending any device or aid to a patient. It is important to match the correct product with the patient's specific needs. Also, take the time to instruct patients on the proper use of their device. Oral irrigation should not be used when a periodontal abscess or ulcerations are present. Once the problem has been resolved, it then may be appropriate to recommend irrigation therapy.

Rapid Dental Hint

It is important to instruct patients on the proper use of an irrigator. Some patients do not know the proper way to use one.

Irrigation Versus Toothbrushing

Controversy exists over whether irrigation provides an additional benefit over toothbrushing and flossing. Irrigation is not a substitute for toothbrushing or flossing. Toothbrushing plus irrigation may be better than toothbrushing alone in patients with poor oral home care (Flemming et al., 1990). Supragingival irrigation is adequate as an adjunctive therapy to decrease inflammation (e.g., redness and bleeding), but there is no significant reduction in probing depth or gain in clinical attachment. Irrigation distributes antimicrobial agents into interproximal areas better than rinsing. There may be no difference between irrigating with a medicament (chemical agent) or with water, however. In patients with good oral hygiene, daily brushing and flossing remain the most efficient methods for controlling gingivitis.

DENTAL HYGIENE NOTES

Antiseptics deserve continued evaluation, and their importance should not be underestimated. Currently, the most valuable application of antiplaque/antigingivitis agents is as an adjunct to conventional mechanical debridement and oral home care for short- to medium-term usage.

An important factor in the efficacy of any antiplaque/antigingivitis agent is an adequate contact time with the target site. Accordingly, the well-proven success of chlorhexidine is related to its substantivity more than to any unique action on the microbiota (bacteria). It is the function of the dental hygienist to advise patients on the role of oral rinses and dentifrices in the hygienic phase of treatment. The hygienist should use his or her knowledge of clinical studies to decide on the appropriate product for each patient.

KEY POINTS

- Oral rinses and irrigation are types of topical delivery systems.
- Oral rinses are only effective supragingivally and do not have any effect on subgingival plaque.
- Oral irrigation may be useful between maintenance appointments to reduce bacterial reinfection (repopulation).

SELF-QUIZ

1. Which one of the following substances can cause extrinsic tooth staining? (p. 322)
   a. Cetylpyridinium
   b. Alcohol
   c. Phenols
   d. Chlorhexidine

2. All the following are indications for the use of mouthrinses in periodontics except one. Which one is the exception? (p. 321)
   a. Limited manual dexterity
   b. Gingivitis
   c. Periodontitis
   d. Peri-implantitis

3. Which one of the following antimicrobial agents possesses high substantivity to the oral soft tissues? (p. 322)
   a. Cetylpyridinium
   b. Alcohol
   c. Chlorhexidine
   d. Erythromycin
   e. Tetracycline

4. Which one of the following instructions should be given to a patient rinsing with chlorhexidine? (p. 322)
   a. Rinse immediately after brushing.
   b. Rinse immediately before brushing.
   c. Wait about 30 minutes after brushing.
   d. Wait about 1 hour after brushing.

5. Which one of the following antimicrobial mouthrinses contains the highest concentration of alcohol? (p. 323)
   a. Listerine
   b. PerioGard
   c. Scope
   d. Viadent Advanced Care

REFERENCES

Addy, M., and R. Wright. 1978. Comparison of the in vivo and in vitro antibacterial properties of povidone-iodine and chlorhexidine gluconate mouth rinses. *J. Clin. Periodontol.* 5:198–205.

American Academy of Periodontology. 2005. The role of supra- and subgingival irrigation in the treatment of periodontal diseases. *J. Periodontol.* 76:2015–2027.

Barnett, M. L. 2006. The rationale for the daily use of an antimicrobial mouthrinse. *JADA* 137(11 supplement):16S–21S.

Braun, R., and S. Ciancio. 1992. Subgingival delivery by an oral irrigation device. *J. Periodontol.* 63:469–472.

Chaves, E. S., K. S. Kornman, and M. A. Manwell et al., Mechanism of irrigation effects on gingivitis. *J. Periodontol.* 1994; 65(11): 1016–1021.

Cheng, H. R. W., W. K. Leung, & Corbet E. F. 2008. Non-surgical periodontal therapy with adjunctive chlorhexidine use in adults with Down syndrome: A prospective case series. *J. Periodontol.* 79(2):379–385.

Christersson, L. A., O. M. Norderyd, and C. S. Puchalsky, 1993. Topical application of tetracycline HCl in human periodontitis. *J. Clin. Periodontol.* 20:80–95.

Ciancio, S. G. 1990. Powered oral irrigation and control of gingivitis. *Biol. Ther. Dent.* 5:21–24.

Ciancio, S. G. 1993. Alcohol in mouth rinse: Lack of association with cancer. *Biol. Ther. Dent.* 9(1):2–3.

Ciancio, S. G., M. L. Mather, J. J. Zambon, and H. S. Reynolds. 1989. Effect of a chemotherapeutic agent delivered by an oral irrigation device on plaque, gingivitis, and subgingival microflora. *J. Periodontol.* 60:310–315.

Clark, W. B., I. Magnusson, C. B. Walker, and R. G. Marks. 1989. Efficacy of Perimed antibacterial system on established gingivitis I. Clinical results. *J. Clin. Periodontol.* 16:630–635.

Cobb, C. M., R. L. Rodgers, and W. J. Killoy. 1988. Ultrastructural examination of human periodontal pockets following the use of an oral irrigation device in vivo. *J. Periodontol.* 59:155–163.

Eakle, W. S., C. Ford, and R. L. Boyd. 1986. Depth of penetration in periodontal pockets with oral irrigation. *J. Clin. Periodontol.* 13:39–44.

Faveri, M., L. C. Gursky, M. Feres, J.A. Shibli, S.L. Salvador, and L.C. de Figueiredo. 2006. Scaling and randomized, placebo-controlled clinical trial. *J. Clin. Periodontol.* 33:819–828.

Felo, A., O. Shibly, S. G. Ciancio, F. R. Lauciello, and A. Ho. 1997. Effects of subgingival chlorhexidine irrigation on peri-implant maintenance. *Am. J. Dent.* 10:107–110.

Fine, D. H., C. Mendieta, M. L. Barnett, D. Furgang, R. Meyers, et al. 1992. Efficacy of preprocedural rinsing with an antiseptic in reducing viable bacteria in dental aerosols. *J. Periodontol.* 63:821–824.

Flemming, T. F., M. G. Newman, F. M. Doherty, E. Grossman, A. H. Mechkel, and M. B. Bakdash. 1990. Supragingival irrigation with 0.06% chlorhexidine in naturally occurring gingivitis: I. Six-month clinical observations. *J. Periodontol.* 61:112–117.

Flotra, L., P. Gjermo, G. Rölla, and J. Waerhaug. 1972. A 4-month study on the effect of chlorhexidine mouth rinses on 50 soldiers. *Can. J. Dent. Res.* 80:10–16.

Gordon, J. M., I. B. Lamster, and M. C. Sieger. 1985. Efficacy of Listerine antiseptic in inhibiting the development of plaque and gingivitis. *J. Clin. Periodontol.* 12:697–704.

Grossman, E. 1988. Effectiveness of a prebrushing mouthrinse under single-trial and home-use conditions. *Clin. Prev. Dent.* 10:3–9.

Jolkovsky, D. L., M. Y. Waki, M. G. Newman, et al. 1990. Clinical and microbiological effects of subgingival and gingival marginal irrigation with chlorhexidine gluconate. *J. Periodontol.* 61:663–669.

Kozlovsky, A., Z. Artzi, O. Moses, et al. 2006. Interaction of chlorhexidine with smooth and rough types of titanium surfaces. *J. Periodontol.* 77(7):1194–1200.

Lamster, I. B., M. C. Alfano, M. C. Seiger, J. M. Gordon. 1983. The effect of Listerine antiseptic on existing plaque and gingivitis. *J. Clin. Prev. Dent.* 5:12–16.

Lavigne, S. E., K. S. Drust-Bay, K. B. Williams, W. J. Killoy, and F. Theisen. 1994. Effects of chlorhexidine on the periodontal status of patients with HA-coated integral dental implants. *Int. J. Oral Maxillofax. Implants.* 9:156–162.

Lobene, R. R. 1969. The effect of a pulsed water pressure cleansing device on oral health. *J. Periodontol.* 40:51–54.

Lobene, R. R., and P. M. Soparkar. 1970, March. The effect of a pulsating water pressure device on gingivitis, plaque and calculus. In *Program and Abstracts of the 48th General Meeting International Association for Dental Research* Chicago, IL.

Löe, H., and C. R. Schiott. 1970. The effect of mouthrinses and topical application of chlorhexidine on the development of dental plaque and gingivitis in man. *J. Periodont. Res.* 5:79–83.

Marshall, M. V., L. P. O. Cancro, and S. F. Fischman. 1995. Hydrogen peroxide: A review of its use in dentistry. *J. Periodontol.* 66:786–796.

Mashimo, P. A., T. Umemoto, J. Slots, R. J. Genco, and S. A. Ellison. 1980. Pathogenicity testing of Macaca arctoides subgingival plaque following chlorhexidine treatment. *J. Periodontol.* 51:190–199.

McCoy, L.C., C.J. Wehler, S.E. Rich, et al. 2008. Adverse events associated with chlorhexidine use. *JADA* 1239:178–183.

Newman, M., M. Cattabriga, D. Etienne, T. Flemmig, M. Sanz, et al. 1994. Effectiveness of adjunctive irrigation in early periodontitis: Multicenter evaluation. *J. Periodontol.* 65:224–229.

Nosel, G., M. Scheidt, R. O'Neal, and T. Van Dyke. 1991. The penetration of lavage solution into the periodontal pocket during ultrasonic instrumentation. *J. Periodontol.* 62:554–557.

Paine, M., J. Slots, and S. Rich. 1998. Fluoride use in periodontal therapy: A review of the literature. *J. Am. Dent. Assoc.* 129:69–77.

Persson, G.R., J. Yeates, R.E. Persson, et al. 2007. The impact of a low-frequency chlorhexidine rinsing schedule on the subgingival microbiota (the TEETH clinical trial). *J. Periodontol.* 78(9):1751–1758.

Pitcher, G. R., H. N. Newman, and J. D. Strahan. 1980. Access to subgingival plaque by disclosing agents using mouth rinsing and direct irrigation. *J. Clin. Periodontol.* 7:300–308.

Poggi, P., R. Rodriguez y Baena, S. Rizzo, and M. T. Rota. 2003. Mouth rinses with alcohol: Cytotoxic effects on human gingival fibroblasts in vitro. *J. Periodontol.* 74: 623–629.

Rees, T. D., and C. E. Orth. 1986. Oral ulcerations with use of hydrogen peroxide. *J. Periodontol.* 57:689–692.

Renton-Harper, P., M. Addy, J. Moran, R. M. Doherty, and R. G. Newcombe. 1996. A comparison of chlorhexidine, cetylpyridinium chloride, triclosan, and C3LG mouth rinse products for plaque inhibition. *J. Periodontol.* 67:486–489.

Roberts, W. R., and M. Addy. 1981. Comparison of in vitro and in vivo antibacterial properties of antiseptic mouth rinses containing chlorhexidine, alexidine, CPC and hexetidine: Relevance to mode of action. *J. Clin. Periodontol.* 8:295–310.

Rölla, G., H. Löe, and R. C. Schiott. 1971. Retention of chlorhexidine in the human oral cavity. *Arch. Oral Biol.* 16:1109–1116.

Sanz, M., M. G. Newman, L. Anderson, and W. Motaska. 1987. A comparison of the effect of a 0.12% chlorhexidine gluconate mouth rinse and placebo on postperiodontal surgical therapy. *J. Dent. Res.* 66:280 (Abstract).

Schiott, C. R., H. Löe, S. B. Jensen, M. Kilian, R. M. Davies, and L. Glavid. 1970. The effect of chlorhexidine mouth rinses on the human oral flora. *J. Periodont. Res.* 5:84–89.

Silverman, S., and R. Wilder. 2006. Antimicrobial mouthrinse as part of a comprehensive oral care regimen. *JADA* 137(11 supplement):22S–26S.

Southard, S. R., C. L. Drisko, W. J. Killoy, C. M. Cobb, and D. E. Tira. 1989. The effect of 2 percent chlorhexidine digluconate irrigation on clinical parameters and the level of *Bacteroides gingivalis* in periodontal pockets. *J. Periodontol.* 60:302–309.

Stabholz, A., J. Kettering, R. Aprecio, G. Zimmerman, P. J. Baker, and U. M. E. Wikesjo. 1993. Antimicrobial properties of human dentin impregnated with tetracycline HCl or chlorhexidine: An in vitro study. *J. Clin. Periodontol.* 20:557–562.

Stoeken, J.E., S. Paraskevas, and G.A. van der Weijden. 2007. The long-term effect of a mouthrinse containing essential oils on dental plaque and gingivitis: A systematic review. *J. Periodontol.* 78(7):1218–1228.

Warrall, S. F., P. J. Knibbs, and H. D. Glenwright. 1987. Methods of reducing contamination of the atmosphere from use of an air polisher. *Br. Dent. J.* 163:118–119.

Weitzman, S. A., A. B. Weitberg, T. P. Stossel, J. Schwartz, and G. Shklar. 1986. Effects of hydrogen peroxide on oral carcinogenesis in hamsters. *J. Periodontol.* 57:685–688.

Winn, D. M., W. J., Blot, J. K. McLaughlin, D. F. Austin, R. S. Greenberg, S. Preston-Martin. 1991. Mouthwash use and oral conditions in the risk of oral and pharyngeal cancer. *Cancer Res.* 51:3044–3047.

Zimmer, S., C. Kolbe, G. Kaiser, T. Drage, M. Ommerborn, and C. Barthel. 2006. Clinical efficacy of flossing versus use of antimicrobial rinses. *J. Periodontol.* 77(8):1380–1385.

Chapter 22

Systemic and Local Drug Delivery Systems: Systemic Antibiotics, Local Drug Devices, and Enzyme Suppression Therapy

Mea A. Weinberg

OUTLINE

Introduction
Selected Drug Information Resources
Rationale for Use of Antibiotics
Delivery Systems
Dental Plaque as a Biofilm
Drug Actions
Systemic Drug Delivery
Local Delivery: Controlled (Sustained)-Release
   Drug Delivery
Precautions/Contraindications
Enzyme Suppression Therapy
Dental Hygiene Notes
Key Points
Self-Quiz
References

EDUCATIONAL OBJECTIVES

Upon completion of this chapter, the reader should be able to:

• Discuss the rationale for the use of antimicrobials in the treatment of the inflammatory periodontal diseases.
• List and discuss the various types of drug delivery systems.
• Describe the different types of controlled-release devices.
• Discuss enzyme suppression therapy.

GOAL: To provide an understanding of current concepts about the adjunctive use of chemical agents in the prevention and treatment of the inflammatory periodontal diseases.

KEY WORDS

adjunctive 336
antibiotic resistance 334
chemotherapeutic
   agents 333
controlled-release
   delivery devices 334
periodontal
   pathogens 333
substantivity 337
systemic drug delivery
   334

INTRODUCTION

The foundation for the treatment of periodontal diseases is mechanical debridement. However, in some patients the adjunctive use of antibiotics, antimicrobial agents or an enzyme suppression drug (e.g., doxycycline 20 mg) is justified. The newest approach in the treatment of inflammatory periodontal diseases is enzyme suppression therapy. Instead of targeting bacteria, enzyme suppression therapy targets the enzyme collagenase which causes destruction of collagen.

The purpose of chemotherapy is to aid the host defenses (body) in controlling and eliminating bacteria that have overwhelmed the host. These chemotherapeutic agents can be administered to the patient via oral rinses, irrigation, systemically in a pill or capsule, or in a controlled-release device placed subgingivally in a pocket. The use of chemotherapeutic agents and enzyme suppression therapy is based on the type of periodontal disease the patient has and the nature of the offending bacteria.

SELECTED DRUG INFORMATION RESOURCES

It is important for the dental hygienist to be aware of the generic names and trade names of drugs. The generic name is the official name of the drug as determined by the United States Adopted Names Council. The trade name of a drug is the registered property of a specific manufacturer and is protected for seventeen years so that the manufacturer has the exclusive rights for that specific drug.

Numerous drug references on the Internet, on personal digital assistants (PDAs), and in books are available. Selected resources include the following:

- *The Physicians' Desk Reference* (PDR®) (Medical Economics Company, Inc., Montvale, NJ). This is published once a year and is essentially a conglomerate of the patient package inserts that the manufacturers supply for each drug.
- *Delmar's Dental Drug Reference* (Delmar Thompson™ Learning, Albany, NY).
- *Mosby's Dental Drug Reference* (Mosby-Year Book, Inc., St. Louis, MO).
- *Drug Information Handbook for Dentistry* (Lexi-Comp, Inc., Hudson, OH).
- *ADA Guide to Dental Therapeutics* (ADA, Chicago).

RATIONALE FOR USE OF ANTIBIOTICS

Although periodontal debridement and periodontal surgery are currently and will always be the foundation for controlling inflammatory periodontal diseases, several factors can substantiate the adjunctive use of chemical or **chemotherapeutic agents** (e.g., antiseptic mouthrinses and antibiotics) (American Academy of Periodontology, 2004; Beikler, Prior, Ehmke, & Flemming, 2004; Haffaje, Socransky, & Gunsolley, 2003; Kaner et al. 2007; Seymour, 2008). An antiseptic is a substance that prevents or inhibits the growth of microorganisms or kills microbes on contact. An antibiotic is a substance that is synthesized by microorgansims that prevents or inhibits the growth of bacteria by either stopping multiplication or killing the bacteria.

Instrumentation often leaves behind significant numbers of periodontal pathogens (Waerhaug, 1978). Repopulation of these pathogens can occur within 60 days of periodontal debridement (Sbordone et al. 1990). In addition, certain **periodontal pathogens** such as *Actinobacillus actinomycetemcomitans* and *Porphyromonas gingivalis* invade the junctional epithelium and connective tissue and elude removal by periodontal debridement (de Graaf, van Winkelhoff, & Goené, 1989; Renvert, Wikström, Dablén, Slots, & Egelberg, 1990). Other periodontal pathogens, such as *Tannerella forsythensis, Prevotella intermedia,* and *Peptostreptococcus micros,* live in nonperiodontal sites such as the tongue, tonsils, saliva, and buccal mucosa (Asikainen, Alaluusua, & Saxén, 1991). These sites are a source for reinfection and must be considered in the overall treatment process. Other factors influencing the use of chemical plaque-control agents include the manual dexterity of the patient.

A number of chemical agents have been studied clinically and shown to be successful in the further suppression of dental plaque in certain types of periodontal diseases when used in conjunction with periodontal debridement and surgery. The role of antimicrobial agents as part of the periodontal treatment plan in certain patients has gained significant importance in recent years since the acknowledgment that periodontal diseases are infectious diseases with specific bacteria as the cause (Loesche, 1976). Based on the specific plaque hypothesis, treatment is geared toward the elimination or reduction of specific bacteria (e.g., *A. actinomycetemcomitans, P. gingivalis, P. intermedia,* and spirochetes). Thus, antimicrobial agents can be instituted as a supplement, not a replacement, during nonsurgical and surgical therapy.

Since there are also beneficial bacteria living in the mouth, it is not desirable nor a goal to eliminate all intra-oral bacteria. Unfortunately, systemic antibiotics used indiscriminately can result in **antibiotic resistance,** in which an antibiotic is ineffective against certain bacteria. This is becoming a worldwide problem.

DELIVERY SYSTEMS

Currently, two systems are available for the delivery of chemotherapeutic agents: local and systemic systems. Topical and controlled (sustained)-release (American Academy Periodontology, 2000) drug devices are types of local delivery systems. Each delivery system has advantages and limitations (Table 22–1 ■).

Topical application delivers the agent or drug to an exposed surface such as the teeth and gingiva. The most common route for the supragingival topical delivery of antimicrobial agents is by a mouthrinse, a dentifrice, or an oral irrigator. Subgingival topical delivery of antimicrobial agents is by oral irrigation or the use of controlled-release devices.

Controlled-release delivery devices are placed directly into the periodontal pocket and are designed to release a drug slowly over 24 hours for prolonged drug action. Antimicrobials are delivered into the periodontal pocket by fibers, gels, chips, powder, ointments, acrylic strips, or collagen films.

Systemic drug delivery involves taking a tablet or a capsule orally with subsequent distribution of the agent through the circulation to the subgingival pocket area.

Choice of the delivery system is based on the target site. For instance, if gingivitis were being treated, oral rinses or irrigation would be chosen for supragingival plaque control. If, on the other hand, a certain type of periodontitis is being treated, the target site is the base of the periodontal pocket. Since oral rinses do not reach subgingivally, the delivery system of choice would be either oral irrigation or systemic or controlled-release delivery.

DENTAL PLAQUE AS A BIOFILM

As mentioned earlier, dental plaque exists as a biofilm. A plaque or oral biofilm is defined as "matrix-enclosed bacterial populations adherent to each other and/or to surfaces or interfaces" (Costerton et al., 1994). Plaque biofilms are of varying thicknesses, and in order to penetrate the biofilm, antibiotic concentrations must be several times greater than that needed to kill bacteria in a

test tube (laboratory conditions) (Kleinfelder, Müller, & Lange, 1999). Subgingival biofilms cannot be removed by toothbrushing, flossing, or the use of antimicrobial agents. It is necessary to physically remove the biofilm by instrumentation, and then the antimicrobial agent can be administered. For this reason, administration of antimicrobial agents should never be the sole treatment and always should be as an adjunct to periodontal debridement and/or periodontal surgery. The biofilm structure also may account for the rapid rebound or repopulation of the pathogenic bacteria, which occurs frequently after the use of antimicrobial agents (Page, Offenbacher, Schroeder, Seymour, & Kornman, 1997).

DRUG ACTIONS

When considering the use of chemotherapeutic agents, the dental hygienist should be aware of the pharmacokinetics and pharmacodynamics of each drug. Pharmacokinetics involves knowledge of the drug's absorption, distribution, metabolism, and excretion. Pharmacodynamics relates to the drug's mechanism of action. In addition, any adverse effects (Seymour & Rudralingham, 2008), drug–drug, and drug–food interactions should be noted, and the patient should be informed.

SYSTEMIC DRUG DELIVERY
Indications

Systemic drug delivery through oral administration has several advantages and disadvantages (see Table 22–1)(Seymour & Hogg, 2008; Walker & Karpinia, 2002) . Antibiotics generally are unnecessary and inappropriate for reducing plaque levels and treating gingivitis, with the exception of necrotizing periodontal diseases.

Systemic antibiotics are useful as adjuncts in periodontal treatment for patients with aggressive periodontitis, all types of refractory periodontitis, and immunodeficiency diseases. Patients with refractory periodontal diseases usually harbor persistent subgingival pathogens that are likely to be resistant to conventional treatment. In localized aggressive periodontitis patients, *A. actinomycetemcomitans* invades the gingival connective tissue and thus evades removal by mechanical instrumentation. Antibiotics will benefit patients with a periodontal abscess when there is accompanied systemic signs such as fever or lymphadenopathy. A recent study reported that there may be no benefit in using antibiotics

Table 22–1 Main Features of Drug Delivery Systems

Delivery System	Target Site	Adequate Concentration at Target Site	Stays at Target Site Long Enough	Reaches the GCF	Advantages
Systemic: tablets, capsules	Periodontal pocket; epithelium and connective tissue; nonperiodontal sites (e.g., saliva, tongue, buccal mucosa, tonsils)	Fair concentrations reached due to some dilution by the time it reaches pocket area; frequent dosing is necessary to maintain therapeutic levels	No	Yes	Reaches all intraoral sites where bacterial reservoirs are found
Topical: oral rinses	Supragingival	Adequate concentrations, but therapeutic level dramatically declines by being washed out by saliva	No	No	No systemic adverse effects; no antibiotic resistance develops
Topical: dentifrices	Supragingival	Adequate concentrations, but therapeutic level dramatically declines by being washed out by saliva	No	No	No systemic adverse effects; high patient compliance
Topical: subgingival irrigation	Periodontal pocket	Adequate concentrations, but therapeutic level dramatically declines by being washed out by GCF	No	No	No systemic adverse effects
Controlled-release: powder, gel, chip	Periodontal pocket	Adequate concentrations; therapeutic levels are relatively constant for several days	Yes	Yes	Maintains therapeutic levels in the GCF for several days; no systemic adverse effects; concentrates in pocket without dilution through entire body; possible development of bacterial resistance to the antibiotic (more studies needed)

for the sole purpose of preventing post-surgical infections (Powell, et al., 2005). Bacterial invasion (spirochetes) of periodontal tissues seen in NUG also evades mechanical removal with instruments.

Selection

Adjunctive systemic antibiotics may be used during initial and/or surgical therapy. In patients with refractory or recurrent periodontitis it may be advantageous to perform microbiologic testing to determine the presence of specific bacteria. Reevaluation with microbiologic testing 1 to 3 months after antimicrobial therapy may be done to verify elimination or suppression of the pathogens. However, the expense of this procedure may preclude its generalized use. Long-term use (1 to 2 months or longer) of systemic antibiotics is considered to be without foundation.

Proper selection and dosing of the appropriate antibiotic are necessary to avoid untoward reactions and antibiotic resistance. Many categories of antibiotics are available, and several are indicated in periodontal infections (Box 22-1). The dental hygienist must be familiar with both the generic and brand or trade names of each drug.

Good oral hygiene is still mandatory and will foster a positive clinical response when patients are prescribed systemic antibiotics. As mentioned earlier, periodontal debridement must be performed before the administration of any antimicrobial agent. This will remove the biofilm that protects subgingival microorganisms, except in cases where the bacteria have invaded the soft tissue. Systemic antibiotics are given in certain situations and are always used as a supplement or adjunct to conventional periodontal debridement and oral hygiene self-care. Antibiotics should never be given as the only treatment regimen. Antibiotics are classified as being either bacteriostatic, which means they suppress the multiplication of the bacteria, or bactericidal, which means they kill the bacteria.

Adverse Drug Events

Heightened public interest in adverse drug events has motivated the government to require pharmaceutical companies to provide adverse drug reaction (ADR) information (Smith, 1999). The requirement is to provide information on the percentage of adverse drug reactions caused by antibiotics in both hospital and nonhospital settings.

ADRs can range from mild reactions that disappear when the antibiotic is discontinued to severe reactions that are life-threatening, disabling, or result in hospitalization (Smith, 1999). Table 22–2 ■ lists common adverse effects associated with antimicrobial agents.

Systemic Antibiotics

Tetracyclines

Tetracyclines as a group are bacteriostatic, inhibiting bacterial growth and multiplication by inhibiting protein synthesis. Two semisynthetic analogues of tetracycline, doxycycline hyclate and minocycline HCl, are broad-spectrum antibiotics, affecting both gram-positive and gram-negative microorganisms. Doxycycline and minocycline have been used in the treatment of *Actinobacillus actinomycetemcomitans* infections in localized aggressive periodontitis and refractory periodontitis. Mandell, Tripodi, Savitt, Goodson, and Socransky (1986) reported that while surgery and treatment with tetracycline were superior in localized aggressive periodontitis patients, it appeared that there was a possibility of reinfection with or incomplete elimination of *A. actinomycetemcomitans*.

Anticollagenase Feature Tetracyclines have both antibacterial and nonantibacterial properties. Besides affecting bacterial growth, they also affect the host response by inhibiting the production and secretion of collagenase by cells in the body such as polymorpho-

---

Box 22–1   Classification of Systemic Antibiotics Used in Periodontics

Tetracyclines
- Tetracycline HCl
- Doxycycline hyclate
- Minocycline HCl

Penicillins (Beta-lactams)
- Penicillin VK
- Amoxicillin trihydrate
- Amoxicillin
- + clavulanic acid

Nitroimadazoles
- Metronidazole

Azalides (derivative of erythromycin)
- Azithromycin dihydrate

Lincomycins
- Clindamycin HCl

Fluoroquinolones
- Ciprofloxacin HCl

Table 22–2	Classification of Adverse Effects of Systemic Antimicrobial Agents
Adverse Effect	*Features*
Hypersensitivity reactions	Involves allergic reactions to the antibiotic (e.g., rashes).
Gastrointestinal disturbances	Very common; includes nausea, vomiting, and diarrhea. Pseudomembranous colitis is the most severe gastrointestinal complication that requires immediate discontinuation of the antibiotic. Although initially believed to be a complication associated primarily with clindamycin, most oral and injectable antibiotics may produce this side effect.
Hepatotoxicity	Liver disease can occur with commonly administered antibiotics such as erythromycin, amoxicillin-clavulanic acid, and quinolones.
Photosensitivity reactions	Occurs with fluoroquinolones and tetracyclines (less with minocycline). Seen as an exaggerated sunburn. Patients should not be exposed to sun when taking these antibiotics.
Fungal infection	Fungal infections can occur especially with use of broad-spectrum antibiotics, which destroy bacteria, allowing fungi (*Candida albicans*) to overgrow, which may produce gastrointestinal irritation, stomatitis, and vaginal infection. Acidophilus (available in a soft gel tablet) or yogurt taken in conjunction with the antibiotic (except tetracycline) will replace some of the bacteria, thereby possibly preventing a fungal infection.

Source: Data from Hersh & Moore, 2008.

nuclear leukocytes (PMNs) (Golub, Ramanurthy, McNamara, Greenwald, & Rifkin, 1984). Collagenase is an enzyme responsible for the destruction of collagen, which makes up the connective tissue of the periodontium. Tetracyclines also were found to inhibit bone resorption by affecting osteoclast function (Rifkin, Vernillo, & Golub, 1993). This anticollagenase property does not depend on the drug's antibacterial actions.

Did You Know?

Doxycycline is unique because it is the only antibiotic that is also has nonantibiotic properties.

Concentration in Gingival Crevicular Fluid
Another property of tetracyclines is their ability to concentrate in the gingival crevicular fluid (GCF) at two to four times blood levels following multiple doses (Gordon, Walker, Murphy, Goodson, & Socransky, 1981). Doxycycline (Pascale et al., 1986) and minocycline also concentrate in higher levels in the GCF than in serum. Tetracyclines exhibit higher **substantivity** than other antibiotics (Baker, Evans, Coburn, & Genco, 1983; Stabholz et al., 1993), which allows binding to root surfaces with a slow release into the GCF. The binding of tetracy-

clines to calcium ions in the GCF enhances their substantivity. These properties allow the drug to maintain high therapeutic levels in the GCF. It is advantageous for a drug to concentrate in high levels in the GCF because the GCF bathes the subgingival pocket area where the periodontal pathogens live.

Adverse Effects, Drug–Drug and Drug–Food Interactions Common adverse effects of tetracyclines include esophageal ulcers (Segelnick & Weinberg, 2008), nausea, vomiting, and diarrhea. Gastrointestinal (stomach) upset is much less with the semisynthetic drugs because they are more highly absorbed from the gastrointestinal tract. Instructions to the patient on how to take tetraycyclines is important to avoid these adverse effects. Taking doxycycline (or any tetracycline) with plenty of water and in an upright position will help avoid the development of esophageal ulcers (Segelnick & Weinberg, 2008). Tetracyclines stain newly formed teeth during enamel deposition and should not be used during the last half of pregnancy or in children up to 8 years of age. A complex is formed with calcium orthophosphate that produces a yellow-gray fluorescent discoloration. Photosensitivity is another adverse effect, resulting in exaggerated sunburn when patients are exposed to the sun.

Tetracyclines, except doxycycline and minocycline, should not be taken concomitantly with dairy products

Rapid Dental Hint

Doxycycline should be taken with plenty of water in an upright or sitting position. Patients should not lie down for a few hours after taking it.

because tetracycline binds to calcium, inhibiting its absorption. Tetracycline should be taken on an empty stomach (1 hour before or 2 hours after meals) because food delays its absorption. Doxycycline and minocycline can be taken without regard to meals. Absorption of all tetracyclines into the bloodstream is delayed with antacids. Tetracyclines, as well as other antibiotics, interfere with the metabolism of oral contraceptives. Estrogens, a component in oral contraceptives, must be metabolized (broken down) to its active form in the stomach by bacteria. Most antibiotics kill or stop the growth of these bacteria, inhibiting estrogen breakdown. Patients must use other forms of birth control if they are taking antibiotics concomitantly. Tetracyclines or any other bacteriostatic drug should not be given together with bactericidal antibiotics such as penicillin, metronidazole, or ciprofloxacin that would interfere with the bactericidal action of that drug. In order for a bactericidal drug to work, the bacteria need to be multiplying.

Penicillins (Beta-lactams)

Penicillins as a group are bactericidal, and their mechanism of action is to inhibit bacterial cell wall synthesis. Penicillin VK has limited activity against gram-negative periodontal pathogens. It is indicated primarily in certain acute periodontal infections such as abscesses. Amoxicillin, a broad-spectrum penicillin, is used frequently in periodontics. Some bacteria produce enzymes called beta-lactamases that inactivate the penicillin molecule. To overcome this vulnerability, a beta-lactamase inhibitor such as clavulanic acid is combined with amoxicillin (Augmentin).

Adverse Effects, Drug–Drug and Drug–Food Interactions Approximately 5 to 10% of individuals are allergic to penicillin. It is best to take this antibiotic with food to decrease gastrointestinal upset. Severe gastrointestinal upset (e.g., nausea, vomiting, and diarrhea) occurs as a result of the acid component. Food does not interfere with absorption of amoxicillin into the bloodstream. Penicillins should not be taken together with bacteriostatic antibiotics because for a bactericidal antibiotic to work, the bacteria need to be multiplying, and this

would be inhibited if a bacteriostatic antibiotic were administered concomitantly with penicillin.

Cephalosporins

Cephalosporins are not considered to be the drug of choice for most types of dental infections, including periodontal diseases. These antibiotics do not provide an advantage over amoxicillin or penicillin.

Nitroimadazoles

Mechanism of Action and Indications Metronidazole is specifically effective against obligate or strict anaerobic (live in a pure nonoxygen environment) microorganisms. Metronidazole penetrates well into the GCF, but not as high as the tetracyclines. Metronidazole is bactericidal, and its mechanism of action is to inhibit bacterial DNA synthesis.

Metronidazole is indicated in the treatment of necrotizing gingivitis (NUG). Metronidazole is also indicated when barrier membranes are used during guided tissue regeneration surgery. *P. gingivalis,* a strict anaerobe, is the primary bacteria that colonize on porous membrane material. It has been reported in both professional journals and in the lay press that periodontal debridement in conjunction with metronidazole may reduce the need for periodontal surgery (Loesche, Giordano, Soehren, & Kaciroti, 1996), but this remains controversial. Metronidazole in combination with amoxicillin or Augmentin may be effective against refactory and aggressive forms of periodontitis associated with *Actinobacillus actinomycetemcomitans* and *P. gingivalis* infection. However, a recent study of 21 patients with moderate, untreated periodontal diseases evaluated the benefits of amoxicillin and amoxicillin plus clavulanic acid after initial therapy. Patients received periodontal debridement twice during the study. After the second debridement, patients were assigned randomly to either the group that received the drug combination or the placebo group. Results indicated no added benefit when amoxicillin and Augmentin were taken after initial therapy (Winkel et al., 1999).

Adverse Effects and Drug–Drug Interactions Antibiotic resistance to metronidazole is rare, but there are numerous adverse effects. Gastrointestinal upset is seen frequently, especially nausea. A metallic taste in the mouth has been reported, as well as darkened urine. Consumption of alcohol beverages, including use of alcohol-containing mouthrinses, while taking metronidazole results in a disulfiram-like reaction. Disulfiram is a drug given to wean alcoholics off alcohol by acting to deter further ingestion of alcohol. It works by inhibition of the enzyme aldehyde dehydrogenase, causing a buildup of acetaldehyde, a toxic by-product of ethanol metabolism (Garey & Rodvold, 1999). Within 5 to 10 minutes after metronidazole is taken with alcohol, serious non-life-threatening adverse effects occur, including headache, flushing, nausea, vomiting, and cramps. The reaction usually lasts for up to 1 hour; however, it may continue for a few days after discontinuation of the medication (Walker, 1996). Alcohol should not be consumed during metronidazole therapy and for at least three days after discontinuing the drug. Metronidazole is contraindicated in patients taking anticoagulants (e.g., warfarin), lithium (a drug used for manic depression), and cimetadine (an antiulcer drug).

Macrolides

Erythromycin, a macrolide antibiotic, is not used in the treatment of periodontal diseases because it is primarily effective against gram-positive microorganisms and does not penetrate gram-negative bacterial cells. Erythromycin also does not penetrate the GCF to effective levels. Erythromycins are bacteriostatic and inhibit bacterial protein synthesis. Adverse effects include severe gastrointestinal disturbances, including nausea, vomiting, and diarrhea.

Second-Generation Drugs: Azalides   The newer second-generation erythromycins, referred to as azilides, have a broader spectrum of action with fewer adverse effects. Azithromycin dihydrate shows promising results in periodontics. Azithromycin has several unique features. Azithromycin concentrates in phagocytes such as PMNs and macrophages, which contribute to its distribution into inflamed periodontal tissues (gingival connective tissue) in greater amounts than in plasma (Dastoor et al., 2007;Malizia, Tejada, Ghelardi, Senesi, & Gabriele, 1997). In addition, a post-antibiotic effect is seen, whereby high antibiotic levels remain after the drug is discontinued (Malizia et al., 1997).

Adverse Effects, Drug–Drug and Drug–Food Interactions   All erythromycins, except for azithromycin, should not be taken with cholesterol-lowering "statin" drugs (such as lovastatin and simvastatin) because erythromycin and clarithromycin inhibit the metabolism of these drugs, resulting in high blood levels. Concurrent use of erythromycins and theophylline (an antiasthma drug) increases blood levels of theophylline.

Rapid Dental Hint

Patients can eat yogurt or take acidophilus tablets immediately before taking the antibiotic to avoid fungal infections when taking antibiotics.

Capsules of azithromycin should be taken on an empty stomach, but tablets can be taken with food.

Lincomycins

Clindamycin HCl penetrates well into the GCF and is active against most periodontal pathogens, except *A. actinomycetemcomitans* and *Eikenella corrodens,* and is especially useful in treating refractory periodontitis. Clindamycin HCl inhibits bacterial protein synthesis and is bacteriostatic. Although the development of pseudomembranous colitis has been associated with the use of clindamycin, it can occur with any antibiotic. Suppression of normal intestinal bacteria allows the overgrowth of *Clostridium difficile,* which produces a toxin that causes severe watery diarrhea and fever. The antibiotic should be discontinued as soon as such signs appear. Clindamycin can be taken with food.

Did You Know?

Any antibiotic can cause pseuomembranous colitis, not just clindamycin.

Quinolones

Quinolones are bactericidal because they inhibit bacterial DNA replication. Quinolones (e.g, ciprofloxacin, levofloxacin) are not actually antibiotics, however, because they are totally synthetic. Antibiotics are chemical substances produced by bacteria; some antibiotics can be semisynthetic, which means that they are a mixture of natural and synthetic substances. Nevertheless, they are frequently referred to as broad-spectrum antimicrobials with good activity against facultative gram-negative anaerobes. Adverse effects include dizziness, convulsions, headache, hallucinations, and joint and cartilage damage. Ciprofloxacin should not be given to children younger than 18 years of age because of its effect on cell growth. Ciprofloxacin should not be administered with theophylline or caffeine because it inhibits their metabolism, resulting in increased blood levels. Dairy products and antacids delay absorption. Food does not slow absorption.

Antibiotic Resistance

Bacterial resistance to antibiotics raises serious questions for healthcare providers. The danger is that an antibiotic will not be effective if administered later on for a truly life-threatening bacterial infection because the bacteria have become resistant to that antibiotic. Thus, antibiotic resistance can lead to an increase in the incidence of disease. Patients often stop their antibiotic treatment prematurely, believing that if they feel better, it is not necessary to take the full course. Patients also self-medicate with leftover antibiotics from a previous infection. Patients may request antibiotics or other medications because they believe they will be beneficial. Many practitioners comply with such patient requests without evaluating the situation clinically, and many practitioners simply overprescribe antibiotics.

Therefore, it is extremely important to use antibiotics and antimicrobials conservatively, only when indicated, and with the narrowest possible spectrum of activity. Prolonged or repetitive courses of antibiotic treatment should be avoided. Antibiotics are an adjunct to periodontal debridment.

LOCAL DELIVERY: CONTROLLED (SUSTAINED)-RELEASE DRUG DELIVERY

The development of site-specific, controlled (sustained)-release delivery systems has provided a further option for antimicrobial therapy by allowing therapeutic levels of a drug to be maintained in the periodontal pocket for prolonged periods of time (Bonito, Lux, & Lohr, 2005). The decision to use local drug delivery during active treatment or maintenance is based upon clinical findings, clinical response to therapy, desired clinical outcomes, and the patient's dental and medical history (Greenstein, 2006). If the drug is released from the device past 24 hours, it is called a controlled-release device; if the drug is released within 24 hours, it is called a sustained-release device. Many devices are available in the United States and Europe that incorporate an antimicrobial agent into a specific material (a polymer) that is placed into the periodontal pocket. The active ingredient is then released from the material, which subsequently exerts its antibacterial activity on subgingival bacteria over several days. Then the material is absorbed (dissolves). The concentration of antimicrobials administered in a controlled (sustained)-release device does not enter the bloodstream and thus does not trigger adverse effects. Types of materials used to incorporate antimicrobial drugs include fibers, gels, chips, collagen film, and acrylic strips. Controlled (sustained)-release drug therapy is used as an adjunct to periodontal debridement and should not replace conventional mechanical therapy. In fact, the American Academy of Periodontology reported in the 2003 Annals that it "would be premature to conclude that insertion of sustained-release antimicrobial systems is as effective as scaling and root planing in all populations of patients" (Hanes & Purvis, 2003). They are indicated for use in recurrent pockets of 5 mm or greater that continue to bleed on probing. The intended results with these devices are gains in clinical attachment levels and reductions in probing depths and bleeding on probing.

The first controlled-release device approved in the United States in the early 1990s was Actisite, which was an ethylene vinyl acetate flexible fiber impregnated with 12.7 mg of tetracycline HCl. It was placed subgingivally into the periodontal pocket, where the tetracycline is released slowly over 7 to 10 days. It is no longer available.

Currently in the United States, PerioChip, Atridox, and Arestin are available commercially. Other controlled-release systems are available in Europe that have not been approved for use in the United States.

Absorbable Controlled (Sustained)-Release Devices

Chlorhexidine Gluconate Chip

The PerioChip (Dexcel Pharma) is a gelatin maxtrix (bovine origin) containing 2.5 mg of chlorhexidine gluconate. This product received Food and Drug Administration approval in June 1998. PerioChip is indicated for use as an adjunct to instrumentation in maintenance patients with pockets 5 mm or larger that bleed recurrently on probing (Jeffcoat et al., 1998; Paolantonio et al., 2008). A recent clinical study comparing the efficacy of periodontal debridement alone with that of periodontal debridement plus PerioChip revealed statistically significant reductions in probing depth and gains in clinical attachment in the periodontal debridement plus PerioChip group. However, the magnitude of these changes was small (0.3 mm), so the results are not clinically significant (Jeffcoat et al., 1998). In this study, mechanical debridement was limited to only 1 hour in patients with moderately advanced peridontitis (5 to 8 mm pockets), which does not seem realistic.

After periodontal debridement, the chip is placed into the periodontal pocket. In contact with subgingival fluids it becomes sticky and binds to the epithelium lining the pocket, so no periodontal dressing is indicated. Its antibacterial action occurs when chlorhexidine is released over 7 to 10 days, after which the chip resorbs and does not have to be removed. Up to eight chips can be inserted into pockets in one visit. Another round of treatment can be done at 3 months.

Doxycycline Hyclate Gel

Atridox is composed of 10% (42.5 mg) doxycycline hyclate in a gel formulation that is biodegradable and subsequently will resorb. The ingredients are available in two syringes (powder and liquid) that are mixed together (Figure 22–1 ■) and injected into the pocket around the entire tooth (Figure 22–2 ■). The gel form allows for ease of flow, readily adapting to subgingival root morphology. When the gel comes in contact with gingival fluid in the pocket, it solidifies to a wax-like substance.

Atridox is indicated as an adjunct to scaling and root planing procedures in patients with chronic periodontitis (Novak et al., 2008). Local anesthesia is not required. Results of therapy are to promote attachment level gain, to reduce pocket depths, and to reduce bleeding on probing. Atridox may also be used in patients who refuse to have periodontal debridement or periodontal surgery, and who are medically, physically, or emotionally compromised.

A randomized, controlled clinical study (Garrett, Johnson, & Stoller, 1998) comparing Atridox alone (all patients had a history of periodontal debridement at least two months before the study) and periodontal debridement alone reported that Atridox produced clinical results comparable with periodontal debridement alone.

■ **FIGURE 22–1** Atridox® is prepared by joining/interlocking the two syringes. (Courtesy of CollaGenex Pharm., Newton, PA)

Both groups showed a statistically significant reduction in pocket depths (an average of 1.3 mm) and gains in attachment levels (average of 0.8 mm).

Levels of doxycycline in the pocket (GCF) peaked at 2 hours after placement into the pocket, and effective drug levels were maintained at 28 days (Stoller, Johnson, Trapnell, Harrold, & Garrett, 1998). Although, within a few days levels of doxycycline has peaked.

Minocycline Hydrocholoride Microspheres

The most recently FDA-approved sustained-release device is Arestin. Arestin microspheres (OraPharm) are a

■ **FIGURE 22–2** After pumping the materials between the two joined syringes, a cannula is connected to the syringe to apply into the pocket. (Courtesy of CollaGenex Pharm., Newton, PA)

Rapid Dental Hint

It is important to remove biofilms with debridement before antibiotics/antimicrobials are administered because biofilms act as a barrier to the penetration of the drug.

sustained-release product containing the antibiotic minocycline hydrochloride. Minocycline is a type of tetracycline but it is longer acting and has a broader spectrum of antibiotic activity. Each cartridge of Arestin contains 1 mg of minocycline (Figure 22–3 ■). Arestin is indicated as an adjunct to scaling and root planing procedures for the reduction of pocket depth in patients with chronic localized periodontitis. Studies have shown that scaling and root planing followed by the application of Arestin resulted in a greater percentage reduction in pocket depths (>2mm) at 9 months compared to scaling and root planing alone (Tomasi, Koutouzis, & Wennström, 2008).

Many periodontal pathogens, including *Porphyromonas gingivalis, Prevotella intermedia, Fusobacterium*

Rapid Dental Hint

The patient does not need to be anesthetized when applying Atridox or Arestin.

nucleatum, Eikenella corrodens, and *Actinobacillus actinomycetemcomitans,* are susceptible to minocycline.

Did You Know?

These controlled-release medicaments are used for localized chronic periodontitis sites.

(a)

(b)

(c)

■ **FIGURE 22–3** Arestin™ being administered into a pocket. Arestin is a powder containing minocycline.

Other Products

Some controlled-release products are available in other countries. Elyzol (Dumex, Copenhagen, Denmark) is a 25% metronidazole gel that is injected into the pocket. Periocline (Sunstar Corp., Osaka, Japan) and Dentomycin (Cyanamid International, Wayne, NJ) are a 2% minocycline gel.

PRECAUTIONS/CONTRAINDICATIONS

Subgingival placement of devices containing antibiotics or antimicrobials is not recommended in an acutely abscessed periodontal pocket. Any antibiotic product should be used with caution in patients having a history of predisposition to oral candidasis because antibiotics suppress the growth of or kill bacteria, which allows for the growth of other microorganisms such as fungi.

The use of tetraycycline and its analogs, doxyccline and minocycline, should not be used during tooth development, which includes the last half of pregnancy, infancy, and childhood up to the age of 8 years.

ENZYME-SUPPRESSION THERAPY

Although bacteria are the culprits in initiating inflammatory periodontal diseases, the inflammatory mediators, including cytokines and prostaglandins produced by the host (body) cells in response to the bacteria, are partly responsible for periodontal tissue breakdown. When produced in excess, inflammatory mediators induce destruction of healthy periodontal tissues. For example, prostaglandins facilitate bone resorption by stimulating the activity of osteoclasts.

Matrix Metalloproteinases

Host cells, including PMNs and fibroblasts, also respond to bacterial products by synthesizing and secreting matrix metalloproteinases (MMPs) in the host connective tissue. The MMPs are a family of enzymes that work together to break down connective tissue proteins, including collagen. MMPs that cause the breakdown of the periodontium include collagenase and gelatinase.

In healthy oral tissues, as part of the normal turnover of connective tissue, fibroblasts synthesize and secrete collagenase, which removes "old" collagen while new collagen is laid down. However, in the presence of disease (bacterial infection), PMNs produce collagenase in excessive amounts, which destroys periodontal tissues (collagen). Thus, the third approach to therapy is to inhibit the collagenase synthesized and released by PMNs. Antibiotics are aimed at reducing or eliminating the periodontal pathogens but do not target the enzyme-producing PMNs.

Subantimicrobial-Dose Doxycycline (SDD)

Golub and colleagues (1984) found that tetracyclines, especially doxycycline, have anticollagenase properties and inhibit collagenase activity. This group of investigators discovered that by using only 20-mg tablets of doxycycline, instead of the customary 50 or 100 mg tablets, collagenase would be inhibited. At these subantimicrobial doses, doxycycline only has anticollagenase activity and no antibacterial action. Doxycycline 20 mg is indicated as an adjunct to periodontal debridement to promote attachment level gain and to reduce pocket depths in patients with chronic periodontitis. A recent study reported that adjunctive subantimicrobial doxycycline in chronic periodontitis reduced gingival crevicular fluid (GCF) collagenase inducers levels and clinical periodontal parameters more than the placebo (Emingil, Atilla, Sorsa, & Tervahartiala, 2008). It is intended to improve the clinical outcome of periodontal debridement. This drug should be taken twice daily. Efficacy beyond nine months of continuous dosing and safety beyond twelve months of continuous dosing have not been established.

A recent clinical study (Preshaw et al., 2008) reported that a modified-release subantimicrobial dose doxycycline (40 mg) that is taken once daily rather than twice with the 20 mg formulation resulted in significantly greater clinical benefits than scaling and root planing alone in periodontitis patients.

In a large-scale clinical study, patients received debridement and either doxycycline 20 mg or a placebo twice a day for nine months. The results of the study showed that after three months of daily use, reductions in probing depth and improvements in attachment levels were statistically greater with SDD and debridement than with placebo and debridement (Ciancio & Ashley, 1998). Reductions in probing depth from baseline were up to 38% greater with SDD in tooth sites with mild to moderate periodontitis (probing depths of 4 to 6 mm) and severe periodontitis (probing depths of 7 mm or more). Improvements in attachment from baseline were up to 54% greater with the SDD than with placebo in severely diseased sites. Although treatment differences in the per-patient mean change in probing depth and clinical attachment level were statistically significant, these differences were relatively small. However, the frequency of probing depth reduction of 2 mm or more was greater in the doxycycline group than in the placebo group.

 Rapid Dental Hint

Since doxycycline 20 mg is still doxycycline, the same precautions and contraindications as with tetracyclines must be followed with doxycycline 20 mg.

DENTAL HYGIENE NOTES

The multifaceted approach to treating periodontal diseases uses mechanical instrumentation, which reduces the bacterial load, and locally and systemically administered antibiotics and host-modulating pharmacotherapies as treatment adjuncts.

Treatment of patients with gingivitis or chronic periodontitis is related to reducing the number of bacteria to a level conducive to health (Loesche, 1976). This may involve periodontal debridement, periodontal surgery, and oral rinses and oral irrigation. Frequently, patients are overtreated using systemic antibiotics, which can lead to the development of bacteria that become resistant to antibiotics. Systemic antibiotics are contraindicated in patients with gingivitis or chronic periodontitis.

Antibiotic resistance of bacteria has enormous clinical and societal implications. In essence, when bacteria become resistant to an antibiotic, that antibiotic becomes ineffective. Although the prudent use of antibiotics will continue to be a valuable treatment option for certain forms of periodontal disease, the abuse and misuse of antibiotics must be addressed and monitored to prevent antibiotic resistance.

Systemic antibiotics are indicated in about 20% of patients with periodontitis (Loesche, 1976) where specific bacteria including *A. actinomycetemcomitans, P. gingivalis, P. intermedia,* and spirochetes (Loesche, 1976; Slots, 1986) have invaded the soft tissues. Treatment including systemic antibiotics is needed to elimi-

nate the bacteria in the tissues because periodontal debridment is ineffective. Examples include patients with localized aggressive periodontitis, necrotizing periodontal diseases, and refractory forms of periodontal diseases. In addition, patients with a compromised immune system, such as AIDS patients, can benefit from the use of antimicrobial agents.

The controlled (sustained) drug devices may be useful in the adjunctive treatment of chronic periodontitis. The clinician's decision to use local antimicrobial agents remains the matter of individual clinical judgement. Even though scaling and root planing disrupts the subgingival biofilms that cause periodontitis, the placement of sustained-release antimicrobial devices subgingivally may help in slowing the rapid return of the biofilm and thus may slow the progression of disease.

As advances are made in the development of new antimicrobial and antibiotic agents, the oral healthcare team will continue to play an integral part in ensuring that these agents are used appropriately. No data are available to support the long-term effectiveness of the newly approved controlled-release devices. Although many studies on site-specific drug therapy and submicrobial-dose doxycycline report statistically significant reductions in probing depths and improvements in attachment levels, the clinical benefit may not be significant. Further clinical studies are needed to determine clinical significance.

KEY POINTS

- Systemic antibiotics are indicated in certain inflammatory periodontal diseases, such as localized or generalized aggressive periodontitis, and refractory forms of periodontal diseases.
- Systemic antibiotics should are not indicated for chronic periodontitis.
- Controlled-release drug devices that slowly release antimicrobial agents are used in site-specific (recurrent) areas in chronic localized periodontitis.
- Enzyme-suppression therapy involves the inhibition of collagenase that is synthesized and released by neutrophils.
- Dental practitioners should contribute to limiting antibiotic use to prevent drug resistance.

SELF-QUIZ

1. All the following results are possible after site-specific chemotherapy except one. Which one is the exception? (p. 340)
   a. Reduction in probing depth
   b. Gain in clinical attachment
   c. Reduction in bleeding
   d. Formation of alveolar bone
2. Which one of the following procedures most effectively removes supra/subgingival dental biofilms? (p. 333)
   a. Oral irrigation
   b. Systemic antibiotics
   c. Periodontal debridement
   d. Controlled-release drugs
3. Which of the following controlled-release devices is in a gel form? (p. 341)
   a. Arestin
   b. Atridox
   c. Actisite
   d. PerioChip
4. Which of the following agents is the active ingredient in Arestin? (p. 342)
   a. Tetracycline HCl
   b. Minocycline HCl
   c. Doxycycline hyclate
   d. Chlorhexidine gluconate
5. Which one of the following antimicrobial agents possesses high substantivity to the root surface? (p. 337)
   a. Cetylpyridinium
   b. Sanguinarine
   c. Tetracycline
   d. Erythromycin
   e. Chlorhexidine
6. All the following are ways a dental practitioner can contribute to limiting antibiotic resistance except one. Which one is the exception? (p. 340)
   a. Prescribe drug at the first sign of purulent exudate.
   b. Avoid prolonged course of the medication.
   c. Instruct the patient on proper use.
   d. Prescribe an antibiotic with the narrowest possible spectrum of activity.

7. All the following properties of tetracyclines favor its use in periodontics except one. Which one is the exception? (pp. 336, 337)
   a. Substantivity
   b. Antifungal
   c. Antibacterial
   d. Anticollagenase
8. Which one of the following indications is for site-specific drug delivery? (p. 340)
   a. Probing depths of less than 4 mm
   b. Pockets with suppuration and bleeding
   c. Nonresponding bleeding sites with probing depths of 5 mm or more
   d. Sites with bone loss, suppuration, bleeding, and probing depths of less than 5 mm
9. Which of the following is an adverse effect that may occur when taking antibiotics? (pp. 336, 340)
   a. Bacterial resistance
   b. Mucosa inflammation
   c. Bone degeneration
   d. Tissue mucositis
10. Which of the following drugs is used in chronic periodontitis to suppress the production and secretion of host cell collagenase? (pp. 336, 337, 343)
    a. Minocycline
    b. Doxycycline
    c. Tetracycline
    d. Metronidazole
    e. Penicillin V

REFERENCES

American Academy of Periodontology. 2000. The role of controlled drug delivery for periodontitis. Position paper. *J. Periodontol.* 71:125–140.

American Academy of Periodontology. 2004. Systemic antibiotics in periodontics. *J Periodontol.*;75:1553–1565.

Asikainen, S., S. Alaluusua, and L. Saxén. 1991. Recovery of *A. actinomycetemcomitans* from teeth, tongue, and saliva. *J. Periodontol.* 62:203–206.

Baker, P., T. Evans, R. Coburn, and R. Genco. 1983. Tetracycline and its derivatives strongly bind to and are released from the tooth surface in active form. *J. Periodontol.* 54:580–585.

Beikler, T., K. Prior, B. Ehmke, and T. F. Flemming. 2004. Specific antibiotics in the treatment of periodontitis – a proposed strategy. *J. Periodontol.* 75:169–175.

Bonito, A. J., L. Lux, and K. N. Lohr. 2005. Impact of local adjuncts to scaling and root planing in periodontal disease therapy: A systematic review. *J. Periodontol.* 76(8):1227–1236.

Ciancio, S. G., and R. Ashley. 1998. Safety and efficacy of subantimicrobial-dose doxycycline therapy in patients with adult periodontitis. *Adv. Dent. Res.* 12:27–31.

Costerton, J. W., Z. Lewandowski, D. DeBeer, D. Caldwell, D. Korber, and G. James. 1994. Biofilms, the customized microniche. *J. Bacteriol.* 176:2137–2142.

Dastoor, S. F., S. Travan, R. F. Neiva, et al. 2007. Effect of adjunctive systemic azithromycin with periodontal surgery in the treatment of chronic periodontitis in smokers: A pilot study. *J. Periodontol.* 78:1887–1896.

de Graaf, J., A. J. van Winkelhoff, and R. J. Goené. 1989. The role *of Actinobacillus actinomycetemcomitans* in periodontal disease. *Infection* 17:269–271.

Emingil, G., G. Atilla, T. Sorsa, and T. Tervahartiala. 2008. The effect of adjunctive subantimicrobial dose doxycycline therapy on GCF levels in chronic periodontitis. *J. Periodontol.* 79(3):469–576.

Garey, K. W., and K. A. Rodvold. 1999. Disulfiram reactions and anti-infective agents. *Infect Med.* 16(11): 741–744.

Garrett, S., L. Johnson, and N. Stoller. 1998. The influence of subgingival calculus levels on outcomes following treatment of periodontitis with subgingivally delivered doxycycline or periodontal debridement. *J. Dent. Res.* 77:923 (Abstract 2336).

Golub, L. M., N. S. Ramamurthy, T. F. McNamara, R. A. Greenwald, and B. R. Rifkin. 1984. Tetracyclines inhibit tissue collagenase activity: A new mechanism in the treatment of periodontal diseases. *J. Periodont. Res.* 19:651–655.

Gordon, J. M., C. B. Walker, J. C. Murphy, J. M. Goodson, and S. S. Socransky. 1981. Tetracycline: Levels achievable in gingival crevice fluid and in vitro effect on subgingival organisms: 1. Concentrations in crevicular fluid after repeated doses. *J. Periodontol.* 52:609–612.

Greenstein, G. 2006. Local drug delivery in the treatment of periodontal diseases: Assessing the clinical significance of the results. *J. Periodontol.* 77(4):565–578.

Haffajee, A. D., S. S. Socransky, and J. C. Gunsolley. 2003. Systemic anti-infective periodontal therapy. A systematic review. *Ann. Periodontol.* 8(1):115–181.

Hanes, P.J., and J.P. Purvis. 2003. Local anti-infective therapy: Pharmacological agents. A systematic review. *Ann Periodontol.* 8:79–98.

Hersh, E. V., and P. A. Moore. 2008. Adverse drug interactions in dentistry. *Periodontology 2000* 46(1):109–142.

Jeffcoat, M. K., K. S. Bray, S. G. Ciancio, A. R. Dentino, D. H. Fine, et al. 1998. Adjunctive use of a subgingival controlled-release chlorhexidine chip reduces probing depth and improves attachment level compared with periodontal debridement alone. *J. Periodontol.* 69:989–997.

Kaner, D., C. Christan, T. Dietrich, et al. 2007. Timing affects the clinical outcome of adjunctive systemic antibiotic therapy for generalized aggressive periodontitis. *J. Periodontol.* 78:1201–1208.

Kleinfelder, J., R. Müller, and D. Lange. 1999. Antibiotic susceptibility of putative periodontal pathogens in advanced periodontitis patients. *J. Clin. Periodontol.* 26:347–352.

Loesche, W. 1976. Chemotherapy of dental plaque infections. *Oral Sci. Rev.* 9:65–107.

Loesche, W. J., J. Giordano, S. Soehren, and N. Kaciroti. 1996. The nonsurgical treatment of patients with periodontal disease. *Oral Surg. Oral Med. Oral Pathol.* 81:533–543.

Malizia, T., M. R. Tejada, E. Ghelardi, S. Senesi, and M. Gabriele. 1997. Periodontal tissue disposition of azithromycin. *J. Periodontol.* 68:1206–1209.

Mandell, R. L., L. S. Tripodi, E. Savitt, J. M. Goodson, and S. S. Socransky. 1986. The effect of treatment on *Aa* in local juvenile periodontitis. *J. Periodontol.* 57:94–97.

Novak, M. J., D. R. Dawson, I. Magnusson, et al. 2008. Combining host modulation and topical antimicrobial therapy in the management of moderate to severe periodontitis: A randomized multicenter trial. *J. Periodontol.* 79(1):33–41.

Page, R. C., S. Offenbacher, H. E. Schroeder, G. J. Seymour, and K. S. Kornman. 1997. Advances in the pathogenesis of periodontitis: Summary of developments, clinical implications and future directions. *Periodontology 2000* 14:216–248.

Paolantonio, M., M. D'Angelo, R. F. Grassi, et al. 2008. Clinical and microbiologic effects of subgingival controlled-release delivery of chlorhexidine chip in the treatment of periodontitis: A multicenter study. *J. Periodontol.* 79(2):271–282.

Pascale, D., J. Gordon, I. Lamster, P. Mann, M. Seiger, and W. Arndt. 1986. Concentration of doxycycline in human gingival fluid. *J. Clin. Periodontol.* 13:841–844.

Powell, C. A., B. L. Mealey, D. E. Deas, H. T. McDonnell, and A. J. Moritz 2005. Post-surgical infections: Prevalence associated with various periodontal surgical procedures. *J. Periodontol.* 76: 329–333.

Preshaw, P. M., M. J. Novak, J. Mellonig, et al. 2008. Modified-release subantimicrobial dose doxycycline enhances scaling and root planing in subjects with periodontal disease. *J. Periodontol.* 79:440–452.

Renvert, S., M. Wikström, G. Dahlén, J. Slots, and J. Egelberg. 1990. On the inability of root debridement and periodontal surgery to eliminate *Actinobacillus actinomycemtemcomitans* from periodontal pockets. *J. Clin. Periodontol.* 17:351–355.

Rifkin, B. R., A. T. Vernillo, and L. M. Golub. 1993. Blocking periodontal disease progression by inhibiting tissue destructive enzymes: A potential therapeutic role of tetracyclines and their chemically modified analogs. *J. Periodontol.* 64:819–827.

Sbordone L, Ramaglia L, Gulletta E, Iacono V. Recolonization of the subgingival microflora after scaling and root planing in human periodontis. *J. Periodontol* 1990. 61(9): 579–584

Segelnick, S., and M. A. Weinberg. 2008. Recognizing doxy-cycline-induced esophageal ulcers in dental practice: A case report and review. *JADA* 139:581–585.

Seymour, R. A. 2008. Pharmacology and therapeutics in den-tistry. *Periodontology 2000* 46(1):7–8.

Seymour, R. A., and S. D. Hogg. 2008. Antibiotics and chemo-prophylaxis. *Periodontology 2000* 46(1):80–108.

Seymour, R. A., and M. R. Rudralingham. 2008. Oral and dental adverse drug reactions. *Periodontology 2000* 46(1):9–26.

Slots, J. 1986. Bacterial specificity in adult periodontitis: A summary of recent work. *J. Clin. Periodontol.* 13:912–917.

Smith, C. 1999, May. Adverse effects of antibiotics. *U.S. Pharmacist:*46–60.

Stabholz, A., J. Kettering, R. Aprecio, G. Zimmerman, P. J. Baker, and U. M. E. Wikesjo. 1993. Antimicrobial proper-ties of human dentin impregnated with tetracycline HCl or chlorhexidine: An in vitro study. *J. Clin. Periodontol.* 20:557–562.

Stoller, N., L. Johnson, S. Trapnell, C. Harrold, and S. Garrett. 1998. The pharmacokinetic profile of a biodegradable controlled-release delivery system containing doxycycline compared to systemically delivered doxycycline in gingival crevicular fluid, saliva, and serum. *J. Periodontol.* 69:1085–1091.

Tomasi, C., T. Koutouzis, and J. L. Wennström. 2008. Locally delivered doxycycline as an adjunct to mechanical debride-ment at retreatment of periodontal pockets. *J. Periodontol.* 79(3):431–439.

Waerhaug, J. 1978. Healing of the dentoepithelial junction fol-lowing subgingival plaque control: II. As observed on ex-tracted teeth. *J. Periodontol.* 49:119–134.

Walker, C. B. 1996. Selected antimicrobial agents: Mechanism of action, side effects and drug interactions. *Periodontology 2000* 10:12–28.

Walker, C., and K. Karpinia 2002. Rationale for use of antibi-otics in periodontics. *J. Periodontol.* 73(10): 1188–1196.

Winkel, E., A. van Winkelhoff, D. Barendregt, G. van der Wei-jden, M. Timmerman, and U. van der Velden. 1999. Clinical and microbiological effects of initial periodontal therapy in conjunction with amoxicillin and clavulanic acid in patient with adult periodontitis. *J. Clin. Periodontol.* 26:461–468.

Chapter 23

Healing After Nonsurgical Periodontal Therapy

Mea A. Weinberg

Cynthia Fong

OUTLINE

Introduction
Nonsurgical Periodontal Therapy
Terminology
Periodontal Debridement
Healing Response and the Outcome of Therapy
Reevaluation of Initial Therapy
Dental Hygiene Notes
Key Points
Self-Quiz
References

GOAL: To provide an understanding of tissue healing after nonsurgical therapy.

EDUCATIONAL OBJECTIVES

Upon completion of this chapter, the reader should be able to:

- Discuss the rationale for periodontal debridement.
- Explain the clinical outcomes of periodontal debridement.
- Discuss the effects of nonsurgical treatment on the subgingival microbiota.
- Describe the effects of combined oral hygiene self-care with subgingival periodontal debridement on clinical attachment loss.
- Describe the healing response in gingivitis and periodontitis after periodontal debridement.
- Discuss the rationale for reevaluation of initial therapy.

KEY WORDS

deplaquing **349**
gain in clinical
    attachment **351**
inflammatory
    periodontal diseases
    350
periodontal debridement
    349
periodontal therapy
    353

prophylaxis **349**
reevaluation **357**
root planing **349**
scaling **349**
soft tissue healing **350**
subgingival debridement
    349
supragingival
    debridement **349**

INTRODUCTION

Because periodontal disease activity is site-specific within the same mouth and differs between individuals, choice of treatment is determined on a site-to-site basis and/or on a patient-to-patient basis. The critical factor in the success of periodontal therapy is not only the thoroughness of the professional debridement but also the achievement of a high standard of oral hygiene self-care.

NONSURGICAL PERIODONTAL THERAPY

The traditional emphasis of the initial phase of periodontal therapy or nonsurgical therapy is control of the supragingival microbial plaque and disruption or removal of subgingival gram-negative microbiota, thus delaying the repopulation of pathogenic microorganisms (Magnusson, Lindhe, Yoneyama, & Liljenberg, 1984). Subgingival plaque originates either from an apical extension of growing supragingival plaque (Waerhaug, 1978) and/or from incomplete subgingival instrumentation. In either case, it is essential to control the supragingival microbial activity through oral hygiene self-care and subgingival plaque removal by professional mechanical instrumentation (Cobb, 1996; Dahlen, Lindhe, Sato, Hanamura, & Okamoto, 1992; Katsanoulas, Renee, & Attström, 1992; Sbordone, Ramaglia, Gulletta, & Iacono, 1990). Subgingival debridement decreases the number of periodontal pathogens such as *Porphyromonas gingivalis* and *Prevotella intermedia* in subgingival plaque and shifts the plaque composition to a predominately gram-positive aerobic species associated with periodontal health.

Thus, nonsurgical therapy is based on returning the gingival tissue to a healthy, noninflamed state that can be maintained easily by the patient and the practitioner.

TERMINOLOGY

The traditional therapy for removing supragingival and subgingival plaque, its by-products and toxins, and calculus has been scaling and root planing. **Scaling** is defined as the mechanical removal of supragingival and subgingival dental plaque, calculus, and stains (tooth-accumulated materials) from the crown and root surfaces. Thus, scaling is performed both supragingivally and subgingivally. Subgingival scaling removes the adherent plaque and calculus attached to the root surface. Subgingival calculus is mineralized plaque that often adheres tenaciously to root surfaces and thus is very difficult to

remove. **Root planing** is defined as a "definitive treatment procedure designed to remove cementum or surface dentin that is rough, impregnated with calculus, or contaminated with toxins or microorganisms" (Ciancio, 1989). Extensive root planing is not needed to obtain healthy tissue. Bacterial enzymes and by-products can be removed with ultrasonic instruments.

Over the past few years, the term **periodontal debridement** has emerged in the literature, and it is defined as the removal of any foreign material, including dental plaque, its by-products and toxins, calculus, and diseased or dead tissue, from the coronal tooth surfaces, root surfaces, sulcus or pocket, and periodontium (e.g., supporting bone). Thus, the difference between periodontal debridement and scaling and root planing is that it encompasses more than just the root surfaces. It includes the pocket space, the pocket wall, and the underlying tissues (O'Hehir, 1999). Rather than total removal of cementum and the attainment of smooth root surfaces, conservation of cementum and the achievement of a good tissue healing response through control of bacterial infection are the objectives of periodontal debridement (O'Hehir, 1999). **Supragingival debridement** (also referred to as supragingival scaling) is the mechanical removal of dental plaque and calculus from tooth surfaces above the gingival margin. **Subgingival debridement** or subgingival scaling and root planing is the mechanical removal of dental plaque and calculus from tooth surfaces below the gingival margin. The term "deep scaling" has been used to denote subgingival scaling and root planing.

Deplaquing describes the mechanical disruption of nonattached, free-floating subgingival plaque and its by-products from the sulcus or pocket. Deplaquing is recommended at reevaluation and maintenance appointments.

There are numerous definitions of oral **prophylaxis** in the literature. The American Dental Hygienist's Association (ADHA, 1995) reversed a change made to the prophylaxis definition published in the Current Dental Terminology (CDT)-4, which stated that prophylaxis was a scaling and/or polishing procedure to remove coronal plaque, calculus, and stains. The change to this definition involved removal of the term "/or", thereby restoring the 1992 ADA Current Dental Terminology definition, which reads "scaling and polishing." The American Academy of Periodontology provides the most comprehensive definition of oral prophylaxis. An oral prophylaxis is the removal of plaque, calculus, and stains from the exposed and unexposed surfaces of the teeth by scaling and polishing as a preventive measure for the control of local irritants (American Academy of Periodontology, 2003).

Polishing is performed to remove stains from the teeth and has not been shown to have any therapeutic benefits. For this reason, the American Dental Hygienist's Association's position on polishing is that it is a procedure that should be performed selectively when teeth have extrinsic stains (American Dental Hygienist's Association, 1995).

In some states, dental hygienists are permitted to perform closed gingival curettage or soft tissue curettage. According to the American Academy of Periodontology, curettage is not an accepted procedure in periodontics. Curettage involves removal of the diseased lining of the soft tissue pocket wall (soft tissue debridement), including the junctional epithelium and the underlying inflamed connective tissue. The goal of gingival curettage is to reduce or eliminate periodontal inflammation. Indications for performing curettage include the presence of inflamed gingival tissues and shallow suprabony pockets. However, the benefits of soft tissue curettage are questionable, and as a separate procedure, it has no justifiable application during active therapy for chronic periodontitis (Ciancio, 1989). Kalkwarf (1989) demonstrated that the healing effects of curettage were not any better than scaling and root planing alone. It is noteworthy, however, that some inadvertent gingival curettage does occur as a result of scaling and root planing procedures.

PERIODONTAL DEBRIDEMENT

Treatment of **inflammatory periodontal diseases** (e.g., gingivitis and periodontitis) has evolved significantly during the past decades. It was once thought that a primary goal of traditional scaling and root planing was the achievement of smooth root surfaces that were free of deposits. This intent was based on the assumption that bacteria would attach to rough surfaces (e.g., calculus and irregular root topography) and interfere with **soft tissue healing** (Adriaens & Adriaens, 2004). It is now known that bacteria adhere to any surface, rough or smooth. Therefore, evaluation of successful periodontal debridement depends primarily on the soft tissue response. The clinical significance of root surface roughness or smoothness is still undetermined (Jacobson, Blomlöf, & Lindskog, 1994), but the dental hygienist nevertheless, to achieve root smoothness, should strive to remove as much subgingival calculus as possible because it can affect plaque accumulation. Oberholzer and Rateitschak (1996)

concluded that striving for total root smoothness during periodontal surgery seems to be unnecessary; however, the value of a cleaned tooth surface cannot be minimized in periodontal tissue healing response.

Mechanical nonsurgical therapy consisting of oral hygiene self-care and periodontal instrumentation is intended to prevent, arrest, control, or eliminate periodontal diseases in order to ultimately maintain the teeth in a functional state of health (Cobb, 1996). Currently, periodontal debridement remains the foundation of nonsurgical periodontal therapy.

Combined Personal and Professional Debridement

Periodontal instrumentation is performed during the initial or preliminary phase of periodontal therapy. The beneficial effects of periodontal debridement combined with oral hygiene self-care in the treatment and prevention of periodontal diseases have been well documented. These include reduction of clinical inflammation, establishment of more beneficial microorganisms and less pathogenic microorganisms, reduction in probing depths, and a gain in attachment (American Academy of Periodontology, 1997; Kaldahl et al., 1996).

One clinical study reported that in the presence of supragingival plaque, a subgingival microbiota containing greater than 5% spirochetes and motile rods, was reestablished 4 to 8 weeks after periodontal debridement. Sites devoid of supragingival plaque following supervised oral hygiene and mechanical instrumentation had less than 5% gram-negative bacteria (Magnusson et al., 1984). A more recent investigation studied the effects of supragingival plaque control alone and plaque control combined with scaling and root planing on clinical attachment loss over a three-year period (Westfelt, Rylander, Dahlen, & Lindhe, 1998). Results showed a reduction in bleeding scores following the combined treatment of plaque control and scaling and root planing. Plaque scores were reduced in both groups. Increased attachment loss of 2 mm or more was low in the combined treatment group. This study demonstrated that supragingival plaque control is not enough to prevent further attachment loss in periodontitis patients.

Rationale and Indications for Periodontal Debridement

The purpose of periodontal debridement is to treat and resolve inflammation in the periodontal soft tissues by removing the irritants, which are the supragingival and subgingival plaque and calculus. In conjunction with oral hygiene self-care, which also decreases supragingival plaque accumulation, repopulation of subgingival pathogenic microbiota is delayed and shifts the composition of pocket material from a pathogenic gram-negative microbiota to gram-positive species, which are more conducive to periodontal health.

Periodontal debridement is indicated at sites showing (1) signs of gingival inflammation, (2) elevated levels of bacterial pathogens, and (3) progressive attachment or alveolar bone loss (Cobb, 1996). Various forms of instrumentation are used, including hand-activated instrumentation and power-driven instrumentation (e.g., sonic and ultrasonic instrumentation).

Outcomes of Periodontal Debridement

The ultimate long-term outcome or end point for nonsurgical periodontal debridement is preservation of the form and function of the dentition (Cobb, 1996). Determining the effects of nonsurgical periodontal treatment requires the use of measurable clinical end points. Most clinical studies, as well as private practices, measure the probing depths, gain or loss of clinical attachment (measuring the clinical attachment levels), and alveolar bone height and document bleeding on probing, visual signs of gingival inflammation, and changes in subgingingival microbiota (Cobb, 1996; Suvan, 2005).

Probing Depths/Clinical Attachment Level

Root planing is contraindicated in sites that do not have periodontal pockets. A landmark clinical study showed that root planing teeth with initially shallow probing depths of less than 3 mm slightly decreased or did not alter probing depths, but loss of clinical attachment did occur (Lindhe, Socransky, Nyman, & Haffajee, 1982). A more recent study found that scaling and root planing performed with hand instruments produce a mean attachment loss of 0.76 mm, observed immediately following the procedure (Alves et al., 2004). Taking into consideration a number of clinical studies over the past years, Cobb (1996) determined that thorough debridement of moderately deep pockets (4 to 6 mm) usually results in a mean reduction in probing depth of 1.29 mm and a mean gain in clinical attachment of 0.55 mm, whereas sites with deeper probing depth (7 mm or more) showed a mean reduction in probing depth of 2.16 mm and a gain in clinical attachment of 1.29 mm. Care in selecting sites that will benefit from subgingival debridement is essential in the prevention of clinical attachment loss.

Subgingival Microbiota

Periodontal debridement of pockets causes profound shifts in the composition of the subgingival microbiota (Umeda et al., 2004). After subgingival debridement, the number of gram-negative microorganisms decreases, especially spirochetes, and the number of gram-positive rods and cocci increases. However, this therapy may be ineffective in eliminating *Actinobacillus actinomycetemcomitans* from affected subgingival sites (Cobb, 1996) because it invades soft tissue (Renvert, Wikström, Dahlen, Slots, & Egelberg, 1990).

Unfortunately, shifts in microbiotal composition are transient, and usually the pocket area becomes repopulated with subgingival microorganisms within days to months. Since the subgingival microbiota originate in supragingival areas (Waerhaug, 1978), regular and effective plaque control and periodontal debridement are absolutely critical for long-term control of inflammatory periodontal diseases (Cobb, 1996).

> **Did You Know?**
>
> It may take days or up to six months before bacteria repopulate the periodontal sites.

Bleeding on Probing

Periodontal debridement has predictably reduced the levels of inflammation. A vast number of clinical studies conducted over recent years have shown that periodontal debridement has reduced bleeding in approximately 57% of sites (Cobb, 1996).

Tissue Consistency

Reduction of the fluid and cellular components of an inflammatory lesion in the lamina propria should result in an increased proportion of collagen fibers, which, when combined with reattachment of the junctional epithelium or the formation of a long junctional epithelium, will produce increased resistance to passage of the probe tip. This results in an apparent **gain in clinical attachment.**

Treatment Sequence

The treatment sequence for periodontal debridement varies depending on clinical findings and diagnosis. The first step after the dental hygiene diagnosis and treatment plan is oral hygiene self-care instructions specifically designed for the patient's needs.

Most patients undergoing subgingival debridement require topical and/or local anesthesia (Palmer & Floyd, 1995). However, the patient must not have any allergy or sensitivity to the agent used. Two types of topical anesthetics are available: amide types, such as 5 or 10% lidocaine, and ester types, such as benzocaine (varied concentrations are available, but usually it is 20%). Oraquix is a combination lidocaine/prilocaine (2.5%/2.5%) gel that is FDA approved for subgingival anesthesia. The possibility of allergic reactions is greater with lidocaine because it shows greater absorption into the systemic circulation than benzocaine. When a topical anesthetic is used, best results are obtained when a small amount is applied on a cotton-tip applicator, the tissues are dried prior to application of the agent, and the applicator is held in contact with the mucous membranes for 1 to 2 minutes. Alternatives include the use of an anesthetic patch, an anesthetic rinse, or electronic anesthesia. Topical anesthetic sprays should not be used because high doses of the agent can be absorbed into the circulatory system.

Local anesthesia is best applied by quadrant. It is recommended to treat one or two quadrants during a single visit depending on the number of teeth present as well as the degree of difficulty of the intervention. When two quadrants are treated during the same appointment, usual practice is to treat the upper and lower quadrants on either the right or the left side of the face. Both mandibular quadrants should not be treated during the same appointment so as to avoid patient discomfort and to prevent an inability on the part of the patient to control his or her mandible with both sides anesthetized.

Posttreatment care focuses on the prevention of dental plaque formation. A long-term plaque-free dentition is an unrealistic goal, and for this reason, periodic periodontal maintenance visits are required to monitor and identify disease recurrence (Westfelt, 1996).

Periodontal Debridement Procedures

Before debridement procedures are started, it is necessary to obtain a written informed consent from the patient. The procedure and its expected outcomes are explained to the patient. It is important for the patient to understand that the decreased probing depths primarily due to gingival shrinkage may cause gingival recession and "longer looking" teeth and that teeth may respond with hyper-

sensitivity to cold, toothbrushing, or sweets. Such hypersensitivity is usually not permanent, but it may cause pain and discomfort that lasts for a few weeks to months.

Subgingival Debridement

Calculus Removal As periodontal debridement is started on a patient, the primary goal is to remove gross deposits from supragingival and subgingival tooth surfaces. The ultimate goal of subgingival debridement is to render a root surface free of plaque, calculus, and endotoxins to enable soft tissue healing. Complete calculus removal is essentially not attainable (Kepic, O'Leary, & Kafrawy, 1990), and total root smoothness is not necessary for adequate tissue healing. Clinical studies have shown that practitioners who spent an average of 12 to 15 minutes to complete the debridement of each tooth with hand and ultrasonic instruments fail to remove calculus from all surfaces. After debridement, about 47% of all nonfurcated surfaces and 63% of 6 mm or larger pockets showed residual calculus. Surgical access reduced the frequency of residual calculus to 20 and 38%, respectively. Teeth with furcations had a higher frequency of residual calculus, and surgical access did not provide any additional benefit (Buchanan & Robertson, 1987; Caffesse, Sweeney, & Smith, 1986; Fleischer, Mellonig, Brayer, Gray, & Barnett, 1989).

While total elimination of causative factors is an appropriate treatment goal, reduction of dental plaque and calculus below threshold levels appears to control the disease process and improve clinical signs of inflammation (Robertson, 1990), producing significant reductions in gingivitis, tooth loss, attachment loss, severity of disease, and probing depths (American Academy of Periodontology, 1997). Thus, if periodontal debridement can achieve elimination of inflammation and disease progression, then no further treatment is necessary. If periodontal debridement fails to achieve these objectives, then periodontal surgery may be necessary.

Root Surface Characteristics With the development of a gram-negative bacterial flora in the gingival crevice, events occur that eventually cause breakdown of the attachment apparatus. If elimination or disruption of the subgingival bacteria is not accomplished, rapid growth and maturation occur. During growth and after the death of subgingival gram-negative microorganisms, endotoxins or lipooligosaccharides are released from their cell walls. Endotoxins are highly toxic compounds that are capable of penetrating the junctional epithelium and entering the connective tissue, resulting in destruction of periodontal tissues. This causes loss of connective tissue attachment from the root surface, apical migration of the junctional epithelium, and bone loss. A periodontal pocket forms, and the root surface (cementum) becomes contaminated when exposed to this new subgingival pocket environment. The cementum is sufficiently porous to allow superficial binding of endotoxins and colonization of dental plaque and calculus onto the altered root surfaces. Cementum that is rough and impregnated with calculus or contaminated with toxins or microorganisms and dentin is referred to as contaminated, altered, or necrotic cementum.

Cementum Removal   The periodontal literature offers no firm conclusions about either the feasibility of or the need for removal of all contaminated cementum. In the past it was thought that the presence of cementum-bound endotoxins inhibited tissue healing after periodontal debridement. Much investigation has been directed toward the elimination of this contaminated or necrotic cementum. *It is the consensus that endotoxins found on diseased root surfaces are weakly and superficially bound and that 99% may be removed by brushing* (Moore, Wilson, & Kieser, 1986; Nakib, Bissada, Simmelnik, & Goldstine, 1982). The primary reason for removing the superficial layer of cementum by subgingival debridement is to remove plaque and calculus from the irregularities on the root surface. Extensive subgingival debridement for a prolonged amount of time is unnecessary (Cheetham, Wilson, & Kieser, 1988), and total removal of cementum is not the goal because the attachment of new soft tissue to the root surface is enhanced by the presence of cementum (Somerman, Archer, Shteyer, & Foster, 1987). O'Leary and Kafrawy (1983) concluded that total removal of cementum under routine clinical conditions is not a realistic objective of therapy. Smart, Wilson, Davies, and Kieser (1990), using ultrasonic instrumentation, showed that contaminated root surfaces could be rendered comparable to healthy teeth. Therefore, the key to **periodontal therapy** is the removal of plaque and calculus in order to reduce the number of oral bacteria below the threshold level capable of initiating inflammation (American Academy of Periodontology, 1997). Precisely how much cementum is removed as a result of root planing is uncertain.

Therefore, it is important to attain relatively smooth root surfaces only for the purpose of reducing plaque retention without excessive and unnecessary removal of cementum and dentin. The therapeutic goal of debridement therapy is to control bacterial infection as opposed to simply removing deposits from root surfaces.

Adverse Effects of Periodontal Debridement

Subgingival debridement may cause soft tissue recession, making the teeth look longer and exposing the root surface to the oral environment. This may result in dentinal hypersensitivity as a result of removal of the thin outer layer of cementum and exposure of the underlying dentin. Usually, teeth are not sensitive immediately after the periodontal debridement; hypersensitivity may take about three to four days to appear. Root sensitivity occurs in approximately half of the patients following subgingival scaling and root planing (von Troil, Needleman, & Sanz, 2002). The intensity of root sensitivity increases for a few weeks after therapy, after which it decreases. In clinical practice, it may be recommended that patients should be made aware of the potential for root sensitivity prior to treatment (von Troil, Needleman, & Sanz, 2002). Treatment of dentinal hypersensitivity is discussed in Chapter 22.

Limitations of Periodontal Debridement

Pocket Depth

The effectiveness of periodontal debridement depends on the effectiveness of the mechanical removal of dental plaque and calculus. Root debridement does not always remove all plaque and calculus from subgingival tooth surfaces. Studies have shown that considerable amounts (54 to 57%) of calculus remain on the root surfaces of teeth with moderate or advanced pockets and that more residual calculus is found on tooth surfaces with increasing probing depths (Wylam, Mealey, Mills, Waldrop, & Moskowicz, 1993). There was no significant difference whether an anterior or a posterior tooth was debrided (Sherman et al., 1990).

Current conclusions about the effectiveness of periodontal debridement in deeper pockets are conflicting, and there is as yet no agreement on whether nonsurgical instrumentation is effective in advanced periodontal lesions (Forabosco, Galetti, Spinato, Colao, & Casolari, 1996). The most frequently lost teeth in patients receiving comprehensive periodontal treatment are the molars. Explanations for this relate to the difficulty in achieving adequate daily plaque removal and the difficulty in properly debriding molars. Stambaugh, Dragoo, Smith, and Carasali (1981) found that the average probing depth for "efficient" removal of plaque, calculus, and necrotic cementum was 3.73 mm. Rateitschak, Schwarz, Guggenheim, Duggelin, and Rateitschak (1992) found that surfaces where curets could reach usually were free of plaque and calculus, but in deep pockets the curet did not reach the base of the pocket. Consequently, modified curets with longer shanks were developed to increase treatment effectiveness in deeper pockets.

Furcations and Root Anatomy

Access for adequate instrumentation in the furcation area is often difficult, if not impossible, given the special anatomic characteristics of multirooted teeth (Fleischer et al., 1989; Greene, 1995). Pathogenic microbiota frequently persists in furcation lesions (Loos, Claffey, & Egelberg, 1988). Narrow furcation openings make periodontal debridement a challenge. Fifty-eight percent of molars have furcation entrance diameters that are smaller than the smallest diameter of a relatively new curet, which is 0.75 mm (Bower, 1979a; Parashis, Anagnon-Vareltzides, & Demetriou, 1990).

Knowledge about the morphology of the furcation area and the variations in root form and structure is important for effective instrumentation. Root concavities, which are depressions found on the proximal root surfaces, are plaque and calculus traps, making instrumentation extremely difficult. For instance, a deep mesial concavity is found on the maxillary first premolar. On the maxillary first molars, the mesiobuccal root has the greatest incidence of concavities, whereas both the mesio- and distobuccal roots of the mandibular first molars have concavities (Bower, 1979b; Figure 23–1 ■). Moreover, any other root also may have root concavities. Another limitation is that the smallest width of the blade of a curet is still larger than the average width of a furcation entrance, which makes it difficult to place a curet effectively into a furcation (Hou et al. 1994)(Figure 23–2 ■).

Time Spent and Clinician Skill

Controversy exists over how much time should be spent on subgingival debridement. Subgingival debridement is dependent on both technique and operator skill. Since endotoxins are just weakly bound to the root surface (Moore et al., 1986), it is not necessary to spend a great deal of time debriding. However, a considerable amount of time still should be spent in effectively removing subgingival plaque, calculus, and necrotic cementum. If this procedure is done incorrectly, root gouging may occur, resulting in the production of grooves and pits in the root surface.

■ **FIGURE 23–1**   Root morphology. Root concavities in the maxillary molar decrease the effectiveness of debridement.

■ **FIGURE 23–2**   It is difficult to effectively scale in furcations because the narrowest width of a curet is still wider than the average width of a furcation entrance.

A clinical study (Anderson, Palmer, Bye, Smith, & Caffesse, 1996) evaluating single versus multiple episodes of subgingival instrumentation to determine effectiveness concluded that there was no significant difference between the two treatments. It was suggested that calculus remaining after one thorough episode of instrumentation is not likely to be removed by repeated instrumentation. How much time is enough? Most researchers suggest that periodontal debridement should take at least 10 minutes per tooth (Lowenguth & Greenstein, 1995). Coldiron, Yukna, Weir, and Caudill (1990) found that cementum removal was generally achieved on periodontally healthy roots with 20 strokes of a curet, but residual calculus remained. Thus, vigorous root planing is not needed and the best way to determine how much root planing should be performed is to monitor tissue healing. If the gingival tissues are still inflamed after initial therapy, then more periodontal debridement is required.

The results of a clinical study assessing periodontal debridement forces in periodontally involved molars show a broad range of forces being applied by the practitioner (Zappa, Röthlisberger, Simona, & Case, 1993). Additionally, the quality of periodontal debridement done on a molar may be primarily determined by the attitude of the practitioner, who subjectively treats the tooth according to his or her habits, rather than according to the characteristics of the root surfaces being treated (Zappa et al., 1993).

Most studies confirm that the more experienced the clinician, the more calculus-free the root surfaces were in deeper pockets and in hard-to-reach areas such as furcations (Brayer, Mellonig, Dunlap, Marinak, & Carson, 1989).

HEALING RESPONSE AND THE OUTCOME OF THERAPY
Diseased Periodontal Unit

When a periodontal probe is inserted into the pocket of a diseased and inflamed pocket, the probe penetrates the tissue apical to the junctional (pocket) epithelium, giving deeper probe readings. This occurs because the connective tissue of the gingival tissue contains less collagen and more inflammatory cells. Once the periodontium is treated, the thin junctional epithelium is closely adapted to the tooth or root surface, and collagen replaces the inflammatory cells in the connective tissue. This is responsible for the increased resistance to probing force so that the probe tip stops at a more coronal level of the junctional epithelium than when inflammation was present resulting in shallower probing depth readings.

Healing Periodontal Unit

An expected outcome of debridement is tissue healing. Healing results in tissue repair, shrinkage of gingival tissue, and the renewal of epithelial cells in contact with tooth surfaces (Caffesse, Mota, & Morrison, 1995; Caton, Nyman, & Zander, 1980).

Generally, the same healing features of periodontal tissues are seen following debridement of any chronically inflamed site. Initially, following debridement, there is an acute inflammatory reaction due to the traumatic nature of the therapy. This inflammation subsides within 24 to 48 hours. Over the next week, there is a gradual reduction of inflammatory cells, epithelial tissue healing, and finally, connective tissue maturation with collagen deposition.

Gingivitis: Healing after Periodontal Debridement

Histologically, in gingivitis, once dental plaque and calculus are removed, the pocket epithelium will reform into junctional epithelium and contact the adjacent tooth surface as it was in health. This happens because the basal cells of the junctional epithelium grow out and contact the tooth surface and develop into a new junctional epithelium. Reattachment of "old" junctional epithelium does not occur. Then, the apical part of the junctional epithelium moves apically until the first gingival connective tissue fibers embedded in cementum are reached. This new junctional epithelium is sometimes referred to as a "long junctional epithelium." Also, the inflammatory cells in the gingival connective tissue are replaced by collagen; these improvements result in an *apparent* "gain in clinical attachment." The formation of a new long junctional epithelium is explained in detailed below.

Clinically, there is a reduction in or elimination of inflammation (e.g., bleeding) and the elimination of edema, both of which result in tissue shrinkage and occasionally gingival recession. Gingiva that is fibrotic will not shrink, as does edematous tissue. The gingiva often returns to its salmon pink color. The greatest reduction in probing depths occurs after four to eight weeks (Segelnick & Weinberg, 2006) and is primarily due to (1) tissue shrinkage, which may result in gingival recession,

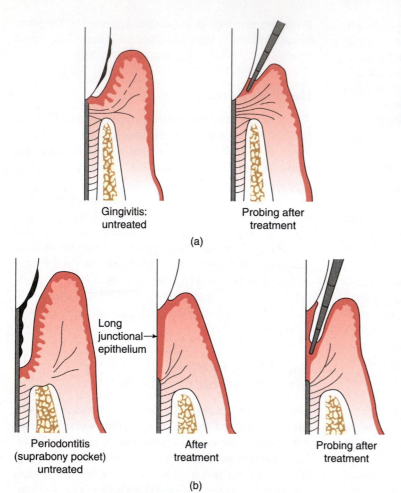

Gingivitis:
untreated

Probing after
treatment

(a)

Long
junctional →
epithelium

Periodontitis
(suprabony pocket)
untreated

After
treatment

Probing after
treatment

(b)

■ **FIGURE 23–3**   Healing of the gingival tissues after subgingival debridement. (a) In gingivitis, the tissues will heal, with approximation of the junctional epithelium to the tooth surface. (b) In periodontitis, after root planing, the tissues heal by formation of a long junctional epithelial attachment to the root surface.

and (2) reformation of collagen, which results in greater resistance to probing (Figure 23–3a ■). The reductions obtained in probing depths as a result of nonsurgical therapy are in the range of 1 to 2 mm.

Periodontitis: Healing after Periodontal Debridement

Histologically, in periodontitis, after the removal of dental plaque, calculus, and necrotic cementum, some healing will occur. Healing will most likely occur by repair or new attachment rather than regeneration, which is formation of new bone, collagen fibers, cementum, and periodontal ligament. Healing by regeneration occurs during periodontal surgery using guided tissue regeneration procedures (discussed in Chapter 25). Essentially, all types of successful periodontal debridement usually heal by new attachment or long junctional epithelium.

Histologically, repair of the root epithelial interface has been described as a long junctional epithelial attachment that prevents the formation of a new connective tissue attachment (Cobb, 1996). Research has shown, however, that the presence of a long junctional epithelium does not represent an area of less resistance to infection (Beaumont, O'Leary, & Kafrawy, 1984; Caffesse et al., 1986). However, patients who are erratic in their compliance with oral hygiene self-care do not do as well with a long junctional epithelium as patients with complete compliance (Wilson, Schoen, & Fallon, 1989).

The same scenario that occurs with healing of gingivitis sites also occurs with periodontitis sites. The pocket epithelium transforms back into junctional epithelium, which begins to come in contact with the root surface between the gingival connective tissue and the root (Figure 23–3b). The formation of a long junctional epithelium results in closure of the pocket. This reestablishment of the junctional epithelium most likely occurs within one (Caton & Zander, 1979) or two (Waerhaug, 1978) weeks. The inflammatory cells in the gingival connective tissue are replaced by collagen, but a long junctional epithelium prevents the formation of a gingival connective tissue attachment (gingival fibers). The greatest reduction in probing depths and an *apparent* gain in clinical attachment level can be measured after 4 to 8 weeks (Segelnick & Weinberg, 2006), although true gains in clinical attachment are seen primarily after periodontal surgery, if at all (that is why the term "apparent" is used). Gains in clinical attachment level after treatment do not necessarily mean that new gingival connective tissue attachment has been achieved (Armitage, 1996). It may simply indicate that the probe is more resistant to penetration once the gingival collagen has reformed and that the probe tip when placed into the gingival crevice stops at a more *coronal* location of the junctional epithelium. This gives the appearance of a gain in clinical attachment when there actually may not be. A true gain in clinical attachment after periodontal treatment indicates that a new connective tissue attachment (collagen fibers inserting) to the root has occurred.

Residual or undetected calculus that instrumentation has failed to remove is often present. Despite incomplete calculus removal, Sherman and colleagues (1990) showed that sites still could respond favorably. Haffajee and colleagues (1997) found that periodontal debridement demonstrated clinical improvement in subjects with chronic periodontitis even though only modest changes in subgingival microbiota were seen. This suggests potential targets for therapy and indicates that radical alterations in subgingival microbiota may not be necessary.

Did You Know?

It takes a lot longer for connective tissue fibers to reform than for junctional epithelium to readapt to the root surface.

REEVALUATION OF INITIAL THERAPY

Reevaluation of initial therapy involves the assessment of treatment performed. Box 23-1 outlines different steps that should be performed on a patient during a reevaluation visit. These findings are compared with the initial clinical findings that were documented before the patient started periodontal debridement.

Box 23-1   Reevaluation Measurements

- Oral hygiene status
- Soft tissue status
- Probing depths
- Clinical attachment levels (CALs)
- Bleeding on probing
- Tooth mobility
- Furcation involvement
- Plaque index

 Rapid Dental Hint

Remember that when measuring clinical attachment level, you use the cemento-enamel junction (CEJ) as your reference point to take the measurement.

Tissue Response

After appropriate initial therapy, a planned **reevaluation** should assess the current state of health or disease. The treatment sequence for the reevaluation appointment consists of a medical history update, a soft tissue examination, a plaque index, determination of the presence of bleeding, an oral hygiene self-care evaluation, and periodontal probing. Pretreatment findings are compared with the current status of the patient. It is important to evaluate and emphasize the patient's oral hygiene self-care techniques. Controversy exists regarding the recommended time interval between the initial therapy and the reevaluation appointment. Recommendations range from a minimum of four to a maximum of eight weeks after periodontal debridement to allow for tissue healing, although waiting longer than six weeks may augment the healing response (Segelnick & Weinberg, 2006). Key points concerning the appropriate time to perform a reevaluation are summarized in Box 23-2 (Segelnick & Weinberg, 2006).

In the absence of improved plaque control, Magnusson et al. (1984) and Mousques, Listgarten, and Phillips (1980) observed that a subgingival microbiota containing large numbers of pathogenic spirochetes and motile rods repopulated within four to eight weeks.

If results of initial therapy show improvement, but with some residual 5 mm probing depths, the patient should be placed on periodontal maintenance and reevaluated in six months. Reevaluation at regular intervals is essential to alert the dental hygienist to areas where plaque control has failed and inflammation has returned.

Box 23–2 **Reevaluation of Initial Therapy**

- After scaling and root planing, there is reestablishment of the junctional epithelium to the tooth surface in one to two weeks; reevaluation before two weeks is too early.
- After scaling and root planing, the repair of connective tissue continues for four to eight weeks.
- Subgingival microbial repopulation occurs within a few months (two months) after instrumentation of periodontal pockets in the absence of improved plaque control.
- Longer than two months may be too long to wait for the reevaluation because pathogenic bacteria have already repopulated periodontal pockets.

Unstable sites should be retreated or monitored closely for signs of attachment loss. At the reevaluation appointment, a decision is made regarding whether the patient qualifies for surgical intervention, continues with initial therapy, or is placed on a periodontal maintenance schedule. Factors that may influence this decision include the overall treatment plan, including restorative procedures, as well as the desires of the patient.

Reevaluation includes an examination of the gingival tissues. If inflammation persists, which is apparent clinically as bleeding on probing and redness, the cause needs to be determined. Persistent inflammation may result from incomplete debridement, patient noncompliance with home care, or a systemic disease. The desired microbial response is a change in the composition of the bacteria found within the pocket from a pathogenic gram-negative species (e.g., spirochetes, *P. gingivalis, P. intermedia*) to a more beneficial gram-positive species such as cocci or nonmotile bacteria (Mousques, et al., 1980).

Ultrasonic versus Hand-Activated Instrumentation

Studies comparing hand- and power-driven scalers are difficult to assess because of the wide variety of study de-

Rapid Dental Hint

Shallower probing depth readings happen because healing occurs with a long junctional epithelium.

signs. With the advent of modified periodontal inserts, subgingival root debridement became possible. Most studies have had comparable results with hand- and power-driven scalers when considering residual plaque and calculus. The ultimate determinant of treatment success with power-driven scalers (e.g., ultrasonics and sonics) is observation of the response of the tissues. Posttreatment evaluation consists of monitoring the soft tissue response and determining the critical levels of periodontal pathogenic organisms present within the gingival crevice. Thus, the outcome of scaling and root planing is similar for hand-activated instrumentation and power-driven scalers.

It has been documented that ultrasonic scalers with modified tips produced smoother roots with less damage, better access to the base of the pocket, and superior plaque and calculus removal than hand-activated instruments and also required less time (Dragoo, 1992; Kocher & Plagmann, 1997).

Comparing manual and ultrasonic instrumentation of deep pockets (6–9 mm), it was found that both methods were equal in reducing total microbial counts and colony-forming units (Oosterwal, Matee, Mikx, van't Hof, & Renggli, 1987). However, Leon and Vogel (1987) found that ultrasonic instrumentation was more effective at reducing spirochetes and motile rods when treating advanced bone loss in furcations. Thus, the tissue healing response is similar with manual and ultrasonic instrumentation.

Lasers

The use of lasers in periodontics for scaling and root planing is very controversial. Each laser has a different wavelength, either the Nd:YAG or Er:YAG wavelengths, which is used for different procedures. There is much concern about using lasers because damage to periodontal tissues can result depending on the wavelength and power, and the periodontal procedure that the laser was used for. The American Academy of Periodontology states that there is limited evidence suggesting that lasers used in an adjunctive capacity to scaling and root planing may provide some additional benefit (Cobb, 2006).

DENTAL HYGIENE NOTES

The philosophy of periodontal therapy has changed over the past decade as a result of further understanding of the disease process. Therapy is based on up-to-date clinical and microbial studies. The decision to perform periodontal debridement as a definitive treatment should depend on the severity of periodontal disease, the inflammatory status of the gingiva, the treatment objectives of the dental hygienist, treatment time, and the skill of the operator (Lowenguth & Greenstein, 1995).

Selection of the proper instrument involves considering the following factors: the amount of calculus, the type of tissue tone (e.g., firm, edematous, or hard and fibrotic), probing depths (or type of disease present), root morphology, and location of the calculus. Root smoothness is no longer the main criterion for periodontal instrumentation, although all detectable deposits should be removed so as to achieve a successful soft tissue response. The primary goal of periodontal debridement is to make the root and the soft tissue biologically compatible (Wilson et al., 1989). In most cases, periodontal debridement improves clinical parameters, decreasing both gingival inflammation (evidenced by less bleeding) and probing depths. Improvements in microbial parameters are transient, and the microbiota soon return to pretreatment levels. Therefore, the patient requires continuous maintenance or plaque control. Both periodontal debridement and daily plaque removal by the patient are equally important for the maintenance of periodontal health and will continue to be the standard of periodontal therapy. Healing after nonsurgical therapy (scaling/root planing) is clinical/histologically complete at about three to six months after final instrumentation. Clinically, there should be fewer bleeding sites, more soft tissue recession, and a gain of clinical attachment as seen by an increased resistance of the probe.

KEY POINTS

- Successful periodontal treatment, maintenance of periodontal health, and the regeneration of periodontal tissues depend on the removal of supra- and subgingival deposits.
- Oral hygiene self-care and periodontal debridement are indicated in the treatment of inflammatory periodontal diseases to reduce inflammation and microbial levels. The clinical end point to periodontal debridement is a good tissue healing response.
- Periodontal debridement has been shown to disrupt or alter the subgingival microbiota, thus slowing down repopulation.
- Although meticulous debridement may remove some cementum, the intentional, aggressive removal of diseased cementum does not seem to be necessary; endotoxins are loosely attached to the root surface and can be removed easily.
- The type of healing occurring after subgingival debridement is a long junctional epithelium attach-

ment to the root surface, which is considered to be a type of repair.
- Reevaluation of initial therapy should be performed between four and eight weeks after completion of scaling and root planing.

SELF-QUIZ

1. Which one of the following healing responses is seen in gingivitis after periodontal debridement? (p. 355)
   a. Formation of new bone, cementum, and periodontal ligament
   b. Formation of new cementum and periodontal ligament
   c. Repair with a long junctional epithelium
   d. Reattachment of the alveolar mucosa
2. Which one of the following healing responses is seen in periodontitis after periodontal debridement? (p. 356)
   a. Reattachment of the sulcular epithelium
   b. Reattachment of the desmosomes
   c. Formation of new bone, cementum, and periodontal ligament
   d. Formation of a long junctional epithelium
3. Which one of the following definitions describes a gain in clinical attachment after periodontal debridement? (p. 355)
   a. Bone fill and formation of new cementum
   b. Improved gingival tone and reattachment of the sulcular epithelium
   c. Improved gingival tone and increased mature collagen fibers
   d. Gingival recession, bone fill, and establishment of a new periodontal ligament attachment
4. After periodontal debridement (reevaluation), on which one of the following does clinical success depend? (p. 357)
   a. Amount of time spent on the procedure
   b. Number of quadrants completed
   c. Total removal of calculus
   d. Tissue response
5. Which one of the following benefits is seen after subgingival debridement? (p. 351)
   a. disruption of the gram-negative microbial flora
   b. repopulation of gram-negative anaerobic flora
   c. removal of gram-positive facultative flora
   d. interference with attachment of Gram-positive anaerobic flora to root surfaces

REFERENCES

Adriaens, P. A., and L. M. Adriaens 2004. Effects of nonsurgical periodontal therapy on hard and soft tissues. *Periodontology 2000* 36(1):121–145.

Alves, R.V., L. Machion, M. Z. Casati, F. H. Nociti, Jr., A.W. Sallum, and E. A. Sallum 2004. Attachment loss after scaling and root planing with different instruments – a clinical study. *J Clin Periodontol* 31: 12–15.

American Academy of Periodontology. 1997. Treatment of gingivitis and periodontitis. *J. Periodontol.* 68:1246–1253.

American Academy of Periodontology. 2003. *Glossary of periodontal terms,* 4th ed. Chicago: Author.

American Dental Hygienist's Association. 1995. *A position paper on selective tooth polishing.* Chicago: Author.

Anderson, G. B., J. Palmer, F. Bye, B. Smith, and R. Caffesse. 1996. Effectiveness of subgingival scaling and root planing: Single versus multiple episodes of instrumentation. *J. Periodontol.* 67:367–373.

Armitage, G. C. 1996. Periodontal diseases: Diagnosis. *Ann. Periodontol.* 1:37–215.

Beaumont, R., T. O'Leary, and A. Kafrawy. 1984. Relative resistance of long junctional epithelial adhesions and connective tissue attachments to plaque-induced inflammation. *J. Periodontol.* 55:213–223.

Bower, R. C. 1979a. Furcation morphology relative to periodontal treatment: Furcation entrance architecture. *J. Periodontol.* 50:23–27.

Bower, R. C. 1979b. Furcation morphology relative to periodontal treatment: Furcation root surface anatomy. *J. Periodontol.* 50:366–374.

Brayer, W. K., J. T. Mellonig, R. M. Dunlap, K. W. Marinak, and R. E. Carson. 1989. Scaling and root planing effectiveness: The effect of root surface access and operator experience. *J. Periodontol.* 60:67–72.

Buchanan, S. A., and P. S. Robertson. 1987. Calculus removal by scaling and root planing with and without surgical access. *J. Periodontol.* 58:159–163.

Caffesse, R. G., L. F. Mota, and E. D. Morrison. 1995. The rationale for periodontal therapy. *Periodontology 2000.* 9:7–13.

Caffesse, R. G., P. L. Sweeney, and B. A. Smith. 1986. Scaling and root planing with and without periodontal flap surgery. *J. Clin. Periodontol.* 13:205–210.

Caton, J., S. Nyman, and H. Zander. 1980. Histometric evaluation of periodontal surgery: II. Connective tissue attachment after four regenerative procedures. *J. Clin. Periodontol.* 7:224–231.

Caton, J., and H. Zander. 1979. The attachment between tooth and gingival tissues after periodontic root planing and soft tissue curettage. *J. Periodontol.* 50:462–466.

Cheetham, W. A., M. Wilson, and J. B. Kieser. 1988. Root surface debridement: An in vitro assessment. *J. Clin. Periodontol.* 15:288–292.

Ciancio, S. G. 1989. Non-surgical periodontal treatment. In eds. M. Nevins, W. Becker, and K. Kornman, *Proceedings of the World Workshop in Clinical Periodontics,* Vol. 2, 1–22. Chicago: American Academy of Periodontology.

Cobb, C. M. Lasers in Periodontics: A review of the literature. *J. Periodontol.* 2006; 77:545–564.

Cobb, C. M. 1996. Non-surgical pocket therapy: Mechanical. *Ann. Periodontol.* 1:443–490.

Coldiron, N. B., R. A. Yukna, J. Weir, and R. F. Caudill. 1990. A quantitative study of cementum removal with hand curettes. *J. Periodontol.* 61:293–299.

Dahlen, G., J. Lindhe, K. Sato, H. Hanamura, and H. Okamoto. 1992. The effect of supragingival plaque control on the subgingival microbiota in subjects with periodontal disease. *J. Clin. Periodontol.* 19:802–809.

Dragoo, M. R. 1992. A clinical evaluation of hand and ultrasonic instruments on subgingival debridement: I. With unmodified and modified ultrasonic scalers. *Int. J. Periodont. Rest. Dent.* 12:310–323.

Fleischer, H. C., J. T. Mellonig, W. K. Brayer, J. L. Gray, and J. D. Barnett. 1989. Scaling and root planing efficacy in multirooted teeth. *J. Periodontol.* 60:402–409.

Forabosco, A., R. Galetti, S. Spinato, P. Colao, and C. Casolari. 1996. A comparative study of a surgical method and scaling and root planing using Odontoson. *J. Clin. Periodontol.* 23:611–614.

Greene, P. R. 1995. Non-surgical periodontal therapy: Essential and adjunctive methods. *Br. Dent. J.* 179:28–34.

Haffajee, A. D., M. A. Cugini, S. Dibart, C. Smith, L. R. Kent, Jr., and S. S. Socransky. 1997. The effect of scaling and root planing on the clinical and microbiological parameters of periodontal diseases. *J. Clin. Periodontol.* 24:324–334.

Jacobson, L., J. Blomlöf, and S. Lindskog. 1994. Root surface texture after different scaling modalities. *Scand. J. Dent. Res.* 102:156–160.

Kaldahl, W. B., K. L. Kalkwarf, D. Kashinath, D. Patil, M. P. Molvar, and J. K. Dyer. 1996. Long-term evaluation of periodontal therapy: I. Response to four therapeutic modalities. *J. Periodontol.* 67:93–102.

Kalkwarf, K. L. 1989. Tissue attachment. In eds. M. Nevins, W. Becker, and K. Kornman, *Proceedings of the World Workshop in Clinical Periodontics,* Vol. 5, 1–21. Chicago: American Academy of Periodontology.

Katsanoulas, T., I. Renee, and R. Attström. 1992. The effect of supragingival plaque control on the composition of the subgingival flora in periodontal pockets. *J. Clin. Periodontol.* 19:760–765.

Kepic, T. J., T. J. O'Leary, and A. H. Kafrawy. 1990. Total calculus removal: An attainable objective? *J. Periodontol.* 61:16–20.

Kocher, T., and H. C. Plagmann. 1997. The diamond-coated sonic scaler tip: Part II: Loss of substance and alteration of root surface texture after different scaling modalities. *Int. J. Periodontics Restorative Dent.* 17(5):484–493.

Leon, L. E., and R.I. Vogel. 1987. A comparison of the effectiveness of hand scaling and ultrasonic debridement in furcations as evaluated by differential dark-field microscopy. *J. Periodontol.* 58:86–94.

Lindhe, J., S. S. Socransky, S. Nyman, and A. Haffajee. 1982. Critical probing depth. *J. Clin. Periodontol.* 9: 323–336.

Loos, B., N. Claffey, and J. Egelberg. 1988. Clinical and microbiological effects of subgingival debridement in periodontal furcation pockets. *J. Clin. Periodontol.* 15:453–463.

Lowenguth, R. A., and G. Greenstein. 1995. Clinical and microbiological response to nonsurgical mechanical periodontal therapy. *Periodontology 2000* 9:14–22.

Magnusson, I., J. Lindhe, T. Yoneyama, and B. Liljenberg. 1984. Recolonization of a subgingival microbiota following scaling in deep pockets. *J. Clin. Periodontol.* 11:193–207.

Moore, J., M. Wilson, and J. B. Kieser. 1986. The distribution of bacterial lipopolysaccharide (endotoxins) in relation to periodontal involved root surfaces. *J. Clin. Periodontol.* 13:748–751.

Mousques, T., M. A. Listgarten, and R. W. Phillips. 1980. Effect of scaling and root planing on the composition of the human subgingival microbial flora. *J. Periodont. Res.* 15:144–151.

Nakib, N. M., N. F. Bissada, J. W. Simmelink, and S. N. Goldstine. 1982. Endotoxin penetration into root cementum of periodontally healthy and diseased human teeth. *J. Periodontol.* 53:368–378.

Oberholzer, R., and K. H. Rateitschak. 1996. Root cleaning or root smoothing: An in vivo study. *J. Clin. Periodontol.* 23:326–330.

O'Hehir, T. E. 1999. Debridement 5 scaling and root planing plus. *RDH.* 14, 62.

O'Leary, T. J., and A. D. Kafrawy. 1983. Total cementum removal: A realistic objective. *J. Periodontol.* 54:221–226.

Oosterwaal, P. J., M. I. Matee, F. H. Mikx, M. A. van't Hof, and H. H. Renggli. 1987. The effect of subgingival debridement with hand and ultrasonic instruments on the subgingival microbflora. *J Clin Periodontol.* 14:528–533.

Palmer, R. M., and F. D. Floyd. 1995. Periodontology: A clinical approach: 3. Non-surgical treatment and maintenance. *Br. Dent. J.* 178:263–268.

Parashis, A. O., A. Anagnou-Vareltzides, and N. Demetriou. 1990. Calculus removal from multirooted teeth with and without surgical access: II. Comparison between external and furcation surfaces and effect of furcation entrance width. *J. Clin. Periodontol.* 20:294–298.

Rateitschak, P., J. Schwarz, R. Guggenheim, M. Duggelin, and K. Rateitschak. 1992. Nonsurgical periodontal treatment: Where are the limits? An SEM study. *J. Clin. Periodontol.* 19:240–244.

Renvert, S., M. Wikström, G. Dahlen, J. Slots, and J. Egelberg. 1990. Effect of subgingival debridement on the elimination of *Actinobacillus actinomycetemcomitans* and *Bacteroides gingivalis* from periodontal pockets. *J. Clin. Periodontol.* 17:345–350.

Robertson, P. B. 1990. The residual calculus paradox. *J. Periodontol.* 61:65–66.

Sbordone, L., L. Ramaglia, E. Gulletta, and V. Iacono. 1990. Recolonization of the subgingival microbiota after scaling and root planing in human periodontitis. *J. Periodontol.* 61:579–584.

Segelnick, S., and M.A. Weinberg 2006. Reevaluation of initial therapy: When is the appropriate time? *J. Periodontol.* 77:1598–1601.

Sherman, P. R., L. H. Hutchens, Jr., L. G. Jewson, J. M. Moriarty, G. W. Greco, and W. T. McFall, Jr. 1990. The effectiveness of subgingival scaling and root planing: I. Clinical detection of residual calculus. *J. Periodontol.* 61:3–8.

Smart, G. J., M. Wilson, E. H. Davies, and J. B. Kieser. 1990. The assessment of ultrasonic root surface debridement by determination of residual endotoxins levels. *J. Clin. Periodontol.* 17:174–178.

Somerman, M. J., S. Y. Archer, A. Shteyer, and R. A. Foster. 1987. Protein production by human gingival fibroblasts is enhanced by guanidine EDTA extracts of cementum. *J. Periodont. Res.* 22:75–77.

Stambaugh, R. V., M. Dragoo, D. M. Smith, and L. Carasali. 1981. The limits of subgingival scaling. *Int. J. Periodont. Restor. Dent.* 1(5):31–41.

Suvan, J.E. 2005. Effectiveness of mechanical nonsurgical pocket therapy. *Periodontology 2000* 37(1):48–71.

Umeda, M., Y. Takeuchi, K. Noguchi, Y. Huang, G. Koshy, and I. Ishikawa 2004. Effects of nonsurgical periodontal therapy on the microbiota. *Periodontology 2000* 36(1):98–120.

von Troil, B., I. Needleman, and M. Sanz. 2002. A systematic review of the prevalence of root sensitivity following periodontal therapy. *J. Clin. Periodontol.* 29(Suppl. 3):173–177.

Waerhaug, J. 1978. Healing of the dentoepithelial junction following subgingival plaque control: II. As observed on extracted teeth. *J. Periodontol.* 49:119–134.

Westfelt, E. 1996. Rationale of mechanical plaque control. *J. Clin. Periodontol.* 23:263–267.

Westfelt, E., H. Rylander, G. Dahlen, and J. Lindhe. 1998. The effect of supragingival plaque control on the progression of advanced periodontal disease. *J. Clin. Periodontol.* 25:536–541.

Wilson, T. G., Jr., J. Schoen, and P. Fallon. 1989. Removing toothborne dental deposits: Mechanical means by the professional. In ed. T. G. Wilson, Jr., *Dental maintenance for patients with periodontal diseases,* 67–96. Chicago: Quintessence.

Wylam, J. M., B. L. Mealey, M. P. Mills, T. C. Waldrop, and D. C. Moskowicz. 1993. The clinical effectiveness of open versus closed scaling and root planing on multirooted teeth. *J. Periodontol.* 64:1023–1028.

Zappa, U., J. P. Röthlisberger, C. Simona, and D. Case. 1993. In vivo scaling and root planing forces in molars. *J. Periodontol.* 64:349–354.

Chapter 24

Principles of Periodontal Surgery: Gingivectomy, Osseous Resection, and Periodontal Plastic Surgery

Mea A. Weinberg

OUTLINE

Introduction
Objectives, Indications, and Contraindications
  of Periodontal Surgery
Preoperative Preparation
Requirements for Periodontal Surgery
Types of Periodontal Surgery
Procedures for Pocket Reduction/Elimination
Procedures for Treating Osseous Defects
Periodontal Plastic Surgery
Sutures
Periodontal Dressing
Surgical and Postoperative Care
Effects of Surgical Procedures
Dental Hygiene Notes
Key Points
Self-Quiz
References

EDUCATIONAL OBJECTIVES

Upon completion of this chapter, the reader should be able to:

- Discuss the rationale for periodontal surgical therapy.
- Describe the indications and contraindications for periodontal surgical therapy.
- Compare and contrast the different surgical treatment modalities.
- Demonstrate postoperative care following periodontal surgery.
- Identify and explain the management of postoperative complications.
- Discuss surgical wound healing and how soon after surgery a reevaluation can be performed.

GOAL: To provide an understanding of the basic indications and principles of periodontal surgery and postoperative care.

KEY WORDS

flap surgery 368
gingivectomy 363
healing responses 365
mucogingival surgery
  363

periodontal dressing
  372
periodontal surgery 363
postoperative care 372

INTRODUCTION

The term *surgery* is a generic word to describe the branch of medical science concerned with the treatment of diseases or injuries by manual or operative means. Periodontal debridement (scaling and root planing) meets this definition, but it is not considered surgery. The term *periodontal surgery,* as used in the dental literature, is applied only to surgical procedures used to treat periodontal diseases or to modify the morphology of soft tissues and bone.

Different surgical procedures have been used to treat gingivitis and periodontitis, as well as to gain access to the underlying root surface and supporting bone.

OBJECTIVES, INDICATIONS, AND CONTRAINDICATIONS OF PERIODONTAL SURGERY

Over the past several years, subgingival scaling and root planing techniques and local and systemic antibiotic periodontal therapy have improved dramatically. Nevertheless, periodontal surgery remains a valid option for many patients. It is imperative for the dental hygienist to have a thorough knowledge of various basic periodontal surgical procedures as well as a clear understanding of the indications and contraindications of these procedures. This is particularly important upon consideration of the limitations of scaling and root planning. Egelberg (1995) reviewed these limitations, which include the fact that complete removal of subgingival calculus may not be predictably attainable after subgingival root planing. This was demonstrated in one study in which pockets with initial probing depths of ≥ 5 mm showed inadequately debrided root 65% of the time (Greenstein, 2000).

The primary objectives of periodontal surgery include the following (Palcanis, 1996):

- Reduction in the pocket depth, which allows the patient and the dental practitioner access for plaque control.
- In patients with very deep pockets and bone loss, to gain access to the root and underlying bone to achieve more effective removal of calculus and subgingival bacterial biofilm so as to maintain periodontal attachment levels and perhaps even gain "new attachment." New attachment is defined as the union of connective tissue with a root surface that has been deprived previously of its original attachment apparatus (American Academy of Periodontology, 2001).

- To regenerate periodontal tissues lost due to the disease.
- To arrest disease progression.
- To create an oral environment that is maintainable by both the patient and the dental team.

After the surgical procedures have been performed, the therapeutic end points of clinical success are measured by the attainment of stable or improved clinical attachment levels, minimal inflammation (bleeding on probing), and reduced and stable probing depths (Palcanis, 1996).

Indications for periodontal surgery include the following:

- Pocket elimination/reduction on teeth with gingival/periodontal pockets.
- Correction of mucogingival defects (e.g., for root coverage, increasing the zone of keratinized/attached gingiva, augmentation of alveolar ridges).
- To improve aesthetics—that is, aesthetic crown lengthening.
- Creation of a favorable restorative environment such as lengthening of the clinical crown.
- Placement of dental implants.
- Incision and drainage of a gingival or periodontal abscess.
- Regeneration of the attachment apparatus that was destroyed as a result of periodontal disease.

Periodontal surgical therapy is contraindicated or at least delayed for the following reasons:

- Systemic diseases that cannot be controlled by medications or otherwise, such as diabetes mellitus, cardiovascular conditions (e.g., hypertension).
- Systemic diseases that are associated with excessive bleeding, such as leukemia, hemophilia, and renal (kidney) dialysis (consult with the patient's physician).
- Patients taking anticoagulation medication (warfarin, heparin), which could result in extensive and difficult to control bleeding.
- Patients who are unable to undergo periodontal surgery.
- Patients taking intravenous bisphosphonates are not candidates for periodontal surgery.
- For patients taking oral bisphosphonates, use professional and clinical judgment; contact physician.

- Patients who are noncompliant with plaque control or periodontal maintenance appointments.
- Concern for cosmetic outcome (e.g., postsurgical gingival shrinkage), especially in anterior areas.
- Treating teeth that have hopeless prognoses.

Did You Know?

John M. Riggs originated a surgical technique for the treatment of pyorrhea alveolaris (periodontal disease) and contributed it to the Pennsylvania Journal of Dental Science in 1876. He was referred to as the "Father of Periodontal Surgery."

PREOPERATIVE PREPARATION

Preoperative management involving patient preparation for surgery includes removal of soft and hard deposits, reinforcement of oral hygiene self-care, selective occlusal adjustment, and selective adjunctive antimicrobial or antibiotic agents. It is important to complete initial therapy because this may eliminate the need for surgery or at least reduce or eliminate gingival inflammation, which will increase the manageability of the tissues during surgery and allow for better healing. Evaluation for surgery is done at a minimum of four to six weeks after completion of the initial phase of therapy. At this time, a soft tissue examination will determine the tissue healing or response to the initial therapy. An evaluation of the patient's oral hygiene status also is made. If there is residual calculus, additional sessions of periodontal debridement may be necessary. A complete periodontal charting is done, including identification and cause of bleeding sites and sites with clinical attachment loss (Carranza, 1996).

REQUIREMENTS FOR PERIODONTAL SURGERY

Specific requirements must be met before surgery is performed. Any uncontrolled or poorly controlled systemic disease (i.e., diabetes) should be addressed by referring the patient to his or her physician prior to surgery. Elimination of plaque-retentive restorations should be performed before surgery (e.g., overhanging margins of restorations or over-contoured restorations) (Flores-de-Jacoby & Mengel, 1995). Any carious lesions should be repaired and hope-

less teeth extracted. Necessary endodontic treatment should be performed prior to periodontal therapy. The hygienist and dentist should recommend a smoking cessation program to the patient prior to surgery. Smoking seems to alter the inflammatory response during healing. Risk factors such as smoking have been shown to delay wound healing after surgery (Boström, Linder, & Bergström, 1998; Persson, 2003; Preber & Bergström, 1990), and this may need to be addressed with the patient.

TYPES OF PERIODONTAL SURGERY

There are many types of surgical procedures, and selection of the appropriate surgery depends on the pattern of bone loss (e.g., horizontal versus vertical or a combination of both) and the presence of mucogingival involvement. Periodontal surgery usually is done in quadrants or sextants depending on the number of teeth involved and the decision of the surgeon. Most important, the practitioner and the patient should be aware of the limitations of periodontal surgery (Box 24–1).

Lang and Löe (1993) proposed a convenient classification of periodontal surgical procedures. It includes five categories:

1. Procedures for supragingival pocket reduction or elimination (gingivectomy).
2. Procedures for gaining access to root surfaces for debridement (periodontal flap surgery).
3. Procedures for treatment of osseous defects (flap surgery with osseous reduction).
4. Procedures for correcting mucogingival defects (periodontal plastic surgery).
5. Procedures for regeneration of lost periodontium (periodontal regeneration).

Box 24–1   Limitations of Periodontal Surgery

- Periodontal surgery does not compensate for the patient's poor plaque control.
- Some adverse effects from surgery include gingival recession, which may compromise aesthetics to some degree.
- It will not routinely produce miraculous and complete regeneration of all lost periodontal tissues.

Healing Following Periodontal Surgery

There are four types of **healing responses** of periodontal tissues that can occur after periodontal treatment (Carranza, 1996). Repair is the healing of periodontal tissues with tissues that do not replicate the original lost periodontium. After periodontal debridement and periodontal surgery, instead of the gingival connective tissue attaching to the tooth, the junctional epithelium reforms on the root surface by migrating along the root surface, forming a long junctional epithelium attachment. Another example of repair is scar formation, in which the new tissue formed is considered epithelium and connective tissue but does not replicate the original tissue that was lost or damaged. Reattachment is the reunion of epithelial or connective tissue to a root surface that was not damaged by periodontal disease. This would occur after an incision, or injury, or where a surgical flap has to be extended to a tooth with a healthy periodontium for better access. New attachment is the union of connective tissue or epithelium with a root surface that was deprived of its original attachment apparatus. Regeneration is the reformation of the periodontal tissues that were destroyed by periodontal disease with the formation of new cementum, periodontal ligament, and bone. This is the ideal treatment result and is the goal of various surgical procedures. However, it is not always attained. Rather, a partial regeneration or new attachment is more often obtained. Epithelium is the first tissue to move or migrate into the wound area. Epithelium migrates up to 0.5 mm a day, which is faster than connective tissue or bone cells. This can interfere with the formation of a new attachment or regeneration. General postoperative instructions are given in Box 24–2.

Box 24–2   General Postoperative Instructions

Discomfort	Usually, minimal discomfort is expected, especially after the anesthesia wears off. If you have been given a prescription, fill it and take the medication as directed. Aspirin should not be used. If discomfort persists, call the office.
Swelling	If swelling occurs, it will peak 48 to 72 hours after the surgery. You may use an ice pack on the outside of your face, 20 minutes on and 20 minutes off, for the next two hours. If swelling occurs after the first day, a moistened heated towel may be used on the area. If excessive swelling occurs, call the office.
Bleeding	There may be occasional blood stains in the saliva for the first four or five hours. This is not unusual; do not be alarmed. If bleeding continues, do not rinse to stop bleeding. Apply firm pressure using a moistened gauze pad or fresh tea bag for 20 minutes, without interruption. Repeat as necessary. If the bleeding does not stop, call the office.
Physical activity	It is recommended that you rest and limit your activities for the rest of the day. Avoid excessive exertion (jogging, swimming, tennis, etc.) for the next week.
Eating	Limit your diet to soft foods on the day of the surgery. Do not drink hot liquids (tea, coffee, soup) for 24 hours following surgery. Do not chew on the area where the surgery was performed. Avoid alcoholic beverages for one week following the surgery.
Sutures	If sutures were used, avoid that area. They will be removed approximately seven to fourteen days following surgery.
Dressing	To help minimize irritation, a periodontal dressing may be placed around the surgical area. It will harden within about two hours and should not be removed. It is of no concern if a few pieces of the dressing break off. However, if the dressing seems to be loose or has come off, contact the office for instructions.
Smoking	Do not smoke. Smoking may negatively affect the healing process, which may result in a poor outcome.
Home care	The most important element required for good healing is meticulous oral hygiene. If a dressing is placed, avoid pressing down on it. Use a soft or ultrasoft toothbrush to carefully clean the occlusal surface and the surface of the dressing. If no dressing was placed, gently use a soft or ultrasoft toothbrush to cleanse the area. Do not floss the surgical site. Brush and floss the untreated areas as usual. Do not rinse on the day of the surgery. On the second day, use the prescribed mouthrinse as directed.
Medications	In some cases, analgesics and/or antibiotics will be prescribed. Use prescribed medications as directed.

PROCEDURES FOR POCKET REDUCTION/ELIMINATION

Gingivectomy/Gingivoplasty

Definition

Gingivectomy is the excision or removal of the soft tissue walls (gingiva) in order to eliminate a pocket. Gingivoplasty, on the other hand, refers to surgical reshaping or recontouring of the oral surface of the gingiva without removing any portion of the gingiva that is attached to the tooth.

Indications

The main objectives of gingivectomy/gingivoplasty procedures are to reduce or eliminate suprabony periodontal pockets that are associated with horizontal patterns of bone loss and to eliminate pseudopockets (gingival enlargement) induced by certain medications, such as phenytoin, cyclosporine, valproic acid, and nifedipine (Bosco et al., 2006). Enlarged gingiva and interdental papillae seen in mouth breathers also can be treated with these techniques. Oftentimes, localized or generalized gingival enlargement is seen during pregnancy, which may or may not resolve postpartum. Surgery in these cases, unless the gingival overgrowth becomes infected or interferes with chewing, is delayed until a reevaluation is made postpartum. Frequently, the gingival enlargement will recur, and gingivectomy procedures may have to be repeated. Less frequently, lengthening of the clinical crown can be achieved using gingivectomy.

Contraindications

Contraindications for gingivectomy include lack of attached gingiva and the presence of infrabony pockets associated with vertical bone loss.

Technique

After the patient receives local anesthesia, the gingivectomy is begun by marking the base of the pockets with a periodontal probe or other instrument. Incisions are made with a surgical blade angled at 45 degrees to the gingiva slightly coronal to the base of the pocket (Figure 24–1 ■). Incisions are not made into the sulcus, but rather on the outer epithelium, with the blade directed in an occlusal or incisal direction rather than apically. Root debridement is performed followed by gingivoplasty to reestablish a physiologic gingiva. After hemostasis is obtained (bleeding is controlled), the area is dried, and a periodontal dressing is placed. The patient is given postoperative instructions. Postoperative instructions to the patient for this procedure are given in Table 24–1 ■. This includes care of the surgical wound, oral hygiene measures taken during initial healing, and reporting adverse signs and symptoms. The patient then returns in seven to ten days for a postoperative visit.

Healing

Epithelialization of the wound surface starts within a few days of surgery and usually takes seven to fourteen days depending on the size of the wound. Soft tissue healing

(a)

(b)

■ **FIGURE 24–1** (a) Clinical picture of a gingivectomy procedure. A 38-year-old patient with pseudopockets (gingival enlargement) due to phenytoin therapy. The incision is made apical to the bleeding points, which demarcate the base of the pocket. (b) After the incision is made, the tissue is removed, exposing the underlying bleeding connective tissue.

Table 24–1	Surgical Care Procedures	
Surgical Procedure	**Postoperative Care**	**Reevaluation Procedures**
Gingivectomy	1. Instruct patient not to brush the area where the periodontal dressing is located.	1. Periodontal probing should not be done until a minimum of six weeks after surgery.
	2. The area will heal by secondary intention; the wound is open and exposed because there is no flap and no sutures. This area is similar to a scraped knee or pizza burn on the palate. It will be sore.	2. Final prosthetic restorations should not be completed until six weeks or more after surgery.
	3. Avoid smoking, if possible.	
	4. At postoperative visit, carefully remove the dressing, irrigate with sterile water or saline and wipe off the white film (this consists of dead epithelial cells).	
	5. Reapply dressing if needed.	3. Supragingival scaling can be done after one week, but subgingival periodontal debridement should not be performed until six weeks after surgery.
	6. After the first postoperative visit, the patient may start to brush the teeth around the surgical site gently with a roll technique. Bleeding will occur but will gradually lessen. The patient should continue to brush even if light bleeding is seen.	
Flap surgery (with or without osseous resection)	1. Instruct patient not to brush the area where the periodontal dressing is located.	1. Periodontal probing should not be done until a minimum of three months after surgery.
	2. Apply ice pack.	
	3. At postoperative visit, carefully remove the dressing and sutures, irrigate with sterile water or saline and wipe off the white film (this consists of dead epithelial cells).	2. Final prosthetic restorations should not be completed until a minimum of three months after surgery.
	4. Reapply dressing if needed; patient may start to brush surgical site gently with a roll technique. Bleeding will occur but will gradually lessen. The patient should continue to brush even if bleeding is seen.	3. Supragingival scaling can be done after one week, but subgingival periodontal debridement should not be performed until three months after surgery.
	5. Avoid smoking, if possible.	

Table 24–1	Surgical Care Procedures (cont.)	
Surgical Procedure	**Postoperative Care**	**Reevaluation Procedures**
Mucogingival surgery (soft tissue grafts)	1. Instruct patient not to brush the area where the periodontal dressing is located.	1. Gingival grafts with root coverage would be reevaluated a minimum of six months after surgery.
	2. At postoperative visit, carefully remove the dressing and sutures at the donor site, irrigate with sterile water or saline and wipe off the white film (this consists of dead epithelial cells).	2. Gingival grafts without root coverage can be reevaluated a minimum of two months after surgery.
	3. Avoid smoking.	
	4. Reapply dressing if needed; patient may start to brush surgical site gently with a roll technique. Advise the patient not to hit the gums with the toothbrush. The patient should discontinue brushing if bleeding is seen and only rinse the area with warm water.	

is completed within four to five weeks, although clinically it may appear healed within two weeks. Clinically, it is important to avoid probing the area until the connective tissue has healed.

Did You Know?

The use of lasers in periodontal therapy is FDA approved only for sulcular debridement and not for surgery. Lasers deliver wavelengths. Using a laser instead of a scalpel is intended to increase coagulation (blood clotting) allowing for a dry surgical field and better visualization. (See American Academy of Periodontology, 2006.)

Periodontal Flap Surgery

A flap is defined as that loosened portion of the gingiva, alveolar mucosa, and/or periosteum that is separated from the underlying structures except at its base, from which the flap receives its blood supply. Flaps are the most commonly used periodontal surgical procedure. Flap procedures are designed to gain access to the underlying bone and root surface for the purpose of debridement, bone recontouring, or regeneration. Generally, a flap is made by an incision with a surgical blade or knife into the pocket (intracrevicular) or slightly subgingival to the gingival margin (internal bevel incision). The amount of attached gingiva present and the depth of the pockets primarily determine the type of incision made. The flap is then reflected away from the tooth with an instrument called a periosteal elevator to expose the underlying tooth and root surface.

Flap Classification

Flaps are classified on the basis of tissue components included in the flap and the positioning of the flap at the end of the procedure. In a full-thickness or mucoperiosteal flap, the gingiva, alveolar mucosa, and periosteum are reflected from the root and the underlying bone surfaces (Figure 24–2a ■). A partial- or split-thickness flap is a flap in which the periosteum and some connective tissue are left attached to the bone and is not included in the flap (Figure 24–3 ■). Partial-thickness flaps are used when the bone is thin and exposure to the environment is not desirable, since this would increase the chances of bone resorption. It is controversial if a partial-thickness flap results in less bone resorption. When the bone needs to be visualized, a full-thickness flap is required.

Based on the final positioning of the flap at the end of the surgical procedure, flaps are classified as replaced (e.g., modified Widman), apically positioned, coronally

(a)   (b)

■ **FIGURE 24–2**   (a) Full-thickness flap consists of the full thickness of mucosa and underlying connective tissue (periosteum) exposing the underlying bone. (b) Replaced flap postoperative.

(Gürgan, Orug, & Akkaya, 2004), and laterally positioned. The most frequently used periodontal flap procedures are the modified Widman flap and apically positioned flap.

Modified Widman Flap

Ramfjord and Nissle (1974) described the modified Widman flap (MWF) as a flap for better visualization of the area.

■ **FIGURE 24–3**   Split- or partial-thickness flap consists of the mucosa and submucosa but not the periosteum. Periosteum is left on the bone.

Objective   The specific objective of the MWF is to gain access to root surfaces for improved periodontal debridement and a reduction in inflammation and pocket depths.

Indications   The procedure is indicated for deep pockets, infrabony pockets, and where aesthetics is important, such as in the anterior region. An advantage of this procedure is direct visualization with debridement of deep pockets. Widman flap procedures also allow complete removal of pocket epithelium, and since the flaps can be placed in close approximation, healing takes place by primary intention. Healing of wounds occurs by primary, secondary, or tertiary intention. Primary intention occurs where the wound heals by fibrous adhesion (edges of flap approximate each other) without the formation of granulation tissue. A gingivectomy wound heals by secondary intention where the wound is left open. Healing by tertiary intention is usually used in surgical wounds complicated by infection whereby they must heal by contraction of the wound edges.

Contraindications   The MWF is contraindicated if there are bony defects that need to be recontoured or regenerated.

Technique   After adequate anesthesia is obtained, incisions are made through the crest of the gingiva approximately 1 mm from the margin (Figures 24–4 ■, 24–5 ■). This is called an inverse bevel incision. This

(a)

(b)

(c)

(d)

■ **FIGURE 24–4** Preoperative measurements on the maxillary canine: (a) 7 mm pocket on the mesiofacial and (b) 5 mm pocket depth on the mesiopalatal. (c) Buccal and palatal flaps allowed access to the underlying root and bone for root and defect debridement. (d) Flaps are replaced to their original position and sutured.

incision is scalloped and extended as far interproximally as possible to preserve the interdental papillae. Gingival tissues are then reflected only far enough to allow the surgeon direct vision of the root surfaces and the crest of bone. After complete debridement of plaque, calculus, and diseased tissue from the root surfaces and bony defects, the flaps are readapted to cover the crest of bone; flaps are replaced to their original position before the surgery. In some cases, bone recontouring is required for better flap adaptation. Interrupted interproximal sutures are then placed, and the surgical area is covered with a periodontal dressing. The patient receives postoperative instructions (Table 24–1). The dressing and sutures are removed after one week, and the patient is placed on a chlorhexidine mouthrinse.

Healing Following traditional flap surgery, the debrided root surface becomes repopulated with epithelial cells that form a long junctional epithelium along the root surface with no new connective tissue attachment (gingival fibers inserting into the cementum) (Figure 24–2b).

Apically Positioned Flap

An apically positioned flap is a full-thickness or split-thickness flap made with an internal bevel incision that following suturing is apically positioned at or near the level of the alveolar crest.

Objective The main objective is to surgically reduce or eliminate deep pockets by apically positioning the gingival complex while retaining the entire width of gingiva.

■ FIGURE 24–5 (a) Preoperative: Note amalgam overhang on the mesial of the premolar. The canine and lateral incisor were being prepared for crowns. (b) Intrasulcular incisions were placed and full-thickness flaps were reflected. The amalgam was recontoured. (c) The flaps were replaced and sutured to the original position.

Indications This procedure is used to (1) eliminate moderate or deep pockets by positioning the gingival tissue apically, (2) lengthen the clinical crown for restorative/prosthetic procedures, and (3) increase the zone of attached gingiva.

Contraindications The apically positioned flap is contraindicated where aesthetics is a concern, such as in the anterior region, where root exposure would be unaesthetic. This type of surgery is also contraindicated in patients at high risk for root caries. It is also contraindicated in areas of advanced bone loss.

Technique (Figures 24–6 ■, 24–7 ■) The apically positioned flap can be used on buccal surfaces of both mandibular and maxillary arches as well as on the mandibular lingual surface. The palatal gingiva cannot

be displaced or moved because it is composed entirely of keratinized gingiva without alveolar mucosa, which is what gives the flap its flexibility.

After obtaining adequate local anesthesia, a reverse (internal) bevel incision is made from the gingival margin to the crest of bone. The location of the initial incision in relation to the gingival margin depends on the width and thickness of the attached gingiva, as well as the depth of the pocket. The incision is scalloped interproximally to obtain optimal coverage of alveolar bone when the flaps are sutured. Vertical releasing incisions at the ends of the initial incision may be placed for flexibility and easier positioning of the flap apically. Next, a split-thickness flap is raised (coronally, a full-thickness flap is necessary if bone is to be contoured), and the incised gingival

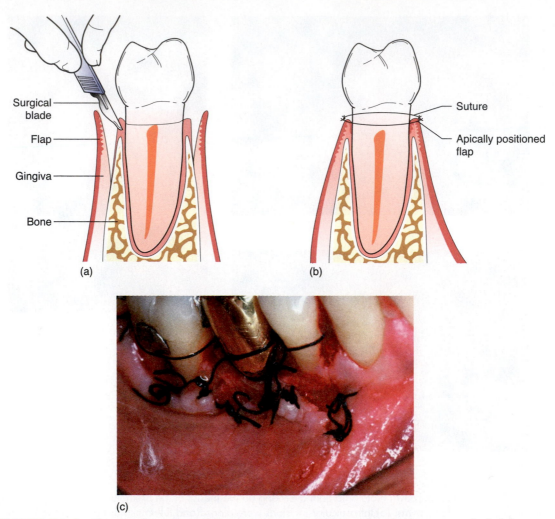

(a)   (b)

(c)

■ **FIGURE 24–6**   The apically positioned flap procedure. (a) An inverse bevel incision is made slightly api-cal to the free gingival margin and the flap is reflected from the alveolar process. (b) The flap is positioned apically and it is sutured. This procedure attempts to help eliminate or reduce the soft tissue pocket depth. Api-cally positioned flap eliminates deep pockets and increases the zone of attached gingiva. (c) In this case, the split-thickness flap is sutured apically exposing the tissue and bone, which when healed allows for an in-creased width of attached gingiva.

tissue collar is removed with a curet. Using power-driven scalers and hand instruments, diseased tissue is removed, and root and bony defect debridement is performed.

If bony defects are present, the bone can be recon-toured. Bone recontouring is done with a high-speed handpiece and/or hand chisels to establish a harmonious relationship between the gingiva and the bone. The flap is then positioned apically to cover the bone and is su-tured. A **periodontal dressing** can be applied.

Healing   The attachment or closure of the soft tissue to the root surface in the apically positioned flap is by a long junctional epithelium, with no new connec-tive tissue attachment. Complete healing occurs within 30 to 35 days. **Postoperative care** procedures are reviewed in Table 24–1 (Figure 24–2b).

Rapid Dental Hint

When removing the periodontal dressing, sometimes the sutures get embedded. Do not pull on the dressing. Carefully hold the dressing and see where the suture is buried and then cut the suture with scissors.

■ FIGURE 24–7 The apically positioned flap procedure. (a) Preoperative: Note mucogingival defects (no attached gingiva) on the anterior teeth. (b) An inverse bevel incision was made. (c) Split-thickness flap was reflected. (d) Apically positioned flap was sutured. (e) One week post-op: Note that the position of the flap allows for the underlying tissue to be exposed. This allows for new keratinized gingiva to granulate in.

PROCEDURES FOR TREATING OSSEOUS DEFECTS

Periodontal Flap Surgery with Osseous Resection

Periodontitis is a disease that involves loss of connective tissue attachment and loss of alveolar bone. This loss creates osseous defects and deformities leading to an uneven gingival architecture, which makes it difficult for the patient and the dental hygienist to maintain a healthy dentition. Osseous surgery is periodontal surgery involving modification of the bone supporting the teeth in order to eliminate pockets and obtain optimal physiologic gingival contours. The elimination or modification of bone defects can be either by resection or recontouring, which is removing bone, or by adding bone, which is termed periodontal regeneration (Figure 24–8 ■). Whether to perform osseous resection or periodontal regeneration depends on the type of osseous defect. This is reviewed in the following paragraph. Periodontal regeneration is discussed in Chapter 25.

Classification of Osseous Defects

The surgical approach (e.g., resection or regeneration) depends on the pattern of bone loss. There are two types of bone loss: horizontal and vertical.

In a suprabony pocket, the base of the pocket is coronal to the alveolar crest and the pattern of bone destruction is horizontal, where the bone height is reduced evenly between two adjacent teeth, creating flat interproximal bone or a horizontal pattern of bone loss (Figure 24–9 ■). On the other hand, in infrabony pockets, the base of the osseous defect is apical to the crest of the alveolar bone. The pattern of bone destruction is vertical (angular), where the bone is "scooped out" along the side of the root.

Intraosseous or infrabony (vertical) defects are classified according to the number of remaining osseous walls and by their predominant morphology: one-, two-, and three-wall defects (Figure 24–10 ■). Most infrabony defects are a combination of one–two- or two–three-wall morphology. Most infrabony defects are interproximal,

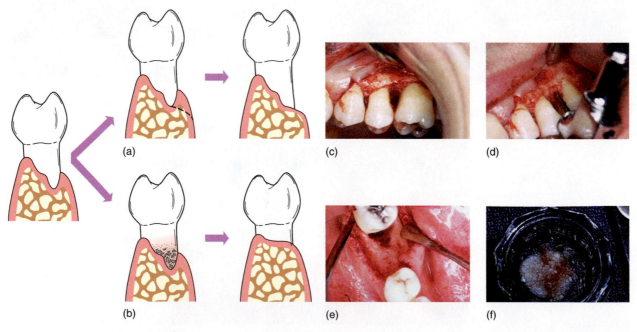

■ **FIGURE 24–8**   A periodontal bony defect is treated either by (a) reshaping or recontouring the bone (top diagram) or (b) filling in the defect (bottom diagram) with bone or a bone substitute (regeneration). (c) Flap reflected showing a two-wall bony defect inbetween the premolar and molar. (d) A high-speed round bur is used to do osseous recontouring to eliminate the defect. (e) This three-wall bony defect (the buccal, lingual, and mesial walls remain) on the mesial surface of the molar is best treated with a regenerative procedure. (f) Bone in the dappen dish is used to place into the infrabony defect.

(a)

(b)

(c)

■ **FIGURE 24–9**   (a) Horizontal pattern of bone loss between the premolars and second premolar and first molar. Interproximal bone (arrows) is destroyed on both sides of adjacent teeth equally. (b) *Left side:* Dry skull specimen showing furcation involvement (F) and vertical pattern of bone loss on the mesial aspect of the first molar. Note that the interproximal bone is not flat as with horizontal bone loss. (c) *Right side:* After the gingiva has been reflected from the tooth and bone, a vertical defect is seen on the mesial aspect of the first molar.

but they can be located on the direct facial or lingual surface. A crater is a specific type of two-wall defect in which the remaining osseous walls are the facial and lingual walls. A hemiseptal defect is a type of one-wall defect in which the remaining wall is usually the facial or lingual. A circumferential defect is a three-wall defect that wraps around the line angle of the tooth to involve the lingual or facial surface. Only by probing through the soft tissue pocket (bone sounding), but more precisely by surgical entry, can a determination of the type of infrabony defect be made.

Ostectomy and Osteoplasty

Ostectomy and osteoplasty are the two types of osseous recontouring during osseous surgery (Figure 24–11 ■). Ostectomy is the removal of supporting bone or bone that is in contact with the root, and osteoplasty is the reshaping or recontouring of nonsupporting bone or bone that is not in contact with the root (e.g., bony ledges) to achieve physiologic contours.

Objectives   The objectives of osseous resective surgery are to create optimal physiologic contours that reduce bony ledges or irregular contours in order to permit

(a)

(b)

(c)

(d)

■ **FIGURE 24–10**   (a) X-ray of three-wall defect; surgical entry. Note that the distal bony wall against the molar is destroyed. Thus, three walls remain: buccal, lingual, and mesial. (b) Surgical entry of a three-wall defect—the buccal, lingual, and distal walls remain. (c) Probing distal of canine. (d) Surgical entry shows a deep three-wall bony defect.

primary flap closure and to eliminate infrabony pockets by eliminating the bony walls of the defect.

Indications   Indications for osseous resective surgery include the following: (1) to permit optimal flap adaptation by removing bony ledges or exostosis, (2) to eliminate shallow infrabony pockets (1 to 2 mm deep), (3) to open furcations for easier maintenance, and (4) to lengthen crowns for restorative procedures (e.g., crowns).

Contraindications   Osseous resective surgery is contraindicated in the following situations: (1) Patients with advanced periodontitis (teeth in these patients already have compromised bone support; additional resection of tooth-supporting structures would be contraindicated); (2) aesthetics (removal of bone in aesthetic areas, especially the anterior maxillary area, will result in

an aesthetically unacceptable appearance); (3) isolated deep vertical defects (attempts to reduce or eliminate such defects would result in removing too much supporting bone from the adjacent tooth); and (4) the existence of local anatomic factors, such as the external oblique ridge, maxillary sinus, and flat palate limits achieving the intended results from osseous resection.

Technique   (Figure 24–12 ■) The patient receives local anesthesia. The flap is reflected from the root and bone. When the flaps are elevated, the alveolar crest and marginal bone are inspected. If the marginal bone is thick with ledges, osteoplasty is performed with burs on a high-speed handpiece with copious irrigation. If infrabony defects are present, ostectomy is performed with burs and hand instruments to flatten the interproximal bone. A

■ FIGURE 24–11 (a) Ostectomy removes bone attached to the tooth, which is called supporting bone. (b) Osteoplasty is the reshaping of the nonsupporting bone.

question arises to how much bone should be removed. The answer is enough bone is removed to eliminate or significantly reduce the depth of the defect but not enough to compromise the tooth or adjacent teeth. These procedures will create a harmonious environment for the alveolar process and the overlying gingiva. The apically positioned flap is the technique of choice when pocket elimination is anticipated. If desired, periodontal dressing may be placed over the surgical area. Postoperative instructions are given (Table 24–1).

Healing The soft tissue attachment to the root surface is by a long junctional epithelium. Healing also results in gingival recession with root exposure. Healing is complete by two to three months.

Rapid Dental Hint

A vertical releasing incision is used to gain better access during surgery.

Did You Know?

In 1949, Schluger was one of the first researchers that described the principles of resective osseous surgery.

Crown-Lengthening Procedures

Crown lengthening or crown extension is a surgical procedure designed to expose more tooth structure for restorative purposes (e.g., placement of a crown or other restoration) (Deas et al., 2004). Indications for crown lengthening are as follows: (1) a tooth that is fractured close to the gingival margin and/or alveolar crest and (2) subgingival caries.

Before surgery is performed, the concept of the biologic width must be considered. Biologic width is the soft tissue dimension that is occupied by the junctional epithelium and the gingival connective tissue attachment (gingival fibers). The average length of the junctional epithelium is 0.97 mm, and the average length of the gingival fibers is 1.07 mm, making the dimension of the biologic width approximately 2.04 mm. Thus, the biologic width is the soft tissue attachment from the base of the sulcus to the crest of alveolar bone. There must be enough length of root surface to allow for these two attachments. This distance is necessary for gingival health. The margin of a crown or other restoration should not be placed within this space. When a margin is placed less than 2 mm from the alveolar crest, it causes gingival inflammation and damage to the attachment apparatus. Bone resorption will then take place to reestablish this biologic width. Thus, if a tooth is fractured, a radiograph will indicate how close the most coronal part of the remaining tooth structure is to the alveolar bone. Osseous resective surgery may be indicated to create more exposed tooth structure and allow for reestablishment of soft tissue attachments and proper placement of restorative margins (Perez, Smukler, & Nunn, 2007) (Figure 24–13 ■).

Root Resection

In patients with substantial furcation involvements (class III or IV) with extensive bone loss around the roots of molar teeth and defective, decayed, or resorbed roots, root resection or hemisection may be indicated. Root resection or amputation is defined as the removal of a root while leaving the crown on a multirooted tooth (Figure 24–14 ■). Root resection is usually done on maxillary molars. Hemisection is the surgical sectioning and removal of one root and the crown portion and is usually done on mandibular molars that have a furcation involvement with severe bone loss around the root. If a molar is adequately stable with sufficient bony support but displays a class III or IV furcation involvement, a bisection or bicuspidization procedure can be done. This involves

■ FIGURE 24–12   (a) A horizontal and vertical releasing incision is made on the facial surface. (b) A full-thickness flap is reflected away from the bone. There is a furcation involvement on the first molar. Note the two bony protuberances called exostoses (singular: exostosis) on the facial surface. A two-wall bony crater exists between the premolar and molar. (c) Osteoplasty removed the exostoses, resulting in a thin, smooth, bony surface. Ostectomy removed the bony crater. (d) An apically positioned flap. The flap is moved in an apical position to the crest of bone to eliminate the depth of the pocket.

the sectioning or cutting of the molar in half, creating two separate teeth. Endodontics (root canal therapy) must be done before any of these procedures. The long-term survival of resected teeth is not predictable (Blomlof, Jansson, Ehnevid, & Lindskog, 1997).

PERIODONTAL PLASTIC SURGERY

The mucogingival relationship is important in sustaining the health of the gingival attachment. Mucogingival surgery is a periodontal surgical procedure used to correct defects in the morphology, position, and/or amount of gingiva.

Indications

Historically, the use of mucogingival surgical procedures was limited to treatment of gingival recession. A certain amount of attached gingiva was considered necessary to maintain gingival health and prevent further recession. However, several studies have shown that periodontal health can be maintained regardless of the width of attached gingiva (Salkin, Freedman, Stein, & Bassiouny,

(a)

(b)

(c)

■ FIGURE 24–13   (a) The premolar fractured due to caries. (b) Flap is elevated, and surgical removal of bone was necessary to lengthen the crown so a crown could be placed without impinging on the biologic width. (c) The flap was positioned apically and sutured.

Root resection
pre-surgical defect

(a)

Root amp

Root resection
affected root removed

(b)

■ FIGURE 24–14   Root resection: Surgical blade used to reflect the flap; buccal furcation involvement with bone loss of the mesiobuccal root of the mandibular first molar allows for the surgical resection of the mesiobuccal root.

1987; Wennström & Lindhe, 1983). Therefore, gingival augmentation is used in sites with inadequate width and thickness of attached gingiva that exhibit persistent inflammation (bleeding) or progressive recession and sites with inadequate dimensions of gingiva that have subgingival restorations or orthodontics. In sites where crown margins are to be placed subgingivally, recession with exposure of the crown margins may occur when there is inadequate gingival dimensions. Other indications for mucogingival procedures include (1) elimination of frenum and muscle pull at or near the gingival margin (Figure 24–15 ■), (2) areas in which the base of a periodontal pocket extends to or beyond the mucogingival junction, (3) deepening of the buccal vestibule, (4) aesthetic reasons (e.g., to cover exposed roots), and (5) modifications of edentulous ridges prior to prosthetic reconstruction.

Rapid Dental Hint

To recognize a mucogingival defect, probe the site and check where the mucogingival junction is located. If there is minimal to no attached gingiva and inflammation is present, the site should be assessed for mucogingival surgery to correct the defect. The patient should be referred to a periodontist.

Classification of Gingival Recession

The original classification of gingival recession by Sullivan and Atkins (1985) was later expanded by Miller (1985) (Figure 24–16 ■). The Miller classification includes: I: soft tissue recession not extending to the

(a)

(b)

(c)

■ **FIGURE 24–15** Frenectomy: (a) Note the lack of attached gingiva on the central incisors and the high frenum attachment that was pulling on the gingival margin. (b) A frenectomy using a split-thickness flap was performed. The frenectomy cuts the frenum, allowing it to relocate further apically. (c) One month postoperative.

■ FIGURE 24–16   P. D. Miller's classification of gingival recession.

mucogingival junction; II: isolated soft tissue recession that extends to or beyond the mucogingival junction with intact interdental papillae and no bone loss; III: soft tissue recession extending beyond the mucogingival junction with bone or soft tissue loss in the interdental area and; IV: extensive soft tissue recession and bone loss or soft tissue loss in the interdental area with malpositioned teeth.

> **Did You Know?**
>
> Smokers have less desirable long-term results following periodontal plastic surgery than nonsmokers.

Types of Soft Tissue Grafts

Mucogingival defects are corrected using different types of soft tissue grafts. In addition, guided tissue regeneration procedures also may be used for this purpose.

Pedicle Graft or Laterally Positioned Flap

The pedicle graft, as the name implies, is used to move gingiva from an adjacent tooth or edentulous area to a prepared recipient site on another tooth with an inadequate amount of attached gingiva. The pedicle graft is "freed" on three aspects but retains its attachment (blood supply) from its base. This procedure requires sufficient width and thickness of gingiva to be present in the donor site. There should be no underlying bone dehiscence or fenestration. The pedicle graft is best used for single-site recession for root coverage and augmentation (increasing the amount) of attached gingiva.

Technique   (Figure 24–17 ■) A V-shaped incision is made around the recipient site. Incised tissue is removed, and root planing of the root surface is performed. A full- or split-thickness flap is elevated on the tooth away from the defect and rotated to cover the defect. The flap is sutured, and pressure is applied (this is done with all soft tissue grafts) for about 4 to 5 minutes, ensuring that no blood clot has formed under the graft. A periodontal dressing to protect the flap can be placed. If a periodontal dressing is not used, the patient should not brush the area. Postoperative instructions are given to the patient (see Table 24–1), and the patient returns one to two weeks later. At the first postoperative visit, the sutures and the dressing are removed, and the area either may be left uncovered or may be redressed for an additional week.

Healing   Usually, clinical healing occurs in about one month. However, complete maturation can take up to one year.

Double Papillae Flap

The double papillae flap is a modification of the laterally positioned flap. The papillae from each side of the tooth with the defect are reflected and rotated over the midfacial aspect of the recipient tooth and sutured.

Free Gingival Soft Tissue Graft

Unlike a pedicle graft, a free gingival graft (FGG) has a donor site located away from the grafted site. Thus, the blood supply is not attached to the graft but depends on the recipient bed. The most common site for donor tissue is the palate, but in many cases, edentulous areas also can be used. Free gingival grafts are more predictable for augmentation of attached gingiva than for root coverage because significant shrinkage of the graft occurs during healing. Thicker free gingival grafts can be used for root coverage because there is less tissue shrinkage. Often, after a frenectomy a free gingival graft is placed at the site to prevent frenum reattachment.

Technique   (Figure 24–18 ■) After local anesthesia is administered on the palate and the recipient area,

■ **FIGURE 24–17** (a) Lateral incisor with severe gingival recession with root exposure. (b) A laterally positioned flap was used to move gingiva from the right central incisor to the left central incisor. An anchor suture is around the lateral incisor. (c) Two months healing shows good root coverage and increased width of attached gingiva.

split-thickness flaps are reflected at the recipient site. A piece of gingiva about 1.5 mm thick is obtained from an intraoral area. Although the most common donor site is the hard palate, edentulous areas also can be used. The donor tissue (graft) is placed on the recipient bed, and the graft is sutured in place, usually with absorbable sutures, making sure that it does not move, since this will interfere with the establishment of a blood supply from the recipient bed and the graft may fail. A periodontal dressing may be applied. Postoperative instructions are given, and the patient returns in one week (see Table 24–1). Smoking is strictly prohibited because soft tissue grafts are more likely to fail if the patient smokes. This was demonstrated by Miller (1987), where he found a

100% correlation between failure to obtain root coverage and heaving smoking. A major disadvantage of free gingival grafts is the poor color match between the graft and the existing gingiva.

Healing The graft will swell initially, then shrinkage occurs (Figure 24–18d). The graft receives blood and nutrients from the underlying connective tissue. Complete healing with keratinization occurs in about one month.

Subepithelial Connective Tissue Graft

The subepithelial connective tissue graft is the procedure of choice for root coverage of single or multiple teeth. The subepithelial connective tissue graft was first de-

(a)   (b)   (c)   (d)

■ **FIGURE 24–18**   (a) Mandibular central and right lateral incisors have no attached gingiva (Miller classification III) (b) A free gingival graft was harvested from the palate and (c) sutured into place at the recipient site. (d) Posttreatment healing of the grafted site. Increased width of attached gingiva was achieved. Note that root coverage was not obtained using this type of grafting procedure.

scribed by Langer and Calagna (1982) as having several advantages over the other grafts: (1) There is no open wound on the palate as in a free gingival graft, (2) the graft has a better blood supply coming from both the underlying connective tissue and the overlaying flap, and (3) better aesthetics and tissue and color blend are seen.

Indications   The subepithelial connective tissue graft may be used for both single and multiple adjacent

Rapid Dental Hint

The free gingival graft donor site will heal by secondary intention (open wound). It may be painful.

teeth with gingival recession and root exposure (Chambrone & Chambrone, 2006). It is limited by the amount of donor tissue able to be harvested.

Technique   (Figures 24–19 ■, 24–20 ■) After local anesthesia is obtained, a split-thickness flap is raised at the recipient site using a surgical blade. A flap is raised at the donor site on the palate, and connective tissue is harvested while leaving the epithelium on the outside of the flap. This palatal flap is sutured into place. The connective tissue is placed on the recipient site and sutured in place with absorbable sutures. A periodontal dressing may be applied. Postoperative instructions are given to the patient, and the patient returns in one to two weeks (see Table 24–1). At one to two weeks, the dressing and

■ FIGURE 24–19 (a) Pretreatment view of the mandibular right central incisor area. There is gingival recession and exposed root surfaces (Miller classification II). A connective tissue graft was selected to cover the root surfaces. (b) The subepithelial connective tissue graft was harvested from the palate. Incisions were made, and the epithelium was reflected. Note the vascular connective tissue underlying the epithelium. (c and d) The graft was sutured to the recipient site and the flap sutured. (e) Flap at donor site is sutured. (Courtesy of Dr. Jesse Sorrentino, New York University College of Dentistry)

(a)

(b)

(c)

(d)

■ **FIGURE 24–20**   (a) Pretreatment view of the maxillary canine. Miller classification II. Gingival recession occurs beyond the mucogingival junction. The patient complained that the area was sensitive to cold and was not aesthetic. (b) Incisions made on the palate to obtain subepithelial connective tissue. This is the donor site. (c) The connective tissue graft is sutured in placed and then covered by the flap. (d) Healing at two weeks. (Courtesy of Dr. James B. Fine, Columbia University College of Dental Medicine)

sutures are removed, and the area is either left uncovered or redressed for another week.

Healing   Healing occurs through a double blood supply. Both the connective tissue from the recipient site and the overlying flap aid in healing of the soft tissue graft. Complete healing occurs in approximately one month (Figure 24–20d).

Guided Tissue Regeneration for Root Coverage

Guided tissue regeneration (GTR) will be discussed further in Chapter 25. Essentially, GTR involves the use of a barrier membrane that is designed to prevent the gingival tissue from establishing contact with the root surface, creating a space for the formation of a new at-

tachment and new bone rather than a long junctional epithelial attachment. This concept was intended originally for the treatment of class II buccal furcation defects and certain infrabony defects. A newer application is for the treatment of gingival recession and for root coverage (Pini Prato et al., 1992).

Alloderm® is a biomaterial that is processed from human tissue. The process removes all epidermal and dermal cells (acellular dermal matrix), while preserving the remaining biological dermal matrix. All cells are removed to remove the risk of rejection or inflammation. This material is indicated for recession defects and for periodontal sites that have little to no attached gingiva where the goal is to increase the amount of keratinized/attached gingiva and to obtain root coverage (Gapski, Parks, & Wang, 2005; Tal, Moses, Zohar, Meir, & Nemcovsky, 2002).

AlloDerm is used in a similar way that a tissue graft from the patient's mouth (e.g., free gingival graft or connective tissue graft) is used except there is no harvesting of donor tissue (e.g., palatal tissue) and thus less pain is involved. At the time of surgery, AlloDerm is rehydrated in sterile saline before it is sutured in place on the recipient bed. AlloDerm acts like a scaffold to support regeneration of the patient's own tissue. Six to eight months postsurgery, AlloDerm becomes integrated into the patient's own soft tissue. A surgical case using AlloDerm is presented in Figure 24–21 ■.

A clinical study showed that treatment with a coronally positioned graft plus AlloDerm significantly in-creased gingival thickness when compared with a coronally positioned flap alone. Coverage of a recession defect was significantly improved with the use AlloDerm (Woodyard et al., 2004).

Technique After local anesthesia is obtained, a full-thickness flap is raised at the recipient site. Root planing is completed on the root surface. A barrier membrane is placed over the recession and bone and sutured. The flap is positioned coronally covering both the membrane and the enamel. If the membrane is resorbable, it is not removed and will resorb in about six to eight weeks after surgery. The flap sutures are removed after two to four weeks. Patients should not brush the area for at least six weeks and are recommended to rinse with chlorhexidine gluconate.

(a)

(b)

(c)

(d)

■ **FIGURE 24–21** (a) Preoperative view of the mandibular right quadrant. Note the gingival recession (Miller Classification I). (b) Flap reflected exposing underlying bone. (c) Placement of AlloDerm at recipient site. Flap sutured in place, covering the AlloDerm. (d) Three weeks post-op. Note the root coverage obtained.

SUTURES

Sutures are used to co-apt or closely adapt a flap to a tooth surface until the wound has healed sufficiently to withstand normal functional stresses. Closure of the wound provides good hemostasis and covers exposed bone. Suture material is broadly classified as absorbable or nonabsorbable and synthetic or nonsynthetic. Absorbable sutures are absorbed by the healing tissues by the breakdown process of hydrolysis (process by which water gradually penetrates the suture filaments, causing the breakdown of the suture's polymer chain) or proteolysis (process by which the suture filaments are absorbed by protein [salivary] enzymes and then digested by body enzymes). Nonabsorbable sutures do not get absorbed and remain in the tissues until removed (Table 24–2 ■).

Absorbable Sutures

Surgical gut is a natural material from the intestines of sheep or cows and is absorbable. Surgical gut is not too strong and is hard to handle, getting knotted easily. Chromic gut is plain gut that has been treated with chromic salts, which make it more resistant to absorption. Through proteolysis, enzymes in saliva will absorb surgical gut sutures within seven to ten days and chromic gut in about fourteen days. However, depending upon the patient's saliva, sutures may still be seen up to two to four weeks later.

The other type of absorbable suture is synthetic. These sutures are easier to handle, the knot will not loosen easily, and they cause less tissue irritation and inflammation than surgical gut because of the more reliable, constant rate of absorption through hydrolysis. Resorption of sutures begins between ten and fifteen days and is usually completed in twenty-eight to seventy days.

Nonabsorbable Sutures

Silk, a type of nonabsorbable natural suture, is the most frequently used suture material because of its ease in handling and superior visibility. Silk sutures can elicit tissue inflammation, so they should be removed not later than ten days after surgery. If sutures need to be left in place for several weeks, absorbable sutures are recommended.

Table 24–2	Suture Materials Used in Periodontics	
Material	**Synthetic/Nonsynthetic**	**Product Name**
Nonabsorbable Sutures		
Silk	Nonsynthetic (natural)	PERMA-HAND
		Black Silk
Nylon	Synthetic	Ethilon
Polyester	Synthetic	Ethibond
		Green polyester
e-PTFE (expanded polytetrafluoroethylene)	Synthetic	Gore-Tex
Absorbable Sutures		
Plain gut	Natural	Plain gut
Chromic gut	Natural	Chromic gut
PGA (Polyglycolic acid)	Synthetic	Absorbex
PGA-FA (FA refers to fast absorption)	Synthetic	PGA-FA
Poliglecaprone 25	Synthetic	Monocryl
Polygalactin 910	Synthetic	Vicryl

Rapid Dental Hint

It is important to obtain hemostasis (stoppage of bleeding) before suturing.

Needles

Needle and suture material come in various sizes. Needles also are classified according to their shape and curvature. Needles are available in a 1/4-, 3/8-, 1/2-, and 5/8-inch circle, with 3/8- or 1/2-inch being employed most commonly in periodontal surgery. Suture size is classified numerically. An increase in the number indicates a decrease in the diameter of the suture. Thus 4-0 and 3-0 sutures are used most often in periodontal flap surgery. The 6-0 and 5-0 sutures are smaller and are used in more delicate mucogingival surgical procedures such as soft tissue grafts (Hutchens, 1995).

Suturing Techniques

Suturing technique varies among surgeons. Basically, there are different ways to tie the suture. The most common and simplest suture is the interrupted suture, which is tied with a square or surgeon's knot (Figure 24–22 ■). After the needle engages the buccal and lingual gingiva,

Did You Know?

Natural materials doctors used in ancient times were flax, hair, grass, cotton, silk, pig bristles, and animal gut.

■ **FIGURE 24–22** Interrupted (simple loop) sutures (interproximal) using 4-0 silk.

it should be tied on the buccal rather than the lingual so that it is easier to remove and the sutures are in a more protected area. When tying a suture, leave about a 2 mm end. Other types of sutures include continuous sutures, mattress sutures, and sling sutures (Figure 24–23 ■). Mattress technique is usually used in areas where tension-free flap closure cannot be accomplished (Silverstein, 1999). Mattress suturing techniques generally are used to resist muscle pull and to adapt the tissue flaps tightly to the underlying structures (e.g., bone graft, tissue graft, alveolar ridge, regenerative membrane, or dental implant) (Silverstein and Kurtzman, 2005). Continuous sutures can be used to attach two surgical flap edges or to secure multiple interproximal papillae of one flap independently of the other flap (Silverstein and Kurtzman, 2005). The disadvantage of using continuous sutures is that there is only

(a)

(b)

■ **FIGURE 24–23** (a) Horizontal mattress suture using 4-0 silk. (b) Continuous suture using one knot.

Rapid Dental Hint

Remember to knot the suture from the buccal because it is easier to see and remove later.

one knot and if the knot or loop breaks the entire surgical site will be compromised.

The number of sutures placed should be documented in the chart. When the patient returns for the postoperative visit, count the number of sutures before removing them. This will verify that all sutures were removed. Sutures should be removed by gently holding the knot with collage pliers in your nondominant hand while using scissors to cut the suture by the knot. The suture is then gently pulled through the tissue to remove it.

Did You Know?

Suture manufacturing comes under the control of the Food and Drug Administration (FDA) because sutures are classified as medical devices.

PERIODONTAL DRESSING

In today's clinical practice, periodontal dressings are of the noneugenol type that does not cause irritation or burning to the tissue or bone. The primary purpose of using a periodontal dressing over a surgical area is for patient comfort. Periodontal dressings also protect the wound area after surgery. Some practitioners prefer not to use a dressing because the dressing creates an anaerobic (nonoxygen) area under itself that favors the growth of pathogenic microorganisms. However, this theory has not been proven.

The most widely used noneugenol dressing is a COE-pak® (GC America, Inc., Alsip, IL). It is supplied in two tubes: the accelerator tube and the base tube. Equal amounts of dressing from each tube are mixed for 30 to 45 seconds. In the hard and fast set, the working time is about 5 to 8 minutes; in the regular set, it is 10 to 15 minutes. The material is then formed into a strip. Hemostasis should be achieved before the dressing is applied, and the area should be dried. The end of the facial strip is wrapped around the distal aspect of the last tooth and meets with the lingual strip. Finger pressure is applied interproximally to wedge the dressing into place. A dressing placed on a surgical site should not overextend onto the gingiva, vestibule, or occlusal surfaces (Figure 24–24). Any excess dressing should be trimmed with a curet.

A light-cured periodontal dressing is available (Barricaid™, Dentsply International, Inc., Milford, DE). It is transparent and is used frequently on anterior areas where aesthetics are a concern. The material is first applied to the area (which does not necessarily have to be completely dry) and then is light-cured.

Rapid Dental Hint

Sometimes putting petrolatum (Vaseline) on your fingers will help prevent the dressing from sticking.

SURGICAL AND POSTOPERATIVE CARE

The dental hygienist plays an important role in the postoperative care of patients.

Surgical Complications

Syncope is defined as a temporary loss of consciousness caused by a loss of blood flow to the brain. Patients have been known to faint before, during, or after surgical procedures. If a patient faints, treatment should be stopped and the patient positioned with the head lower than the body. The patient's vital signs, including blood pressure, respiration, and pulse, should be monitored. Oxygen can be administered if necessary. Causes for patient syncope include fear or anxiety about the procedure, the site of blood, pain, or low blood sugar.

■ **FIGURE 24–24** Placement of a periodontal dressing. The packing should not interfere with occlusion or impinge on the gingiva.

Immediately after the administration of a local anesthetic containing epinephrine, patients may complain of a fast heartbeat or begin to shake or shiver. This is caused by the inadvertent injection of the anesthetic solution into a vein rather than a nerve. Keep the patient calm by reassuring that this will pass very soon and in most cases the patient will be fine. To prevent this situation, it is essential to aspirate while injecting.

During periodontal surgery, bleeding will occur because blood vessels are severed and the diseased tissue is vascular. Small blood vessels will be severed or broken when making incisions. However, it is important not to severe certain arteries such as the greater palatine artery in the maxillary palatal area. Once the diseased tissue is removed and the flaps are raised, bleeding should diminish. Excessive bleeding is controlled by finding the source of the bleeding and applying pressure by administering a vasoconstrictor (e.g., lidocaine 2% with 1:50,000 epinephrine) or by tying the offending artery.

It is important to avoid unnecessary or excessive hemorrhaging or bleeding. The patient's medical history should be evaluated carefully and updated to help avoid these situations. For example, a patient may be taking aspirin every day or even several times a week as a preventive measure for stroke. Aspirin (acetylsalicylic acid) binds to platelets and inhibits the formation of prostaglandins, resulting in a prolonged bleeding time that lasts for approximately seven days, until new platelets are formed. A similar situation occurs with nonsteroidal anti-inflammatory drugs such as ibuprofen. It is best to consult with such a patient's physician before performing surgery for patients taking these drugs.

Postoperative Complications

After periodontal surgery, the patient is given a number of written suggestions and instructions. These instructions must be reviewed carefully with the patient before he or she is allowed to leave the office. An example of postoperative patient instructions is given in Table 24–1. During the first postoperative week, the patient may experience swelling, pain, and sensitivity; these are usually mild and transient. Swelling generally can be controlled by the use of ice packs for the first day. An ice pack should be applied extraorally 20 minutes on and 20 minutes off for the first day. If swelling continues, the patient should switch to warm packs. Swelling can be due to soft tissue inflammation from the surgical procedure or an infection. If swelling continues, advise the pa-

tient to return to the office. Pain is usually due to swelling. If there is severe pain, the patient should return to the office. The patient may be given systemic antibiotics and analgesics (pain medication). The dental hygienist should confirm that the patient is taking the appropriate medications as prescribed. The patient should be asked if he or she is taking any over-the-counter medications, vitamins, or herbal remedies.

The patient may complain of seeing blood in the mouth for a few hours after the surgery. Most of the time this is residual blood in the saliva probably remaining on the tongue after surgery. If there is frank bleeding coming from the surgical site, the patient should apply pressure to the site and return to the office as soon as possible. Rinsing should not be done because it will prevent a blood clot from forming.

Oral Hygiene Instructions

Maintenance of the surgical area is important, and the dental hygienist must instruct the client on proper care (see Table 24–1). It has been demonstrated that regardless of the type of surgery performed (i.e., gingivectomy, MWF, or osseous recontouring), all will fail and probing depths recur if plaque control is not meticulously controlled following surgery (Nyman, Lindhe, & Rosling, 1977). Vigorous toothbrushing and flossing should not be done until healing is complete, yet it must be stressed to patients that removal of dental plaque is important for healing. The period of time the patient refrains from toothbrushing varies with each surgeon. While a periodontal dressing is in place, the patient should not brush that area. Rinsing with chlorhexidine gluconate is recommended. After the dressing and sutures are removed, patients are instructed to brush gently with a roll technique. Gradually, as healing occurs, regular brushing can be resumed. After surgery, the interdental papillae are usually absent or blunted, creating large gingival embrasures. Plaque removal in these areas is best accomplished with an interdental brush (single-tuft brush). Also, plaque removal on teeth with Class III/IV furcation involvement is best with a single-tuft brush. If no large interdental spaces develop after surgery, the patient can continue to use dental floss or a small interdental brush.

Postoperative Visit Management

The dental hygienist may be called on to attend to a patient at the first postoperative visit. Box 24–2 describes various reevaluation procedures that may be performed at this visit. At the seven- to ten-day postoperative visit, the dressing and sutures are removed. After the dressing is carefully removed, the number of sutures are counted and compared with the number of documented sutures placed at the time of the surgery. Frequently, parts of or all of the periodontal dressing may have come off during the week. When the dressing is removed, care must be taken not to pull the sutures. If the sutures are being pulled by the dressing, cut the interfering sutures before the dressing is further removed. Once the dressing is removed, a white layer can be seen on the tissue surface. This represents dead epithelial cells. A moistened (with water, saline, or chlorhexidine) cotton-tipped applicator is used to carefully cleanse the area. Following suture removal, the area is again thoroughly irrigated with water or saline. Only supragingival debridement should be performed; subgingival debridement should be postponed until complete healing has occurred. The decision to apply another dressing to the area depends on the amount of discomfort the patient is experiencing and the rate of healing.

EFFECTS OF SURGICAL PROCEDURES

As a consequence of surgery, several problems may arise. Patients should be informed about these adverse side effects before surgery. All patients also should sign an informed consent form.

Tooth Mobility

Tooth mobility may increase immediately after surgery and may not return to preoperative levels for as long as six months. The patient should be told that this is a normal consequence of surgery. Increased tooth mobility is due to the extension of inflammation into the periodontal ligament and to the surgical manipulation. The occlusion should be checked to verify that there is no occlusal trauma. Any occlusal interferences should be eliminated. Check for fremitus to help determine occlusal interferences.

Gingival Recession: Dentinal Hypersensitivity and Root Caries

Gingival recession with longer clinical crowns may occur after surgery. With exposure of the root surface, the patient may experience dentinal hypersensitivity and can develop root caries due to demineralization.

Maintaining adequate plaque control can reduce both the sensitivity and risk for root caries. For immediate hypersensitivity relief, an in-office application of DentinBloc® (Colgate Oral Pharmaceuticals, New York) or Seal and Protect® (Dentsply, Pa) is done. Other in-office desensitizing products are available, including chemical agents (oxalates, fluorides), sealants, and bonding agents. Reducing plaque accumulation is important for reducing hypersensitivity.

It is also helpful for the patient to use at home a dentifrice containing potassium nitrate (Sensodyne®). Unfortunately, the use of dentifrices is controversial, and they may take several weeks to have a positive effect. Once the patient has relief from the hypersensitivity, he or she can start to use the regular dentifrice but should return to the desensitizing dentifrice if the sensitivity returns. An over-the-counter 0.4% stannous fluoride gel (Gel-Kam®, Colgate Oral Pharmaceuticals) that is applied to the toothbrush may reduce dentinal hypersensitivity and prevent demineralization of the exposed root surfaces. A 0.63% stannous fluoride oral rinse (Gel-Kam® Oral Care Rinse, Colgate Oral Pharmaceuticals) is available by prescription for patient use at home. Adverse effects of stannous fluoride include staining of the dentin and stinging of the soft tissue.

DENTAL HYGIENE NOTES

The range of treatment alternatives for periodontitis is wide. The type of treatment depends on a number of factors, including the patient's level of plaque control, the type of gingival or periodontal pocket, and the type of periodontal defect. Careful assessment and planning of a case are important in the overall surgical treatment.

KEY POINTS

- Periodontal flap surgery is indicated for increasing access to the underlying root and bone in deeper periodontal pockets.
- The patient must be able to maintain excellent plaque control before periodontal surgery is performed.
- The therapeutic clinical end point of success for surgical pocket therapy is an oral environment that is easily maintainable by the patient and the clinician; there should be minimal inflammation (bleeding) and minimal probing depths.
- Cigarette smoking adversely affects the outcome of surgery.

SELF-QUIZ

1. All of the following factors are indications for periodontal surgery except one: (p. 363)
   a. Maintain teeth with a hopeless prognosis
   b. Pocket elimination
   c. Arrest disease progression
   d. Gain access to underlying bone

2. Which one of the following healing responses is usually seen after periodontal flap surgery? (p. 365)
   a. New bone, cementum, and periodontal ligament
   b. New bone and cementum
   c. Long junctional epithelium
   d. Connective tissue attachment

3. Which one of the following surgical procedures is indicated for gingival enlargement in a patient who is taking phenytoin? (pp. 364, 366)
   a. Mucogingival
   b. Gingivectomy
   c. Periodontal flap
   d. Excisional new attachment

4. When placing sutures, the knot is usually tied on the palatal surface because this is a protected area. (p. 388)
   a. Both the statement and the reason are correct and related.
   b. Both the statement and the reason are correct but not related.
   c. The statement is correct, but the reason is not.
   d. The statement is not correct, but the reason is correct.
   e. Neither the statement nor the reason is correct.

5. After periodontal surgery, which one of the following hygiene aids is best recommended to clean exposed furcations? (p. 390)
   a. Dental floss
   b. Manual toothbrush
   c. Powered toothbrush
   d. Single-tuft brush

6. Which one of the following surgical procedures is best recommended for augmenting the amount of attached gingiva and covering exposed root surfaces before a patient undergoes orthodontic treatment? (pp. 382–385)
   a. Gingivectomy
   b. Connective tissue graft
   c. Modified Widman flap
   d. Crown lengthening

7. Which one of the following immediate measures should be advised to a patient who calls the office two days after periodontal surgery and states that he or she has bleeding from the surgical site? (pp. 389–390)
   a. Rinse with warm saltwater
   b. Lie down on a couch
   c. Remove the packing
   d. Apply pressure

8. Which of the following is the primary objective of periodontal flap surgery? (p. 363)
   a. Gain access to the bone and root surface
   b. Augment the amount of free gingiva
   c. Provide easy-to-maintain areas
   d. Allow for healing by regeneration

9. A patient has experienced some root sensitivity in the area of flap surgery. Which one of the following recommendations can the dental hygienist make to alleviate the pain? (p. 391)
   a. Floss the area
   b. Rinse with a nonfluoride mouthrinse
   c. Rinse and brush with a baking soda solution
   d. Meticulous plaque control

10. All the following adverse effects the patient should be informed about before periodontal surgery is performed except one. Which one is the exception? (p. 391)
    a. Dental hypersensitivity
    b. Gingival recession
    c. Tooth mobility
    d. Root caries
    e. Open bite

REFERENCES

American Academy of Periodontology. 2001. *Glossary of periodontal terms,* 4th ed. Chicago: Author.

American Academy of Periodontology. 2006. Position paper: Lasers in periodontics: A review of the literature. *J. Periodontol.* 77:545–564.

Blomlof, L., L. Jansson, H. Ehnevid, and S. Lindskog. 1997. Prognosis and mortality of root-resected molars. *Int. J. Periodontics Restorative Dent.* 17(2):190–201.

Bosco, A. F., S. Bonfante, D. S. Luize, G. M. D. Bosco, and V. G. Garcia. 2006. Periodontal plastic surgery associated with treatment for the removal of gingival overgrowth. *J. Periodontol.* 77(5):922–928.

Boström, L., L. E. Linder, and J. Bergström. 1998. Influence of smoking on the outcome of periodontal surgery: A 5-year follow-up. *J. Clin. Periodontol.* 25:194–201.

Carranza, F. A., Jr. 1996. The surgical phase of therapy. In eds. F. A. Carranza, Jr., and M. G. Newman, *Clinical periodontology,* 565–569, 584–587. Philadelphia: W. B. Saunders.

Chambrone, L.A., and I. Chambrone. 2006. Subepithelial connective tissue grafts in the treatment of multiple recession-type defects. *J. Periodontol.* 77(5):909–916.

Deas, D. E., A. J. Moritz, H. T. McDonnell, et al. 2004. Osseous surgery for crown lengthening: A 6-month clinical study. *J. Periodontol.* 75(9):1288–1294.

Egelberg, J. 1995. Effectiveness of subgingival scaling and root planning. In *Periodontics the scientic way. Synopses of human clinical studies,* 2nd ed., 71–90. Malmo, Sweden: OdontosSience.

Flores-de-Jacoby, L., and R. Mengel. 1995. Conventional surgical procedures. *Periodontology 2000.* 9:38–54.

Gapski, R., C. A. Parks, and H. L. Wang. 2005. Acellular dermal matrix for mucogingival surgery: A meta-analysis. *J. Periodontol.* 76(11):1814–1822.

Greenstein, G. 2000. Nonsurgical periodontal therapy in 2000. A literature review. *J. Am. Dent. Assoc.* 131:1580–1592.

Gürgan, C. A., A. M. Oruç, and M. Akkaya. 2004. Alterations in location of the mucogingival junction 5 years after coronally positioned flap surgery. *J. Periodontol.* 75(6):893–901.

Hutchens, J. L., Jr. 1995. Periodontal suturing: A review of needles, material, and techniques. *Postgrad. Dent.* 2(4):3–14.

Lang, N. P., and H. Löe. 1993. Clinical management of periodontal diseases. *Periodontology 2000* 2:128–139.

Langer, B., and L. Calagna. 1982. The subepithelial connective tissue graft: A new approach to the enhancement of anterior cosmetics. *Int. J. Periodont. Rest. Dent.* 2:22–23.

Miller, P. D. 1985. A classification of marginal tissue recession. *Int. J. Periodont. Rest. Dent.* 5:15–37.

Miller, P. D. 1987. Root coverage with free gingival grafts. Factors associated with incomplete coverage. *J. Periodontol.* 58:674–681.

Nyman, S., J. Lindhe, and B. Rosling. 1977. Periodontal surgery in plaque infected dentitions. *J. Clin. Periodontol.* 4:240–249.

Palcanis, K. G. 1996. Surgical pocket therapy. *Ann. Periodontol.* 1:589–617.

Perez, J. R., H. Smukler, and M. E. Nunn. 2007. Clinical evaluation of the supraosseous gingivae before and after crown lengthening. *J. Periodontol.* 78(6):1023–1030.

Persson, G. R., L. A. Mand, J. Martin, and R. Page. 2003. Assessing periodontal disease risk. *J Am Dent Assoc.* 134(5):575–582.

Pini Prato, G., C. Clauser, P. Cortellini, C. Tinti, G. Vincenzi, and U. Pagliaro. 1992. Guided tissue regeneration versus mucogingival surgery in the treatment of human buccal gingival recession. *J. Periodontol.* 63:919–928.

Preber, H., and J. Bergström. 1990. Effect of cigarette smoking on periodontal healing following surgical therapy. *J. Clin. Periodontol.* 17:324–328.

Ramfjord, S. P., and R. R. Nissle. 1974. The modified Widman flap. *J. Periodontol.* 45:601–607.

Salkin, L. M., A. L. Freedman, M. D. Stein, and N. A. Bassiouny. 1987. A longitudinal study of untreated mucogingival defects. *J. Periodontol.* 58:164–166.

Silverstein, L. H. 1999. *Principles of dental suturing: The complete guide to surgical closure.* Mahwah, NJ: Montage Media.

Silverstein, L. H., and G. M. Kurtzman. 2005. A review of dental suturing for optimal soft-tissue management. *Compendium* 2(3):163–169.

Sullivan, H. C., and J. H. Atkins. 1968. Free autogenous gingival grafts: I. Principles of successful grafting. *Periodontics* 16:121–129.

Tal, H., O. Moses, R. Zohar, H. Meir, and C. Nemcovsky. 2002. Root coverage of advanced gingival recession: A comparative study between acellular dermal matrix allograft and subepithelial connective tissue grafts. *J. Periodontol.* 73:1405–1411.

Wennström, J. L., and J. Lindhe. 1983. Role of attached gingiva for maintenance of periodontal health. *J. Clin. Periodontol.* 10:206–221.

Woodyard J. G., H. Greenwell, M. Hill, C. Drisdo, J. M. Iasella, J. Scheetz. 2004. The clinical effects of acellular dermal matrix on gingival thickness and root coverage compared to coronally positioned flap alone. *J. Periodontol.* 75:44–56.

Principles of Periodontal Surgery: Periodontal Regeneration

Stuart J. Froum

OUTLINE

Introduction
Periodontal Regenerative Surgery
Biologics and Devices
Bone Grafts and Bone Substitutes:
   Surgical Procedure
Guided Tissue Regeneration
Regenerative Surgery: Postoperative Care
Root Surface Treatment
Risk Factors for Regenerative Therapy
Dental Hygiene Notes
Key Points
Self-Quiz
References

GOAL: To provide an understanding of the basic principles of periodontal surgical regeneration.

KEY WORDS

allograft **396**
alloplast **396**
autograft **396**
barrier membrane **404**
bone grafts **396**
bone substitutes **396**
growth factors **398**

guided tissue
   regeneration (GTR)
   395
periodontal
   regeneration **395**
xenograft **396**

EDUCATIONAL OBJECTIVES

Upon completion of this chapter, the reader should be able to:

- Describe the process of periodontal regeneration, including the type and origin of cells involved in the regenerative process.
- Describe the different bone grafts and bone substitutes that are used in periodontal regeneration.
- Discuss the role of enamel matrix protein derivatives and growth factors in regeneration of bony defects.
- Compare and contrast the different clinical procedures used to attain periodontal regeneration.

INTRODUCTION

The goals of periodontal therapy have long included arresting the disease process, preventing disease recurrence, and providing for the regeneration of periodontium lost as a result of the disease. Over the past four decades, great strides have been made in the field of periodontal regeneration. **Periodontal regeneration** is defined as healing after periodontal surgery that results in the reconstruction of lost tissues, including supporting alveolar bone, cementum, and a functionally oriented periodontal ligament (American Academy of Periodontology, 2001). Guided bone regeneration is defined as healing after periodontal surgery that results in the formation of only new bone and includes use of a barrier membrane. This procedure is usually performed to increase the height or width of bone before implant placement and is discussed in Chapter 26. This chapter provides a review of the various regenerative therapies and materials currently in use today (Box 25–1). Future directions in this ever-changing field also will be discussed. Techniques currently in use include open flap debridement, the use of bone grafts and bone substitutes, guided tissue regeneration, combination techniques, and root surface treatment, and the use of biomimetics and growth factors.

Box 25–1 Procedures Used to Enhance Periodontal Regeneration

- Bone and bone substitute grafting to fill the periodontal defect
- Prevention or retardation of junctional epithelial downgrowth and selective cell repopulation: Guided tissue regeneration (GTR)
- Guided bone regeneration (GBR)
- Acid conditioning of the root surface
- Application of enamel matrix protein derivatives
- Growth factor application to promote specific cell proliferation

---

PERIODONTAL REGENERATIVE SURGERY
Objectives

Once inflammation of the gingiva is resolved with initial therapy (e.g., periodontal debridement and oral hygiene self-care instruction), the periodontitis component still must be treated. Periodontitis is characterized by apical migration of the junctional epithelium resulting in periodontal pocket formation, loss of clinical attachment (connective tissue fibers attached to the tooth surface), and alveolar bone loss. **Periodontal tissue regeneration** involves surgery using bone grafts, bone substitute materials, and/or barrier membranes and modulators of tissue healing are aimed at regenerating the periodontal attachment apparatus lost due to periodontitis (Froum, Gomez, & Breault, 2001).

The primary goal of regenerating lost attachment is the preservation of the natural tooth . Secondary goals of using such bone-replacement materials as bone grafts and bone substitutes in infrabony defects include the following: (1) a reduction in probing depths, (2) a gain in clinical attachment level (this refers to a reduction in probing depth caused by decreased penetration of the probe at the base of the pocket), (3) filling of the osseous defects with new bone, and (4) regeneration of new supporting alveolar bone, new cementum, and a functionally oriented periodontal ligament (Brunsvold & Mellonig, 1993; Laurell et al., 2006; Schallhorn, 1977). The latter can only be determined by histologic examination of the healed periodontal tissues.

Regenerative surgery significantly differs from osseous resective procedures, in which the osseous (bony) walls are removed surgically to eliminate the intraosseous component of the defect. Often, the morphology of the defect requires the removal of too much bone to obtain complete elimination of the defect (parabolic interdental bone), which would further compromise the affected tooth. Periodontal regenerative surgery involves "adding" bone (bone fill) into the intraosseous defect instead of its removal. Certain bony defects are more amenable to regeneration than others (Table 25–1 ■). The type of periodontal defects that respond best to the use of bone grafts include three-wall, two-wall, and combination-type intraosseous defects. This is because the remaining bony walls contain and hold the bone graft in the defect. The depth and width of these infrabony type defects influence the amount of bone and connective tissue attachment gain. For example, an infrabony defect that is deep and narrow will most likely achieve better regeneration than a defect that is deep and wide (Tonetti, Pini Prato, & Cortellini, 1993). Moreover, the additional surrounding bony walls provide more surface area upon which bone can form. Horizontal patterns of bone loss, loss of buccal or lingual plates of bone, and furcation defects cannot be treated predictably with bone graft and bone substitute materials alone. Furcation defects are more

Table 25–1	Bony Defects: Response to Regeneration	
Defects That Heal Best After Regeneration		**Defects with a Lower Chance for Regeneration**
Three-wall infrabony defect		One-wall infrabony defect
Class II buccal furcation involvement on mandibular molars		Class III furcation involvement
Deeper bony defects (deeper than 3 mm)		Shallower bony defects

Rapid Dental Hint

To diagnosis an infrabony defect, the clinician must probe the area and evaluate the radiographs.

predictably treated with GTR. Class II buccal furcation defects on the mandibular molars are most predictable types of furcation defects for periodontal regeneration.

The following are different types of regenerative techniques.

Rapid Dental Hint

Remember that an "infrabony" defect is the generic term used for a vertical defect in the alveolar bone while an "intrabony" defect is a special type of three-wall defect with cancellous bone between the cortical lining and the cortical plate.

Rapid Dental Hint

Class II buccal furcation defects and three-wall vertical bony defects are most amenable to regenerative procedures.

Surgery: Open Flap Debridement

As a surgical technique, open flap debridement (OFD), in which a flap is reflected and the roots and pocket area are debrided without the addition of any bone or bone substitute material, has been used primarily as a control for comparison in assessing other treatment modalities (Laurell, Gottlow, Zybetz, & Persson, 1998). In most histologic studies, open flap debridement resulted in repair rather than regeneration of periodontal tissues. A greater recurrence of probing depth over time has been shown with open flap debridement alone (Smith, Ammons, & van Belle, 1980) when compared with traditional osseous resective procedures. A review of the literature shows that OFD results in an average clinical attachment level gain of 1.5 mm and average bone fill of 1.1 mm (Stahl, Froum, Kushner, 1982).

Surgery: Bone Grafts and Bone Substitutes

Bone grafts and their substitutes are classified into four categories: **autografts, allografts, alloplasts,** and **xenografts. Bone grafts** refer to naturally occurring autografts and allografts (Hanes, 2007). Despite the benefits of autografts and allografts, the limitations of each have necessitated the pursuit of alternatives. Many of these alternatives, or **bone substitutes** (also referred to as bone replacement materials), can be synthetic (manufactured, not naturally occurring) materials (alloplasts), including natural and synthetic polymers and ceramics or natural and recombinant growth factors (Christgau et al., 2006) or materials processed from the bone of other species (xenografts). Table 25–2 ■ describes the different types of bone graft materials.

Autografts (Autogenous Grafts)

Autogenous bone is living bone derived directly from the patient's own body. This has shown the best potential of any of the bone fill material for periodontal regeneration and bone fill. This bone is often mixed with the patient's blood. However, when a sufficient amount of bone is not available intraorally, or if the patient does not want bone obtained from extraoral sites such as the hip, other materials must be considered. Autogenous bone has long been considered to be the gold standard of grafting materials in terms of stimulating new bone formation.

A bone blend is a mixture of cancellous and cortical bone. When cortical bone is mixed with the patient's blood, it becomes an osseous coagulum.

Allografts (Allogeneic Grafts)

Allografts such as demineralized freeze-dried bone (DFDBA) obtained from human cadavers have demonstrated bone-forming properties. Bone allografts are obtained from bone banks. The issue of safety (e.g., nontransmission of hepatitis, HIV, and other known diseases) when using allografts has been well established, thus minimizing this factor as a concern (Marx & Carlson, 1993; Mellonig, Preuett, & Moyer, 1992). Controlled clinical studies have shown greater bone fill in sites treated with DFDBA than in nongrafted controls, with DFDBA reporting a mean bone fill of 2.6 mm (65% defect fill) compared with 1.3 mm (30% defect fill) in nongrafted controls (Mellonig, 1984). A recent review of the literature concluded that both autogenous bone and DFDBA support the formation of a new attachment apparatus (Reynolds, Aichelmann-Reidy, Branch-Mays, & Gunsolley, 2003).

Alloplasts (Alloplastic Grafts)

Alloplastic bone substitutes are manufactured synthetic materials. They are classified as implant material. Alloplasts (implants) are differentiated from grafts, which are defined as "any tissue or organ used for implantation or transplantation" (Hallmon, Carranza, Drisko, Rapley, & Robinson, 1996). Advantages of alloplasts include zero risk of disease transmission as compared with allografts and no additional surgical sites required in the mouth or body to harvest bone (as with autografts). However, alloplasts are not as effective in forming bone as are graft materials. Alloplasts are inert (nonliving) materials acting as a bone

Rapid Dental Hint

Bone grafts and substitutes are indicated for infrabony (vertical) defects, and not for sites with horizontal bone loss.

"filler" in the defect, and when effective, they act as a scaffold for bone to form around them. (Osteoconductive)

A number of alloplastic materials have been introduced in an attempt to create a readily available material for bone fill of infrabony periodontal defects. Synthetic alloplasts may be divided into ceramic and nonceramic categories. These may be further divided into absorbable and nonabsorbable materials. Absorbable materials will absorb or dissolve (it may take years) and be replaced with new bone, whereas nonabsorbable grafts may never absorb. Ceramic alloplasts are materials that include calcium phosphate such as hydroxyapatite and tricalcium phosphate. The most commonly used ceramic materials are nonporous hydroxyapatite, porous hydroxyapatite, and tricalcium phosphate. Frequently, these materials result in a repair that evidences a long junctional epithelium to the root surface and/or adhesion of connective tissue fibers oriented parallel to the root (Yukna, 1993).

Bioactive glass is another type of alloplast. In a clinical study of the treatment of infrabony periodontal defects, a bioactive glass showed significant clinical superiority in gain of clinical attachment and defect fill compared with sites that were treated with open flap debridement alone (Froum, Weinberg, & Tarnow 1998).

Table 25–2	Types of Bone Grafts/Bone Replacement Materials
Name	**Features**
Autografts	Bone harvested from one part of the body and grafted to another part of the same patient's body. The bone can be obtained from an intraoral site such as the maxillary tuberosity area, edentulous area, chin, ramus, healing extraction site, or mandibular torus during implant placement or an extraoral site (e.g., tibia, femur). Osteogenic
Allografts	Bone material obtained from other individuals of the same species but genetically different. Donors include human cadavers. Allografts are obtained from bone banks. The main forms of bone allografts used in clinical practice are demineralized freeze-dried bone (DFDBA) and freeze-dried bone (FDBA). Osteoinductive
Alloplasts	Made of biocompatible, inorganic, inert materials including synthetic hydroxyapatite, calcium sulfate, bioactive glass, and tricalcium phosphate. Osteoconductive
Xenografts	A type of natural bone substitute derived from a genetically different species (e.g., bovine). Osteoinductive

Bioactive glass particles contain silicon dioxide, sodium oxide, calcium oxide, and phosphorus pentoxide. Advantages of this material include the ability to bond to both hard and soft tissue (Hench, 1988), its cohesiveness (Hench & West, 1996), and its ability to inhibit the apical migration of junctional epithelium (Fetner, Martigan, & Low, 1994). One human histological study showed the clinical improvement to be a repair rather than a regenerative response (Nevins et al., 2000).

While many of these materials serve as scaffolds or fillers that allow bone from the surrounding area to grow over and into them, to date alloplasts have failed to demonstrate human histologic evidence of new cementum and a functionally oriented periodontal ligament. From a clinical standpoint, these materials appear to be biocompatible, nontoxic, nonallergenic, noncarcinogenic, and noninflammatory.

Xenografts (Xenogeneic Grafts)

Heterografts or xenografts are taken from a donor of another species. Bio-Oss (Osteohealth Co., Shirley, NY) and Osteograf/N (CeraMed Dental, Lakewood, CO) are types of natural bone mineral obtained from the cow (bovine). This bone is anorganic and deproteinated. A histological study showed that Bio-Oss used in periodontal osseous defects has the potential to regenerate lost periodontal support (Camelo et al., 1998). The safety of these materials has also been demonstrated in regard to causing mad cow disease.

Properties of Bone Grafts and Bone Substitutes

Bone grafts and bone replacement materials are divided into their properties of osteogenesis, osteoinduction, and osteoconduction. Osteogenic bone contains bone cells called osteoblasts that make new bone and obtain a bone fill in the defect. Autogenous bone (e.g., bone from the host—intraoral or extraoral) is an example of osteogenic bone and it is considered the gold standard that bone alternatives must meet. Autogenous bone directly lays down new bone during wound healing after it is placed in the periodontal defect. This is ideal; however, there are many limitations to autogenous bone including limited amounts obtained and donor site morbidity.

Osteoinductive agents are bone grafts and bone graft substitutes, generally proteins, which induce the transformation of immature stem cells into bone-producing osteoblasts which make new bone through growth factors that are found only in living bone (Fox, 1997). This bone does not contain osteoblasts as autogenous bone. Examples of osteoinductive agents include de-

mineralized freeze-dried bone (DFDBA) from cadavers, bone morphogenic proteins (BMPs), and growth factors (platelet derived growth factor).

This differs from alloplastic grafts, which, when placed into a periodontal defect, at best function as osteoconductive material. In these situations, the alloplastic graft acts as a scaffold or framework to allow bone cells from the surrounding bone in the defect to lay down bone against its surface. Additionally, the porous surface of the graft material provides for bone in growth from bone adjacent to the bone material. Such osteoconductive materials require the presence of existing bone, and the more bone there is (greater number of bony walls in an intraosseous defect), the greater is the chance of a successful bone fill (Fox, 1997). These materials are not osteoinductive and do not produce new bone. The size and shape of the bone substitute particles influence their osteoconductive capacity. Eventually, the particles of material are either replaced by bone growing over them or incorporated into the new bone.

BIOLOGICS AND DEVICES

Biologics is a rapidly developing field that is generating new clinical studies. Wound healing is a complex, well-orchestrated sequence of events. In studying the dynamics of cell-to-cell and cell-to-tissue interaction, scientists discovered the presence of growth factors. Attempts have been made to use these factors to enhance wound healing (repair and regeneration).

Growth factors are naturally occurring proteins that mediate or regulate cellular events such as cell proliferation. Growth factors are found only in living tissue in cells such as bone, platelets, and macrophages. The most widely studied growth factor has been platelet-derived growth factor (PDGF). Platelet derived growth factor is a potent wound healing growth factor and stimulates the proliferation and recruitment of periodontal ligament cells and bone cells. The incorporation of PDGF in bone allograft (product is available as GEM21—Osteohealth, NY) may induce periodontal regeneration during wound healing when placed in a periodontal defect (Lynch et al., 2006; McGuire et al., 2006).

Other proteins called bone morphogenic proteins (BMPs) are normally found in bone and can induce new bone formation. Recently a bone graft material composed of recombinant (genetically manufactured) BMP-2 and a bovine collagen sponge (available as Infuse Bone Graft—Medtronic, TN) has been used in periodontal defects to stimulate bone formation in the bony defect.

There are still questions about the concentration of growth factors when they are used by themselves or in combination with other factors. The variability of growth factor responses locally and systemically is still unknown (Nevins, et al., 2007).

Another material referred to as enamel matrix proteins (amelogenins) are retrieved from the developing teeth in pigs (porcine). This product, Emdogain (Straumann, Switzerland, Chicago), is used in periodontal regenerative techniques. Clinical studies have shown improved clinical results and gain in clinical attachment and bone fill in sites treated with Emdogain versus open flap debridement (Froum, Weinberg, Rosenberg, & Tarnow, 2001). Multi-center studies have been performed with this material and verify the safety of multiple uses in the same patient (no allergies or immunologic problems) (Froum, Weinberg, Novak, Mailhot et al., 2004). After flap reflection and debridement, EDTA (ethylenediaminetetraacetic acid) is ap-

plied to the root surface to remove the smear layer. This is then washed off with sterile water or saline. Emdogain is applied to the root surface which promotes attachment of certain cells that will eventually encourage the formation of cellular cementum and bone. Emdogain is available in a premixed, one-vial preparation. After flap reflection and debridement of the infrabony defect, Emdogain is syringed onto the root surface and the flap is sutured.

BONE GRAFTS AND BONE SUBSTITUTES: SURGICAL PROCEDURE

For bone grafting, intracrevicular incisions are made, and a gingival flap is reflected. The root surface and osseous defect are debrided to remove all granulomatous (diseased) tissue (Table 25–3 ■). A combination of

Table 25–3	Common Bone Grafts and Bone Substitutes		
For Periodontal Defects	*Composition*	*Supplied*	*Company*
Puros	Cadaver (allograft)	Cancellous particles, cortical particles, corticocancellous block	Zimmer Dental, Carlsbad, CA
MinerOss	Cadaver (allograft)	Cortical and cancellous chips	Biohorizons Alabama
Bio-Oss	Bovine (xenograft)	Particles	Geistlich Biomaterials, Switzerland
Osteo-graf	Hydroxyapatite (alloplast)	Particles	Dentsply, York, PA/Friadent/Ceramed
SynthoGraft	Pure phase beta-tricalcium phosphate (alloplast)	Particles	Synthograft, Boston
Perioglas, Biogran	Bioactive glass (calcium, phosphorus, sodium, silicon) (alloplast)	Particles	NovaBone Products, Jacksonville, FL; Implant Innovations Inc. ("3i"), a Biomet Company, Warsaw, IN
Capset	Calcium sulfate (plaster of Paris) (alloplast)	Particles	LifeCore Biomedicals, Chaska, MN
DFDBA (demineralized freeze dried bone)	Cadaver (allograft)	Particles	many
Demineralized and mineralized cortical bone	Cadaver (allograft)	Particles	many
Regenafil	Cadaver (allograft)	Powder/fluid	Exactech Inc., FL
OrthoBlast II	Demineralized bone matrix (DBM) and cancellous bone in a reverse phase medium (allograft)	Putty and paste	Isotis Orthobiologics, Irvine, CA
Dynablast	Demineralized bone matrix with cancellous bone (allograft)	Putty and paste	Keystone Dental, MA

(continued)

Table 25–3   Common Bone Grafts and Bone Substitutes (cont.)

For Periodontal Defects	Composition	Supplied	Company
GEM 21S	Bioactive protein (highly purified recombinant human platelet derived growth factor, rhPDGF-BB) and a biocompatible osteoconductive matrix (beta-tricalcium phosphate, β-TCP)	Particles and liquid	Osteohealth, New York
PepGen P-15	Synthetic P-15 peptide, bovine hydroxyapatite	Flow, particles, putty	Dentsply/Friadent/CeraMed
Emdogain	Enamel matrix derivative; porcine	Gel	Straumann, Andover, MA

For Ridge Augmentation—Implant	Composition	Supplied	Company
Infuse	Recombinant human bone morphogenic protein 2 (rhBMP)	Apply to an absorbable collagen sponge carrier	Medtronic, TN
DFDBA, FDBA (bone allografts)	Cadaver	Block	many
Bio-Oss Cortical Block	Bovine	Block	Geistlich Biomaterials, Switzerland
Regenaform	Cadaver	Thermoplastic/moldable	Exactech, FL

power-driven and hand instruments is commonly used to ensure that all calculus and plaque as well as altered cementum are removed from the root surface (Brunsvold & Mellonig, 1993). The defect is filled and packed with bone or a bone replacement material. The flap is replaced and sutured in an attempt to fully cover the material (Figures 25–1 ■, 25–2 ■, 25–3 ■). A periodontal dressing may be placed if desired. The patient returns seven to fourteen days later for suture removal, light debridement, and oral hygiene instruction during the first postoperative visit.

RDH   Rapid Dental Hint

Many bone materials are either mixed with the patient's blood or sterile saline before it is placed in the defect. Some products such as Emdogain are already premixed.

GUIDED TISSUE REGENERATION

Cells Involved in Regeneration

The periodontal unit can be divided into five tissue components: the gingival epithelium, the gingival connective tissue, the periodontal ligament (PDL), the supporting alveolar bone, and cementum. In 1976 it was theorized that the type of tissue that predominates in the healing wound after periodontal surgery determines whether the response is either repair (e.g., long junctional epithelial attachment or connective tissue adherence) or regeneration (e.g., new bone, new cementum, and new periodontal ligament) (Melcher, 1976; Zeichner-David, 2006).

Did You Know?

Hydroxyapatite for bone grafting comes from coral from the ocean.

■ **FIGURE 25–1**   (a) A 6-mm combination one-two-three-wall intraosseous defect on the mandibular second molar. (b) After flaps are reflected and the roots and defect thoroughly debrided, demineralized freeze-dried bone autograft (DFDBA) (c,d) was placed into the defect and the flap sutured to cover the bone (e).

(a)

(b)

(c)

(d)

■ **FIGURE 25–2**   (a) A 9-mm intraosseous periodontal defect is present on the mesial aspect of the maxillary cuspid. (b) Following reflection of a periodontal flap and defect and root debridement, a bone blend is mixed consisting of autogenous bone and the patient's blood and (c) placed into the defect. (d) The replaced flap is sutured with silk sutures to cover the graft material.

Epithelium is the fastest growing tissue, migrating at a rate of 0.5 to 1.0 mm per day. A periodontal wound in which unimpeded epithelial migration is allowed to occur results in repair with a long junctional epithelium. This type of healing occurs after open flap debridement and osseous resective surgical procedures. Regeneration does not occur when either gingival (junctional) epithelium or gingival connective tissues (e.g., tissue inside the flap) contact the root surface during healing. In order for regeneration to occur, cells capable of forming new cementum, PDL, and supporting alveolar bone must migrate into the periodontal osseous defect and produce these tissues. It is believed that these cells come from the PDL (osteoblasts, fiberblasts, and cementoblasts) and/or alveolar bone remaining around the tooth (Melcher, McCulloch, Cheong, Nemeth, & Shiga, 1987). In order for these cells to migrate into the periodontal defect, apical epithelial migration must be delayed, and the gingival connective tissue from the gingival flap must be excluded. If the flap makes contact with the tooth surface, a long junctional epithelium forms along the root and may prevent the necessary regenerative cells from gaining access to the periodontal defect. This concept led to the theory of selective cell repopulation or **guided tissue regeneration** (GTR) (Gottlow, Nyman, Karring, & Wennström, 1986; Nyman, Gottlow, Karring, & Lindhe, 1982).

This concept has been the basis for clinical techniques using barrier membranes inserted between the gingival flap and the root surface. The membrane maintains a

■ **FIGURE 25–3** (a) Probing between the mandibular second premolar and first molar. (b) Probing of the deep defect after flap reflection. (c) After thorough tooth and root debridement, Perioglas® was placed into the defect and the flaps were sutured with silk sutures to cover the graft material. (d) Flap sutured with interrupted sutures. (e) Reentry of the site six months later shows that the bony defect has been filled in with new bone (also there is slight crestal resorption). The inter-proximal bone is flat, not cratered. Compare with Figure 25–3b.

(a)

(b)

(c)

(d)

■ **FIGURE 25–4**   Schematic illustration of a guided tissue regeneration procedure. (a) The periodontal defect with the junctional epithelium on the root surface. (b) After a flap is raised and the defect debrided, a barrier membrane is placed over the defect to create a space for the defect to heal. The periodontal ligament and bone cells attempt to migrate coronally (arrows) into the defect to produce new cementum, periodontal ligament, and supporting alveolar bone. The flap is then sutured over the membrane covering it. (c) Healing by regeneration. (d) The result of therapy after healing.

"space" between the tooth and the flap. This procedure is designed to retard apical migration of the junctional epithelium and exclude the gingival connective tissue cells from making contact with the root surface and defect. This then allows cells originating from the PDL space and/or alveolar bone cells to migrate coronally into the defect to form new bone, cementum, and attachment (Figure 25–4 ■).

Surgical Procedure

Barrier membranes have been used in the treatment of Grade II buccal furcation defects in both maxillary and mandibular molars and in two- and three-wall interproximal infrabony periodontal defects as well as for guided bone regeneration (GBR) applications. Optimal results are obtained in patients who are healthy nonsmokers who demonstrate good oral home care.

Clinically, GTR techniques are performed by making intrasulcular incisions and full-thickness flap reflection. Following debridement of the periodontal defect and the root surface, a membrane barrier is placed on the tooth so as to cover the periodontal bony defect (Figures 25–5 ■, 25–6 ■). The membrane is situated between the inner flap and the tooth and bone. The flap is sutured so that the membrane is fully covered and not exposed to the oral cavity. Frequently, a bone graft is first placed into the periodontal defect to prevent the membrane from collapsing into the defect and to aid in regeneration.

Types of Barrier Membranes

Nonabsorbable Membranes

Membranes are classified as nonabsorbable or absorbable. Nonabsorbable membranes were the first to be used and studied clinically. Since the body does not absorb (degrade) a nonabsorbable membrane, it has to be removed. A second surgical procedure, therefore, is performed a minimum of six to eight weeks later to remove the barrier. The most commonly used nonabsorbable barrier membrane is expanded polytetrafluoroethylene (e-PTFE). Examples of an e-PTFE membrane are Gore-Tex® and Gore-Tex® Regenerative Membrane Titanium Reinforced, in which the titanium

enhances the space creating ability of the membrane (Gore Associates, Flagstaff, AZ). Similar nonabsorbable barriers are TefGen-FD™ and TefGen-RE™ (Lifecore Biomedical, Chaska, MN), which are less porous than Gore-Tex®, and thus may limit the amount of connective tissue ingrowth.

Most studies using nonabsorbable membranes in infrabony defects showed positive results. Over the past two decades, studies of infrabony defects in human beings treated with e-PTFE barriers showed definitive clinical gains in new attachment, with three-wall defects having the greatest improvement (Gottlow et al., 1986). A twelve-month study of one-, two-, and three-wall infrabony defects treated with e-PTFE barriers showed a 93% fill of three-wall defects, an 82% fill of two-wall defects, and a 39% fill of one-wall defects (Cortellini, Pini Prato, & Tonetti, 1993a, 1993b).

Absorbable Membranes

Absorbable membranes appeared half a decade after nonabsorbable membranes. These membranes have various compositions, including collagen (Bornstein, Bosshardt, & Buser, 2007). Absorbable membranes offer a distinct advantage over nonabsorbable barriers in that there is no need for a second surgery to retrieve the membrane. Macrophages, a type of phagocyte, are always involved in the degradation process. The barrier must remain in place a minimum of three to four weeks (Minabe, 1991) for proper wound healing. Several membranes are available commercially (Table 25–4 ■).

The general consensus seems to be that furcation closure in a horizontal dimension is better with absorbable membranes (Garrett, 1996). The clinician must choose the appropriate barrier for the appropriate defect. Although nonabsorbable barriers do not have breakdown products that can interfere with tissue healing, the need for a second procedure to remove the membrane is a distinct disadvantage to wound healing.

The membrane should be covered completely by the flap to prevent bacterial colonization on the outer part of the membrane. Membrane exposure may lead to early infection and poor results. Unfortunately, membrane exposure to the oral cavity occurs with both barrier types. Tissue management when membrane exposure occurs with nonabsorbable barriers may be a problem. Bacteria from the oral cavity may contaminate the exposed membrane by attaching to it. If complete flap closure is not possible, absorbable membranes may be the best choice.

■ **FIGURE 25–5**   Bone + membrane: infrabony defect on the canine. Flaps are reflected and surgical debridement performed until the defect is visualized. Bio-Oss is placed into the defect and BioGide placed on top of the bone graft. Then the flaps are sutured to cover both the bone and membrane.

■ **FIGURE 25–6**   Mandibular right quadrant: initial incisions on the buccal (a) and lingual (b). (c) Full-thickness flap is reflected showing circumferential bony defects (bone destruction from the interproximal to the lingual surface) and furcation involvement. (d) After debridement, the bony defects are grafted with DFDBA (demineralized freeze-dried bone) and (e) an absorbable membrane is sutured over the defect. (f) The flaps are sutured. (g) One week postoperative; sutures removed and (h) four weeks postoperative with the membrane still in place. (Courtesy of Dr. James B. Fine, Columbia University College of Dental Medicine)

Table 25–4	**Absorbable Barrier Membranes**	
Material	*Product*	*Manufacturer*
Synthetic: Polyglycolic acid, polylactic acid, and trimethylene carbonate	Gore OsseoQuest	W.L. Gore, Flagstaff, AZ; distributed by Nobel Biocare, Yorba Linda, CA
	Gore Resolut XT	W.L. Gore
Synthetic: Polyglycolic acid and trimethylene carbonate	Gore Resolut Adapt	W.L. Gore, Flagstaff, AZ; distributed by Nobel Biocare, Yorba Linda, CA
	Gore Resolut Adapt LT	
Synthetic: PLA (poly-DL-lactide)	Epi-Guide	Curasan Inc., NC
	Atrisorb FreeFlow	Tolmar, Fort Collins, CO
	Atrisorb-D FreeFlow (with 4% doxycycline)	Tolmar
Natural: Collagen (bovine)	BioMend	Zimmer Dental, Carlsbad, CA
(bovine)	BioMend Extend	Zimmer Dental
(porcine)	BioGide	Geistlich, Switzerland; distributed by Osteohealth Company, Shirley, NY
(bovine)	OsseoGuard	Biomet 3i, Warsaw, IN
(porcine)	Ossix Plus	OraPharma, Warminster, PA

Although GTR using nonabsorbable and absorbable membranes has revolutionized clinical practice, the technique is not as yet predictable for class II, class III, and horizontal bone defects. More research in regeneration of furcation and interproximal defects is needed.

Barrier membranes need to be secured around the tooth to hold them in place and prevent them from moving. Either sutures or bone tacks can be used to attach and immobilize the membrane. A mallet is used to secure the tacks in place. The bone tacks are either stainless steel or titanium. Most are nonabsorbable, thus a second surgery is needed to remove the tacks. Osteo-Pin (Osteohealth, Shirley, NY) is a bioabsorbable fixation pin that does not need to be removed.

Several bacteria, including *A. actinomycetemcomitans* and *P. gingivalis,* have been shown to attach to bioabsorbable membranes, which could cause a bacterial infection. Additionally, these bacteria produce and release proteolytic bacterial enzymes that may take part in the degradation of collagen barrier membranes such as Bio-Gide and Biomend (Sela et al., 2003).

REGENERATIVE SURGERY: POSTOPERATIVE CARE

The patient's oral home care is of utmost importance for a desirable outcome. The dental hygienist should provide the patient with thorough home care instructions. Guidelines for postoperative care are outlined in Table 25–5 ■ (Becker & Becker, 1993; Garret & Bogle, 1993; Yukna, 1993). An antimicrobial mouthrinse such as chlorhexidine gluconate may be prescribed. The patient may be prescribed an antibiotic before and after the surgery to prevent infection. The first postoperative visit is within seven to fourteen days.

Professional maintenance and plaque control have been repeatedly shown to correlate with successful clinical results of regenerative therapies including open flap debridement (Froum et al., 1982; Nyman, Lindhe, &

Rapid Dental Hint

Do not probe or do subgingival scaling for at least six months in areas that have a bone graft or barrier membrane placed either around a tooth or implant.

Table 25–5	Periodontal Regenerative Surgery: Postoperative Care	
Surgical Procedure	**Postoperative Home Care**	**In-Office Reevaluation Procedures**
Bone grafting	• If a periodontal dressing is placed, instruct the patient not to brush the area. Instruct the patient to rinse with 0.12% chlorhexidine gluconate twice a day. • Following suture removal the patient may start to brush (soft or ultrasoft brush) surgical site gently with a circular technique. Bleeding may occur but will gradually lessen, and the patient should continue to brush. • If an antibiotic was prescribed, instruct the patient to continue until all medication is finished.	• At the postoperative visit (seven to fourteen days), carefully remove the dressing (cut sutures if embedded in dressing), wipe off the white film (this consists of dead epithelial cells); and irrigate the area with sterile water or saline. • Reapply dressing if needed (especially if sutures and dressing are removed before ten days). • Periodontal probing should not be done prior to six months after surgery. • Final prosthetic restorations should not be completed until six months or more after surgery. • Initial appointments for professional plaque removal should be every two to three weeks for the first month, then every month for four visits, followed by every three months (alternate with visits to the general dentist).
Guided tissue regeneration	• A periodontal dressing is usually not placed. Instruct the patient not to floss or brush around the surgical area for six weeks after the surgery. However, a soft or ultrasoft toothbrush may be used for coronal brushing of the surgical area. • Rinse with 0.12% chlorhexidine gluconate twice a day, and use cotton swabs saturated with chlorhexidine around the surgical area. • Instruct the patient to continue to take the prescribed antibiotic until finished.	• At the first postoperative visit (one to two weeks), the surgical area is inspected. • The patient should be seen every two to three weeks for supragingival scaling and tooth polishing with sterile water. • Between four and six weeks, the membrane-attached sutures are removed. • At 8 to 12 weeks, an incision is made to remove the nonabsorbable membrane. • Periodontal probing should not be done prior to six months after surgery. • Final prosthestic restorations should not be completed prior to six months after surgery.

Source: Yukna, 1993; Becker & Becker, 1993; Garrett & Bogle, 1993.

Rosling, 1977; Rosling, Nyman, & Lindhe, 1976), bone grafting (Rosen, Reynolds, & Bowers, 2000), and guided tissue regeneration (Cortellini, Pini Prato, & Tonetti, 1994). The hygienist thus plays a key role in the short- and long-term success of regenerative therapy.

Complications can occur during the healing period after GTR surgery. Some complications (Becker & Becker, 1993) are outlined in Table 25–6 ■.

ROOT SURFACE TREATMENT

Animal studies have shown that the root surface becomes contaminated by bacteria, bacterial by-products, and endotoxins that will prevent connective tissue attachment and regeneration (Garrett, 1977). The classic method of scaling and root planing, while effective in removing endotoxins from the root (Smart, Wilson, Davies, & Kieser, 1990), in most cases will not result in new connective

Table 25–6	Complications After Periodontal Regenerative Surgery
Complication	**Procedures to Follow**
Membrane becomes uncovered	Instruct the patient to call the office. Most often the membrane will become exposed within a few weeks after surgery. If there is no infection, instruct patient to keep optimal oral hygiene. Monitor the area. Instruct the patient not to disrupt the membrane. Bacteria associated with exposed membranes include *A. actinomycetemcomitans* and *P. gingivalis.* Aggressive antimicrobial therapy may be necessary, including chlorhexidine mouthrinses and antibiotics such as metronidazole alone or combined with amoxicillin.
Gingival recession at the surgical site	If recession occurs, it will usually happen within one to three weeks after surgery. Since increased plaque accumulation may result, optimal plaque control is stressed.
Pus	If an infection develops, it is most likely at the fourth and fifth postoperative visit. Remove the membrane and place the patient on an antibiotic. If the patient is already on an antibiotic, change to another antibiotic in a different classification.

tissue attachment, but rather a long junctional epithelium. Use of an acid solution such as citric acid or tetracycline HCl has been studied to determine if a new connective tissue attachment results. The proposed purposes of using acidic solutions on contaminated root surfaces are to detoxify the root and expose collagen fibers for a connective tissue attachment. However, two recent reviews of periodontal regeneration studies with and without the use of citric acid root conditioning showed no clinical advantage to its use (Garrett, 1996; Mariotti, 2003).

RISK FACTORS FOR REGENERATIVE THERAPY

The same contraindications for any surgical periodontal therapy apply to regenerative therapies. These include any acute or chronic uncontrolled systemic diseases that put the patient at risk (e.g., diabetes mellitus), inadequate plaque control, and smoking (especially more than one pack per day). Smoking has been shown to have a negative influence on the results of regenerative therapy. Using GTR therapy, smokers had less than 50% gain in attachment levels compared to results in nonsmokers (Tonetti, Pino Prato, & Cortellini, 1996). Of the failures with GTR, the majority (80%) occurred in smokers (Rosenberg, Dent, & Cutles, 1984).

DENTAL HYGIENE NOTES

Today, the role of periodontics in dentistry focuses not only on arresting the progression of inflammatory periodontal diseases but also on the regeneration of periodon-

tal structures (cementum, PDL, supporting alveolar bone) that were destroyed by disease. Periodontal regenerative therapy uses bone replacement materials and guided tissue regeneration (GTR) techniques. The use of growth factors (e.g., bone morphogenic proteins, platelet-derived growth factor, and tissue modifiers) holds great promise. These factors most likely will be the next addition to periodontal regenerative techniques.

KEY POINTS

- Periodontal regeneration is defined as healing after periodontal surgery that results in the reproduction of cementum, PDL, and supporting alveolar bone that was lost or destroyed by periodontal diseases.
- Ideally, after periodontal surgery, healing by regeneration is preferred over repair.
- Periodontal regenerative techniques include the use of bone grafts, synthetic bone substitutes, guided tissue regeneration (GTR), and a combination of these.
- Bone-replacement materials may contribute to new bone formation or serve as a filler material for bone formation that starts from the adjacent bone and grows into the defect.
- GTR is used to delay apical migration of the junctional epithelium and exclude gingival connective tissue (inner flap) from the surgical site. The goal is to allow periodontal regenerative cells to repopulate the wound first.
- A barrier membrane is placed over the osseous defect and root to create a space for the migration of

cells from the PDL and alveolar bone to repopulate the wound.

SELF-QUIZ

1. During periodontal surgery, bone is taken from a mandibular torus and placed into a three-wall periodontal osseous defect. Which one of the following types of bone graft is this? (pp. 396, 397)
   a. Allograft
   b. Autograft
   c. Alloplast
   d. Xenograft

2. Cells coming from which one of the following structures is required for successful periodontal regeneration? (p. 400)
   a. Periodontal ligament
   b. Alveolar bone
   c. Gingival connective tissue
   d. Gingival epithelial

3. Guided tissue regeneration (GTR) focuses on the isolation or exclusion of what type of tissue cells? (p. 400)
   a. Junctional epithelial and gingival connective tissue
   b. Alveolar bone and sulcular epithelium
   c. Connective tissue and alveolar bone
   d. Alveolar bone and junctional epithelial

4. Which one of the following types of material is BioMend membrane? (p. 407)
   a. Polytetrafluoroethylene (e-PTFE)
   b. Poly-DL-lactide (PLA)
   c. Polylactic acid/polyglycolate (PLA/PGA)
   d. Bovine collagen

5. After surgical placement of a barrier membrane around an intraosseous defect, it is important to cover the membrane with the flap because (p. 405)
   a. brushing the area is easier.
   b. bacterial colonization can be prevented.
   c. aesthetics are enhanced.
   d. tooth mobility is reduced to pretreatment levels.

6. Which one of the following defects heals best when treated with bone grafts or bone substitutes? (p. 395)
   a. One-wall
   b. Two-wall
   c. Three-wall
   d. Class III furcations
   e. Horizontal bone loss

7. All the following are objectives of using bone grafts or bone-replacement materials in the treatment of infrabony defects except one. Which one is the exception? (p. 395)
   a. Reduction in probing depth
   b. Reduction of bleeding
   c. Gain in clinical attachment
   d. Fill of the defect
   e. Regeneration of the attachment apparatus

8. Which one of the following materials is a type of allograft? (p. 397)
   a. Bone from the patient's chin
   b. Demineralized freeze-dried bone
   c. Bone from the patient's hip
   d. Enamel matrix protein derivatives
   e. Bioactive glass particles

9. All the following complications may be seen after placement of barrier membranes except one. Which one is the least likely? (p. 409)
   a. Suppuration
   b. Gingival overgrowth
   c. Soft tissue recession
   d. Membrane exposure

10. All the following postoperative instructions apply to a patient after a regenerative procedure using a barrier membrane except one. Which one is the exception? (pp. 407–408)
    a. Floss the surgical area.
    b. Rinse the area frequently with diluted saltwater.
    c. Use an antimicrobial mouthrinse.
    d. Take antibiotics as prescribed.

REFERENCES

American Academy of Periodontology. 2000. Tissue Banking of bone allografts used in Periodontal Regeneration. *J Periodontol* 72:834–838.

Becker, W., and B. E. Becker. 1993. Clinical applications of guided tissue regeneration: Surgical considerations. *Periodontology 2000* 1:46–53.

Bornstein, M.M., D. Bosshardt, and D. Buser. 2007, October. Effect of two different bioabsorbable collagen membranes on guided bone regeneration: A comparative histomorphometric study in the dog mandible. *J. Periodontol.* 78(10):1943–1953.

Brunsvold, M. A., and J. T. Mellonig. 1993. Bone grafts and periodontal regeneration. *Periodontology 2000* 1:80–91.

Camelo, M., M. L. Nevins, R. K. Schenk, M. Simion, G. Rasperini, et al. 1998. Clinical, radiographic, and histological evaluation of human periodontal defects treated with

Bio-Oss and Bio-Guide. *Int J. Periodontics Restorative Dent.* 18:321–331.

Christgau, M., D. Moder, K-A. Hiller, A. Dada, G. Schmitz, and G. Schmalz. 2006. Growth factors and cytokines in autologous platelet concentrate and their correlation to periodontal regeneration outcomes. *J. Clin. Periodontol.* 33:837–845.

Cortellini, P., G. Pini Prato, and M. S. Tonetti. 1993a. Periodontal regeneration in human intrabony defects: I. Clinical measures. *J. Periodontol.* 64:254–260.

Cortellini, P., G. Pini Prato, and M. S. Tonetti. 1993b. Periodontal regeneration in human intrabony defects: II. Reentry procedures and bone measurements. *J. Periodontol.* 64:261–268.

Cortellini, P., G. Pini Prato, and M. Tonetti. 1994. Periodontal regeneration of human infrabony defects (V). Effect of oral hygiene on long-term stability. *J. Clin. Periodontol.* 21:606–610.

Fetner, A. E., M. S. Martigan, and S. B. Low. 1994. Periodontal repair using Perioglas® in nonhuman primates: Clinical and histologic observations. *Compend. Contin. Ed. Dent.* 15:932–939.

Fox, J. S. 1997. Bone grafting materials for dental applications: A practical guide. *Compend. Contin. Ed. Dent.* 18:1013–1038.

Froum S. J., M. Coran, B. Thaller, L. Kushner, I. W. Scopp, and S. S. Stahl. 1982. Periodontal healing following open flap debridement. *J. Periodontol.* 53:8–14.

Froum S. J., C. Gomez, and M. R. Breault. 2001. Current concepts of periodontal regeneration. *NYSDJ* 68(9):14–22.

Froum, S. J., M. A. Weinberg, J. Novak, J. Mailhot, J. Mellonig, et al. 2004. A multicenter study evaluating the sensitization potential of enamel matrix derivative after treatment of two infrabony defects. *J. Periodontol.* 75:1001–1008.

Froum, S. J, M. A. Weinberg, E. Rosenberg, and D. Tarnow. 2001. A comparative study utilizing open flap debridement with and without enamel matrix derivative in the treatment of periodontal intrabony defects: A 12-month re-entry study. *J. Periodontol.* 72:25–34.

Froum, S. J., M. A. Weinberg, and D. Tarnow. 1998. Comparison of bioactive glass synthetic bone graft particles and open debridement in the treatment of human periodontal defects: A clinical study. *J. Periodontol.* 69:698–709.

Garrett, S. 1977. Root planing: A perspective. *J. Periodontol.* 48:553–557.

Garrett, S. 1996. Periodontal regeneration around natural teeth. *Ann Periodontol.* 1:621–666.

Garrett, S., and G. Bogle. 1993. Periodontal regeneration: A review of flap management. *Periodontology 2000* 1:100–108.

Giannobile W.V., and M. Somerman. 2003. Growth and amelogenin-like factors in periodontal wound healing. A systematic review. *Ann. Periodontol.* 8:193–204.

Gottlow, J., S. Nyman, T. Karring, and J. Wennström. 1986. New attachment formation in the human periodontium by guided tissue regeneration: Case reports. *J. Clin. Periodontol.* 13:604–616.

Hallmon, W. W., F. A. Carranza, Jr., C. L. Drisko, J. W. Rapley, and P. Robinson. 1996. Surgical therapy. In *Periodontal literature review,* 167–194. Chicago: American Academy of Periodontology.

Hanes, P.J. 2007, November. Bone replacement grafts for the treatment of periodontal intrabony defects. *Oral Maxillofac. Surg. Clin. North Am.* 19(4):499–512, vi.

Hench, L. L. 1988. Bioactive ceramics. *Ann. N.Y. Acad. Sci.* 523:54–71.

Hench, L. L., and J. K. West. 1996. Biological application of bioactive glasses. *Life Chem. Rep.* 13:187–241.

Laurell, L., M. Bose, F. Graziani, M. Tonetti, and T. Berglundh. 2006. The structure of periodontal tissues formed following guided tissue regeneration therapy of intra-bony defects in the monkey. *J. Clin. Periodontol.* 33:596–603.

Lynch, S., L. Wisner-Lynch, M. Nevins, M. L. Nevins. 2006. A new era in periodontal and periimplant regeneration: Use of growth factor enhanced matrices incorporating rhPDGF. *Compend. Contin. Educ. Dent.* 27(12):672–679.

Mariotti, A. 2003. Efficacy of chemical root surface modifiers in the treatment of periodontal disease. A systematic review. *Ann. Periodontol.* 8:205–226.

Marx, R. E., and E. R. Carlson. 1993. Tissue banking safety: Caveats and precaution for the oral and maxillofacial surgeon. *J. Oral Maxillofac. Surg.* 51:1372–1379.

McGuire, M. K., and E. T. Scheyer. 2006. Comparison of recombinant human platelet-derived growth factor-BB plus beta tricalcium phosphate and a collagen membrane to subepithelial connective tissue grafting for the treatment of recession defects: A case series. *Int. J. Periodont. Restor. Dent.* 26(2):127–33.

Melcher, A. H. 1976. On the repair potential of the periodontal tissues. *J. Periodontol.* 47:256–260.

Melcher, A. H., C. A. G. McCulloch, T. Cheong, E. Nemeth, and A. Shiga. 1987. Cells from bone synthesize cementum-like and bone-like tissues in vitro and may migrate into periodontal ligament in vivo. *J. Periodontol. Res.* 22:246–247.

Mellonig, J. T. 1984. Decalcified freeze-dried bone allograft as an implant material in human periodontal defects. *Int. J. Periodont. Restor. Dent.* 4(6):41–55.

Mellonig, J. T., A. B. Preuett, and M. P. Moyer. 1992. HIV inactivation in a bone allograft. *J. Periodontol.* 63:979–983.

Minabe, M. 1991. A critical review of the biologic rationale for guided tissue regeneration. *J. Periodontol.* 62:171–179.

Nevins, M., J. Hanratty, and S.E. Lynch. 2007, October. Clinical results using recombinant human platelet-derived growth factor and mineralized freeze-dried bone allograft in periodontal defects. *Int. J. Periodont. Restor. Dent.* 27(5):421–427.

Nevins, M. L., M. Camelo, M. Nevins, C. J. King, R. J. Oringer, et al. 2000. Human histologic evaluation of bioactive ceramic in the treatment of periodontal osseous defects. *Int. J. Periodont. Restor. Dent.* 20:459–467.

Nyman, S., J. Gottlow, T. Karring, and J. Lindhe. 1982. The regenerative potential of the periodontal ligament: An experimental study in the monkey. *J. Clin. Periodontol.* 9:257–265.

Nyman, S., J. Lindhe, and B., Rosling. 1977. Periodontal surgery in plaque-infected dentitions. *J. Clin. Periodontol.* 4:240–249.

Reynolds, M. A., M. E. Aichelmann-Reidy, G. L. Branch-Mays, and J. C. Gunsolley. 2003. The efficacy of bone replacement grafts in the treatment of periodontal osseous defects. A systematic review. 8:227–265.

Rosen, P. S., M. A. Reynolds, and G. M. Bowers. 2000. The treatment of intrabony defects with bone grafts. *Periodontology 2000* 22:88–103.

Rosenberg, E. S., H. D. Dent, and S. H. Cutles. 1994. The effect of cigarette smoking on the long-term success of guided tissue regeneration: A preliminary study. *Ann. Royal Aust. Coll. Dent. Surg.* 112:89–93.

Rosling, B., S. Nyman, and J. Lindhe. 1976. The effect of systematic plaque control on bone regeneration in infrabony pockets. *J. Clin. Periodontol.* 3:38–53.

Schallhorn, R. G. 1977. Present status of osseous grafting procedures. *J. Periodontol.* 48:570–576.

Sela, M.N., D. Kohavi, E. Krausz, D. Steinberg, and G. Rosen. 2003. Enzymatic degradation of collagen-guided tissue. Regeneration membranes by periodontal bacteria. *Clin. Oral Impl. Res.* 4, 263–268.

Slavkin, H. C., and A. Boyde. 1975. Cementum: An epithelial secretory product? *J. Dent. Res.* 53:157 (Abstract 409).

Smart, G. J., M. Wilson, E. H. Davies, and J. B. Kieser. 1990. The assessment of ultrasonic root surface debridement by determination of residual endotoxin levels. *J. Clin. Periodontol.* 17:174–178.

Smith, D., W. Ammons, and G. van Belle. 1980. A longitudinal study of periodontal status comparing osseous recontouring with flap curettage: II. Results after 6 months. *J. Periodontol.* 51:367–375.

Stahl, S. S., S. J. Froum, L. Kushner. 1982. Periodontal healing following open debridement flap procedures. II. Histologic observations. *J. Periodontol.* 53(1):15–21.

Tonetti, M., G. Pini Prato, and P. Cortellini. 1993. Periodontal regeneration of human infrabony defects. IV. Determinants of the healing response. *J. Periodontol.* 64:934–940.

Tonetti M., G. Pini Prato, and P. Cortellini. 1996. Factors affecting the healing response of intrabony defects following guided tissue regeneration and access flap surgery. *J. Clin. Periodontol.* 23:548–556.

Yukna, R. 1993. Synthetic bone grafts in periodontics. *Periodontology 2000* 1:93–99.

Zeichner-David, M. 2006. Regeneration of periodontal tissues: Cementogenesis revisted. *Periodontology 2000* 41(1):196–217.

Chapter 26

Implantology

Suzanne K. Farrar

Jeanne St. Germain

Raymond A. Yukna

OUTLINE
Introduction
Age, Systemic, and Social Factors
Components of Dental Implants
Types of Dental Implants
Surgical Procedure
Implants Versus Teeth
Bacteriology
Implant Maintenance Program
Dental Hygiene Notes
Key Points
Self-Quiz
References

EDUCATIONAL OBJECTIVES

Upon completion of this chapter, the reader should be able to:

- Define the role of the dental hygienist in the management of patients with dental implants.
- Explain the various types of dental implants currently in use.
- Discuss the general sequence of implant placement, uncovering, and restoration.
- Compare the tissues around natural teeth and dental implants.
- Discuss the steps in evaluating tissue conditions around dental implants.
- Describe proper instrument selection and therapeutic steps for in-office maintenance procedures.
- Choose appropriate home-care techniques for patients with dental implants.

GOAL: To provide an understanding of dental implants and the establishment of proper implant evaluation procedures and maintenance.

KEY WORDS

endosseous implants 415

dental implant 414

nonmetallic materials 433

osseointegration 416

perimucosal seal 423

peri-implant diseases 430

INTRODUCTION

The dental hygienist plays a critical role in implant dentistry, providing valuable information on treatment and maintenance. The dental hygienist should know the types of implants used in his or her dental office. It is usually beneficial to have before and after pictures of patients who have undergone implant procedures in the office to show prospective patients potential end results.

A potential implant patient must be well educated about the entire procedure, especially the need for follow-up care. Although most implants now have a success rate of over 90%, they still require maintenance and routine care for long-term survival.

AGE, SYSTEMIC, AND SOCIAL FACTORS

The age of the patient has not shown to have an effect on the success or failure of implants (Dao, Anderson, & Zarb, 1993).

Implant therapy may not be an option for patients with certain systemic diseases or adverse risk factors. Systemic diseases such as reduced immune defense (HIV/AIDS) and uncontrolled diabetes mellitus can cause an increased susceptibility to infection and interfere with wound healing. Similarly, social risk factors such as smoking, excessive alcohol intake, drug abuse, and stress have been shown to be associated with an increased frequency of implant infections, including failure (Bain, 1996). Consultation with a patient's physician is required if a patient has disturbances of blood coagulation (including anticoagulation therapy), is on long-term steroids, or has a cancer that requires chemotherapy (Belser et al., 1996). An alternate method of replacing missing teeth should be pursued for such patients, such as fixed partial dentures, removable partial dentures, or complete dentures.

Patients taking intravenous bisphosphonates for cancer, osteoporosis, multiple myeloma, or other medical condition are not candidates for implant surgery. Implant surgery is a precipitating factor associated with ONJ whereby there is *poor or delayed wound healing* in patients taking bisphosphonates.

According to the most current JADA report (Edwards et al., 2008), patients taking oral bisphosphonates can have implant surgery, but the patient may be at increased risk of developing osteonecrosis of the jaw when extensive implant placement is necessary or bone augmentation surgery can be performed (Fugazzotto, Lightfoot, Jaffin, & Kumar, 2007; Grant, Amenedo, Freeman, & Kraut, 2008; Marx, Cilla, & Ulloa, 2007; Cartsos, Zhu, & Zavras 2008; Marx, 2007; Marx, Sawatari, Fortin, & Broumand, 2005). Thus, patients on long-term oral bisphosphonates should still be treated with caution (Wang, Weber, McCauley, 2007).

COMPONENTS OF DENTAL IMPLANTS

The components of a **dental implant** include the following (Figure 26–1 ■):

1. The implant body or fixture is the part that is surgically placed into the bone.
2. The abutment (or metal post) is the part that is attached to the implant body and will be fitted with a restoration that can be placed on top of it.
3. The superstructure is the prosthetic replacement (e.g., crown or denture) that is either screwed or cemented to the abutment.

TYPES OF DENTAL IMPLANTS

Several types of implants have been used to replace teeth or support prostheses over the centuries. A few types have been developed that provide the predictable success rates that clinicians and patients expect (Albrektsson & Sennerby, 1991; Brånemark, Zarb, & Albrektsson, 1985).

Implant success and survival rates are affected by the anatomic region of the jaw, the quality of bone, and the length and width of the implant (Cochran, 1996). Minimal criteria for a successful implant should include absence of clinical mobility, absence of persistent and/or irreversible signs and symptoms of pain or infections, no peri-implant radiolucency, no irreversible mechanical failures (e.g., implant fractures), support and/or retention of functional restoration(s), and lack of progressive bone loss beyond physiologic remodeling (0.2 mm per year after the first year of loading [occlusal function]). There are four types of implants: endosseous, subperiosteal, transosteal, and endodontic.

Endosseous Implants

Endosseous means "within the bone." **Endosseous implants** have several different shapes, including blade,

(a)

Superstructure (prosthesis)

Abutment

Implant

Bone

(b)

Core-Vent   Nobelpharma   IMZ   ISIS

ITI Hollow   TPS Screw   Steri - OSS   Integral

(c)

■ **FIGURE 26–1**   (a) Parts of a dental implant. Osseointegration occurs with direct anchorage of bone to the implant. Diagrammatic (b) and clinical (c) examples of different types of root-form dental implants showing different shapes, surfaces, and coatings.

cylinder, and screw types, with each manufacturer having its own designs. These are the most commonly used implants, and they are placed in edentulous areas of the maxilla or mandible (endosseous). Blade-type implants

were popular in the 1960s and 1970s and were associated with a fibrous type of attachment to bone (connective tissue found between the implant and bone). They have been replaced generally by root-form implants, which are associated with a direct bony attachment called osseointegration (see Figures 26–1b and 26–1c).

Rapid Dental Hint

There are many types of dental implant systems available. These systems are based on their shapes and the relation to the patient's bone.

Osseointegration

Osseointegration is a term introduced by Brånemark and coworkers in 1969 to describe the direct contact of a load-carrying dental implant (inert metal) with bone without any intervening connective tissue. Thus, the implant becomes an integral part of the bone and is, in effect, ankylosed, as seen at the light microscopic level (Brånemark et al., 1969). Osseointegration has revolutionized implant dentistry and made it the mainstream form of therapy it is today.

Osseointegrated description has been expanded by the same group of investigators to characterize the long-term success of an osseointegrated implant. Success rates have been reported to be greater than 90% in both fully edentulous and partially edentulous patients. Such success requires full occlusal function without pain and, most important, after an initial marginal bone height loss in the first year of 1 to 2 mm at the bone crest, a crestal bone height loss of no more than 0.1 to 0.2 mm per year. Inflammation of the gingiva around the implant neck is acceptable as long as it is contoured and does not affect the bone or jeopardize long-term implant success rates (Smith & Zarb, 1989).

The implant fixture that initially showed long-term success was made of machined pure titanium with a screw shape. The titanium surface oxidizes into a thin nonreactive titanium oxide layer to which bone adheres, at least at the light-microscopic level. This type of bone-implant interface is called osseointegration. While almost all dental implants today are titanium based (pure titanium or titanium alloy), some are coated, sprayed, or otherwise treated to create a rough surface, thus produc-

ing more surface area for the bone to contact or adhere to (see Figures 26–1b, 26–1c). The coatings used are usually acid-etched and sprayed, a titanium plasma spray, titanium beads, grit blasted-acid etched, or calcium-phosphate ceramics (hydroxyapatite and others). Some research has shown that the initial bone bonding to hydroxyapatite may be greater and stronger than the bonding to titanium (Weinlander, 1991). Endosseous implants are the predominant type (>90%) used in current practice (Figure 26–2a ■).

Subperiosteal Implants

Subperiosteal means "under the periosteum." Subperiosteal implants are individually designed cast-metal frames that fit intimately over the bone and under the periosteum and gingiva. Resting on the bone for support, the frame may or may not be fixed by screws to the bone. Posts protrude through the gingiva as anchors for the replacement teeth (Figure 26–2b). Currently, this type of implant is not used frequently except if there is insufficient bone mass for a root-type implant that cannot be corrected with surgery.

Transosteal Implants

Transosteal means "through the bone." Transosteal implants are mandibular denture anchors placed all the way through the mandible from under the chin into the mouth. They are commonly called mandibular staple implants. A curved, flat plate fits under the anterior mandible and usually has five to seven pins. The pins are anchor screws to hold the plate, and the posts are drilled parallel through the mandibular alveolar ridge by means of a jaw-fixation jig with parallel drilling sleeves. This implant has a good success record and is used for very severely resorbed mandibles. However, complications may be more common, and there is greater risk of tissue damage and infection.

(a)

(b)

■ **FIGURE 26–2** (a) Panoramic radiograph of root-form dental implants in mandible. (b) Panoramic radiograph of supraperiosteal dental implants on mandible.

Endodontic Implants

Endodontic implants are placed "in and through the tooth." They are also called endodontic stabilizers because they consist of a long, wide post inserted into the prepared root canal space that purposely extends at least a centimeter beyond the apex. The rationale is that this extension will stabilize the tooth and improve its usefulness as an abutment. However, this type of implant is not used commonly in the United States and has a poor prognosis because of the potential for root fracture, mechanical retention problems, and root resorption.

SURGICAL PROCEDURE

Surgical protocol for implant placement varies from two-stage surgery, to single-stage surgery, and to single-stage surgery with immediate or early loading.

Dental hygienists should be familiar with the basics of dental implant therapy, including the surgical procedures. While dental implant treatment may sound extensive, involved, and painful, most patients receive their dental implants in an outpatient setting and have few postoperative problems such as bleeding, infection, or pain. The general stages of dental implant treatment are outlined in Figure 26–3 ■.

The patient should be aware that several preoperative steps usually are necessary before the actual implant surgery. The restorative dentist (and the surgeon) should do a full workup on the patient. This includes mounted study casts, a wax-up of the planned restoration, fabrication of a radiographic and surgical guide

stent, and appropriate pretreatment radiographs such as periapicals, panoramic, and computed or linear tomography for a three-dimensional view of the bone. These steps are needed to ensure accurate planning as to implant number, diameter, length, and location based on the restorative needs of the patient, bone quantity and quality, and anatomic structures.

Bone quantity and quality of the maxilla and mandible is also important for implant success. Bone quantity refers to the available bone at the future implant

■ **FIGURE 26–3** Diagram of sequence of dental implant placement using two-stage technique. The body of the implant (fixture) is surgically placed in the bone under the gingiva, allowed to heal for several months, uncovered so that a healing post can be connected to the implant, and the restoration completed.

site. Bone quantity factors that must be evaluated are the bone width (distance between facial and lingual cortical plates of bone; a minimum of 5 mm is recommended), height (measured from the crest of the edentulous ridge to an anatomical structure such as the maxillary sinus or mandibular canal), and length (mesiodistal distance in an edentulous site or the distance between two adjacent implants (recommended distance between two implants is 3 mm). Determination of bone quality is based on bone density (Table 26–1 ■), which reflects the strength of the bone (Lekholm & Zarb, 1985). Types I, II, and III bone offer good strength, while type IV bone has poor strength because this type of bone has a thin cortical plate and low trabecular density.

Implant placement can be done as a two-stage or single-stage procedure in which the implant body is placed in the bone and following a healing period is surgically exposed to prepare the implant for a restoration. In the single-stage procedure the implant body is placed in bone with a portion of the implant body (collar) or abutment (post) left exposed until the time of restoration some time later.

Two-Stage Surgical Procedure

First-Stage Surgery

Once the patient is made comfortable and the areas of implant placement are anesthetized, the surgical guide stent is positioned and the specific implant locations marked. An incision is made through the crest of the gingiva, and flaps are reflected to expose the bone. A specific sequence of drills/burs is used to create a hole of specific diameter and depth for the implant(s) to be used. The drilling is done at relatively slow speed with copious irrigation to keep the bone cool and minimize trauma to the potential bone-healing cells. The root-form implant is then threaded or gently tapped into position so that its top is flush with the top of the bone. A cover screw is placed on top of the implant to seal the screwhole for cleanliness. The gingiva is then sutured to cover the implant(s) (Figure 26–4 ■). The implant surgeon may prescribe analgesics and antibiotics as needed. Sutures are left in place for approximately seven to fourteen days. While most patients would like to have a temporary tooth replacement in the implant area immediately, pressure on top of the implant should be avoided. A fixed temporary restoration relieved over the implant sites often can be placed in the partially edentulous implant patient.

The implants are allowed to heal undisturbed for three to six months in order that osseointegration occurs before second-stage uncovering surgery is performed. The time period needed for osseointegration varies depending on the bone quality or density and therefore is shortest for the mandibular anterior area, which is composed of dense cortical bone (three to four months), and longest for the maxillary posterior area, which is composed of more fragile cancellous bone (five to six months). However, recent advances in implant surfaces

---

Did You Know?

Cortical bone allows for a greater implant-bone contact and implant fixation than cancellous bone because cortical bone has a 80 to 90% volume density of bone matrix versus 20 to 25% for cancellous bone.

Table 26–1	Quality of Bone for Implant Placement	
Type of Bone	**Quality of Bone**	
I	Homogenous cortical (compact) bone	
II	Core of dense trabecular (cancellous) bone with a thick layer of compact bone surrounding it	
III	Thin layer of cortical bone surrounding dense trabecular bone of favorable strength	
IV	Thin layer of cortical bone surrounding a core of low-density trabecular bone	

Source: Lekholm & Zarb, 1985.

(a)

(b)

(c)

(d)

■ **FIGURE 26–4**   Clinical case illustrating implant placement. (a) Initial drill hole (osteotomy) using surgical guide stent. (b) Test pins placed to verify position and angulation of the planned implants. (c) Two implants placed into properly drilled holes to be level with bone crest. (d) Five-year follow-up radiograph illustrating fixed-bridge design for good oral hygiene and maintenance of bone level.

have allowed manufacturers to claim implants can be loaded as early as two months after placement (Avila, Galindo, & Rios, 2007).

Second-Stage Surgery

Second-stage or uncovering surgery is performed to expose the top of the implant to create a permanent opening and replace the cover screw with a temporary healing abutment or post that screws into the implant fixture and protrudes through the gingival tissue into the oral cavity. This surgery is usually performed using local anesthesia. After a small incision is made over the implants, the cover screw is removed, and the healing abutment is placed. The gingiva is then sutured tightly around the protruding

abutment. After two to three weeks of soft tissue healing, the restoration process continues. Impressions of the implant(s) are taken and crowns are fabricated to cement or screw onto the implant abutments. A removable prosthesis can also be attached to the abutment, which allows the patient to remove and clean the tooth.

RDH **Rapid Dental Hint**

A cooling water spray that is used during the osteotomy (drilling the hole in the bone) keeps the temperature of the bone to below 47 degrees Celsius (approximately 117 degrees Fahrenheit).

Single-Stage Surgical Procedure

Some implant systems avoid the second-stage surgery with one-stage implants. Single-stage implants are left exposed but not loaded at the time of surgery. This single-stage surgery still requires a three- to six-month healing time but rather than performing a second surgery, the cover screw or healing abutment is removed and the final restoration (crown) is placed.

Single-Stage Surgical Procedure with Early/Immediate Loading

Implants placed with primary stability can be put into function immediately as long as the forces are controlled and below the critical movement threshold. If primary stability cannot be achieved, then delayed (ex-

tended time for healing) loading is required. This procedure allows the attachment of a temporary prosthesis at the time of implant placement rather than waiting months until healing is complete. Early loading of implants with a dental prosthesis occurs at another visit after the surgery, whereas immediate loading of implants with dental prosthesis/tooth occurs at the same visit as the surgery (Assad, Hassan, Shawky, & Badawy, 2007; Esposito et al., 2007).

 Rapid Dental Hint

For an immediate implant placement, timing of the extraction is important due to the potential for postextraction bone resorption and ridge deformation.

(a)

(b)

(c)

■ **FIGURE 26–5**   (a) Preoperative clinical view of a missing maxillary canine. (b) Radiograph of implant placement to replace maxillary canine. (c) Final clinical view of single tooth implant. (Courtesy of Dr. Stuart J. Froum, New York, New York)

Single-Tooth Replacements

Single-tooth replacement with dental implants is a treatment option for anterior or posterior teeth. Single missing anterior and posterior teeth are generally caused by trauma/injury, congenitally missing, extensive caries, or failed endodontic procedures. In the past, the primary concern with single-tooth placements in the anterior maxilla was with aesthetics and having the single dental implant closely resemble adjacent natural teeth (Figure 26–5 ■). Advancements in clinical application, concepts, and technology have developed into single-tooth replacements with a high rate of success.

Immediate Implant Placement in Extraction Sockets

Implants can also be placed at the same visit that a natural tooth is extracted. Immediately following extraction of a tooth, the implant is placed into the socket. Loading can be performed at a future time or in the same visit. There are a number of considerations for success, including adequate availability of bone, primary stability of the implant, and absence of infection. Drawbacks to this type of surgery include protracted healing time, excessive pain and swelling, and a large ridge defect if the implant fails and has to be removed (Froum, 2005; Froum et al., 2007; Wagenberg & Froum, 2006).

Dental Implant Site Preservation and Development

A tooth that is going to be extracted and later used as an implant site requires intact cortical plates of bone after the extraction for optimal aesthetics and implant function. Atraumatic extraction and socket preservation techniques have been introduced to minimize bone resorption after tooth extraction (John, De Poi, & Blanchard, 2007). However, sometimes this is not possible, and the socket needs to be grafted with bone and membrane to preserve the alveolar plates. An implant is usually placed about six months after socket bone grafting (Figure 26–6 ■).

While the surgical procedures outlined above are basic and apply to patients with good bone quantity, quality, and form, additional procedures often must be used to build up the bone or gingival tissues to allow proper implant placement and restoration. These other procedures may include such therapy as guided bone regeneration (with bone grafts and membranes), soft tissue

(a)

■ **FIGURE 26–6** Extraction + graft: The maxillary central incisor was extracted and a bone graft placed in the extraction socket to preserve the bony walls for a future implant.

grafts, sinus bone grafts (sinus lift), distraction osteogenesis, or combinations of these. These additional procedures may extend the total treatment time until the final restoration can be delivered.

Guided bone regeneration (GBR) is a surgical procedure performed to increase the amount of alveolar bone available for the proper placement of a dental implant (Esposito, Grusovin, Coulthard, & Worthington, 2006). The terms *guided tissue regeneration* and *guided bone regeneration* are often used interchangeably in literature, but they are really two different terms—however, based on the same basic principles. Guided bone regeneration describes the formation of only bone, not any other tissue (McAllister & Haghighat, 2007), whereas guided tissue regeneration involves the formation of bone, cementum, and periodontal ligament around teeth. Guided bone regeneration surgery is indicated when there is a volume, height, or width deficiency of the residual ridge that prohibits implantation or optimal implant installation for aesthetic and functional needs (Keith & Salama, 2007; Kfir, Kfir, Eliav, & Kaluski, 2007; Migani & Esposito, 2007). Bone grafting and use of an absorbable (or nonabsorbable) membrane, which is placed over the bone defect site, is used to stimulate the patient's osteoblasts (bone-producing cells) to develop additional alveolar bone mass. This procedure is done about six months prior to placement of dental implants; however, it can be done in conjunction with dental implant placement surgery.

Sinus grafts are needed to increase the height of the posterior alveolus (Figure 26–7 ■). Surgery is performed

(a)

(b)

(c)

(d)

(e)

(f)

(g)

(h)

■ **FIGURE 26–7** Sinus lift procedure: (a,b) Preoperative X-ray and clinical slide of the maxillary right side. This procedure is performed to increase the amount of bone in the maxilla for implant placement. (c) Surgical incision made on the edentulous ridge. (d) Soft tissue in anterior maxilla has been reflected back to expose the bone. An outline of the maxillary sinus area has been made (e) Osteotomy in bone. Bone flap created by osteotomy has been pushed inward with maxillary sinus membrane (referred to as the Schneiderian membrane), creating space that is packed with bone graft material as shown in (f). (g) A membrane is placed over the bone material with bone tacks that hold the membrane in place to prevent movement. These tacks must be removed after healing has occurred. (h) Postoperative X-ray showing increased alveolar ridge height (right). Now implants can be placed.

to expose and elevate the maxillary sinus membrane from the floor of the sinus, and bone graft material is placed into this area. Onlay bone block grafts (bone is placed on the alveolar ridge) are required to augment thin ridges (buccal/lingual dimension) (Fugazzotto & Vlassis, 2007; Wallace et al., 2005).

Distraction osteogenesis is a surgical procedure used to increase the bone height of the alveolar ridges by cutting the bone into two pieces, which are gradually separated by 1 mm a day to form new bone between the cut pieces of bone. This allows for the displacement of bone into the deficient site. This procedure does not require placement of bone grafts. Figure 26–8 ■ reviews a case involving distraction osteogenesis.

Implant patients and dental office personnel must realize the stages and timeline involved in dental implant therapy. Generally, it takes nine to twelve months to arrive at the point of delivery of the desired restoration. Longer times are necessary if implant sites require bone grafts or guided tissue (bone) regeneration procedures prior to implant placement. After the final restoration is placed, patients must commit to long-term professional maintenance and optimal oral hygiene self-care.

Prostheses

The original Brånemark implant system in the 1980s was initially recommended for edentulous (no teeth) patients and used "hybrid" prostheses supported by implants in the anterior area of the maxilla or mandible with the abutments visible when the lips are retracted. The function was good but the appearance of these hybrid prostheses was not highly acceptable and alternative, more aesthetic restorations were needed. Completely edentulous mouths may be treated with fixed prostheses or overdentures, while partially edentulous mouths may be treated with fixed partial prostheses and single-tooth replacements.

Implant-supported overdentures are recommended in edentulous (completely without teeth) patients to provide more stability to the denture and may help stop alveolar ridge resorption. Usually, two mandibular implants

are placed in the canine area and a denture is fabricated to attach to the implants (Figure 26–9 ■).

If the patient is not totally edentulous, fixed dentures (bridges) attached to multiple implants may be a treatment option. Although some studies showed that splinting of implants to natural teeth resulted in intrusion of the natural tooth (Sheets & Earthman, 1993), a recent long-term study showed no higher risk for implant or prosthetic failure for implants splinted to teeth compared to implants splinted only to implants.

IMPLANTS VERSUS TEETH

There are obvious differences between implants and teeth in structure and components (Table 26–2 ■). Implants are not prone to caries, endodontic (pulpal) problems, or root sensitivity, as are teeth. However, implants depend on proper restoration and occlusion, good oral hygiene, and regular maintenance, just as teeth do. Having a healthy soft tissue barrier is very important. Superstructures should be designed to help facilitate this. It has been shown that plaque accumulation and excessive occlusal forces are primary causes for implant failures (Meffert, Langer, & Frutz, 1992).

Anatomy

Implant–Tissue Interface

Natural teeth are surrounded by the periodontium: alveolar and supporting bone, cementum, periodontal ligament, and gingiva. Dental implants are surrounded by peri-implant tissues, including osseointegrated bone surrounding the fixture. There is no periodontal ligament. The abutment, like the crown of a natural tooth, is surrounded by gingiva. After surgery, the gingiva heals around the abutment. During the healing process, a new free gingival margin forms, including a gingival sulcus.

On natural teeth, the junctional epithelium provides a seal at the base of the sulcus against the invasion of bacterial substances. If the seal is disrupted and/or the gingival fibers are destroyed, the junctional epithelium migrates in an apical direction onto the root surface and connective tissue fibers are destroyed, forming a periodontal pocket. The evidence supports the fact that a junctional epithelium, referred to as a **perimucosal seal,** adheres to implant component surfaces and has similar biologic features to the epithelial-tooth interface of a natural tooth.

■ **FIGURE 26–8**   Distraction osteogenesis procedure. (a) Note the reduced alveolar ridge height of the mandible. The mandibular bone height must be lengthened to place dental implants. (b) Surgical procedure starts with raising a flap and exposure of the cortical bone. The area is outlined where the distraction device will be placed. This device is used to transmit controlled torque for elongation of the device thereby affecting distraction osteogenesis. (c) This device for lengthening bone by distraction osteogenesis (separating bone pieces) comprises a telescoping screw assemble. (d) The flap is repositioned to cover the device and sutured. The lead screw is exposed and is left in place until bone healing occurs. (e) Final case complete. (Courtesy of Dr. Stuart J. Froum, New York, New York)

(a)

(b)

(c)

■ **FIGURE 26–9**   Periodontal probing around implants and tissue health. (a) Plastic probe with pressure-limiting mechanisms showing shallow probing depth. Note health of surface tissue. Also note relative lack of keratinized gingiva. (b) Probing access is easier with superstructure removed. Shallow probing depth and good zone of keratinized gingiva. (c) Inflamed tissue with deeper probing depth and bleeding on probing indicating an unhealthy implant site.

On the other hand, the implant–connective tissue interface shows marked differences when compared with the connective tissue in teeth. There is a lack of cementum, and no connective tissue fibers insert into the implant surface. Connective tissue fibers subjacent to the epithelium on implants have been shown to be either parallel or circular in orientation to the implant surface, but they do not insert directly into the implant surface. These circular fibers are likely the first line of defense against bacteria. The arrangement of fibers is sometimes called a pursestring arrangement, and it helps to keep the soft

tissues tightly adapted to the implant (Listgarten, Lang, Schroeder, & Schroeder, 1991).

Keratinized Gingiva

There are conflicting reports concerning the need for keratinized tissue around implants. However, multiple factors may influence the desirability for the presence of keratinized tissue (Bahat, 1996; Nemcovsky & Ofer, 2002). The type of tissue around an implant is essential to create the ideal emergence profile and an aesthetic illusion of a natural tooth (Kois, 2001). The type of tissue

Table 26–2   Biologic Environment

Natural Tooth	Dental Implant
Perpendicular connective tissue (PDL) attachment inserting into cementum	No PDL; parallel connective tissue fibers because there is no cementum for attachment
Cementum	No cementum
Greater blood supply at neck	Less blood supply at neck due to scar formation during healing
Plaque—more confined inflammation	Plaque—more widespread inflammation
Transseptal/supracrestal fibers	No limiting fibers; only circular or parallel
Aggressive or slow bone loss in suprabony or infrabony patterns	Earlier, faster bone loss—circumferential around the implant
Inflammation not found in bone marrow	Inflammation into bone marrow
May show slight mobility	Any mobility means implant failure

that surrounds a dental implant dictates the long-term health of the implant and its ability to withstand peri-implantitis (Nemcovsky & Ofer, 2002).

Blood Supply

Implants have less blood supply near their neck with more of a scar tissue appearance. Lack of a periodontal ligament limits the blood supply to the area to only the periosteal vessels (blood vessels covering the surface of bone) and bone marrow spaces.

Inflammatory Lesion

Dental plaque has been shown to grow faster on titanium than on enamel (Quirynen, Van Steenberghe, Jacobs, Schotte, & Darius, 1991). When plaque accumulation occurs, it results in more widespread inflammation around implants than the confined nature of the inflammatory lesion seen around teeth (Ericsson, Berglund, Marinello, Liljenberg, & Lindhe, 1992; Lekholm, 1986). This is due primarily to a lack of limiting attached connective tissue fibers such as the transseptal and supracrestal fiber groups that are present on teeth. Similarly, natural teeth tend to exhibit slow bone loss, and the inflammation does not usually extend into the bone marrow to any great degree. Infected implants, however, tend to have earlier and more rapid bone loss that extends into the adjacent bone marrow, creating a low-grade osteomyelitis.

BACTERIOLOGY

Neither dental implants nor natural teeth are immune to plaque accumulation. Regular, effective plaque control is imperative for soft tissue health and a good long-term prognosis with both.

Several studies have investigated the amount, rate, and contents of plaque deposits on implants as compared with teeth. Virtually all these studies show that there are no differences in the amount of plaque or the type of bacteria that accumulate on teeth or various implant surfaces. The types of pathogens found on both teeth and implants are similar (Newman & Flemming, 1988; Box 26–1). Peri-implantitis (inflammation of the soft tissues around the implant) and marginal bone loss have been associated with the presence of these pathogens in both partially and fully edentulous patients.

For both implants and teeth, smooth surfaces inhibit and roughened surfaces encourage plaque accumulation. Therefore, in-office maintenance procedures should not roughen the surface of implant components (or teeth). Care should be taken not to locally damage the implant surface with metal ultrasonic or manual instruments. Plastic instruments should be used instead.

In summation, the major difference between implants and teeth, therefore, is the mechanism by which they are attached to the jawbone. Teeth are connected to the bone by means of a connective tissue sling, the periodontal ligament, which is a dynamic, responsive, ad-

---

Box 26–1   Pathogens Associated with Peri-Implantitis

Porphyromonas gingivalis	*Fusobacterium nucleatum*
Campylobacter recta	*Eikenella corrodens*
Tannerella forsythensis	*Eubacterium* species
Prevotella intermedia	*Selemonas* species
Peptostreptococcus micros	Spirochetes
Actinobacillus actinomycetemcomitans	

---

justable attachment mechanism. Implants, by design, become osseointegrated or ankylosed without the cushioning effect of a periodontal ligament. Teeth can move as a result of occlusal or orthodontic forces. Implants do not have any physiologic movement.

IMPLANT MAINTENANCE PROGRAM

Periodontal maintenance procedures (continuing care) provided by the dental hygienist for implant patients include assessment of the entire oral cavity as well as the implant sites. A thorough assessment of plaque and calculus accumulation, as well as evaluation of soft and hard tissues, should be a part of the protocol for each maintenance visit. Box 26–2 reviews these assessment procedures.

The goal for maintenance therapy is to continually monitor the stable condition created by active treatment. Recall appointments should take place at three-month intervals, and the frequency should be increased if that interval is not adequate to maintain oral health.

Some clinicians assumed that patients with a history of tooth loss caused by periodontal disease presented a potentially higher risk for implant failure. However, several publications disproved this assumption demonstrating successful osseointegration in patients with different types of periodontal disease (Ellegaard, Baelum, & Karring, 1997; Mengel, Stelzel, Hasse, & Flores-de-Jacoby, 1996; Nevins & Langer, 1995). However, since the same periodontal microbiota colonizes teeth and implants placed in patients with periodontally compromised teeth, it is essential that optimum oral hygiene and plaque control be maintained prior to and following implant placement.

Box 26–2   Assessment of Dental Implants and Maintenance Procedures (In-Office)

1. Review medical history.
2. Head and neck examination, oral cancer screening.
3. Take radiographs every three months for first year after implant restoration is placed; then yearly to check for bone loss. Place radiographs in sequential mounts.
4. Remove superstructure if necessary and possible.
5. Clean superstructure.
6. Check tissues for surface inflammation.
7. Check for plaque and review oral hygiene practices.
8. Record probing depths using a plastic or nylon periodontal probe.
9. Record bleeding on probing.
10. Clean implant abutments using special nonmetallic instruments.
11. Irrigate with antimicrobial solution if indicated.
12. Replace superstructure, if removed.
13. Have occlusion checked.
14. Review dental hygiene again with superstructure in place.
15. Reschedule for three- or four-month recall, depending on evaluation of tissue and oral hygiene.

Clinical Parameters of Evaluation

Soft Tissue Evaluation

The clinical similarities between the natural dentition and dental implants have led to the use of similar parameters for evaluation of the periodontium and peri-implant tissues (Box 26–3). Clinical similarities provide a means of monitoring and observing peri-implant health status and the effectiveness of treatment. Evaluation of the soft tissue surrounding dental implants is very similar to that of natural tooth structure. A basic assessment begins with the color, contour, and consistency (texture) of the surrounding soft tissue. The presence of erythema, edema, and suppuration, which are the traditional signs of inflammation, should be noted. Thorough documentation of the changes in the soft tissue is important because change may signify current disease activity.

Probing Depth Probing depth also can be used to assess the health of peri-implant tissues. However, the use of periodontal probes for evaluation of the peri-implant condition is highly controversial (Brägger, 1994). Some clinicians feel that probing depth is not an important clinical parameter in the success of an implant (Smith & Zarb, 1989). Concern has been expressed that probing for pockets around an implant may create a pathway for bacteria to attack the peri-implant seal. The probe may carry microorganisms from an infected site and seed a noninfected site. Also, different probing forces allow the probe to penetrate into the connective tissue/bone region easily because of the lack of a connective tissue attachment. Gentle probing is recommended around implants if the practitioner suspects pathology.

Box 26–3 Periodontal Criteria for Success with Dental Implants

- No mobility
- Frequent inspection and debridement
- Shallow, stable pockets
- No bleeding on probing
- Effective oral hygiene
- Patient ability/accessibility
- Keratinized gingiva
- Accurate, secure fit of parts
- No trauma from occlusion
- Change in dental behavior pattern
- Maintenance of biocompatible interface

If probing is performed, four measurements around the circumference of the implant should be recorded. As with natural teeth, minimal probing depth (<4 mm) is preferable (Balshi, 1986; Orton, Steele, & Wolinsky, 1987). Changes in probing depth over a period of time around an implant may be more important as an indicator of disease activity than a single probe depth measurement (Balshi, 1986). The use of a plastic or nylon periodontal probe is recommended to prevent scratching of the titanium components. With some abutment and superstructure designs, accurate probing may be difficult because the probe is prevented from reaching the base of the sulcus; thus the probing depth may be underestimated. A more accurate measurement may be obtained by removing the superstructure, which would allow probe insertion parallel to the long axis of the implant. However, more important than the actual probing depth is detecting early changes in the depth of the pocket. Early detection provides an opportunity for therapeutic intervention before irreversible changes have occurred. Probing level has been demonstrated to correlate highly with the marginal bone level (Quirynen et al., 1991; Figure 26–9).

Bleeding on Probing Controversy also can be found in the literature regarding the use of bleeding on probing as a clinical assessment parameter for implants. As with natural teeth, bleeding on probing can be a significant clinical finding. Despite the apparent healthy look of surface tissues and even shallow probing depths, bleeding on probing is an indication that there is underlying disease (Lekholm, 1986). Any bleeding site (especially if the same site bleeds from visit to visit) should be inspected closely for the presence of irritants, and appropriate therapy should be instituted. However, some researchers find that bleeding may be related to probing force and wounding of the tissue rather than actual inflammation (Esposito, Hirsch, Lekholm, & Thomsen, 1998) and should not be used as an indicator of healthy or diseased peri-implant tissue.

Keratinized Gingiva

As mentioned earlier, the presence of keratinized gingiva adjacent to implants is associated with improved tissue health. As with natural teeth, keratinization improves the strength and stability of the epithelium and promotes long-term implant success. An inadequate zone of keratinized gingiva may lead to increased recession, tissue soreness with toothbrushing or eating, and the ability of metallic components to be seen through mucosal tissues.

Hard Tissue Evaluation

Radiographic Procedures

Implant bone levels are best determined by regular accurate radiographic evaluations. Panoramic radiographs commonly are taken for baseline data following abutment placement; however, individual periapical or vertical bitewing radiographs should be taken using the paralleling technique with a gridded film (film with millimeter markings). Such radiographs are preferable for determining bone height and density. Marginal bone height should be measured both mesially and distally and recorded in relation to a landmark on the implant system. For dental implant success, 0.2 mm or less of bone loss annually along the implant surface is acceptable (Albrektsson, Zarb, Worthington, & Eriksson, 1986). For proper continued evaluation, radiographic examinations are recommended after prosthetic connection, at six and twelve months, and subsequently at one- to three-year intervals.

Mobility

It is recommended that the prosthesis be removed at least once a year to test for implant and abutment mobility. Since the truly osseointegrated implant has no periodontal ligament, there should be zero mobility around healthy implants. Mobility of an implant after an appropriate healing period is a sign of implant failure, indicating lack of osseointegraton. Radiographic examinations together with implant mobility tests seem to be the most reliable parameters in the prognostic assessment of osseointegrated implants (Esposito et al., 1998).

Mobility of the superstructure can be evaluated by wedging a curet between the prosthesis and the abutment head or by traditional mobility detection. If the abutment is loose, the screws may need to be examined and possibly tightened.

Identifying the Problem Implant

While endosseous root-form dental implants are quite successful, with most studies showing greater than 90% long-term success with a variety of systems, some do develop problems. Identification of these problems when they first begin is important for effective management. The two primary reasons for ailing and failing implants are bacterial infection and mechanical trauma.

Criteria for Success

The periodontal criteria for success are similar for dental implants and natural teeth (Box 26–3). The basis of success is frequent inspection and debridement. As with natural teeth, shallow and stable probing depths are desirable at each visit. In addition, there should be no bleeding on probing at any evaluation site. An adequate zone of keratinized gingiva may be advantageous to protect the soft tissue interface (Brånemark et al., 1985). The main difference in success criteria involves mobility. While unchanging mobility within physiologic limits is acceptable with natural teeth, any implant mobility is unacceptable.

Restoratively, the prosthesis must fit accurately and securely. There should be no trauma from occlusion (excessive occlusal force on the implant), especially in lateral excursions. Moreover, there should be no mobility of the superstructure and especially of the implant itself. Radiographically, no radiolucency should be present around the implant, and less than 0.2 mm of bone loss per year should be present.

Perhaps the most important factor in success is to effect a change in the patient's dental behavior pattern. If this occurs, and the preceding technical aspects are achieved, then a biocompatible interface between the implant and the host tissues can be maintained for a long time. These criteria are summarized in Box 26–3 (Smith & Zarb, 1989).

 Rapid Dental Hint

There should be at least 1.5 to 2 mm of interproximal bone between an implant and a natural tooth.

Overloading of Implants

Mechanical failures of both the implant components and prosthetic superstructures have been associated with occlusal overload and ill-fitting restorative frameworks. Since implants do not have a periodontal ligament, occlusal forces placed on the implant are transmitted directly to alveolar bone instead of the periodontal ligament. Thus, excessive occlusal force (overloading) generated either from improper placement/angle of implant, prosthesis design, and/or parafunctional activity may cause loosening and/or fracture of the screws through bending overload (Akca & Iplik-cioglu, 2001).

> ## Did You Know?
> The most obvious sign of implant failure is mobility.

Marginal bone loss around implants also has been associated with implant overload.

Stages of Peri-Implant Disease

Plaque-induced inflammation occurs in a similar fashion around dental implants as around natural teeth. The pathogenesis is very similar for both entities, but there are several differences, as noted earlier in this chapter. **Peri-implant diseases** keep classified as peri-implant mucositis and peri-implantitis.

Peri-implant mucositis is similar to gingivitis; it is a reversible inflammatory reaction with bleeding on probing. There may be slight increased probing depths, but the perimucosal seal is intact.

Peri-implantitis has many of the same clinical manifestations and stages as periodontitis and is characterized by rapid loss of bone that can occur without any classic signs of pain or mobility. Peri-implantitis is an aggressive lesion. It can be graded from slight to severe, and its treatment parallels that of the stages of periodontitis (Figures 26–10 ■, 26–11 ■, 26–12 ■). Slight problems are treated with improved oral hygiene and nonsurgical local therapy (controlled-release antibiotics, mouthrinses) (Ciancio, Lauciello, Shibly, Vitello, & Mather, 1995). Moderate problems usually require systemic antibiotics (Mombelli & Lang, 1992) or flap access surgery. Severe problems require flap surgery for access, with the likelihood of regenerative therapy, including bone-replacement grafts and guided tissue regeneration barriers. The latter has not been shown to be as effective with implants as with natural teeth. The best results in severe cases of peri-implantitis are obtained when the implant has the plaque removed and can be reburied to recapture the lost osseointegration. Sometimes, the problem is so advanced that the implant must be removed.

Superstructure Removal

On some occasions, the prosthetic superstructure supported by an implant must be removed for better access for maintenance of the implant abutment posts. Some superstructures are removable prostheses anyway, and the patient is familiar with their removal and replacement. Others (increasingly common) are fixed prostheses (screw-retained or cemented) and must be removed by dental office personnel.

Since the hygienist may be asked to remove a superstructure, he or she must be familiar with the removal and replacement process (Box 26–4).

Removing the superstructure generally entails unscrewing it from the abutments. This must be done in a systematic way. For example, a patient may have crowns and bridges from tooth 2 to tooth 15 with six implants under this superstructure. The hygienist should have six containers, small cups, or dappen dishes, with markings on them to correspond to the jaw location of the implants. When the screw from implant 2 is removed, it should be placed in the container marked 2. When the screw from implant 6 is removed, it should be placed in the container

(a)

(b)

■ **FIGURE 26–10**   Radiographic evidence of bone loss around dental implants, indicating peri-implantitis.

(a)

(b)

(c)

■ **FIGURE 26–11**   (a) X-ray showing implants with peri-implantitis. There is bone loss around the threads of the implant. (b) Clinical characteristics of these implants. Note the presence of gingival inflammation and swelling. (c) Surgical site with flap reflected showing bone loss around the implants.

marked 6, and so on. The hygienist will want to back the screws off a little at a time, alternating among them, much in the way a tire is removed and replaced on a car. Unscrewing one side, for example, implant screws 2, 4, and 6 all the way, and not unscrewing implant screws 11, 13, and 15, may cause the integrity of the implants and superstructure to be compromised. When removing screws, the hygienist should employ a throat pack (gauze) to block and prevent any loose screws or abutments from being accidentally swallowed by the patient.

Once the superstructure is removed, better access is available to evaluate the soft tissue and gingiva and provide maintenance therapy to the individual implants. The

Did You Know?

The peri-implant sulcus and the surfaces of endosseous dental implants acquire the patient's indigenous periodontal microflora.

(a)

(b)

(c)

■ **FIGURE 26–12**   Peri-implantitis: (a) Surgical exposure of an implant. Bone resorption has occurred on the buccal aspect. Note the dehiscence with exposure of the threads of the implant. (b) Placement of Bio-Oss bone graft in the bony defect and (c) a barrier membrane attached to the bone with bone tacks. (Courtesy of Dr. Stuart J. Froum, New York, New York)

superstructure itself should be thoroughly inspected and cleaned. The hygienist must be aware that the inside of the screw holes always must be kept free of debris or pumice, or the screws may not fit, and the superstructure may not seat properly.

When replacing the superstructure, begin with one implant, and slightly tighten the screw. Then move to the

next implant, and so on, just like replacing a tire on a car. Once all the screws are in position and slightly tightened, the hygienist can begin to tighten them down fully. Since peri-implant bone loss may result from occlusal overload, always make sure the occlusion is checked once the superstructure is in place.

Appropriate Instruments for Implants

Deposits that accumulate on supra- and subgingival surfaces of dental implant components should be removed. Normally, calculus on these surfaces is not as tenacious as on natural teeth because the deposits do not penetrate or interlock with the implant component surfaces (Lang, Mombelli, & Attström, 2003).

RDH   **Rapid Dental Hint**

It is very important for patients to be on a regular recall schedule for maintenance, including plaque control, of the implant-supported prostheses.

Box 26–4   Removal and Replacement of Superstructure

1. Review radiographs and familiarize yourself with the implant location(s).
2. Note location of each implant under super-structure.
3. Have appropriately sized screws and instruments for removal and replacements available.
4. Remove any temporary filling material that may be in the screw hole area.
5. Have small containers, dappen dishes, or envelopes available. When removing the screws use a throat pack.
6. Once screws are removed, place in containers labeled as to location.
7. If removing extensive restorations, loosen screws a little at a time. Then return to each screw and loosen fully.
8. Remove superstructure and examine underside for debris.
9. Clean appropriately, keeping the integrity of the interface with the abutments and the screw holes free of debris.
10. Clean around implant abutments.
11. Replace superstructure.
12. Using correct screws, screw into place using same sequential technique as was used when removing superstructure.
13. Place temporary filling material over screws if indicated.
14. Check occlusion.

■ **FIGURE 26–13**   Several types of nonmetallic scalers and curets for use on dental implant components.

Air-powder abrasive units are effective, but they should not be used directly on implant components for any length of time. The use of ultrasonic- and sonic-powered scalers with metal tips is also contraindicated with implants. Specific plastic or nylon sleeves placed over the tip are available that allow cleaning of implants without scratching (Figure 26–15 ■).

In-Office Irrigation

The purpose of in-office irrigation is to attempt to irrigate to the base of the pocket. Plastic rather than metal irrigation tips or needles should be used when irrigating around implants, and care should be taken not to become too aggressive in forcing the tip into the pocket. Using an irrigation device with an antimicrobial solution at every maintenance visit is considered to be of some benefit by certain practitioners. Irrigation can be used if pathologic changes are present (Meffert et al., 1992). However, this information is anecdotal, and there are not enough controlled clinical studies to support implant irrigation.

DENTAL HYGIENE NOTES

Implant therapy is a rapidly growing part of dental care. With the growing number of implants being placed, the dental team will have an important role in helping attain and preserve the oral health of these patients. Patient education regarding the scope of implant procedures, recommendations for daily home-care regimens, periodic maintenance visits, and regular evaluations are all part of the role of the dental hygienist. The hygienist probably will spend the most time with the patient and can help contribute substantially to the success of dental implant treatment. The dental hygienist has a significant role not only in implant maintenance but also in patient

The nature of the surface of implant components must be considered when deciding which instruments to use during office procedures. Most implant components are titanium, a very tough but easily scratchable metal. Stainless steel and carbon steel instruments used directly on titanium can cause marring and scratching of the surface, resulting in roughness, which can increase plaque adherence. Curets made of **nonmetallic materials,** such as plastic, graphite, Teflon®, or nylon, are recommended, and these are available from several manufacturers (Figures 26–13 ■, 26–14 ■). Cleaning around the tissue surface of the prosthesis and implant abutments also can be performed with gauze or tufted floss.

(a)

(b)

■ **FIGURE 26–14**   Use of nonmetallic curets.

■ **FIGURE 26–15**   Nylon or plastic sleeve for ultrasonic or sonic instruments to prevent scratching of implant components.

motivation and education. It is important to keep in mind that implant therapy is not for everyone. For this reason, it is crucial that the dental hygienist be informed about implant types, the sequence of therapy, and the social and systemic factors that influence implant success.

KEY POINTS

- Controversy exists regarding the use of periodontal probes around healthy implants.

- Progressive bone loss is a pathologic sign that can lead to implant failure.
- The implant should not be mobile; mobility indicates lack of osseointegration and implant failure.
- Different prosthetic designs are used for final implant restorations.
- Implant placement can be done as a single- or second-stage procedure.
- Metal (e.g., stainless steel) instruments should never be used on dental implants; use only Teflon®, wood, nylon, graphite, rubber, or plastic instruments.

SELF-QUIZ

1. All the following systemic conditions are precautions or contraindications to implant placement except one. Which one is the exception? (p. 414)
   a. Uncontrolled diabetes mellitus
   b. Controlled hypertension
   c. Smoking
   d. AIDS
2. Which one of the following types of dental implants is used most commonly today to support prostheses? (pp. 414–415)
   a. Submucosal
   b. Subperiosteal
   c. Endosseous
   d. Transosteal

3. Which one of the following similarities is common between dental implants and natural teeth? (p. 423)
   a. Bone interface
   b. Microbial flora
   c. Connective tissue attachment
   d. Probing depths topography

4. The presence of keratized gingiva is important around implants because it may improve tissue health. (p. 428)
   a. Both the statement and the reason are correct and related.
   b. Both the statement and the reason are correct but not related.
   c. The statement is correct, but the reason is not.
   d. The statement is not correct, but the reason is correct.

5. In which one of the following drugs a patient is taking is implant placement a contraindication? (p. 414)
   a. IV bisphosphonate
   b. Aspirin
   c. Acetaminophen
   d. Vitamin D

6. All the following types of instruments are used to clean implant abutments except one. Which one is the exception? (p. 433)
   a. Teflon®
   b. Stainless steel
   c. Nickel
   d. Wood

7. Which one of the following factors is the major criterion for success of an implant? (p. 428)
   a. Inflammation
   b. Mobility
   c. Bleeding
   d. Bone level

8. Which one of the following parameters is most reliable in the assessment of the prognosis for osseointegrated implants? (pp. 427–428)
   a. Color and contour of the gingiva
   b. Bleeding on probing and mobility
   c. Radiographic changes and mobility
   d. Periodontal probing and color of the gingiva

9. Which one of the following signs indicates implant failure? (p. 429)
   a. Deep probing depths
   b. Edematous tissue
   c. Bleeding
   d. Mobility

10. Oral irrigation should be used routinely around dental implants because there is no periodontal ligament attachment to an implant, allowing for easy access of the irrigant to the implant surface. (p. 433)
    a. Both the statement and the reason are correct and related.
    b. Both the statement and the reason are correct but not related.
    c. The statement is correct, but the reason is not.
    d. The statement is not correct, but the reason is correct.
    e. Neither the statement nor the reason is correct.

REFERENCES

Akca, K., and H. Iplikcioglu. 2001. Finite element stress analysis of the influence of staggered versus straight placement of dental implants. *Int. J. Oral Maxillofac. Implants* 16:722–730.

Albrektsson, T., and L. Sennerby. 1991. State of the art in oral implants. *J. Clin. Periodontal.* 16:474–481.

Albrektsson, T., G. Zarb, P. Worthington, and A. R. Eriksson. 1986. The long-term efficacy of currently used dental implants: A review and proposed criteria of success. *Int. J. Oral Maxillofac. Implants* 1:11–25.

Assad, A. S., S. A. Hassan, Y. M. Shawky, and M. M. Badawy. 2007, June. Clinical and radiographic evaluation of implant-retained mandibular overdentures with immediate loading. *Implant Dent.* 16(2):212–223.

Avila, G., P. Galindo, and H. Rios. 2007. Immediate implant loading: Current status from available literature. *Implant Dent.* 16(3):235–245.

Bain, C. A. 1996. Smoking and implant failure: Benefits of a smoking cessation protocol. *Int. J. Oral Maxillofac. Implants* 11:756–759.

Bahat, O. 1996. Interrelations of soft and hard tissues for osseointegrated implants. *Compend. Contin. Educ. Dent.* 12:1161–1170.

Balshi, T. J. 1986. Hygiene maintenance procedures for patients treated with the tissue integrated prosthesis (osseointegration). *Quintessence Int.* 17:95–102.

Belser, U., R. Mericske-Stern, D. Buser, J. P. Bernard, D. Hess, and J. P. Martinet. 1996. Preoperative diagnosis and treatment planning. In eds. A. Schroeder, F. Sutter, D. Buser, and G. Krekeler, *Oral Implantology,* 231–255. New York: Thieme Medical.

Brägger, U. 1994. Maintenance, monitoring, therapy of implant failures. In eds. N. P. Lang and T. Karring, *Proceedings of the 1st European Workshop on Periodontology.* Chicago: Quintessence.

Brånemark, P. I., U. Breine, R. Adell, O. Hansson, J. Lindström, and A. Ohlsson. 1969. Intraosseous anchorage of dental prosthesis. *Scand. J. Plast. Reconstr. Surg.* 3:81–100.

Brånemark, P. I., G. Zarb, and T. Albrektsson. 1985. *Tissue-integrated prosthesis osseointegration in clinical dentistry.* Chicago: Quintessence.

Cartsos, V. M., S. Zhu, and A. Zavras. 2008. Bisphosphonate use and the risk of adverse jaw outcomes. *JADA* 139(1):23–30.

Ciancio, S. G., C. Lauciello, O. Shibly, M. Vitello, and M. Mather. 1995. The effect of an antiseptic mouthrinse on implant maintenance: Plaque and peri-implant gingival tissues. *J. Peridontol.* 66:962–965.

Cochran, D. 1996. Implant therapy. I. *Ann. Periodontol.* 1:707–820.

Dao, T. T., J. D. Anderson, and G. A. Zarb. 1993. Is osteoporosis a risk factor for osseointegration of dental implants? *Int. J. Oral Maxillofac. Implants.* 8:137–144.

Edwards, B. J., J. W. Hellstein, and P. L. Jacobson. Updated recommendations for managing the care of patients receiving oral bisphosphonate therapy: An advisory statement from the American Dental Association Council on Scientific Affairs. *J Am Dent Assoc.* 2008; 139; 1674–1677.

Ellegaard, B., V. Baelum, and T. Karring. 1997. Implant therapy in periodontally compromised patients. *Clin. Oral Implants Res.* 8:180–188.

Ericsson, I., N. T. Berglund, C. Marinello, B. Liljenberg, and J. Lindhe. 1992. Long-standing plaque and gingivitis at implants and teeth in the dog. *Clin. Oral Implant Res.* 3:99–103.

Esposito, M., M. G. Grusovin, P. Coulthard, and H. V. Worthington. 2006. The efficacy of various bone augmentation procedures for dental implants: A Cochrane systematic review of randomized controlled clinical trials. *Int. J. Oral Maxillofac. Implants* 21(5):696–710.

Esposito, M., M. G. Grusovin, M. Willings, et al. 2007. The effectiveness of immediate, early, and conventional loading of dental implants: A Cochrane systematic review of randomized controlled clinical trials. *Int. J. Oral Maxillofac. Implants* 22(6):893–904.

Esposito, M., J. M. Hirsch, U. Lekholm, and P. Thomsen. 1998. Biological factors contributing to failures of osseointegrated oral implants: I. Success criteria and epidemiology. *Eur. J. Oral Sci.* 106:527–551.

Froum, S. J. 2005, July. Immediate placement of implants into extraction sockets: Rationale, outcomes, technique. *Alpha Omegan* 98(2):20–35.

Froum, S. J., S. C. Cho, H. Francisco, et al. 2007. Immediate implant placement and provisionalization—two case reports. *Pract. Proced. Aesthet. Dent.* 19(10):621–628.

Fugazzotto, P. A., W. S. Lightfoot, R. Jaffin, and A. Kumar. 2007, September. Implant placement with or without simultaneous tooth extraction in patients taking oral bisphosphonates: Postoperative healing, early follow-up, and the incidence of complications in two private practices. *J. Periodontol.* 78(9):1664–1669.

Fugazzotto, P. A., and J. Vlassis. 2007. Report of 1633 implants in 814 augmented sinus areas in function for up to 180 months. *Impl. Dent.* 16(4):369–378.

Grant, B. T., C. Amenedo, K. Freeman, and R. A. Kraut. 2008. Outcomes of placing dental implants in patients taking oral bisphosphonates: A review of 115 cases. *J. Oral Maxillofac. Surg.* 66(2):223–230.

John, V., R. De Poi, and S. Blanchard. 2007, December. Socket preservation as a precursor of future implant placement: Review of the literature and case reports. *Compend. Contin. Educ. Dent.* 28(12):646–53; quiz, 654, 671.

Keith, J. D., Jr., and M. A. Salama. 2007, November. Ridge preservation and augmentation using regenerative materials to enhance implant predictability and esthetics. *Compend. Contin. Educ. Dent.* 28(11):614–21; quiz, 622–4.

Kfir, E., V. Kfir, E. Eliav, and E. Kaluski. 2007. Minimally invasive guided bone regneration. *J. Oral Implantol.* 33:205–210.

Kois, J. C. 2001. Predictable single tooth peri-implant esthetics: Five diagnostic keys. *Compend. Contin. Educ. Dent.* 3: 199–206.

Lang, N. P., A. Mombelli, and R. Attström. 2003. Dental plaque and calculus. In *Clinical periodontology and implant dentistry*, 4th ed., 81–105. Oxford, UK: Blackwell Publishing.

Lekholm, M. 1986. Marginal tissue reactions at osseointegrated titanium fixtures. *Int. J. Oral Maxillofac. Implants* 15:53–61.

Lekholm, M., and G. A. Zarb. 1985. Patient selection. In eds. P-I. Brånemark, G. A. Zarb, & T. Albrektsson. *Tissue integrated prosthesis. Osseointegration in clinical dentistry*, 199–209. Chicago: Quintessence.

Listgarten, M. A., N. P. Lang, H. E. Schroeder, and A. Schroeder. 1991. Periodontal tissues and their counterparts around endosseous implants. *Clin. Oral Implant Res.* 2:1–19.

Marx, R. E. 2007. *Oral and intravenous bisphsphonate-induced osteonecrosis of the jaws: History, etiology, prevention, and treatment.* Chicago, IL: Quintessence, 15.

Marx, R. E., J. E. Cillo, Jr., and J. J. Ulloa. 2007, December. Oral bisphosphonate-induced osteonecrosis: Risk factors, prediction of risk using serum CTx testing, prevention, and treatment. *J. Oral Maxillofac. Surg.* 65(12):2397–2410.

Marx, R.E., Y. Sawatari, M. Fortin, and V. Broumand. 2005. Bisphosphonate-induced exposed bone (osteonecrosis/osteopetrosis) of the jaws: Risk factors, recognition, prevention, and treatment. *J. Oral Maxillofac. Surg.* 63:1567–157.

McAllister, B.S., and K. Haghighat. 2007. Bone augmentation techniques. *J. Periodontol.* 78;377–396.

Meffert, R., B. Langer, and M. Frutz. 1992. Dental implants: A review. *J. Periodontol.* 63:859–870.

Mengel, R., Stelzel, M. Hasse, C. and Flores-de-Jacoby, L. 1996. Osseointegrated implants in patients treated for generalized severe adult periodontitis. An interim report. *J. Periodontol.* 67:782–787.

Migani, M., and M. Esposito. 2007, May-June. Vertical ridge augmentation with autogenous bone grafts: Resorbable barriers supported by osteosynthesis plates versus titanium-reinforced barriers. A preliminary report of a blinded, randomized controlled clinical trial. *Int. J. Oral Maxillofac. Implants* 22(3):373–382.

Mombelli, A., and N. P. Lang. 1992. Antimicrobial treatment of peri-implant infections. *Clin. Oral Implants Res.* 3:162–168.

Nemcovsky, C. E., and M. Ofer. 2002. Rotated palatal flap. A surgical approach to increase keratinized tissue width in maxillary implant uncovering: Technique and clinical evaluation. *Int. J. Periodont. Restor. Dent.* 22:607–612.

Nevins, M., and B. Langer. 1995. The successful use of osseointegrated implants for the treatment of the recalcitrant periodontal patient. *J. Periodontol.* 66:150–157.

Newman, M., and T. Flemming. 1988. Periodontal considerations of implants and implant associated microbiota. *J. Dent. Ed.* 52:737–744.

Orton, G. S., D. L. Steele, and L. E. Wolinsky. 1987. The dental professional's role in monitoring and maintenance of tissue-integrated prosthesis. *Int. J. Oral Maxillofac. Implants* 4:305–310.

Quirynen, M., D. van Steenberghe, R. Jacobs, A. Schotte, and P. Darius. 1991. The reliability of pocket probing around screw-type implants. *Clin. Oral Implant Res.* 2:186–192.

Sheets, C. G., and J. C. Earthman. 1993. Natural tooth intrusion and reversal in implant-assisted prostheses. *J. Prost. Dent.* 70:513–520.

Smith, D., and G. Zarb. 1989. Criteria for success of osseointegrated endosseous implants. *J. Prosthet. Dent.* 62:567–572.

Wagenberg, B., and S.J. Froum. 2006, January-February. A retrospective study of 1925 consecutively placed immediate implants from 1988 to 2004. *Int. J. Oral Maxillofac. Implants* 21(1):71–80.

Wallace, S. S., S. J. Froum, S. C. Cho, et al. 2005, December. Sinus augmentation utilizing anorganic bovine bone (Bio-Oss) with absorbable and nonabsorbable membranes placed over the lateral window: Histomorphometric and clinical analyses. *Int. J. Periodont. Restor. Dent.* 25(6):551–559.

Wang, H. L., D. Weber, and L. K. McCauley. 2007. Effect of long-term oral bisphosphonates on implant wound healing: Literature review and a case report. *J. Periodontol.* 78(3):584–594.

Weinlander, M. 1991. Bone growth around dental implants. *Dent. Clin. North Am.* 35:585–601.

Chapter 27

Periodontal Emergencies

Mea A. Weinberg

OUTLINE
Introduction
Necrotizing Periodontal Diseases
Primary Herpetic Gingivostomatitis
Dental Hygiene Notes
Key Points
Self-Quiz
References

EDUCATIONAL OBJECTIVES

Upon completion of this chapter, the reader should be able to:

• Define the role of the dental hygienist in the treatment of abscesses.
• Define the role of the dental hygienist in the treatment of necrotizing ulcerative gingivititis.
• Define the role of the dental hygienist in the treatment of primary herpetic gingivostomatitis.
• Define the role of the dental hygienist in the treatment of pericoronitis.

GOAL: To provide an understanding of the etiology, identifying features, and therapy of different emergency infections.

KEY WORDS

gingival abscess **439**
necrotizing ulcerative
    diseases **441**
operculum **441**
periodontal abscess
    439
primary herpetic
    gingivostomatitis
    442

INTRODUCTION

Chapter 11 reviewed the different types of abscesses of the periodontium. This chapter reviews the treatment of these abscesses as well as other common periodontal emergencies that may be encountered in the dental office (Minsk, 2006).

As mentioned in Chapter 11, an abscess is defined as an infection originating from the tooth or periodontium. Pain and swelling from an abscess usually brings the patient into the dental office as an emergency visit. Classification of abscesses is based upon the location of the infection. For example, a gingival abscess is an infection located in the gingival tissue, usually the free (marginal) gingiva; a periodontal abscess is an infection located within the tissues adjacent to the periodontal pocket; and a pericoronal abscess is an infection located within the tissue around the crown of a partially erupted tooth, usually the last tooth in the arch. Treatment of an abscess is based upon the origin of the abscess.

Gingival Abscess

To review, a **gingival abscess** is an acute infection characterized by a localized, painful edema at the free gingival margin. Foreign objects such as popcorn kernels, fish bones, or seeds that become lodged in the gingival crevice are responsible for many gingival abscesses. Since the abscess develops fairly rapidly (within 24 to 48 hours), the patient often knows the cause. Calculus is usually *not* the etiologic factor. Often, there are no signs of periodontitis (Corbet, 2004).

The differential diagnosis of a gingival abscess is a periodontal abscess or endodontic abscess. The gingival abscess is usually located more coronally than the periodontal or endodontic abscess. The gingival abscess is usually found just within the gingival sulcus, whereas the periodontal abscess is usually found at the lateral side (corresponding to a deep pocket), and the endodontic abscess is usually found at the apical area of the root. Treatment requires removal of the etiologic agent by periodontal debridement (Table 27–1 ■). Since the gingiva may be friable, careful tissue manipulation is advised. It is best to place the finger of the nondominant hand on the tissue to support it. Local anesthesia may be helpful, but the injection should never be directly into the infection as the infection may spread. Scaling establishes drainage through the gingival crevice. The patient can be placed on a warm saline rinse (1/4 teaspoonful of salt to 8 oz of warm water; rinse every one to two hours for several days). Make sure the patient is not hypertensive (because of the salt). The patient should be instructed to use a soft-bristled toothbrush. If treated adequately, the condition will resolve within 24 hours or so. Systemic antibiotics are not recommended, as there is no systemic infection.

Periodontal Abscess

A **periodontal abscess,** also called a lateral abscess, is a localized purulent nidus of acute inflammation within the periodontal tissues. A periodontal abscess develops as a result of a bacterial infection that eventually leads to the formation of pus (suppuration). Periodontal abscesses show typical clinical features associated with untreated periodontitis (Jaramillo et al., 2005). Gram-negative anaerobic rods are the most common bacteria isolated in the exudate of periodontal abscesses (Herrera, Roldan, & Sanz, 2000; Meng, 1999). Thus, a periodontal abscess contains bacteria, bacterial by-products, inflammatory

Table 27–1	Treatment Steps for Gingival and Periodontal Abscesses	
Gingival	*Periodontal*
First probe the site: shallow	First probe the site: deep
Periodontal health	Periodontitis
Location is submarginal	Location is base of pocket
Incision and drainage: debride and irrigate area	Incision and drainage: debridement and irrigation
Rinse with warm water and salt	May require periodontal surgery for pocket elimination or extraction
No antibiotics required	Systemic antibiotics if lymphadenopathy is present

cells, tissue breakdown products, and serum. In the gingival connective tissues an inflammatory reaction occurs due to the bacteria and bacterial by-products, resulting in the connective tissue becoming infiltrated with inflammatory cells (e.g., neutrophils, macrophages). As a result of the inflammatory infiltrate, there is destruction or breakdown of the gingival connective tissues (e.g., collagen). The bacterial mass becomes encapsulated with the resultant pus formation.

Periodontal abscess formation is often seen in deep periodontal pockets (Figures 27–1 ■, 27–2 ■) and in furcation sites. Such patients usually have a number of sites with chronic periodontitis. Periodontal abscesses can occur as a result of inadvertent embedding of a foreign body subgingivally (calculus fragment, popcorn husk, seeds, shellfish fragments, etc.) that obstructs the normal sulcular drainage of gingival crevicular fluid and inflammatory by-products of chronic periodontitis. To reestablish drainage, a fistula may form that drains pus through the otherwise intact surface of the gingiva or mucosa.

The periodontal abscess presents as a shiny, swollen, discolored mass on the gingiva or mucosa. Finger pressure may produce purulent drainage. The involved tooth is often tender to percussion, mobile, and may feel high to the patient. Patients usually complain of pain. Occasionally, patients may demonstrate localized lymphadenopathy and fever.

It is important to rule out a pulpal etiology prior to addressing the periodontal condition. To help confirm the diagnosis, an endodontic gutta percha point is placed

■ **FIGURE 27–2** Draining periodontal abscess in a child.

into the fistula and positioned until resistance is felt. A radiograph is taken with the gutta percha point in place. The end of the point will end at the origin of the abscess. This will help to distinguish between a periodontal and endodontic abscess.

Treatment of a periodontal abscess consists of two phases (Herrera et al., 2000). The first phase involves management of the acute signs and symptoms. Different therapies have been suggested for the acute lesion, including incision and drainage, scaling and root planing, administration of systemic antibiotics, periodontal surgery, and tooth extraction (see Table 27–1). Some clinicians prefer to wait until the acute lesion has subsided followed by scaling and root planing (López-Píriz, Aguilar, & Giménez, 2007), or periodontal surgery. Treatment consists of establishing drainage and removing any foreign causative agent. When giving infiltration anesthesia, the abscess should never be directly injected into because the infection could spread. Drainage is initially obtained through the pocket entrance either with a periodontal probe or a curet. Then, subgingival debridement reestablishes drainage and removes any foreign body. Antibiotics may be prescribed if systemic involvement (e.g., fever and/or lymphadenopathy) is suspected. The

■ **FIGURE 27–1** Periodontal abscess involving the mandibular molar area. Initial treatment involved scaling and root planing and then referral to a periodontist.

Did You Know?

Abscesses are polymicrobial in nature. *Fusobacterium nucleatum* is found in severe infections.

successfully treated patient will notice improvement within 24 hours of treatment. If symptoms fail to improve promptly, surgical access to the affected root surface may be necessary.

Once acute symptoms resolve, the second phase of treatment is performed to treat the underlying original or residual periodontal lesion. This may consist of periodontal surgery to eliminate the deep periodontal pocket.

Rapid Dental Hint

Always know the origin of the infection; is the infection coming from the pulp or from the periodontal tissues?

Pericoronal Abscess

The gingival flap (or **operculum**) overlying the erupting tooth (third molar) usually disappears once the tooth fully erupts, but many of these teeth remain partially erupted (Figure 27–3 ■). Food and debris accumulate under the operculum, leading to a localized purulent infection within the tissue surrounding the partially erupted crown (Meng, 1999). Trimus is another common symptom.

Treatment initially is toward controlling the infection. Irrigation with saline, iodine solution, or water is common therapy to flush out the food and debris found under the operculum. This area is very sensitive, so care must be taken when manipulating the tissues. If the infection is severe or systemic involvement (e.g., lymphadenopathy) is suspected, systemic antibiotics such as penicillin are indicated. Ultimately, extraction of the erupting tooth may be necessary but is better performed when the patient no longer has acute local infection or trismus.

NECROTIZING PERIODONTAL DISEASES

Necrotizing periodontal diseases is composed of necrotizing ulcerative gingivitis (NUG) and necrotizing ulcerative peridontitis (NUP). These diseases are bacterial infections of the periodontium with specific etiologies, clinical features, and microbial profile. It is important to distinguish between NUG and primary herpetic gingivostomatitis. The latter is highly contagious, and both are seen most commonly in young adult populations. Both are painful and can occur simultaneously. Patients with primary herpetic gingivostomatitis usually have a fever and show small ulcerations on the hard palate and attached gingiva remote from the gingival margins. NUG

■ **FIGURE 27–3**   Periocoronitis. (Courtesy of Dr. Michael Turner, New York University College of Dentistry.)

patients are often afebrile, and have a characteristic fetid mouth odor and ulcerated and necrotic papillae and marginal gingiva. The ulcers are covered with a grayish layer of necrotic tissue, cells, and bacteria. Risk factors for NUG include stress, smoking, poor oral hygiene, and malnutrition. Extreme pain is usually the reason for the patient's seeking treatment.

NUG is treated by addressing its causes. Since NUG is an infectious disease, treatment involves systemic antibiotics and mechanical debridement when the patient is out of pain (Table 27–2 ■). The pain is usually so intense that the patient has trouble eating. The signs and symptoms of NUG are reduced when the microbial concentration is reduced. Systemic analgesics may also be used in the initial treatment due to the pain. If left untreated, extensive gingival tissue destruction can occur. Even with treatment, recurrent lesions may occur.

Treatment of necrotizing ulcerative gingivitis is divided into two phases: acute and maintenance. The objective of the acute phase is to eliminate disease activity. Treatment on the first day consists of data collection (e.g., medical/dental history, chief complaint, etc.) and making the correct diagnosis. Initial supragingival debridement should be performed, if the patient can tolerate it. Usually, the patient is in too much pain, and the first step is to place the patient on a systemic analgesic (e.g., ibuprofen; make sure there are no drug/drug or drug/disease interactions) to eliminate the pain and a systemic antibiotic to eliminate the bacterial infection.

If antibiotics are indicated, metronidazole (250 mg three times a day), tetracycline, or penicillin are used.

Table 27–2	Treatment Steps for Necrotizing Ulcerative Gingivitis
First appointment	Supragingival debridement, if the patient can tolerate it. If not, get the patient out of pain: Give a systemic analgesic. Use of systemic antibiotic is controversial. Instead of brushing, rinse twice daily with either chlorhexidine, warm water/hydrogen peroxide, or an oxygenating agent.
Second appointment (day 1–2)	When patient is out of pain, supragingival debridement (power-driven scalers) is started.
Third appointment (successive days)	Continued periodontal debridement under topical/local anesthesia. Oral hygiene instructions given (ultrasoft toothbrush gently). Control of other risk factors (e.g., smoking cessation).
Fourth appointment	Maintenance phase: Referral to periodontist to surgically correct gingival architecture.
Fifth appointment	Two-month periodontal maintenance.

Although symptoms diminish within 24 hours, the antibiotic should still be taken for the prescribed time. Toothbrushing should be avoided and instead patients are instructed to rinse twice daily with a mixture of 1 tablespoon of 3% hydrogen peroxide in 1/2 glass of warm water, an oxygenating rinse such as GlyOxide (Wennström & Lindhe, 1979) or chlorhexidine; brushing is usually impossible due to extreme oral pain. The patient is advised to avoid alcohol and tobacco, eat a balanced diet, and rest. Within one day the patient should see much improvement with alleviation of pain and the infection under control. The patient then returns to the office for supragingival debridement with ultrasonic or sonic scalers and hand instrumentation (anesthesia is given) and adequate water spray. Depending on the patient's tolerance, complete debridement may take a few visits. When debridement is finished, the patient will return in a few days so that a gingival examination can be done to evaluate the gingival architecture. When gingival tissues have healed, plaque control instructions are given and instruction on the elimination of other risk factors such as smoking cessation. The patient is instructed to use a soft toothbrush and interproximal devices.

When the acute phase is completed, the maintenance phase begins. The patient is placed on a two-month maintenance schedule. Once the necrotic gingiva has healed, the gingival craters may persist and act as plaque traps. Referral to a periodontist for surgical correction of gingival craters is recommended.

Patients with necrotizing ulcerative periodontitis (NUP) have the same gingival features as seen in NUG except there is also loss of attachment and bone destruction. Many NUP patients are immunosuppressed (low neutrophil levels; e.g., HIV). In NUP patients, treatment is aimed at periodontal debridement, improved oral hygiene self-care, and frequent use of an antiplaque rinse or irrigant such as chlorhexidine gluconate. Oral fungal infections are sometimes present, and these may require antifungal medication. Referral to a periodontist is recommended.

HIV-related oral lesions may not fully respond to therapy. Periodontal debridement may expose necrotic bone that should be removed. Local anesthesia, pain medication, and antibiotics may be necessary. Frequent periodontal maintenance visits are recommended. Oral care should be provided in collaboration with the patient's physician. Referral to a periodontist should be considered.

PRIMARY HERPETIC GINGIVOSTOMATITIS

Primary herpetic gingivostomatitis is a condition of the oral mucosa characterized by a *previous* infection with herpes virus (HSV 1), which is mainly a disease of infants and children and clinically detectable in about 90% of patients. After a brief prodromal period (one to two days before development of blisters) of fever,

Rapid Dental Hint

Patients with NUG are in severe pain. Do not attempt to do a debridement, even with ultrasonics, until they receive an analgesic to ease their pain.

headache, nausea, vomiting, and malaise, many small blisters (vesicles) form on the mucosa inside the lower lip. Vesicles also appear on the hard palate and tongue. These blisters quickly break and form painful, yellowish-gray ulcers, which form in groups surrounded by a red halo (inflammation). Rarely are the vesicles present at the time of the office visit because they quickly rupture. One of the most important distinguishing features, which is diagnostic for primary herpetic gingivostomatitis, is the presence of a generalized acute gingivitis. The gingival papillae are intact and not necrotic as in NUG. The gingiva is red (erythematous), and swollen (edematous). Submandibular lymphadenopathy is present. The patients do not have a past history of recurrent herpes labialis. When this disease is present in adults, it may be more difficult to diagnose because the typical signs and symptoms may not be present. Most patients develop the infection through direct contact with another person with active recurrent lesions (e.g., through kissing). Symptoms usually last for one to two weeks. However, a differential diagnosis (determination of which two or more diseases with similar symptoms is the one from which a patient is suffering) would be aphthous stomatitis (canker sores). Aphthous stomatitis occurs only on unattached mucosa, and there is a history of recurrence. Usually, there is no associated fever, whereas the ulcers in primary herpetic gingivostomatitis occur on both unattached and attached mucosa.

Treatment of primary herpetic gingivostomatitis in both children and adults is primarily palliative. The intense oral pain makes eating and drinking difficult. Dehydration must be prevented with frequent drinking of liquids. Rinsing with viscous xylocaine 2% before eating and drinking may be helpful to anesthetize the area. Antipyretics such as acetaminophen are recommended to reduce the fever and pain. Antiviral drugs such as acyclovir (Zovirax®; 400 mg four times daily for one to two weeks is recommended) are used to reduce the duration of the infection.

DENTAL HYGIENE NOTES

An abscess is an infection originating from the tooth or periodontium. It is important to determine the point of origin so that proper treatment is given. Treatment involves removal of the irritant, if possible, and establishing drainage. Once the acute infection is managed, further treatment of the underlying lesion may be necessary.

Treatment of necrotizing ulcerative gingivitis involves elimination of the bacterial infection with systemic antibiotics. Since the condition is very painful, once the patient is out of pain, then mechanical debridement can be started.

A differential diagnosis of NUG is primary herpetic gingivostomatitis. Primary herpetic gingivostomatitis is treated with antiviral drugs, fluids, and acetaminophen.

KEY POINTS

- Abscesses are bacterial infections.
- It is important to determine the origin of the abscess.
- Establish incision and drainage of the infection.
- Systemic antibiotics are only needed if there is systemic involvement.
- Necrotizing ulcerative gingivitis is confined to gingival tissues.
- Five to ten percent of patients initially infected with the herpes simplex virus develop primary herpetic gingivostomatitis.

SELF-QUIZ

1. Which of the following is usually the first treatment in the management of the acute periodontal abscess? (p. 440)
   a. Site-specific antibiotics
   b. Supragingival scaling
   c. Incision and drainage
   d. Leave alone until it becomes chronic
2. Which of the following diseases is a differential diagnosis of necrotizing ulcerative gingivitis? (p. 441)
   a. Chronic periodontitis
   b. Necrotizing ulcerative periodondititis
   c. Primary herpetic gingivostomatitis
   d. Aphthous ulcers
3. Which of the following is the first step in treating NUG? (p. 442)
   a. Scaling and root planing
   b. Ultrasonic debridement
   c. Systemic antibiotics
   d. Observation
4. Which of the following treatments is used for a patient with a gingival abscess? (p. 439)
   a. Incision and drainage
   b. Systemic antibiotics
   c. Systemic analgesic
   d. Controlled-drug delivery

5. Which of the following is a prominent feature of NUG? (p. 441)
   a. tooth mobility
   b. fetid odor
   c. pain
   d. pus

REFERENCES

Corbet, E. F. 2004. Diagnosis of acute periodontal lesions. *Periodontology 2000* 34:204–216.

Herrera, D., S. Roldàn, and M. Sanz. 2000. The periodontal abscess: A review. *J. Clin. Periodontol.* 27:377–386.

Jaramillo, A., R. M. Arce, D. Herrera, M. Betancourth, J. E. Botero, and A. Contreras. 2005, December. Clinical and microbiological characterization of periodontal abscesses. *J. Clin. Periodontol.* 32(12):1213–1218.

López-Píriz, R., L. Aguilar, and M. J. Giménez. 2007, March 7. Management of odontogenic infection of pulpal and periodontal origin. *Med. Oral. Patol. Oral Cir. Bucal.* 12(2):E154–9.

Meng, H. X. 1999. Periodontal abscess. *Ann. Periodontol.* 4:79–82.

Minsk, L. 2006, January. Diagnosis and treatment of acute periodontal conditions. *Compend. Contin. Educ. Dent.* 27(1):8–11.

Wennström, J., and J. Lindhe. 1979. Effect of hydrogen peroxide on developing plaque and gingivitis in man. *J. Clin. Periodontol.* 6:115–130.

Chapter **28**

Periodontal Maintenance Therapy

Mea A. Weinberg

OUTLINE

Introduction
Refractory Periodontal Diseases/Recurrent
    Periodontal Diseases
Objectives of Periodontal Maintenance
Components of the Periodontal Maintenance Visit
Periodontal Conditions and Smoking
Treatment: Recurrent Periodontal Disease Versus
    a Well-Maintained Periodontium
Chemotherapeutics
Frequency of Intervals
General Dentist-Periodontist Relationship
Patient Adherence
Dental Hygiene Notes
Key Points
Self-Quiz
References

GOAL: To provide an overview of the role periodontal maintenance has in the long-term management of inflammatory periodontal diseases.

KEY WORDS

patient adherence **455**   retreatment **449**
periodontal   secondary prevention
    maintenance **446**   **446**
primary prevention **446**   smoking cessation **451**

EDUCATIONAL OBJECTIVES

Upon completion of this chapter, the reader should be able to:

• List the objectives of periodontal maintenance.
• Describe the components of periodontal maintenance.
• Describe the role of the dental hygienist in periodontal maintenance visits.
• Define the role of the dental hygienist in smoking cessation.
• Identify when retreatment is necessary.
• Explain the factors involved in patient compliance.

INTRODUCTION

Periodontal maintenance also has been referred to as periodontal recall, supportive periodontal care, and continuing care. All these terms are appropriate, but the American Academy of Periodontology (AAP) has adopted the term *periodontal maintenance,* which may be a more up-to-date and inclusive term because it is a branch of periodontal therapy.

It is known generally that after periodontal treatment is completed, patients will exhibit a decrease in plaque control and a recurrence of gingivitis or periodontitis unless they are enrolled in a regular periodontal maintenance program (Axelsson & Lindhe, 1981). Patients must be informed of the need for periodic periodontal maintenance visits throughout their life. Since it cannot be predicted when and if gingivitis will progress into periodontitis, the disease must be monitored, and regular professional removal of dental plaque and calculus must be accomplished.

REFRACTORY PERIODONTAL DISEASES/RECURRENT PERIODONTAL DISEASES

Refractory periodontal disease occurs in treated periodontal patients who fail to respond to periodontal treatment including maintenance therapy and who demonstrate meticulous oral hygiene. Patients may be refractory because of inadequate treatment, presence of systemic disease (e.g., diabetes mellitus), deficient immune response, or persistence of periodontal pathogens. On the other hand, *recurrent periodontal disease* occurs in patients who previously responded well to periodontal therapy but later showed signs of disease reactivation. In this situation, there was a recurrence of the disease. Recurrent disease sites also occur in patients demonstrating meticulous plaque control and on a regular maintenance program.

Treatment for refractory periodontitis may include adjunctive use of antibiotics. Treatment for recurrent disease sites is based on conventional periodontal therapy (e.g., scaling/root planing, surgery, good plaque control and maintenance).

OBJECTIVES OF PERIODONTAL MAINTENANCE

The primary objectives of periodontal maintenance are (American Academy of Periodontology, 2003b) (1) to prevent or minimize the recurrence of periodontal diseases in patients by controlling risk factors known to contribute to the disease process (e.g., dental plaque, calculus); (2) to prevent or reduce the incidence of tooth or implant loss by monitoring the dentition and prosthetic replacements of the natural teeth; (3) to increase the probability of locating and treating other conditions or diseases found in the mouth; and (4) to preserve the health, comfort, and function of the teeth. Periodontal maintenance is also important for monitoring the overall dental health of the patient and to recognize, identify, and manage other diseases or conditions found within or related to the oral cavity (Wilson, 1996b).

Indications for Periodontal Maintenance

Periodontal maintenance is indicated for three types of patients: (1) peridontally healthy patients who have never had periodontal disease as a preventive procedure (this type of care is termed **primary prevention** and applies to a large section of the population), (2) patients after active periodontal therapy to prevent or minimize the recurrence and progression of periodontal disease and tooth loss (this type of care is termed **secondary prevention**), and (3) medically compromised patients or patients who maintain poor oral hygiene and are not considered candidates for periodontal surgery.

COMPONENTS OF THE PERIODONTAL MAINTENANCE VISIT

Patient needs at the periodontal maintenance visit vary widely and are modified on an individual basis. Regardless, standard periodontal maintenance procedures include the following steps (American Academy of Periodontology, 2003b):

1. An update of medical and dental histories.
2. Extraoral and intraoral examinations.
3. Dental examination and gingival and periodontal assessment.
4. Radiographic review.
5. Oral hygiene evaluation (amount of plaque, calculus, and stains).
6. Review of the patient's plaque-control efficacy.
7. Removal of dental plaque from the supragingival and subgingival areas, root debridement where indicated, teeth polishing, and adjunctive chemotherapy if necessary.

The patient's chart should be reviewed for previous periodontal treatments, including periodontal maintenance care, before any current treatment is initiated. Any medications needed before periodontal maintenance, such as antibiotic prophylaxis, can be determined before the patient is seen and acknowledged when the patient arrives at the dental office.

Two aspects emphasized and provided during periodontal maintenance are monitoring and therapy. The preceding examination steps should be performed on every patient at each periodontal maintenance visit but are subject to the judgment of the dentist and the dental hygienist. The clinical findings obtained at the periodontal maintenance visit should be compared with baseline findings. Baseline values are first established at the initial examination and again following active therapy.

Periodontal maintenance is designed to eliminate or reduce primary and secondary risk factors. The primary risk factor for inflammatory periodontal diseases is dental plaque. Secondary factors include plaque-retentive areas such as calculus and restorations with overhangs or defective margins. The patient removes supragingival dental plaque by toothbrushing and flossing, and the dental hygienist or dentist removes both supragingival and subgingival plaque and calculus by mechanical debridement. The dentist should replace or restore defective or failed restorations. Box 28–1 provides a step-by-step review of the components of a periodontal maintenance visit.

Medical and Dental Update

The patient should be asked if there have been any medication or health changes, including hospitalizations, since the last appointment. Review current medications (prescription and over-the-counter) with the patient. Note any changes in dosage or instructions for use. A medical consultation with the patient's physician may be warranted if new illnesses are recognized or if a previous condition has changed significantly. A chief complaint should be noted, and this should be accompanied by a notation of the degree of comfort or discomfort. The patient and the dentist should sign the amended form.

Rapid Dental Hint

Remember to take a medical history at every visit.

Counseling of the patient on risk factors that contribute to periodontal diseases, such as cigarette smoking, stress, nutrition, medications (e.g., calcium channel blockers, phenytoin, cyclosporine, oral contraceptives), and systemic diseases (e.g., diabetes mellitus, AIDS), also should be done during the periodontal maintenance visit (Kerry, 1995). The patient should be informed about the availability of programs for smoking cessation in and outside the office.

Since many patients are on an alternating periodontal maintenance program, seeing both a general dentist and a periodontist, any communication from the last treating office should be reviewed. Any new restorative treatment should be indicated on the chart and evaluated clinically.

Extraoral/Intraoral Examination

An updated examination is performed in the head and neck area and intraoral tissues for the detection of any abnormalities, including enlarged lymph nodes or salivary glands and red, white, or pigmented lesions. If any suspicious lesions are found, the dentist should be informed for further examination or treatment.

Dental Examination

The dental examination at the periodontal maintenance visit includes caries assessment as well as documentation of the status of restorations. Restorations should be charted, noting any defective restorations or failures such as fractures or open margins of amalgams, composites, and crowns. The stability of bridges and removable partial dentures also should be noted. Documentation of tooth loss since the last charting should be recorded, including the cause. A good rule to follow is to always count the number of teeth present.

Gingival and Periodontal Assessment

Gingival Assessment

Initially, a visual examination of the gingival tissues is done to determine the condition of the gingiva. The color, contour, consistency, and surface texture of the gingiva are recorded. Any mucogingival involvement should be noted. If compromised teeth are to receive crowns, augmentation of the attached gingiva may be necessary. If gingival inflammation is found, the location and severity should be noted, as well as etiologic factors (e.g., dental plaque accumulation due to poor oral

Box 28–1	Components of a Periodontal Maintenance Visit	

Examination	*Remarks*
Review and update medical and dental history, take blood pressure, pulse, respiration.	To determine if additional risk factors are responsible for recurrent or progressive periodontal breakdown.

Clinical examination, including
   Extra intraoral examination
   Plaque evaluation/disclosing
   Evaluating the patient's oral hygiene technique
   Dental charting of caries, restorative care
 	
Periodontal charting of probing depths, gingival recession, furcation defects, bleeding on probing, exudation, tooth mobility, fremitus
 	
Implant evaluation: peri-implant tissues, probing depths, bleeding on probing, stability of dental implant (mobility), examination of abutment teeth, occlusal examination
	Changes that should be of concern during a periodontal maintenance visit include sites that have changed from nonbleeding to bleeding, sites that have increased 2 to 3 mm or more in attachment loss or probing depth, and any sites with pus or suppuration.

Radiographic review	Since radiographs only show past activity (e.g., bone loss occurred approximately six months ago, not yesterday or today), it is important to correlate the radiographic findings with clinical probing depths and clinical attachment levels.

Treatment options
   Removal of supragingival and subgingival plaque and calculus
   Selective polishing
   Oral hygiene reinstruction
	These treatment guidelines depend on the type of periodontal patient. Treatment should not be started unless the data collected are appropriately recorded.

Adjunctive therapy
   Antimicrobial therapy
   Occlusal treatment
   Counseling on control of contributing factors such as smoking cessation, stress reduction, and nutrition
   Restorative and prosthetic care
Reevaluation four to eight weeks after debridement
Scheduling of next periodontal maintenance appointment	

hygiene self-care, medication-induced, or resulting from a hormonal imbalance).

Periodontal Assessment

Next, a periodontal evaluation is performed. This includes recording of probing depths, gingival recession, clinical attachment level, furcation involvement, suppuration (pus), and tooth mobility.

Gingival Recession The position of the gingival tissues on the tooth is defined as the location of the gingival margin in relation to the cementoenamel junction (CEJ). Gingival recession that has progressed since the

last appointment must be addressed and treatment options given to the patient. If the recession has remained unchanged, then monitoring is all that is needed. In order to treat gingival recession, the cause must be determined. Etiologic factors include inappropriate toothbrushing technique, attachment loss (disease process), and shrinkage of tissues after initial therapy. Treatment may include educating the patient on proper brushing technique or mucogingival surgery. Common patient complaints concerning gingival recession include poor aesthetics and tooth pain or hypersensitivity with air or cold application. Any dentinal hypersensitivity can be managed in most patients with desensitizing agents (e.g., potassium nitrate, sodium fluoride, or stannous fluoride).

Disease Stability: Probing Depth and Clinical Attachment Level   Monitoring of probing depths and clinical attachment levels (CALs) currently is the most reliable way to determine periodontal disease stability. It may be time-consuming to determine the CAL, but it is an extremely important measurement. Probing depth recordings should be taken at six sites per tooth. If a patient's periodontal condition has deteriorated rapidly since the last periodontal maintenance visit, systemic disease such as diabetes mellitus, smoking, stress, or use of alcohol might be the cause.

Measurement of the CAL is made from the CEJ to the apical extent of the tip of the probe. Such measurements are compared with measurements obtained at the last periodontal maintenance visit. A 2 to 3 mm increase in attachment loss indicates disease progression (Haffajee, Socransky, & Goodson, 1983; Kornman, 1987), and more aggressive treatment or **retreatment** may be justified. A patient with a 3 mm probing depth associated with 6 mm of gingival recession, for example, has 9 mm of attachment loss. In such patients, periodontal maintenance must be discontinued and active periodontal therapy started. However, a patient with a 3 mm probing depth without recession has a 3 mm CAL with no attachment loss, and this is not of great concern.

Bleeding on Probing   Probing depths should be interpreted on a patient-by-patient, site-by-site basis. For example, a 5 mm probing depth that does not bleed on probing is viewed differently from a 5 mm probing depth with bleeding on probing and suppuration. Bleeding on probing in deep pockets indicates inflammation within the connective tissue (Armitage, 1996), whereas bleeding while stroking the lateral wall of the gingival crevice indicates early gingival inflammation (Van der Weijden, Timmerman, Nijbor, Reijerse, & Van der Velden, 1994). Thus, disease stability can be monitored during periodontal maintenance on the basis of bleeding on probing (Lang, Joss, & Tonetti, 1996). Bleeding sites in deep pockets seem to have an increased risk for progression of periodontitis (progressive attachment loss) in patients on periodontal maintenance care (Claffey, Nylund, Kiger, Gorrett, & Egelberg, 1990). The absence of bleeding on probing is a better indicator of gingival health than its presence is of periodontal disease (Lang et al., 1996). However, in patients who smoke, bleeding on probing may not be evident (Dietrich, 2004). One should chart the sites that bleed on probing (e.g., use a red dot over the

Did You Know?

Bleeding indicates that there is inflammation present. The epithelium is avascular, but the underlying connective tissue is very vascular.

site). Thus, sites that bleed warrant more attention during the periodontal maintenance visit and may have to be reinstrumented, whereas nonbleeding sites should be left without repeated subgingival instrumentation (Lang et al., 1996). Bleeding on probing generally is apparent 10 seconds after probing (Lang et al., 1996).

It should be emphasized that the force used while probing (probing force) varies considerably during probing depth measurements, even from tooth to tooth. Therefore, a tooth with healthy periodontium may bleed because "too much" force was used and not because of inflammation. Ideally, a probing force of 0.25 N (25 g) should be used, which clinically represents a "light probing force" (Joss, Adler, & Lang, 1994; Lang et al., 1996), or probe until slight resistance is felt. A nonmetallic probe should be used to probe around implants.

Tooth Mobility   Tooth mobility for each tooth is noted on the chart. Tooth mobility also should be measured and recorded on the chart as Grade I, II, III, or IV (Carranza & Takei, 1996). If there is increasing mobility since the last visit, the cause should be determined and appropriate treatment rendered. The presence of fremitus also should be recorded.

Rapid Dental Hint

Use the Nabers' probe to detect furcation involvement.

Radiographic Review

Radiographs show past bone destruction. It is important to monitor the patient's periodontal status with clinical probing and standardized radiographs taken at appropriate intervals so as to compare with previously taken radiographs. Radiographs should be taken according to the American Dental Association *Guidelines* (American Dental Association, 2004). In a recall periodontal patient with a history of bone loss and periodontal surgery, clinical judgment is used as to the need for and type of radiographic images for the evaluation of periodontal disease.

Imaging may consist of, but is not limited to, selected bitewing and/or periapical images of areas where periodontal disease (other than nonspecific gingivitis) can be identified clinically (American Dental Association, 2004). Sites that have had bone (osseous) grafting or guided tissue regeneration can be evaluated with radiographs at least six months after surgery. The need for bitewing and periapical radiographs depends on the stage and severity of the disease, risk for caries, and presence of implants. Vertical bitewing views are ideal for patients with periodontal disease because they show more of the alveolar bone than do horizontal bitewings.

Oral Hygiene Evaluation and Patient's Plaque-Control Regimen

The next step is to evaluate gross plaque accumulation, determine the quality of oral hygiene self-care procedures, and conduct patient education. A disclosing agent is used for patient education and as a basis for recording a plaque index. Scoring of plaque at a periodontal maintenance appointment may be misleading because patients frequently brush very well just before coming to such an appointment. In any event, monitoring of the plaque level can be used to evaluate the patient's compliance with oral hygiene self-care. The patient's oral hygiene practices are reviewed by asking the patient to brush and use interdental devices while the hygienist watches. The level of patient motivation to perform daily plaque removal must be determined. A patient may understand and show correct technique in the office but may not comply with instructions at home because of lack of interest or time constraints. It is important to recognize such patients and to spend more time explaining to them the importance of performing these tasks.

Dental Implants

Evaluation of a patient with dental implants is essentially the same as that of a patient with natural teeth. However, rather than teeth, the implants and peri-implant tissues are evaluated (Sison, 2003). If inflammation or disease is detected around an implant, the probing depth should be measured and bleeding and suppuration noted. The stability of the abutment teeth and prosthesis also should be noted by recording mobility. An abutment is a tooth or implant used for support and retention of a crown or removable partial denture. The prosthesis is checked for occlusal wear. Any loosened screws should be recorded. Calculus deposits on implant surfaces are not firmly at-tached because the titantium surface of the implant is nonporous which is just the opposite of natural teeth in which the cementum is porous allowing for a firm attachment of calculus. Light, short strokes should be used to prevent trauma to the peri-implant tissues (Sison, 2003).

Because there is a correlation between implant failure and bone characteristics, it is essential to take radiographs periodically. Generally, periapical films are indicated at 6-month to 1-year intervals to determine the height of bone around an implant. The accepted standard for a stable endosseous implant one year after placement is vertical bone loss less than 0.2 mm per year (Albrektsson, Zarb, Worthington, & Eriksson, 1986; American Academy of Periodontology, 1989). Radiographically, an ailing, failing, or failed implant will show varying amounts of alveolar bone loss (Meffert, 1992). Mobility will occur with the failed implant.

 Rapid Dental Hint

Normally, the tissue around the implant should not be probed.

PERIODONTAL CONDITIONS AND SMOKING

The literature supports the conclusion that smokers, especially cigarette smokers, have increased calculus, greater bone loss, and increased pocket depths but have the same levels of plaque accumulation and the same or less gingival inflammation (American Academy of Periodontology, 1996; Haber et al., 1993). It also has been shown that surgical periodontal procedures are less effective for smokers (Bergström, Eliasson, & Preber, 1991). The amount and frequency of tobacco use are essential information when evaluating the risk factors associated with smoking (American Academy of Periodontology, 1996). Since smoking cessation may decrease the progression of periodontal diseases, it is important that the dental hygienist urge periodontal patients who smoke to stop and perhaps recommend an effective smoking-cessation program. The dental hygienist should perform periodic soft tissue evaluations and recognize any deleterious changes in the periodontium. The dental hygienist can provide assistance in guiding patients to stop smoking, yet he or she needs to realistically assess the effects of this habit on the gingival health and the resulting compromised healing. Education and continued support are beneficial factors influencing the patient's decision to stop smoking. A current article reported that regular maintenance treatment in a population of highly motivated patients with chronic periodontitis seemed to be equally successful in preventing progressive periodontal tissue destruction in current smokers and current nonsmokers (Fisher et al., 2008). Additionally, smoking exerts a strong, chronic, and dose-dependent suppressive effect on gingival bleeding on probing (Dietrich, 2004).

Practical Steps to Smoking Cessation

Smoking-cessation programs can be made available in the dental office. The dental office is a logical place to counsel patients on the effects of smoking on the periodontium and the importance of stopping smoking for improved long-term periodontal health and better results after periodontal treatment. Furthermore, it is important to stress to the patient that smoking cessation also can reduce the risk for other medical diseases such as cancer (Christen, McDonald, & Christen, 1991), heart disease, and respiratory disease (e.g., bronchitis). A smoking-cessation program should be a part of comprehensive preventive periodontal care. This includes behavior modification and, if necessary, medications.

The first step in establishing a smoking-cessation program is to get the office staff organized by selecting a director or coordinator such as the dental hygienist. The role of the director is to become familiar with the National Cancer Institute (NCI) manual and parts of the program, organize records and procedures, assist patients by reviewing self-help material with them, and involve the entire dental office team (Stone & Mattana, 1996).

Patients should be reassured that the entire office is going to help them. If a patient shows interest in quitting, then a program can be initiated. If a patient is not interested in quitting, do not force him or her, but rather counsel the patient and give him or her literature to take home. At the next visit ask the patient about smoking cessation again. Once the patient is enrolled in a program (yours or another one), continued maintenance or follow-up visits and communication through phone calls are important.

The role of the dental hygienist includes patient education and counseling in tobacco prevention and cessation. The patient should be informed that smoking influences periodontal conditions such as implant failure (Bain, 1996), oral cancer, and periodontal problems such as loss of clinical attachment (Grossi et al., 1994), impaired wound healing (Grossi et al., 1997; Jones & Triplett, 1992), halitosis, increased calculus formation, black-brown extrinsic staining, and bone loss (Bergström et al., 1991).

A set of guidelines is presented to the patient. Behavior modification should be part of a comprehensive smoking-cessation program. This includes talking to patients about their smoking habits and possibly incorporating hypnosis. Hypnosis has been used for many years in the treatment of habits (Weinberg, 1986). Hypnosis allows patients to be more susceptible to accepting suggestions, such as quitting smoking. This allows the patient to be in full control of the situation, and responsibility is placed on the patient not to smoke (Weinberg, 1986). Patients are put into a situation where they see themselves not smoking anymore. The dentist can perform hypnosis on the patient in the office. The patient is never asleep during this procedure. The patient also can learn self-hypnosis, which can be used anytime and anywhere.

Smoking-Cessation Program

The Smoking, Tobacco, and Cancer Program of the National Cancer Institute (1996) recommends guidelines to help patients to stop using tobacco. The 4A Program consists of the following components that are reviewed with the patient during the initial examination and periodically:

Ask. Inquire whether your patient smokes and, if so, how long he or she has been smoking and how much.

Advise. Inform the patient of the benefits of quitting and the risks associated with continuing the tobacco habit; strongly suggest that your patient should work toward a goal of complete smoking cessation.

Assist. Give the patient behavioral self-monitoring techniques and, as appropriate, pharmacologic intervention such as nicotine gum, nicotine patches, or another agent. Encourage the patient to quit smoking. Let the patient set up a quitting date or discuss different therapies.

Arrange for follow-up. Set up follow-up visits. The patient should return to the office at regular intervals to observe his or her periodontium and to reinforce his or her quitting behavior.

Additionally, another "A" would be to assess for motivation to stop. Patients should be assessed for their reasons for quitting smoking and their thoughts for quitting.

Pharmacologic Agents

Table 28–1 ■ reviews various types of smoking-cessation methods.

Pharmacologic agents include nicotine gum, transdermal nicotine patches, nasal sprays, and a systemic dosage form. The nicotine-replacement drugs (gum or patches) work by replacing the nicotine that is absorbed in the body while smoking and act as a substitute for the cigarette. The manufacturers of these products claim that they help patients quit while lessening any concomitant nicotine cravings (Stone & Mattana, 1996). The efficacy of this method is questionable on a long-term basis. Patients must refrain from smoking while on the gum or patch because nicotine from these products is being introduced into the body. Nicotine therapy should not be used in a patient who continues to smoke. The importance of taking the gum as directed must be stressed to the patient. The gum should be placed between the cheek and gingiva and chewed slowly for about 30 minutes and then thrown away. Currently, the gum is available over-the-counter without a prescription. Nicotine patches are available in different doses that are worn on the skin for variable amounts of time. Indications for use of these products is for the reduction of symptoms associated with smoking cessation, including nicotine craving.

Bupropion HCl (Zyban® Sustained-Release Tablets, Glaxo Wellcome, Research Triangle Park, NC) is an oral medication prescribed by dentists or physicians to help decrease the withdrawal symptoms and the urge to smoke that accompany smoking cessation. Advantages to this form of therapy are that it is nicotine-free and helps the patient to quit while still smoking. Bupropion is also used to treat depression. Adverse side effects include dry mouth (xerostomia) and insomnia (difficulty sleeping). Both nicotine gum and patches and bupropion should be used in conjunction with behavioral modification therapy.

TREATMENT: RECURRENT PERIODONTAL DISEASE VERSUS A WELL-MAINTAINED PERIODONTIUM

Recurrent periodontal disease occurs when signs and symptoms of disease return after having subsided during active treatment. Clinical signs include bleeding on probing, increasing tooth mobility, continued soft tissue attachment loss (including deep pockets), suppuration from the pocket, and radiographic changes. Recurrent occlusal problems include increasing tooth mobility and

fremitus. A good rule to follow may be that when bleeding on probing or the presence of suppuration is seen two to three weeks following the periodontal maintenance appointment, then retreatment is plausible (Ramfjord, 1987). Another reason for retreatment includes a 2 mm or greater increase in probing depth or attachment loss. Specific treatment could include periodontal debridement (scaling and root planing), periodontal surgery, antimicrobial agents, occlusal adjustment, splinting, extractions, or a night guard. After the initial therapy is completed, reevaluation should be performed. If resolution does not occur after retreatment, then a systemic disease component must be considered and the patient referred to a periodontist. See AAP Guidelines for Referral (American Academy of Periodontology, 2006).

In a well-maintained patient in whom inflammation is not present (no bleeding on probing) and for whom soft tissue attachment loss or bone loss is minimal, the following treatment is recommended at a periodontal maintenance visit:

1. Point out any areas in the mouth where the patient is having difficulty with plaque control, and correct the patient's technique, if necessary.
2. Deplaquing may be performed. In patients with little or no subgingival deposits (usually after active treatment), a deplaquing stroke can be used with a curet or ultrasonic or sonic scaler. The tip of the instrument is "floating" within the gingival sulcus, lightly touching the root surface.
3. Selective tooth polishing can be performed. Extrinsic stains may be derived from nicotine, tea, coffee, foods, and chlorhexidine oral rinse.
4. Determine the interval of the next periodontal maintenance visit.

Subgingival instrumentation, including root planing of shallow pockets, has been shown to increase soft tissue attachment loss (Lindhe, Socransky, Nyman, Haffajee, & Westfelt, 1982). Patients with dental implants should be questioned about any difficulty in oral hygiene self-care or discomfort or difficulty in chewing. Plastic periodontal probes, scalers, and curets should be used because stainless steel instruments can scratch the titanium surfaces of implants.

All patients must undergo oral hygiene reinstruction and counseling on control of contributing risk factors such as smoking. Patients should be kept informed of their current periodontal condition and treatment

Table 28–1	Smoking-Cessation Methods: Pharmacologic Therapy	
Product	*Directions for Use*	*Supplied*
Nicotine Gum		
Nicorette® gum (2 mg; 4 mg) (GlaxoSmithKline)	One piece of gum every 1–2 hours for weeks 1–6, every 2–4 hours for weeks 7–9, and every 4–8 hours for weeks 10–12. Do not eat or drink for 15 minutes before chewing a piece of gum.	Over the counter; starter kit has 108 pieces, and refill kits have 48 pieces.
Nicotine Transdermal System		
Nicotrol® (Pharmacia Consumer Products)	Taper patches; up to 6 weeks.	Over the counter; 15 mg, 10 mg, and 5 mg nicotine patch.
Habitrol® (Novartis Consumer, East Hanover, NJ)	One patch daily; 21 mg/day for 6 weeks, then 14 mg/day for 2 weeks, then 7 mg/day for 2 weeks. Maximum therapy is 3 months.	Over the counter; patch containing 7 mg of nicotine, 14 mg, and 21 mg; 7-day supply.
Nicoderm® CQ (GlaxoSmithKline)	One patch daily; taper dosage as recommended by manufacturer (21 mg/day for 6 weeks, then 14 mg/day for 2 weeks, then 7 mg/day for 2 weeks). Maximum therapy is 3 months.	Over the counter; 7 mg patch, 14 mg patch, 21 mg patch; 7-day supply in 7 mg dose.
Prostep® (Lederle, Carolina; Puerto Rico)	One patch daily; 22 mg/day for 4–8 weeks, then 11 mg/day for 2–4 weeks. Maximum therapy is 3 months.	Over the counter; box contains 7 patches that deliver 22 or 11 mg/day.
Nicotine Nasal Spray		
Nicotrol® NS (McNeil Consumer Health Care, Fort Washington, PA)	Start with 2 sprays in each nostril every hour, which may be increased to 80 sprays per day (heavy smokers); maximum therapy is 6 months. Can cause nasal irritation.	Prescription; each spray delivers 0.5 mg nicotine; available in 10 ml bottles.
Nicotine Lozenge		
Commit® (GlaxoSmithKline)	Allow lozenge to dissolve slowly over 20–30 min, swallow as little as possible.	Over the counter; 2 mg and 4 mg lozenge
Nicotine Inhalation System		
Nicotrol® Inhaler (McNeil Consumer Health Care, Fort Washington, PA)	Reduces craving to smoke. Less nicotine per puff is released with the inhaler than with a cigarette. Best effect is achieved by frequent continuous puffing for about 20 minutes. The recommended treatment is up to 3 months and, if needed, a gradual reduction over the next 6–12 weeks. Total treatment should not exceed 6 months.	Prescription; the inhaler uses nicotine cartridges (10 mg/cartridge) that provide about 20 minutes of active puffing, or approximately 80 deep draws.

(continued)

Table 28–1	Smoking-Cessation Methods: Pharmacologic Therapy (cont.)	
Product	*Directions for Use*	**Supplied**
Oral Medications		
Bupropion HCl (Zyban®) Sustained-Release Tablets (Glaxo Wellcome, Research, Triangle Park, NC)	Start initial dose while the patient is still smoking to allow for higher blood levels; initial dose is 150 mg/day for 3 days. Maximum daily dose is 300 mg. Should stop smoking within 2 weeks of initiation of drug therapy. Continue drug therapy for 7–12 weeks after the patient stops smoking. Can be used with nicotine transdermal systems (nicotine patches). It is contraindicated in patients with eating disorders (anorexia, bulimia), seizure disorder, patients undergoing abrupt discontinuation of alcohol or sedatives	Prescription; 150 mg sustained-release tablets.
Varenicline (Chantrix™)	Day 1–3: 0.5 mg once daily; Days 4–7: 0.5 mg twice daily; Day 8–end of treatment: 1 mg twice daily. Common side effects: nausea, sleep disturbance (trouble sleeping or vivid, unusual, or increased dreaming), constipation, gas, and vomiting.	Prescription: 0.5 and 1 mg tablets

options. Consultation may be required with other dentists who will be providing restorative or prosthetic treatment or who will be involved in the periodontal maintenance program.

CHEMOTHERAPEUTICS

Chemotherapeutic agents may be beneficial in certain patients as an adjunct to standard oral hygiene procedures, but they do not replace brushing and flossing. Since chemotherapeutic agents help to prevent repopulation of potential gram-negative periodontal pathogens between periodontal maintenance appointments, medically compromised patients or those exhibiting poor oral hygiene may benefit from such agents. Since periodontitis is a subgingival malady, rinsing with an agent is ineffective. To target subgingival bacteria, oral irrigation may be helpful between periodontal maintenance visits to prevent repopulation of periodontal pathogens

(Jolkovsky et al., 1990). Irrigation with water or a medicament detoxifies and removes unattached dental plaque. Systemic antibiotics are not recommended routinely during periodontal maintenance because of the potential development of bacterial resistance, although antibiotics occasionally may be of some benefit in aggressive and refractory periodontitis cases during periodontal maintenance. Controlled-release drugs such as Arestin, PerioChip, or Atridox may be used in selected recurrent pockets of 5 mm or greater that bleed. Desensitizing agents may be applied at a periodontal maintenance visit to reduce or eliminate dentinal hypersensitivity in patients in whom gingival recession is present.

FREQUENCY OF INTERVALS

Periodontal maintenance intervals are determined on an individual basis according to periodontal disease severity, type of treatment performed, adequacy of oral hygiene self-care, presence of orthodontic and prosthetic appliances, systemic health, and **patient adherence** (compliance) and cooperation (American Academy of Periodontology, 1998). The premise on which a time-interval frame for periodontal maintenance has been based is the repopulation time of periodontal pathogens after the last periodontal debridement. Data suggest that periodontal maintenance intervals of three months or less are indicated for continued suppression of potentially pathogenic microorganisms in susceptible patients (American Academy of Periodontology, 1998). A twelve-month recall interval may be acceptable for patients with limited susceptibility to periodontitis (Rosén et al., 1999). Regardless, the periodontal maintenance interval is determined on a patient-by-patient basis. Figure 28–1 ■ is a schematic flowchart that reviews suggested time intervals for healthy and periodontal patients. Patients can return two to three weeks after periodontal debridement for further observations. Any time during a periodontal maintenance program, a patient may temporarily go back into active therapy.

At the completion of initial therapy (after reevaluation)

PERIODONTAL HEALTH (NO PREVIOUS HISTORY OF PERIODONTAL DISEASES)		GINGIVITIS
Compliant with oral hygiene self-care No extensive restorative or prosthetics No occlusal discrepancies No extensive restorative or prosthetics	No bleeding No periodontally comprised teeth Complaint with oral hygiene self-care hygiene	Generalized or localized bleeding No periodontally compromised teeth Noncomplier or irregular complier
6 months	6 months	3 months or less for the first periodontal maintenance visit; if patient responds to treatment with improvement in oral hygiene then increase interval between visits; if there is no improvement after a few periodontal maintenance visits enroll the patient into active treatment. Risk factors including smoking and systemic diseases (e.g.,diabetes mellitus, medications, hormonal imbalance) must be considered.

SLIGHT TO MODERATE PERIODONTITIS (SURGICAL AND NONSURGICAL PATIENTS)	SEVERE PERIODONTITIS (SURGICAL AND NONSURGICAL PATIENTS)
No teeth with less than 50% bone remaining Localized or no bleeding on probing Localized shallow pockets remain A controlled systemic disease that contributes to periodontal destruction Compliers with oral hygiene self-care	If many of the following factors are present: Many periodontally compromised teeth (>50% bone loss) Generalized deep pockets Occlusal problems Systemic disease (uncontrolled or poorly controlled) that predisposes to periodontal destruction (e.g., diabetes mellitus) Extensive restorative and prosthetic appliances Periodontal surgery not performed for medical, psychological, or financial reasons Noncomplier or irregular complier with oral hygiene self-care
6 months to 1 year	3 months or less depending on the number of risk factors present.

■ **FIGURE 28–1** Schematic illustration describing suggested time intervals for periodontal maintenance.

The time required for the periodontal maintenance visit depends on the number of teeth; disease severity; amount of plaque, calculus, and stains; instrumentation access; presence of extensive prosthetic crowns and bridges; orthodontic appliances; depths of pockets; and patient cooperation. Although periodontal maintenance visits usually are scheduled for 45 to 60 minutes, the amount of time should be individualized (American Academy of Periodontology, 1998).

GENERAL DENTIST–PERIODONTIST RELATIONSHIP

Periodontal patients should be monitored by both their general dentist and their periodontist, but they should be seen by the periodontist at least once a year for a thorough periodontal evaluation. Periodontal maintenance can be performed alternately by the general dentist and the periodontist.

Gingivitis or mild chronic periodontitis patients can receive total care, including chronic periodontal maintenance, by the general dentist. Moderate chronic periodontitis patients should alternate periodontal maintenance visits between the general dentist and the periodontist once active treatment is completed. Severe chronic periodontitis patients should be seen primarily by a periodontist, with annual appointments with the general dentist for general care. Refractory periodontitis and aggressive periodontitis patients should be seen exclusively by the periodontist for all active periodontal treatment.

PATIENT ADHERENCE

An essential aspect of periodontal maintenance therapy is patient adherence. Most patients do not comply with long-term behavioral changes, especially for conditions that are not life-threatening. Wilson (1996a) identifies three types of compliers: full compliers, irregular compliers, and noncompliers. Periodontal maintenance appointments are essential and important for all groups, but noncompliers have less successful surgical outcomes over time. Better communication may contribute to more successful outcomes. Other methods of improving patient adherence include providing positive reinforcement and attempting to better accommodate patient needs (Wilson, 1996a). Furthermore, the severity of the periodontal problem should be stressed because the more threatening a patient perceives a disease, the higher is the adherence.

Wilson, Glover, Schoen, Baus, and Jacobs (1984) reported that of 100 treated patients who were given the opportunity for periodontal maintenance over an eight-year period in a private periodontal office, 34% never returned to the office for periodontal maintenance, and only 16% completed periodontal maintenance. Becker, Becker, and Berg (1984), in a study of 44 patients who refused to participate in periodontal maintenance, found that in the absence of periodontal maintenance, periodontal surgery was of questionable benefit in maintaining periodontal health. The patient dropout rate (43%) was highest in the first year, which, according to the authors, suggested that a patient is more likely to remain compliant in the long-term if he or she is compliant with the maintenance treatment for the first year (Mendoza, Newcomb and Nixon, 1991).

Some common reasons for patient nonadherence with office visits include the expense, the belief by patients that they no longer require treatment because they no longer have any signs of disease, fear of dental treatment (Mendoza, Newcomb, & Nixon, 1991; Wilson, 1996a), or lifestyle changes (e.g., job change or move).

Most longitudinal studies have shown that patients who receive therapy maintain their teeth longer than those who do not. A study by Becker and colleagues (1984) looked at patients in three categories:

1. Patients with untreated moderate to advanced periodontal disease lost an average of 0.33 teeth per year.
2. Patients who had treatment but no periodontal maintenance lost an average of 0.22 teeth per year.
3. Patients who had treatment and periodontal maintenance lost an average of 0.11 teeth per year.

Providing patients with motivational strategies may help to improve compliance. Examples of such approaches include (1) giving patients printed self-care instructions at every periodontal maintenance visit, (2) noting the next periodontal maintenance appointment on the instructions, (3) counseling patients about their condition and the benefit-to-risk ratio of having periodontal maintenance, (4) seeking out patient concerns and responding to them, and (5) sending reminders or calling patients about their next periodontal maintenance visit.

DENTAL HYGIENE NOTES

Professional plaque control, oral hygiene self-care, and periodic periodontal maintenance are and will continue to be the foundation of periodontal therapy. Following periodontal and implant therapy, regular periodontal maintenance can encourage periodontal and peri-implant health. In the majority of patients, periodontal maintenance is started after completion of active periodontal therapy, but it can be used in other phases of treatment. Periodontal maintenance evolved from a dental prophylaxis and now emphasizes treatment of areas with previous attachment loss and areas where clinical signs of inflammation are found (Wilson, 1996a). Since the timing interval for periodontal maintenance appointments is not standardized, the decision is empirical, with no real scientific basis. An interval of three months between periodontal maintenance visits appears to be an effective schedule to follow, but this may vary according to clinical judgment, the periodontal disease severity of the patient, and clinical findings.

A number of risk factors must be identified and monitored during periodontal maintenance. Increases in bleeding, pockets, and tooth loss will occur in high-risk patients. Clinical decisions during maintenance therapy will be influenced by the presence of risk factors, and better knowledge of these risk factors may lead to improved and more efficient risk-management efforts during periodontal maintenance (Tonetti, Muller-Campanile, & Lang, 1998).

Dental hygienists play an important role not only in the mechanical aspects of periodontal maintenance but also in promoting preventive measures and explaining the importance of periodontal maintenance. Properly motivated patients will stay on a regularly scheduled periodontal maintenance regimen.

KEY POINTS

- Reevaluation of initial therapy should be performed between four to eight weeks after completion of scaling and root planing.
- The desired outcome of periodontal maintenance in patients after active therapy is the maintenance of periodontal health.
- Nonadherent with regular periodontal maintenance visits may result in recurrence of progression of disease.
- Despite adequate periodontal maintenance and oral hygiene self-care, some patients may show recurrence or progression of disease, and thus active therapy should be reinstated.

SELF-QUIZ

1. All the following are goals of periodontal maintenance except one. Which one is the exception? (p. 446)
   a. Maintain the patient's oral status and function.
   b. Minimize inflammation and bleeding.
   c. Prevent the recurrence of disease.
   d. Prevent the patient from having surgical therapy.
2. Which one of the following assessments best determines when periodontal disease activity or destruction is occurring? (p. 449)
   a. Clinical attachment level measurement
   b. Bleeding localized to certain teeth
   c. Redness and edema of the gingival tissues
   d. Suppuration
3. The absence of bleeding on probing is a better indicator of gingival health than its presence is of periodontal disease because bleeding only indicates inflammation. (p. 449)
   a. Both the statement and the reason are correct and related.
   b. Both the statement and the reason are correct but not related.
   c. The statement is correct, but the reason is not.
   d. The statement is not correct, but the reason is correct.
   e. Neither the statement nor the reason is correct.
4. Which one of the following procedures is appropriate if a bleeding site with a probing depth of 5 mm is found during a periodontal maintenance visit? (pp. 452, 454)
   a. Reevaluate the site at the next appointment.
   b. Immediately refer the patient to a specialist.
   c. Perform periodontal debridement.
   d. Prescribe systemic antibiotics.
5. All the following risk factors can be controlled during periodontal maintenance therapy except one. Which one is the exception? (pp. 446, 447)
   a. Stress
   b. Smoking
   c. Interproximal plaque accumulation
   d. Genetic susceptibility

6. Which one of the following protocols is most appropriate in a patient who shows generalized recurrence of disease at a periodontal maintenance visit? (p. 452)
   a. Perform periodontal surgery.
   b. Reinstate Phase I therapy.
   c. Insert tetracycline fibers into the sites.
   d. Prescribe a systemic antibiotic in conjunction with periodontal debridement.

7. All the following determine the most appropriate time interval for periodontal maintenance visits except one. Which one is the exception?
   (pp. 454–455)
   a. Medical condition
   b. Level of plaque control
   c. Severity of the disease
   d. Number of medications taken

8. Which one of the following types of pockets is most appropriate for adjunctive controlled-release drug delivery? (p. 454)
   a. Nonbleeding, > 5 mm
   b. Nonbleeding, < 5 mm
   c. Bleeding, ≥ 5 mm
   d. Bleeding, ≤ 5 mm

9. All the following techniques the dental hygienist can use to improve patient adherence to periodontal therapy except one. Which one is the exception? (pp. 455)
   a. Print self-care instructions.
   b. Counsel patients about their condition.
   c. Call the patient every week.
   d. Seek out patient concerns and respond to them.
   e. Send patients reminders about their next visit.

10. All the following components of the 4A Program are introduced during smoking-cessation sessions except one. Which one is the exception?
    (pp. 450–451)
    a. ask
    b. advise
    c. agree
    d. assist
    e. arrange

REFERENCES

Albrektsson, T., G. Zarb, P. Worthington, and A. R. Eriksson. 1986. The long-term efficacy of currently used dental implants: A review and proposed criteria of success. *Int. J. Oral Maxillofac. Implants* 1:11–25.

American Academy of Periodontology. 1989. *Proceedings of the World Workshop in Clinical Periodontics, Consensus report, Discussion section VIII: Implant therapy (VIII-11-18).* Chicago: Author.

American Academy of Periodontology. 1996. Tobacco use and the periodontal patient. *J. Periodontol.* 67:51–56.

American Academy of Periodontology. 1998. Periodontal maintenance (PM). *J. Periodontol.* 69:502–506.

American Academy of Periodontology. 2003b. Periodontal maintenance. *J. Periodontol.* 74:1395–1401.

American Academy of Periodontology. 2006. Guidelines for the management of patients with periodontal diseases. *J. Periodontol* 77:1607–1611.

American Dental Association. 2004, November. *Guidelines for prescribing dental radiographs.* Chicago, IL. American Dental Association

Armitage, G. C. 1996. Manual periodontal probing in supportive periodontal therapy. *Periodontology 2000* 12:33–39.

Axelsson, P., and J. Lindhe. 1981. The significance of maintenance care in the treatment of periodontal disease. *J. Clin. Periodontol.* 8:281–294.

Bain, C. A. 1996. Smoking and implant failure: Benefits of a smoking cessation protocol. *Int. J. Oral Maxillofac. Implants* 11:756–759.

Becker, W., B. E. Becker, and L. E. Berg. 1984. Periodontal treatment without maintenance. A retrospective study in 44 patients. *J. Periodontol.* 55:505–509.

Bergström, J., S. Eliasson, and H. Preber. 1991. Cigarette smoking and periodontal bone loss. *J. Periodontol.* 62:242–246.

Carranza, F. A., and H. H. Takei. 1996. Treatment of furcation involvement and combined periodontal-endodontic therapy. In eds. F. A. Carranza and M. G. Newman, *Clinical periodontology,* 640. Philadelphia: W. B. Saunders.

Christen, A. G., J. L. McDonald, and J. A. Christen. 1991. *The impact of tobacco use and cessation on nonmalignant and precancerous oral and dental diseases and conditions.* Indianapolis: Indiana University School of Dentistry.

Claffey, N., K. Nylund, R. Kiger, S. Garrett, and J. Egelberg. 1990. Diagnostic predictability of scores of plaque, bleeding, suppuration and probing depth for probing attachment loss. 3 1/2 years of observation following initial periodontal therapy. *J. Clin. Periodontol.* 17:108–114.

Dietrich, T. 2004. The effect of cigarette smoking on gingival bleeding. *J. Periodontol.* 75(1):16–22.

Fisher, S., L. Kells, J. P. Picard, S. C. Gelskey, D. L. Singer, et al. 2008. Progression of periodontal disease in a maintenance population of smokers and non-smokers: A 3-year longitudinal study. *J. Periodontol.* 79(3):461–468.

Grossi, S. G., J. J. Zambon, A. W. Ho, G. Koch, R. G. Dunford, et al. 1994. Assessment of risk for periodontal disease: I. Risk indicators for attachment loss. *J. Periodontol.* 65:260–267.

Grossi, S. G., J. Zambon, E. E. Machtei, R. Shifferle, S. Andreana, et al. 1997. Effects of smoking and smoking cessation on healing after mechanical periodontal therapy. *J. Am. Dent. Assoc.* 128:599–607.

Haber, J., J. Wattles, M. Crowby, R. Mandell, K. Joshipura, and R. L. Kent. 1993. Evidence for cigarette smoking as a major risk factor for periodontitis. *J. Periodontol.* 64:16–23.

Haffajee, A. D., S. S. Socransky, and J. M. Goodson. 1983. Comparison of different data analyses for detecting changes in attachment level. *J. Clin. Periodontol.* 10:298–310.

Jolkovsky, D. L., M. Y. Waki, M. G. Newman, J. Otomo-Corgel, M. Madison, et al. 1990. Clinical and microbiological effects of subgingival and gingival marginal irrigation with chlorhexidine gluconate. *J. Periodontol.* 61:663–669.

Jones, J. K., and R. G. Triplett. 1992. The relationship of cigarette smoking to impaired intraoral wound healing: A review of evidence and implications for patient care. *J. Oral Maxillofac. Surg.* 50:237–239.

Joss, A., R. Adler, and N. P. Lang. 1994. Bleeding on probing. A parameter for monitoring periodontal conditions in clinical practice. *J. Clin. Periodontol.* 21:402–408.

Kerry, G. J. 1995. Supportive periodontal treatment. *Periodontology 2000* 11:176–184.

Kornman, K. S. 1987. Nature of periodontal diseases: Assessment and diagnosis. *J. Periodontol. Res.* 22:192–204.

Lang, N. P., A. Joss, and M. S. Tonetti. 1996. Monitoring disease during supportive periodontal treatment by bleeding on probing. *Periodontology 2000* 12:44–48.

Lindhe, J., S. S. Socransky, S. Nyman, A. Haffajee, and E. Westfelt. 1982. "Critical probing depths" in periodontal therapy. *J. Clin. Periodontol.* 9:323–336.

Mendoza, A., G. Newcomb, and K. Nixon. 1991. Compliance with periodontal maintenance. *J. Periodontol.* 62:731–736.

Meffert, R. M. 1992. How to treat ailing and failing implants. *Implant Dent.* 1:25–33.

Mendoza, A., G., Newcomb, K. Nixon, Compliance with supportive periodontal therapy. *J Periodont* 1991;62:731–736.

National Cancer Institute, U.S. Department of Health and Human Services. 1996. In eds. R. E. Mechlenburg, D. Greenspan, D. V. Kleinman, et al. *Tobacco effects in the mouth.* Bethesda, MD: Author.

Ramfjord, S. P. 1987. Maintenance care for treated periodontitis patients. *J. Clin. Periodontol.* 14:433–437.

Rosén, B., G. Olavi, A. Baderstan, A. Rönström, G. Söderholm, and J. Egelberg. 1999. Effect of different frequencies of preventive maintenance treatment on periodontal conditions. *J. Clin. Periodontol.* 26:225–230.

Sison, S. G. 2003, May-June. Implant maintenance and the dental hygienist. *Access* (Supplement issue):1–12.

Stone, C., and D. J. Mattana. 1996, January. The role of the dental team in helping patients stop using tobacco. *J. Mich. Dent. Assoc.:* 58–66.

Tonetti, M., V. Muller-Campanile, and V. Lang. 1998. Changes in the prevalence of residual pockets and tooth loss in treated periodontal patients during a supportive maintenance care program. *J. Clin. Periodontol.* 25:1008–1016.

Van der Weijden, G. A., M. F. Timmerman, A. Nijbor, E. Reijerse, and U. Van der Velden. 1994. Comparison of different approaches to assess bleeding on probing as indicators of gingivitis. *J. Periodontol.* 21:589–594.

Weinberg, A. 1986. *Instructions in hypnosis,* unpublished findings.

Wilson, T. G., Jr., M. E. Glover, J. Schoen, C. Baus, and T. Jacobs. 1984. Compliance with maintenance therapy in a private periodontal practice. *J. Periodontol.* 55:468–473.

Wilson, T. G. 1996a. Compliance and its role in periodontal therapy. *Periodontology 2000* 12:16–23.

Wilson, T. G. 1996b. Supportive periodontal treatment introduction: Definition, extent of need, therapeutic objectives, frequency and efficacy. *Periodontology 2000* 12:11–15.

Appendices

Appendix **A**
Periodontal Information Resources

Appendix **B**
Reading the Literature

Appendix **C**
Antibiotic Prophylaxis

Periodontal Information Resources

Mea A. Weinberg

A great number of scientific and clinical resources on periodontology are available from organizations and various journals. This information should be used for continuing education so that the dental hygienist can keep up with current clinical studies and product availability. The Internet provides an excellent opportunity for dental professionals and patients to obtain information related to all aspects of dental hygiene.

PUBLICATIONS: AMERICAN ACADEMY OF PERIODONTOLOGY

The American Academy of Periodontology (AAP) publishes patient education brochures, practice management resources, journals, and clinical publications. The website for the American Academy of Periodontology is www.perio.org.

The following materials are available:

1. Patient education brochures
2. *2007 Current Procedural Terminology for Periodontics and Insurance Reporting Manual,* 11th ed.
3. *2003 Practice Profile Survey: Characteristics and Trends in Private Periodontal Practice*
4. Practice management resources
   - "Designing Effective Practice Marketing Materials"
   - "Sample Periodontal Office Forms"
   - "Informed Consent for Surgical Periodontics"
5. Study club kits (binders containing slides, lecture script, consensus reports, article reprints, references)
   - "The Periodontal-Systemic Education Kit"
   - "Periodontal Maintenance for Natural Teeth and Implants Study Club Kit"
   - "Periodontal Plastic Surgery"
   - "Implant Dentistry: A Team Approach to Optimal Patient Care" presentation kit
   - "Comprehensive Insurance Workshop: Reporting Periodontal Procedures to Third Parties" (CD-ROM)
   - "Evidence-Based Periodontal Research: Set of Three Scientific Study Club Presentations"
   - "Introduction to Periodontal Surgery for Dental Hygienists" presentation kit
   - "Classification, Epidemiology and Diagnosis of Periodontal Diseases"
   - "The Role of Pharmacotherapeutics in Periodontal Diseases"
   - "Periodic Reevaluation and Supportive Periodontal Therapy"
6. Clinical publications: *Journal of Periodontology* (monthly publication); also available on CD-ROM
7. *Annals of Periodontology*
   - *Annals of Periodontology* (1996 World Workshop in Periodontics), Vol. 1
   - *Annals of Periodontology* (1996 Joint Symposium on Clinical Trial Design and Analysis in Periodontics), Vol. 2
   - *Annals of Periodontology* (1997): New Directions in Periodontal Medicine, Vol. 3.
   - *Annals of Periodontology* (1999): 1999 International Workshop for a Classification of Periodontal Diseases and Conditions, Vol. 4.
   - *Annals of Periodontology* (2003): Proceedings of the Workshop on Contemporary Science in Clinical Periodontics, Vol. 8
   - *Periodontal-Systemic Links: An AAP Literature Compilation* (CD-ROM), 2003

8. *Periodontal Literature Reviews: A Summary of Current Knowledge* (1996)
9. *Periodontal Disease Management* (1993)
   - *2003 Current Procedural Terminology for Periodontics and Insurance Reporting Manual* (9th edition)
   - In-Service Exams (questions given to postgraduate students)
10. Audiotapes from past annual meetings (www.mobiltape.com or 1-800-369-5718).
11. Guidelines
    - Guidelines for the Management of Patients with Periodontal Disease (2006)
    - Guidelines for In-Office Use of Conscious Sedation in Periodontics (2001)
    - Position Statement and Guidelines for Soft Tissue Management Programs (1996)
12. Parameters of care: Various papers on the parameters of care of periodontal diseases (2000)
13. Position papers (some position papers are listed below)
    - "The Role of Supra- and Subgingival Irrigation in the Treatment of Periodontal Diseases" (2005)76:2015-2027.
    - "Periodontal Diseases of Children and Adolescents" (2003)
    - "Diagnosis of Periodontal Diseases" (2003)
    - "Oral Features of Mucocutaneous Disorders" (2003)
    - "Modulation of the Host Response in Periodontal Therapy" (2002)
    - "Dental Implants and Periodontal Therapy" (2000)
    - "The Role of Controlled Drug Delivery for Periodontitis" (1999)
    - "Tobacco Use and the Periodontal Patient" (1999)
    - "The Pathogenesis of Periodontal Diseases" (1999)
    - "Periodontal Disease as a Potential Risk Factor for Systemic Diseases" (1998)
    - "Diabetes and Periodontal Diseases" (1999)
    - "Treatment of Gingivitis and Periodontitis" (1997)
    - "Epidemiology of Periodontal Diseases" (2005)
    - "Implications of Genetic Technology for the Management of Periodontal Diseases" (2005)
    - "Oral and Recorrective Considerations in Periodontal Therapy" (2005)
    - "Periodontal Regeneration" (2005)
    - "Systemic Antibiotics" (2004)
    - "Drug-Associated Gingival Enlargement" (2004)

14. Product and procedure statements
    - "Risk Assessment" (2008)
    - "Bisphosphonates" (2005)
    - "Local Delivery of Sustained or Controlled Release Antimicrobials as Adjunctive Therapy in the Treatment of Periodontitis" (2006)
    - "Periodontal Management of the Pregnant Patient" (2004)
    - "Tooth Extraction During Periodontal Therapy" (2003)
    - "The Use of Conscious Sedation by Periodontists" (2003)
    - "Gingival Curettage" (2002)
    - "Use of Dental Lasers for Excisional New Attachment Procedure (ENAP)"
    - "Periostat® Systemically Delivered Collagenase Inhibitor of Doxycycline Hyclate" (1998)
15. AAP-Commissioned Reviews
    - Bone Augmentation Techniques (2007)
    - Diabetes Mellitus and Periodontal Disease (2006)
    - Lasers in Periodontics (2006)
    - Temporary Anchorage Devices for Tooth Movement (2006)
16. Other associations include:
    - The American Dental Hygiene Association (ADHA). www.adha.org
    - The American Dental Association (ADA). www.ada.org

JOURNALS/BULLETINS

1. *Journal of Periodontology* (American Academy of Periodontology, Chicago; website: www.perio.org).
2. *Journal of Dental Hygiene* (American Dental Hygiene Association, Chicago; website: www.adha.org).
3. *Practical Periodontics and Aesthetic Dentistry* (Montage Media Corp., Mahwah, NJ; 800-899-5350).
4. *Journal of Practical Hygiene* (Montage Media Corp., Mahwah, NJ; 800-899-5350).
5. *Periodontology 2000* (Musksgaard, Copenhagen; e-mail: fsub@mail.munksgaard.dk).
6. *Journal of Clinical Periodontology* (Munksgaard, Copenhagen; e-mail: fsub@mail.munksgaard.dk).
7. *Journal of Periodontal Research* (Munksgaard, Copenhagen; e-mail: fsub@mail.munksgaard.dk).
8. *Perio Reports* (www.PerioReports.com)—research articles are reviewed (*Compendium of Current Research*).

9. *International Journal of Oral and Maxillofacial Implants* (Quintessence Publishers, Carol Stream, IL; e-mail: quintpub@aol.com; www.quintpub.com).
10. *Clinical Oral Implants Research* (Munksgaard International Publishers, ltd., Malden, MA. e-mail: fsub@mail.munksgaard.dk; www.munksgaard.dk).

OTHER WEBSITES

1. www.dentalcare.com (Procter & Gamble)
2. www.colgate.com (Colgate Oral Pharmaceutical)
3. http://jeffline.tju.edu/DHNet (National Center for Dental Hygiene Research)
4. www.oralhealth.org (Oral Health Letter)

Reading the Literature

Trisha E. O'Hehir

ARTICLE CLASSIFICATION

- Clinical trial (in vivo)
- Laboratory study (in vitro)
- Combination studies—part clinical, part laboratory
- Case studies—reports of individual patients and their outcomes
- Epidemiology—incidence and/or prevalence of disease in a population
- Informational
- Review

Research articles include several distinct sections. Each section provides valuable information. These sections do not have to be read in the order they are printed. It depends on what information is being requested. The following is a brief summary of each section.

ABSTRACT

- Brief overview of the entire article
- Hypothesis being tested
- Number of subjects involved
- Methods used
- Results

The last sentence of an abstract often provides the essence of the project. The last sentence is where reading of a research article should begin.

INTRODUCTION

- Lays the groundwork for the project
- Historical information on the subject area
- Past research studies are sited in this area
- Author or authors have to make a case for the project

- Controversies in the area based on previously published work
- Statement of the hypothesis

Most often, a null hypothesis is stated, which says that if the researchers do what they propose, no changes will be seen. The goal of the researchers is to then disprove the null hypothesis. Approaching the hypothesis from the other direction requires stating that the drug, tool, or therapy to be tested will have a specific effect on the test subject, which necessitates quantifying the expected result. Guessing at the outcome before the study begins can be quite difficult. Therefore, disproving a null hypothesis allows for a positive result without the need to estimate the outcome at the start.

Some researchers state their purpose rather than formulating a hypothesis. The following is an example of stating a purpose:

> Thus, this study compares the amount of aerosol produced by a traditional ultrasonic scaler insert and that produced by a new focused style insert. In addition, the effect of using an aerosol reduction device with both types of inserts is evaluated. [Rivera–Hidalgo, F., Barnes, J., and Harrel, S. 1999. Aerosol and splatter production by focused spray and standard ultrasonic inserts. *J. Periodontol.,* 70:473–477]

Here is the same statement of purpose restated as a hypothesis:

> The hypothesis to be tested is that no difference in aerosol spray is expected comparing

traditional and focused-style ultrasonic inserts, used either alone or with an aerosol reduction device.

The goal of the researchers remains the same—to determine if there is a difference, thus disproving the null hypothesis.

METHODS AND MATERIALS

This section is often divided into subsections, providing some of the following information:

- *Study population.* Collection of people, items, or observations to be studied
- *People*
  - *Number of subjects.* Setting a desired outcome in statistical terms allows the statistician to calculate exactly how many subjects are needed.
  - *Random sample.* All subjects of a given population have an equal chance of being selected (e.g., picking names out of a hat or using a table of random numbers to select subjects).
  - *Convenience population.* Sample does not represent the population at large (e.g., dental or dental hygiene students).
  - *Volunteers or paid participants.*
  - *Subject solicitation.* Clinic patients, newspaper ads, etc.
  - *Demographics.* Age, gender, general health, oral health, dental history.
- *Location of the study.* University, clinical practice, community, etc.
- *Study design*
  - Timeline of events, including length of the study.
  - Indices used and any modifications.
- Description of drugs, tools, or techniques to be tested
- Who the examiners were and their preparation for the study.
- Characteristics of the clinical study design
  - *Case control.* Subjects with a certain condition are selected and compared with controls (e.g., subjects without the condition). For example, a group of subjects with oral cancer is compared with a control group without oral cancer for smoking habits over the previous five years.
  - *Crossover.* Each subject receives two or more treatments at different times, and end points are observed after each treatment.

- *Cross-sectional.* End points are observed at one given point in time.
- *Longitudinal.* End points are observed more than once over a period of time.
- *Observational.* Subjects or objects of interest (e.g., teeth) are observed in their natural state with no intervention by researchers.
- *Prospective.* Study subjects selected based on a certain treatment or exposure and observed for a specific outcome over a period of time (e.g., subjects selected based on smoking habits and observed for cancer development over a five-year period).
- *Retrospective.* Study subjects are selected based on a certain outcome, and then data are gathered on previous exposure (e.g., subjects selected based on the presence of oral cancer and studied as to smoking habits during the previous five years).
- *Parallel group.* Experimental groups do not experience the same treatment or products (e.g., a control group and a test group).
- *Randomized.* Subjects or objects of interest (e.g., teeth) are assigned to different treatments or interventions randomly.
- *Split-mouth.* Each subject receives two or more treatments at different sites within the mouth, and outcomes are observed at a given point in time.
- *Details of laboratory tests*
  - How specimens are collected.
  - How they are stored.
  - How the tests are run.
  - What equipment is used.
  - Who does the testing.
- *Statistical analysis.* Selection of mathematical techniques used to assist in the understanding and interpretation of data for the purpose of decision making.
- *Descriptive statistics.* Methods to simply describe data in a numerical way, such as frequency of a given parameter.
- *Inferential statistics.* Methods used to infer something about a population from a sample of observations from that population.

RESULTS

- Factual presentation of the study data.
- Statistics. (Opinions or conclusion are left for the next section.)

Discussion

- Limitations of the study.
- Confirmation of earlier findings.
- Integration of study findings with previously published data.
- Unanswered questions.
- New questions raised by the findings.
- Interesting side findings that do not relate to this hypothesis.
- Subjective opinions of the patients who participated.
- Suggestions for future studies.
- Conclusions that can be drawn from this study.
- Significance of these findings, both statistical and clinical.

Statistical significance might be better stated as "statistical difference," since the difference actually may not be clinically significant.

Appendix C

Antibiotic Prophylaxis

Cardiac conditions associated with the highest risk of adverse outcome from IE for which antibiotic prophylaxis is indicated (Wilson et al., 2007)

- Prosthetic cardiac valve or prosthetic material used for cardiac valve repair.
- Previous infective endocarditis.
- Congenital heart disease (CHD)
  - Unrepaired cyanotic CHD, including palliative shuts and conduits.
  - Completely repaired congenital heart defect with prosthetic material or device, whether placed by surgery or by catheter intervention, during the first six months after the procedure.
  - Repaired CHD with residual defects at the site or adjacent to the site of a prosthetic patch or prosthetic device (which inhibit endothelialization).

- Cardiac transplantation recipients who develop cardiac valvulopathy.

REFERENCES

Wilson, W., K. A. Taubert, M. Gewitz, et al. Prevention of infective endocarditis. Guidelines from the American Heart Association Rheumatic Fever, Endocarditis and Kawasaki Disease Committee, Council on Cardiovascular Disease in the Young, and the Council on Clinical Cardiology, Council on Cardiovascular Surgery and Anesthesia, and the Quality of Care and Outcome Research Interdisciplinary Working Group. *Circulation* 2007; 116:1736–1754.

Prophylactic Antibiotic Regimens for Oral and Dental Procedures		
Situation	*Drug*	*Regimen (single dose taken 30 to 60 min before Dental Procedure*
Standard general prophylaxis	Amoxicillin	Adults: 2.0 g orally; Children: 50 mg/kg orally
Unable to take oral medication	Ampicillin	Adults: 2.0 g intramuscularly (IM) or intravenously (IV); Children: 50 mg/kg IM or IV
	OR	Adults: 1 g IM or IV; Children: 50 mg/kg IM or IV
	Cefazolin* or ceftriaxone*	

(continued)

Prophylactic Antibiotic Regimens for Oral and Dental Procedures (cont.)		
Situation	*Drug*	*Regimen (single dose taken 30 to 60 min before Dental Procedure*
Allergic to penicillins—oral	Cephalexin*	Adults: 2 g; children: 50 mg/kg
	OR	
	Clindamycin	Adults: 600 mg; children: 20 mg/kg
	OR	
	Azithromycin or clarithromycin	Adults: 500 mg; children: 15 mg/kg
Allergic to pencillin and unable to take oral medications	Cefazolin*	Adults: 1.0 g; children: 25 mg/kg IM or IV
	OR	
	Clindamycin	Adults: 600 mg; children: 20 mg/kg IV

*Cephalosporins should not be used in patients with immediate-type hypersensitivity reaction (urticaria, angioedema, or anaphylaxis) to penicillins.

Case Study I

MEDICAL HISTORY

The patient is a 31-year-old female who presents to the clinic and states that she is in perfect health. Her last physical examination was one year ago. The blood pressure is 125/82 and pulse is 72. She is 5 feet 4 inches tall and weighs 125 lbs (56.8 kgs). Medications: She takes Yasmin (an oral contraceptive) and a multivitamin daily.

DENTAL HISTORY

When she was a child, she had regular dental visits. Her "gum" problems started when she was about 12 years old. She said the dentist said she was "losing some bone around some back teeth." But she has not been to a dentist in the last fifteen years. She tries to brush once a day, but if she is too busy she will not brush. She does not floss. She has a sister who also has "gum" problems. At work she has a habit of biting a pencil when under stress. She also notices that her "gums are shrinking."

SOCIAL HISTORY

The patient is married with one child. She denies smoking and consumption of alcohol.

CHIEF COMPLAINT

"My teeth have spaces between them and I feel cold."

ORAL HYGIENE STATUS

The patient has poor oral hygiene. There is generalized supra/subgingival plaque and calculus.

GINGIVAL EXAM

The gingiva is red with rolled margins. The papillae are blunted, pointed, and absent. There is loss of stippling on the mandibular gingiva.

PERIODONTAL EXAM

Probing depths range up to 10 mm. The mandibular right second premolar has 5 mm of gingival recession on the direct facial surface. There is generalized bleeding on probing.

INTERPRETATION

Patient Problem	Basis for Discussion	Questions (Q)/Answers (A)	Chapter Location
Localized bone loss started at 12 years of age.	Patient was young to lose bone.	Q) Why did the patient lose bone at such an early age? A) The periodontal condition is recognized as aggressive periodontitis. Initially, it was localized to the molars and then later it became generalized. The criteria for localized aggressive periodontitis includes clinically healthy patient, rapid attachment loss, and bone destruction and familial. Later in life, this condition became chronic periodontitis. It is not aggressive at this point because there is moderate amounts of plaque and calculus. Q) What is the cause of aggressive periodontitis? A) Bacteria and host response. Elevated levels of *Actinobacillus actinomycetemcomitans* and, in some populations, *Porphyromonas gingivalis* may be elevated. Elevated levels of PGE_2 and IL-1β.	8

INTERPRETATION (cont.)

Patient Problem	Basis for Discussion	Questions (Q)/Answers (A)	Chapter Location
Gingival recession	Patient is sensitive to cold and air.	Q) What is the cause of the gingival recession? A) There are many causes of gingival recession, but in this case it is caused by attachment loss where the gingival fibers are destroyed by collagenase, allowing the junctional epithelium to migrate apically onto the root surface. This is referred to as attachment loss and is the result of the disease process.	8, 16
A lot of diastemas (spaces between teeth).	The chief complaint.	Q) Why are the teeth moving and developing spaces? A) Pathologic migration due to severe bone loss.	8, 16
Patient gets food stuck in between the teeth – in the papilla.	Blunting (tip of papilla is destroyed) of gingival papilla.	Q) Why are the papillae blunted? A) There is a saying in periodontics that "gingiva follows the bone." So, with bone loss the gingiva can become blunted.	7, 15
Patient taking oral contraceptive.	May be a contributing factor to the patients' gingival condition.	Q) Do you think that the oral contraceptive is a contributing factor to the patient's periodontal condition? A) No. Also, with todays formulation of oral contraceptive less hormones are used, thus reducing the incidence of gingivitis.	6

1. Which of the following teeth exhibits a vertical defect?
   a. Maxillary right lateral incisor
   b. Maxillary left canine
   c. Maxillary right central incisor
   d. Mandibular left first molar

2. Which of the following conditions is the cause of the patient's chief complaint?
   a. Attrition
   b. Erosion
   c. Bone loss
   d. Furcation involvement
   e. Medication induced

3. The papillary condition between the mandibular left premolars and first molar is most likely to be caused by
   a. bone loss.
   b. improper flossing.
   c. overzealous toothbrushing.
   d. intrusion of opposing teeth.
   e. extrusion of mandibular teeth.

4. Which of the following factors is the cause of the condition in photo E where the arrow is pointing?
   a. Oral contraceptive
   b. Attachment loss
   c. High frenum
   d. Prominent root

5. Which of the following bacteria is primarily found in this patient?
   a. *Actinobacillus actinomycetemcomitans*
   b. *Streptococcus mutans*
   c. *Streptococcus viridans*
   d. *Clostridium difficle*

6. Which of the following factors is the most likely cause for mobility of the mandibular incisors?
   a. Parafunctional habit
   b. Bone loss
   c. Oral contraceptive
   d. Oral biofilm

7. The amount of clinical attachment loss on the direct facial surface of the mandibular right second premolar is _____ mm.
   a. 1
   b. 2
   c. 4
   d. 5
   e. 6

8. Which of the following teeth has a hopeless prognosis?
   a. Maxillary right second premolar
   b. Maxillary left second molar
   c. Mandibular left first molar
   d. Mandibular left canine

9. Which of the following devices is best used to remove plaque in between the right mandibular lateral and canine?
   a. Dental floss
   b. Floss threader
   c. Toothpick
   d. End-tufted brush

10. Which of the following statements is correct about the right mandibular central incisor?
    a. Adequate bony support
    b. Poor crown to root ratio
    c. Widened periodontal ligament
    d. Extensive caries

DENTAL FINDINGS

Based upon clinical and radiographic findings
Enter / diagram radiographic findings from pg 3B

Date: _____6/15/09_____

Chart #

5	6	7	1	4	1

Probe Depth 1 Date: 6/15/09 X

635	333	857	423	323	322	213	212	213	213	313	857	253	235	385

Probe Depth 2 Date: ___/___/___

1	2	3	4	5	6	7	8	9	10	11	12	13	14	15	16

Facial

CARIES & RESTORATIVE

Missing CM RCT Ponlic Implant

TOP ROW:
Caries Scores:
EO, E1 E2, D1, D2 D3
(see legend on reverse)

BOTTOM ROW:
Fillings: color in Black
Caries: color in Red

DIAGNODENT *readings:*
Chart on reverse side as needed

Palatal

	1	2	3	4	5	6	7	8	9	10	11	12	13	14	15	16

Probe Depth 1 Date: 6/15/09 X

| 232 | 353 | 756 | 452 | 317 | 217 | 212 | 212 | 212 | 212 | 433 | X | 282 | 245 | 535 |

Probe Depth 2 Date: ___/___/___

Probe Depth 1 Date: 6/15/09 X

| 337 | 455 | 323 | 323 | 323 | 345 | 533 | 323 | 323 | 323 | 323 | 323 | 345 | 533 | X |

Probe Depth 2 Date: ___/___/___

32	31	30	29	28	27	26	25	24	23	22	21	20	19	18	17

Lingual

PERIO LEGEND

Suppuration:
5 next to crown

Free Gingival Margin -
black line

Mucogingival Line -
black line

Mobility: +1,+2,+3 *in crown*

Furcation: Class I II III

Spacing: | |

Occlusion:

Facial

32	31	30	29	28	27	26	25	24	23	22	21	20	19	18	17

Probe Depth 1 Date: 6/15/09 X

| 337 | 542 | 212 | 212 | 325 | 324 | 512 | 212 | 224 | 212 | 323 | 323 | 2310 | 623 | X |

Probe Depth 2 Date: ___/___/___

Assessment of Oral hygiene and Gingival Inflammation

	Tooth # (Surface)	3 (B)	9 (B)	12 (B)	19 (L)	25 (L)	28 (L)	Total + 's
Date ___/___/___	Plaque +/-							
	Bleeding +/-							
Date ___/___/___	Plaque +/-							
	Bleeding +/-							

Substitutions:

If 3, 12,19 or 28 is missing, substitute the next most posterior tooth.

If 9 or 25 is missing, substitute the nearest incisor in the arch.

If all incisors are missing from the arch, substitute a cuspid.

Preliminary Clinical Findings Reviewed

Student Name/#: _____

Faculty Signature/#: _____

Final Findings Reviewed

Student Name/#: _____

Faculty Signature/#: _____

(a)

(d)

(b)   (L)

(e)

(c)   (R)

(R)

(L)

Case Study II

MEDICAL HISTORY

The patient is a 66-year-old female who presents to the dental office. She has type 2 diabetes mellitus, hypertension, and hypercholesterolnemia. She does not regularly take her blood glucose levels at home but recently it was 210. The blood pressure is 130/80 and pulse 65. She is 5 feet 7 inches tall and weighs 150 lbs (68.2 kgs). Medications: She takes amlodipine (Norvac), metformin (Glucophage), glyburide (Diabeta), aspirin (325 mg/day), atorvastatin (Lipitor).

DENTAL HISTORY

She has not been to the dentist in many years. At work she has a habit of biting a pencil when under stress.

SOCIAL HISTORY

The patient has one drink of wine every night. She denies smoking.

CHIEF COMPLAINT

"My gums bleed."

ORAL HYGIENE STATUS

The patient has poor oral hygiene. There is generalized supra/subgingival plaque and calculus.

GINGIVAL EXAM

The gingiva is red and edematous with rolled margins. The papillae are bulbous. Gingival clefts are evident.

PERIODONTAL EXAM

Probing depths are deep with numerous furcation involvements. The majority of teeth are mobile.

INTERPRETATION

Patient Problem	Basis for Discussion	Questions (Q)/Answers (A)	Chapter Location
Patient has diabetes.	Affect of diabetes on the periodontium.	Q) Is diabetes a possible risk factor for periodontal disease? A) Yes. Diabetes (poor glycemic control) is associated with increased prevalence and severity of gingivitis and periodontitis. Periodontal destruction is worse due to hyperglycemia (increased levels of blood glucose or sugar). Q) Is periodontal disease a possible risk factor for diabetes? A) Yes. Conversely, periodontitis may increase the risk for worsening glycemic control in diabetic patients and may increase the risk for diabetic complications.	5, 6

INTERPRETATION (cont.)

Patient Problem	Basis for Discussion	Questions (Q)/Answers (A)	Chapter Location
Gingiva is enlarged.	Difficult to brush.	Q) What is causing the gingival enlargement? A) The antihypertensive (amlodipine) is a calcium channel blocker and is causing gingival enlargement. Other drugs such as phenytoin (antiseizure drug) and cyclosporine (immunosuppressant drug) can also cause gingival enlargement. Q) How is the gingival enlargement managed? A) As long as the patient is taking the offending drug there will be gingival enlargement. Meticulous oral hygiene is important.	7
Teeth are mobile and many spaces are developing.	There is a lot of bone loss.	Q) Why are the teeth mobile with development of diastemas? A) There is advanced bone loss (chronic periodontitis) with pathologic migration of the teeth.	8
Gingiva bleeds.	Inflammation is present.	Q) What is causing the bleeding? A) Bleeding is caused by vascular proliferation in the connective tissue. Bleeding on probing occurs when the sulcular epithelium becomes ulcerated, and the probe penetrates the epithelium. The enlarged blood vessels protrude from the underlying connective tissue.	7
Patient bites on pencil.	May be causing trauma and mobility of teeth.	Q) What type of occlusal trauma is seen in this patient? A) Secondary occlusal trauma occurs when normal or abnormal occlusal forces (parafunctional habit such as pencil biting) occurs on teeth with compromised bone levels such as in this patient.	10

1. Which of the following is the most likely cause for the patient's gingival condition?
   a. Amlodipine
   b. Aspirin
   c. Alcohol
   d. Parafunctional habit
   e. Pathologic migration

2. Which of the following factors is most likely the cause for the mobility of the right maxillary central incisor?
   a. Secondary occlusal trauma
   b. Primary occlusal trauma
   c. Gingival enlargement
   d. Aspirin use

3. The discoloration of the gingival tissue in Photo C (arrow) is due to
   a. coffee.
   b. inflammation.
   c. lead of pencil.
   d. melanin.

4. To which of the following classifications of periodontal diseases does this patient belong?
   a. Aggressive periodontitis
   b. Ulcerative gingivitis
   c. Ulcerative periodontitis
   d. Chronic periodontitis

5. Which of the following is the arrow in Photo E pointing to?
   a. Nutrition canal
   b. Dentinal caries
   c. Root caries
   d. Supragingival calculus

6. Which of the following conditions does the arrow point to in the full-mouth-series of X-rays?
   a. Furcation defect
   b. Tooth caries
   c. Supragingival calculus
   d. Periodontal abscess

7. In Photo B, the arrow is pointing to:
   a. tooth caries.
   b. endodontic abscess.
   c. furcation involvement.
   d. gingival recession.

8. Which one of the following oral hygiene devices is best for in between the mandibular central incisors?
   a. Interdental brush
   b. Tufted floss
   c. Extra soft toothbrush
   d. Toothpick-in-holder

9. All of the following are probable risk factors for this patient's periodontal condition EXCEPT which one?
   a. Poor oral hygiene
   b. Amlodipine
   c. Atorvastatin (Lipitor)
   d. Diabetes

10. The pattern of bone loss found between the maxillary central incisors is
    a. vertical.
    b. horizontal.
    c. angular.
    d. circumferential.

DENTAL FINDINGS

Based upon clinical and radiographic findings
Enter / diagram radiographic findings from pg 3B

Date: _7/10/09_

Chart #	8	6	7	4	3	1

Probe Depth 1 Date: 7/10/09	X	X	X	X	545	777	777	777	776	767	545	777	258	745	653	X
Probe Depth 2 Date: __/__/__																
	1	2	3	4	5	6	7	8	9	10	11	12	13	14	15	16

CARIES & RESTORATIVE

Missing CM RCT Ponlic Implant

TOP ROW:
Caries Scores:
EO, E1 E2, D1, D2 D3
(see legend on reverse)

BOTTOM ROW:
Fillings: color in Black
Caries: color in Red

DIAGNODENT *readings:*
Chart on reverse side as needed

Facial

Palatal

	1	2	3	4	5	6	7	8	9	10	11	12	13	14	15	16
Probe Depth 1 Date: 7/10/09	X	X	X	X	444	777	777	776	768	767	444	767	666	656	656	X
Probe Depth 2 Date: __/__/__																

Probe Depth 1 Date: 7/10/09	X	454	454	454	646	666	666	666	545	545	555	535	555	666	666	X
Probe Depth 2 Date: __/__/__																
	32	31	30	29	28	27	26	25	24	23	22	21	20	19	18	17

PERIO LEGEND

Suppuration:
5 next to crown

Free Gingival Margin -
black line

Mucogingival Line -
black line

Mobility: +1,+2,+3 *in crown*

Furcation: Class I II III

Spacing: | |

Occlusion:

Lingual

Facial

	32	31	30	29	28	27	26	25	24	23	22	21	20	19	18	17
Probe Depth 1 Date: 7/10/09	X	454	454	644	666	656	454	545	444	644	454	454	555	666	666	X
Probe Depth 2 Date: __/__/__																

Assessment of Oral hygiene and Gingival Inflammation

	Tooth # (Surface)	3 (B)	9 (B)	12 (B)	19 (L)	25 (L)	28 (L)	Total + 's
Date __/__/__	Plaque +/-							
	Bleeding +/-							
Date __/__/__	Plaque +/-							
	Bleeding +/-							

Substitutions:

If 3, 12,19 or 28 is missing, substitute the next most posterior tooth.

If 9 or 25 is missing, substitute the nearest incisor in the arch.

If all incisors are missing from the arch, substitute a cuspid.

Preliminary Clinical Findings Reviewed

Student Name/#: _____

Faculty Signature/#: _____

Final Findings Reviewed

Student Name/#: _____

Faculty Signature/#: _____

(a)

(b)   (R)

(c)   (L)

(d)

(e)

(f)

(R)

(L)

Case Study III

MEDICAL HISTORY

The patient is a 29-year-old female who presents to the clinic. Her last physical examination was one year ago. The blood pressure is 110/70 and pulse is 68. She is 5 feet 1 inches tall and weighs 100 lbs (45.5 kgs). She has the following conditions

Heart murmur—present since birth. Asthma induced particularly by cold weather; asthma attacks about twice a year. Iron deficiency anemia. Sickle cell trait—patient has been aware of this since birth, no signs of sickle cell anemia.

MEDICATIONS

The patient is taking prednisone, Singulair, Advair and albuterol for asthma. She is also taking Claritin for allergies.

ALLERGIES

Seasonal allergies only

DENTAL HISTORY

Her last dental visit was one year ago for adult prophylaxis. She brushes once per day and does not floss. Patient has herpes labialis outbreaks several times per year. At work she has a habit of biting a pencil when under stress.

CHIEF COMPLAINT

"I have gum disease. The gum disease has led to pain, bleeding, loose teeth, and bad breath, present for a few years."

SOCIAL HISTORY

The patient is single. She is very anxious about treatment. Patient reports no drug abuse, alcohol use, or tobacco use.

FAMILY HISTORY

Cancer and hypertension history in immediate family members.

ORAL HYGIENE STATUS

The patient's oral hygiene is poor.

GINGIVAL EXAM

The gingiva is extremely red, edematous and painful.

PERIODONTAL EXAM

There is deep probing depths with tooth mobility. Generalized bleeding on probing.

INTERPRETATION

Patient Problem	Basis for Discussion	Questions (Q)/Answers (A)	Chapter Location
Gingiva is red and bleeding.	Inflammation; interferes with normal function.	Q) Why is the gingiva red and bleeding? A) Vasodilation—blood vessels become dilated and engorged with blood. This is happening in the gingival connective tissue. Also, because of the microulcerations in the epithelium, the blood vessels come through, resulting in bleeding on probing.	4,7,8
Teeth are moving with spaces developing.	Difficult for patient to function and aesthetically unpleasing.	Q) Why are the teeth moving with development of diastemas? A) Pathologic migration.	8
Severe periodontal destruction.	Prognosis of case is poor because the patient is so young.	Q) What are the underlying factors that are involved in the development of this patient's periodontal condition? A) Chronic periodontitis can occur at any age; classification is no longer based on age. It may affect a variable number of teeth and it has variable rates of progression. The fact that the patient has asthma, sickle cell anemia trait, and is physically challenged are not contributory to the periodontal disease. There is severe attachment loss and bone destruction. One can argue that the case may be an aggressive periodontitis because of the severe periodontal destruction in a young person. There is heavy plaque and calculus deposits. Usually in an aggressive case there are minimal deposits. But according to the American Academy of Periodontology (AAP), aggressive periodontitis has certain criteria that may not all be present, including minimal amount of deposits (this patient has heavy plaque and calculus deposits).	8,18
Taking multiple medications.	Medications may be co-involved in changes to the periodontium.	Q) Do any of her medications affect the periodontium? A) Albuterol is an inhaler for asthma. It can cause oral candidiasis. Thus, tell the patient to rinse her mouth after every use. Systemic steroids (Advair, predisone, and Singular) have not been documented to have any influence on periodontal disease.	6

1. To which of the following classifications of periodontal diseases does this patient belong?
   a. Periodontitis associated with a genetic disorder
   b. Chronic periodontitis
   c. Periodontitis associated with systemic disease
   d. Ulcerative periodontitis

2. Which of the following factors is involved in the etiology of this patient's disease?
   a. Bacteria + immune function
   b. Medication + immune function
   c. Medical condition + medications
   d. Medical condition only

3. The condition between the maxillary right lateral and central incisor is most likely due to
   a. endodontic abscess.
   b. periodontal abscess.
   c. herpetic ulcer.
   d. aphthous ulcer.

4. The arrow in Photo A is pointing to
   a. food debris.
   b. composite restoration.
   c. calculus.
   d. melanin.

5. The arrow in the posterior right mandibular radiograph is pointing to
   a. furcation involvement.
   b. cervical enamel projection.
   c. enamel pearl.
   d. fremitus.

6. Considering the patient's medical history, which of the following statements is true?
   a. The systemic drugs the patient is taking for asthma contribute a lot to her disease.
   b. The patient's oral hygiene neglect is a primary cause of her disease.
   c. The patient's anemia is a secondary cause of her disease.
   d. The patient's herpes lesion is a primary cause of her disease.

7. What is the pattern of bone loss found between the maxillary central incisors?
   a. Vertical
   b. Horizontal
   c. Circumferential
   d. Hemispetal

8. The arrow in the posterior left mandibular radiograph is pointing to:
   a. furcation.
   b. palatogingival groove.
   c. calculus.
   d. radicular bone.

9. Which of the following describes the relationship of the mandibular incisors?
   a. wide interdental septum
   b. long, bulbous roots
   c. crowding
   d. close root proximity

10. The primary histological cause of the gingival condition in this patient is
    a. vasodilation.
    b. vasoconstriction.
    c. fibrosis.
    d. increased stippling.

Date: 7/29/09

DENTAL FINDINGS
Based upon clinical and radiographic findings
Enter / diagram radiographic findings from pg 3B

Chart # | 7 | 7 | 6 | 2 | 3 | 3

Probe Depth 1 Date: __/__/__	X	538	848	746	838	537	737	737	523	523	523	523	756	745	745	X
Probe Depth 2 Date: __/__/__																
	1	2	3	4	5	6	7	8	9	10	11	12	13	14	15	16

CARIES & RESTORATIVE

Missing CM RCT Ponlic Implant

TOP ROW:
Caries Scores:
EO, E1 E2, D1, D2 D3
(see legend on reverse)

BOTTOM ROW:
Fillings: color in Black
Caries: color in Red

DIAGNODENT *readings:*
Chart on reverse side as needed

Facial

Palatal

	1	2	3	4	5	6	7	8	9	10	11	12	13	14	15	16
Probe Depth 1 Date: __/__/__	X	758	586	757	837	835	735	737	535	555	533	858	846	747	745	X
Probe Depth 2 Date: __/__/__																
Probe Depth 1 Date: __/__/__	X	958	757	758	746	657	656	355	535	535	545	646	656	737	526	X
Probe Depth 2 Date: __/__/__																
	32	31	30	29	28	27	26	25	24	23	22	21	20	19	18	17

PERIO LEGEND

Suppuration:
5 next to crown

Free Gingival Margin -
black line

Mucogingival Line -
black line

Mobility: +1,+2,+3 *in crown*

Furcation: Class   I   II   III

Spacing: | |

Occlusion:

Lingual

Facial

	32	31	30	29	28	27	26	25	24	23	22	21	20	19	18	17
Probe Depth 1 Date: __/__/__	X	768	768	857	857	755	535	555	535	556	353	636	645	747	758	X
Probe Depth 2 Date: __/__/__																

Assessment of Oral hygiene and Gingival Inflammation

	Tooth # (Surface)	3 (B)	9 (B)	12 (B)	19 (L)	25 (L)	28 (L)	Total + 's
Date __/__/__	Plaque +/-							
	Bleeding +/-							
Date __/__/__	Plaque +/-							
	Bleeding +/-							

Substitutions:

If 3, 12,19 or 28 is missing, substitute the next most posterior tooth.

If 9 or 25 is missing, substitute the nearest incisor in the arch.

If all incisors are missing from the arch, substitute a cuspid.

Preliminary Clinical Findings Reviewed

Student Name/#: _____

Faculty Signature/#: _____

Final Findings Reviewed

Student Name/#: _____

Faculty Signature/#: _____

(a)

(b)   (R)

(c)   (L)

(d)

(R)   (L)

Case Study IV

MEDICAL HISTORY

The patient is a 66-year-old female who presents to the dental office. Her last physical examination was six months ago. The blood pressure is 130/82 and pulse is 72. She is 5 feet 8 inches tall and weighs 150 lbs (68.2 kgs). Medications: She takes oxybutynin (Ditropan) and alendronate (Fosamax) (has been on it for three years).

DENTAL HISTORY

When she was a child, she had regular dental visits. She has not been to a dentist for the last three years since her regular dentist moved. She previously had periodontal surgery in only three quadrants but knows she needs more treatment. She is interested in implants. She says she tries to brush at least once a day but it does not always happen.

SOCIAL HISTORY

The patient is married with one child. She smokes three cigarettes a day.

CHIEF COMPLAINT

"I have two very loose teeth on lowers."

ORAL HYGIENE STATUS

Poor oral hygiene.

GINGIVAL EXAM

The gingiva is red and fibrotic with localized edematous areas. The papillae are primarily blunted.

PERIODONTAL EXAM

There are deep probing depths with bleeding on probing. There is localized tooth mobility and generalized gingival recession.

INTERPRETATION

Patient Problem	Basis for Discussion	Questions (Q)/Answers (A)	Chapter Location
Patient is taking bisphosphonates.	Bisphosphonates are implicating in causing osteonecrosis of the jaw (ONJ).	Q) What is the appropriate treatment in this patient who is taking oral bisphosphonates? A) Communication between the dental clinician and physician is important. There is a higher incidence of ONJ in patients on IV bisphosphonates. There is still limited information concerning the risk of ONJ in patients taking oral bisphosphonates. Periodontal debridement can be performed on patients taking oral bisphosphonates but precautions must be taken for the development of ONJ.	6
Mandibular central incisors are mobile.	This is the patient's chief complaint, and it must be addressed first.	Q) Why are these teeth mobile? A) Because there is advanced bone loss.	8,16

INTERPRETATION *(cont.)*

Patient Problem	Basis for Discussion	Questions (Q)/Answers (A)	Chapter Location
Teeth have stains.	Aesthetically unpleasing for patient.	Q) Why are the teeth stained? A) Because of smoking.	14
Patient wants implants.	Concern for osteonecrosis of the jaw (ONJ).	Q) Is this patient a candidate for implants? A) Patient is taking oral bisphosphonates for < 3 years can have implants, but it is important to be aware of possible ONJ.	6, 26
Left mandibular first molar has furcation involvement (Buccal II).	Surgical correction of bony defects.	Q) What type of periodontal surgery is indicated for this defect? A) Periodontal regeneration using bone graft and membranes.	25
Patient wants a mouthrinse to help her with oral hygiene.	Is a mouthrinse indicated for adjunctive therapy?	Q) Should you recommend a mouthrinse to this patient? A) Yes, mouthrinses are used as adjuncts to brushing and interdental care.	20, 21

1. Which of the following periodontal procedures is best indicated for this patient?
   a. Local antibiotics (e.g., Arestin)
   b. systemic antibiotics
   c. topical antimicrobial rinse (e.g., chlorhexidine)
   d. periodontal debridement and surgery

2. Which of the following factors is involved in the gingival recession on the mandibular left central incisor?
   a. High frenum
   b. Tooth mobility
   c. Poor toothbrushing habit
   d. Previous periodontal surgery

3. Which of the following teeth has the worst prognosis?
   a. Maxillary right first molar
   b. Maxillary right central incisor
   c. Maxillary left first premolar
   d. Mandibular right first molar

4. The patient requires multiple teeth to be extracted and periodontal surgery. Which of the following factors needs to be considered in this patient before these procedures are performed?
   a. Pulse rate
   b. Bisphosphonate use
   c. Oxybutynin use
   d. Blood pressure

5. Which of the following teeth has a periapical pathology related to an endodontic problem?
   a. Maxillary right lateral incisor
   b. Maxillary left first premolar
   c. Mandibular right first premolar
   d. Mandibular left first molar

6. To which of the following classifications of periodontal diseases does this patient belong?
   a. Chronic periodontitis
   b. Aggressive periodontitis
   c. Periodontitis associated with systemic disease
   d. Ulcerative periodontitis

7. Which of the following factors is involved in this patient's periodontal condition?
   a. Oxybutynin
   b. Alendronate
   c. Poor oral hygiene
   d. Previous periodontal surgery
   e. bisphosphonate

8. The arrow in Photo A points to
   a. dehiscence.
   b. enamel.
   c. milky white stain.
   d. fenestration.

9. Which of the following conditions exists on the dental surface of the maxillary left first premolar?
   a. Widened periodontal ligament
   b. Infrabony defect
   c. Endodontic abscess
   d. Periodontal abscess

10. Which of the following interproximal hygiene devices is best for the area between the left maxillary lateral incisor and canine?
    a. Wooden wedge
    b. Dental floss
    c. Tufted floss
    d. Rubber-tip stimulator

DENTAL FINDINGS

Based upon clinical and radiographic findings
Enter / diagram radiographic findings from pg 3B

Date: ___8/12/09___

Chart #	8	9	3	1	3	1

Probe Depth 1 Date: 8/12/09	X	X	432	314	224	322	322	313	213	213	333	333	433	X	312	X
Probe Depth 2 Date: __/__/__																
	1	2	3	4	5	6	7	8	9	10	11	12	13	14	15	16

CARIES & RESTORATIVE

Missing CM RCT Ponlic Implant

TOP ROW:
Caries Scores:
EO, E1 E2, D1, D2 D3
(see legend on reverse)

BOTTOM ROW:
Fillings: color in Black
Caries: color in Red

DIAGNODENT *readings:*
Chart on reverse side as needed

Facial

Palatal

	1	2	3	4	5	6	7	8	9	10	11	12	13	14	15	16
Probe Depth 1 Date: 8/12/09	X	X	333	333	334	323	212	212	112	123	114	223	313	X	333	X
Probe Depth 2 Date: __/__/__																

Probe Depth 1 Date: 8/12/09	X	X	X	532	557	312	212	434	434	223	223	212	223	5410	524	424
Probe Depth 2 Date: __/__/__																
	32	31	30	29	28	27	26	25	24	23	22	21	20	19	18	17

PERIO LEGEND

Suppuration:
5 next to crown

Free Gingival Magin -
black line

Mucogingival Line -
black line

Mobility: +1,+2,+3 *in crown*

Furcation: Class I II III
△ △ ▲

Spacing: | |

Occlusion:

Lingual

Facial

	32	31	30	29	28	27	26	25	24	23	22	21	20	19	18	17
Probe Depth 1 Date: 8/12/09	X	X	X	343	336	212	212	324	114	212	112	112	318	617	423	425
Probe Depth 2 Date: __/__/__																

Assessment of Oral hygiene and Gingival Inflammation

	Tooth # (Surface)	3 (B)	9 (B)	12 (B)	19 (L)	25 (L)	28 (L)	Total + 's
Date __/__/__	Plaque +/-							
	Bleeding +/-							
Date __/__/__	Plaque +/-							
	Bleeding +/-							

Substitutions:

If 3, 12,19 or 28 is missing, substitute the next most posterior tooth.

If 9 or 25 is missing, substitute the nearest incisor in the arch.

If all incisors are missing from the arch, substitute a cuspid.

Preliminary Clinical Findings Reviewed

Student Name/#: _____

Faculty Signature/#: _____

Final Findings Reviewed

Student Name/#: _____

Faculty Signature/#: _____

(a)

(b)   (L)

(c)   (R)

(d)

(e)

Glossary

A

Abrasion Wearing away of a structure, such as a gingiva or the teeth, through an abnormal mechanical process. Examples would be gingiva or tooth abrasions due to incorrect brushing.

Abutment (tooth) A tooth or implant used for support and retention of a crown or removable partial denture.

Abutment screw A screw that secures (holds) the abutment to the implant.

Accretions Accumulation of foreign materials on the teeth, such as dental plaque, materia alba, and calculus.

Acellular Without cells.

Acellular cementum Cementum that does not contain cementocytes.

Acquired pellicle a thin film derived from salivary glycoproteins which forms over the surface of a clean tooth when it is exposed to saliva.

Adjunctive in addition to (chap 3).

Adhesions molecules on bacteria that attach to the tooth.

Aerobic Utilizing and dependent on oxygen.

Air polishing A controlled stream of sodium bicarbonate used to remove extrinsic tooth stains and dental plaque.

Allograft See Graft, osseous.

Alloplastic See Graft, osseous.

Alveolar bone See Bone, alveolar.

Alveolar crest The most coronal part of the interproximal bone.

Alveolar mucosa See Mucosa, alveolar.

Alveolar process Compact and cancellous bone that surrounds and supports the roots of the teeth.

Anaerobic Non-oxygen utilizing. Oxygen is toxic to these organisms.

Anatomic factors Root size and shape and position of teeth in arch may influence the accumulation of biofilms.

Angle's classification of malocclusion A classification of different types of malocclusion based on the relationship of the anteroposterior relationship of the dental arches.

Class I (neutroocclusion): The mesiobuccal cusp of the maxillary first permanent molar occludes in the buccal groove of the mandibular first molar. Crowding has to be present.

Class II (distoocclusion): The mesiobuccal cusp of the maxillary first permanent molar is mesial to the mandibular first molar; the mandibular dental arch is posterior to the maxillary arch.

Class II, division 1: Labioversion of the maxillary incisors.

Class II, division 2: Linguoversion of the maxillary central incisors.

Class III (mesioocclusion): The mesiobuccal cusp of the maxillary first permanent molar is distal to the mandibular first molar; the mandibular dental arch is anterior to the maxillary arch.

Ankylosis Fusion of the tooth with the alveolar bone without an intervening periodontal ligament.

Antibiotic A soluble substance produced by microorganisms that has the capacity to inhibit the growth of or to kill other organisms.

Antibiotic prophylaxis See Prophylaxis.

Antibiotic resistence See resistance, antibiotics

Antibodies Serum proteins synthesized and released by plasma cells. Antibodies bind to and neutralize bacterial toxins.

Antigen A foreign substance (e.g., bacteria, bacterial toxins, and by-products) that elicits the formation of antibodies.

Antimicrobials Chemical agents that inhibit the growth of or kill a microorganism. The terms antimicrobial and anti-infective are used interchangeably.

Antiseptic An antimicrobial applied to the skin surface or oral mucosa that inhibits the growth and development of microorganisms.

Apical Refers to the apical or anatomic end of the root of a tooth.

Assessment Process of documentation.

Attachment apparatus Comprises the cementum, periodontal ligament, and alveolar and supporting bone.

Attachment level See Clinical attachment level (CAL).

Attachment loss, connective tissue (also referred to as clinical attachment loss) A pathologic process whereby the gingival collagen fibers become detached from the root surfaces with the concomitant apical migration of the apical aspect of the junctional epithelium along the root surface.

Attrition The wearing away of tooth structure by tooth-to-tooth normal or abnormal function.

Autograft See Graft, osseous.

Autoimmune disease Disease caused by the immunologic response against components of the body's own tissues.

Avascular Lacking in blood supply (e.g., tooth enamel, gingival epithelium, cementum).

B

Bacteremia Presence of bacteria in the bloodstream.

Bactericidal The ability of a drug or agent to kill bacteria.

Bacteriostatic Inhibiting the growth of bacteria.

Barrier membrane Material placed over a bone graft (in a periodontal defect) that keeps the bone graft at the site and prevents the growth of epithelial cells into the site.

Bass toothbrushing method See toothbrushing methods.

Bifurcation The anatomic area where roots of a two-rooted tooth separate.

Biodegradable Resorbable.

Biofilm, (plaque, oral, dental) Matrix-enclosed bacterial populations adherent to each other and/or to surfaces or interfaces.

Biologic width The combined height of the gingival connective tissue (1.07 mm) and the junctional epithelium (0.97 mm) present around teeth.

Biota, oral The bacteria and other microorganisms that normally inhabit a bodily organ or part (also called oral flora)

Bisphosphonate chemical that inhibits osteoclasts activity. Used in the treatment of osteoporosis.

Bleeding on probing Bleeding that occurs when the gingival crevice is probed.

Bone A hard type of connective tissue that contains collagen fibers, calcium phosphate, and hydroxyapatite.

Alveolar bone (also called alveolar bone proper): Compact bone that lines the tooth socket (alveolus).

Bundle bone: Alveolar bone with insertion of Sharpey's (principal) fibers.

Cancellous bone (spongy bone): Bone with trabeculae, located between the cortical plates and alveolar bone proper. It makes up the majority of a bone.

Compact bone: Bone that is hard and dense.

Cortical (plate) bone: Compact bone found on the facial and lingual aspects of the alveolar process.

Supporting bone: Surrounds and supports the alveolar bone proper. Is composed of the compact cortical plates of bone and cancellous trabecular bone.

Bone augmentation Correction of a bone defect or deficiency with the placement of a bone graft and/or bone replacement material.

Bone grafting A surgical procedure performed to reestablish bone volume. Placement of a bone graft or bone replacement material into an infrabony defect.

Bone grafts See Grafts, osseous

Bone loss

Horizontal bone loss: An equal amount of bone loss between two teeth.

Vertical bone loss (also called angular bone loss): Bone destruction that does not occur of the entire thickness of the alveolar process. Bone loss affects only a portion of bone surrounding the affected tooth. Examples include one-, two-, and three-wall bony defects. See Periodontal bony defect.

Bone resorption Bone loss.

Bone substitute materials Alternative bone grafting materials to allografts and autografts. Many of these alternatives use a variety of materials, including natural and synthetic polymers, ceramics, and composites.

Bovine (as in bovine bone) Pertaining to cattle (cows).

Broad-spectrum (antibiotic) Antibiotic that affects a wide range of bacteria, including both gram-negative and gram-positive microorganisms.

Bruxism The involuntary and unconscious grinding or clenching of teeth. It is usually triggered by emotional stress, anxiety, or occlusal irregularities and usually results in abnormal wear patterns on the teeth.

Bundle bone See Bone, bundle.

C

Calculus Calcified microbial plaque. It is not viable (living bacteria) and thus is a local contributing risk factor for periodontal diseases. Bacteria embed into the porous surface.

Cancellous bone See Bone, cancellous.

Cellular immunity Immune response coordinated by T-lymphocytes that targets and kills cells infected with microorganisms such as viruses, fungi and certain bacteria.

Cementocytes Cementoblasts from the periodontal ligament that lie close to the root and become surrounded by forming cementum.

Cementoenamel junction The area at which the enamel and cementum are united at the cervical region of the tooth.

Cementum Thin, calcified layer of connective tissue that covers the root of teeth.

Centric occlusion See Occlusion, centric.

Centric relation The most posterior or retruded position of the mandible to the maxilla from which lateral movements of the jaw can be made.

Cervical enamel projection Apical extension of the coronal enamel beyond the CEJ.

Charters' toothbrushing method See toothbrushing methods.

Chemotaxis The process by which cells (PMNs, macrophages) are attracted toward an inflamed area, often by certain substances, including bacterial products, proteins, and interleukins.

Chemotherapeutic agents Drugs used to treat various forms of bacterial diseases and cancers.

Chemotherapeutics The prevention or treatment of a disease by medical visit.

Chief complaint Statement describing the symptom or problem that is the reason for the dental/medical visit.

Cleft, gingival A vertical-shaped slit extending from and into the gingival margin, usually due to the start of pocket formation or improper flossing.

Clinical Pertaining to the signs, symptoms, and course of a condition or disease as observed by a clinician.

Clinical attachment level (CAL) Distance measured from the cementoenamel junction to the location of the tip of the periodontal probe at the most coronal level of the attached periodontal tissues (junctional epithelium).

More reliable marker for disease progression than probing depth measurements.

Clinical attachment loss See Attachment loss, connective tissue.

Clinical connective tissue attachment loss See attachment loss.

Codestructive Another factor besides the primary factor further contributes to destruction (e.g. some believe that occlusal trauma and periodontal inflammation may act as codestructive agents in periodontal disease.

Col A valleylike depression of the interdental gingiva that connects the facial and lingual papillae. It is just below the contact area of the tooth.

Collagen The most abundant protein of skin, bone, and other connective tissues. Synthesized by fibroblasts, osteoblasts, and odontoblasts.

Collagen fibers See Fibers, collagen.

Collagenase Belongs to a family of enzymes called matrix metalloproteinases, which are responsible for the normal turnover of connective tissue and destruction of host (body's) tissue (collagen). Produced and secreted by bacteria and host cells including PMNs and fibroblasts. Collagenase produced and secreted by PMNs is responsible for the host tissue destruction. Collagenase produced and secreted by fibroblasts is responsible for the normal remodeling and turnover of collagen.

Community periodontal index of treatment needs (CPITN) An index used in population studies of periodontal disease designed by the World Health Organization to assess periodontal treatment needs.

Compact bone See Bone, compact.

Complement A sequence of serum proteins that, when activated, attempt to destroy a foreign substance.

Complement system See complement.

Compliance The patient's ability to adhere to the appointment schedule and oral home self-care instructions given by the dental hygienist or dentist.

Computed tomographic (CT) Scan Digitized tomography that results in an enhanced image that is much easier to read than a plane (conventional) tomogram. It measures the amount of energy transmission through an object. It produces a cross-sectional image of a slice of tissue (e.g., bone). Many slices are made of a given edentulous site.

Connective tissue attachment Mechanism of attachment of the connective tissue (gingival fibers) to the tooth or implant surface.

Continuing care See Periodontal maintenance.

Contributing factor Does not initiate the disease process or act independently as an etiologic agent. Helps to allow a condition to become established and/or progress.

Contributory Helping to bring about a result.

Controlled Release delivery device (chap 20) an active agent dispersed. In a biodegradable matrix that slowly is released from that matrix (e.g., Atridox, Arestin, and PerioChip).

Conventional radiograph X-rays taken with films.

Coronal Toward the crown of a tooth.

Cortical bone See Bone, cortical.

Crater Interdental depressions in the gingiva or bone.

C-reactive protein (CRP) A blood marker for inflammation.

Crestal Of or pertaining to the crest or most coronal portion of the alveolar bone.

Curets

> Area-specific curets (also called Gracey curets): Designed to be used on specific tooth surfaces of different teeth. Their design includes one cutting edge per end with a rounded back and toe.

> Universal curets: Designed to be used on the mesial and distal surfaces of teeth without changing the instrument. Their design includes two cutting edges per end with a rounded back and toe.

Curettage, gingival Removal of the ulcerated soft tissue pocket wall.

Cytokines Proteins produced and secreted by host cells including macrophages and lymphocytes. These proteins signal and modify the behavior or actions of these cells and other cells. Examples are the interleukins, such as interleukin-1 (IL-1), which is responsible for bone destruction.

Cytoxic The ability to kill cells, including human cells.

D

Debridement The removal of inflamed, devitalized, or contaminated tissue or foreign material from or adjacent to a lesion.

Dehiscence Loss of radicular bone on a root or implant extending from the crest and proceeding apically.

Dental hygiene diagnosis an analysis of the cause and nature of the periodontal problem.

Dental calculus Calcified plaque.

Dental charting provides a graphic description of the conditions in a patient's mouth, including caries and probing depths.

Dental implant An artificial (usually titanium metal) post that substitutes for a tooth root and to which a prosthesis is attached.

Dental/medical history See Endosseous implant account of a patient's past and present state of health.

Dental plaque Accumulations of bacteria and other microorganisms on tooth surfaces in the area of the sulcus or pocket. Referred to as plaque (dental) biofilm.

Dentifrice A powder, paste, or gel used in conjunction with a toothbrush to aid in the removal of plaque, materia alba, and stain from teeth.

Dentinal hypersensitivity The short, exaggerated, painful response elicited when exposed dentin is subjected to certain thermal, mechanical, or chemical stimuli.

Dentogingival unit Composed of two parts, the gingival connective tissue attachment and the junctional epithelium.

Deplaquing The removal of subgingival dental plaque after the completion of periodontal debridement. It is performed at the reevaluation/supportive periodontal therapy appointments.

Desensitization Reducing or eliminating dentin sensitivity.

Diagnosis

> Dental diagnosis: Refers to the identification and naming of a disease.

> Dental hygiene diagnosis: Identifies certain problems or the patient's response to the disease process that can be treated by a dental hygienist.

Diastema A space between two adjacent teeth in the same dental arch.

Digital imaging X-ray images that use a sensor to transmit the image directly to a computer via a cable link. X-ray image appears on a monitor and can be manipulated electronically to change contrast, orientation, resolution, and size of the image.

Direct digital radiography direct conversion of transmitted x-rays into a digital image.

Disease A process characterized usually by at least two of these criteria: a recognized etiologic agent (or agents), an identifiable group of signs and symptoms, and consistent anatomic alterations.

Disease activity See Periodontal disease activity.

Disease severity See Periodontal disease severity.

Documentation the recording in a permanent format of information derived from activities.

Donor site Area in the mouth or body from which a graft (bone or soft tissue) is harvested.

Drifting Tooth migration as a result of loss of proximal contact of adjacent teeth in a healthy periodontium.

E

Edema An abnormal swelling caused by an accumulation of fluid in a tissue or part.

Edentulous Without teeth.

Enamel matrix derivative (EMD) Protein obtained from amelogenin (enamel matrix precurser of enamel) of the developing tooth. Product called Emdogain.® Indicated for bone grafting.

Endosseous implant Type of implant placed in a hole (osteotomy) drilled in the bone. See Implant, endosseous.

Embrasure The spaces that widen out from the proximal contact area. Each interdental space has four embrasures: facial embrasure, lingual embrasure, an occlusal or incisal embrasure, and a gingival embrasure. An open gingival embrasure is seen frequently in patients with periodontal disease.

Endotoxins Lipooligosaccharide (lipid) complexes formed by gram-negative bacteria. When the bacteria die and break apart (lysis), the endotoxin is released from the cell wall of the bacteria and is capable of having a toxic or harmful effect on the host tissue.

Enzyme A protein substance formed by living cells that acts to speed up metabolic processes or chemical reaction.

Epidemiology The study of the distribution and determinants of illnesses and their associated factors in the human population.

Epithelial ridges Ridgelike projections of epithelium into the underlying lamina propria.

Epithelium (oral) The tissue that lines the intraoral surfaces. It extends into the gingival crevice and adheres to the tooth at the base of the gingival crevice.

Erosion Chemical wearing away of a structure, such as a tooth.

Erythema (erythematous) Redness of the mucous membranes due to inflammation.

Evaluation Judging the value of material based on personal opinions.

Exposure time duration of the process of exposure to radiation.

Extent The number or percent of diseased teeth or sites in an individual.

Extrusion (extrude) Overruption of a tooth from its normal occlusal position in the dental arch.

Exudate A fluid substance formed within tissues as a result of inflammation. It consists of polymorphonuclear leukocytes, degenerated tissues, dead cells, bacteria, and tissue fluid.

F

Facial Pertaining to the face. The facial surfaces of the teeth are called buccal and labial.

Failed implant A dental implant that is mobile; lost failing implant osseointegration. A dental implant that is progressively losing bone around it.

Fenestration Root or implant surface is denuded (loss) of bone but the crestal bone is intact.

Fiber A filament or thread. In periodontics, the term usually refers to collagenous or connective tissue fibers.

Collagen fibers: White fibers composed of collagen. Found within connective tissue of the gingiva and periodontal ligament arranged in bundles or haphazardly distributed. Characterized by its hydroxyproline and hydroxylysine content.

Gingival fibers: (also called gingival connective tissue or supracrestal fiber apparatus) Fibers composed primarily of collagen that radiate from the cementum or bone into the lamina propria. Includes alveogingival, circular, dentogingival, dentoperiosteal, and transseptal.

periodontal ligament fibers: Collagen fibers of the periodontal ligament. Includes alveolar crest, apical, horizontal, interradicular, and oblique.

Fibroblast A cell found within connective tissue that synthesizes collagen and ground substance of connective tissue.

Fibrotic Tissue that is in a state of repair; tissue is hard and not resilient or spongy.

Filtration The use of absorbers for the selective reduction in intensity of radiation of certain wavelengths from a primary X-ray beam.

Flap A part of tissue (gingiva) separated from the underlying tissues except at its base.

Fluorosis, dental Enamel hypoplasia due to the ingestion of water containing excessive amounts of fluoride.

Food impaction The forceful wedging of food into the interproximal space by chewing pressure or tongue or cheek pressure.

Free gingival graft See Graft.

Fremitus Vibrational movement of the tooth under occlusal function.

Frenum A narrow band of alveolar mucosa radiates from a fixed part to a movable part and limits movement of that part. Example: Frenum runs from the gingiva to the lip, cheek, or under the tongue.

Frequency The number of times per second the insert tip moves back and forth during one cycle.

Full-mouth survey The production of the minimal number of radiographic examinations necessary for a radiographic interpretation.

Furcation (also called furca) Anatomic area on multirooted teeth where the root base divides.

Furcation involvement (invasion) Pathologic loss of bone in the furcation of a multirooted tooth.

G

Gain in clinical attachment (also referred to as gain in periodontal attachment) A decrease in probing depths after periodontal therapy due to an increase in resistance of the periodontal probe into the tissue and maybe gingival recession. The inflamed tissue is replaced by firm collagen fibers.

Genetics Inheritance or transmission of a disease or condition from a parent to a child.

Gingiva A part of the masticatory mucosa that is attached to the teeth and alveolar process.

> Attached gingiva: The portion of the gingiva that is firm, dense, and tightly bound down to the underlying periosteum, tooth, and bone.

> Free (marginal) gingiva: The portion of the gingiva that is unattached and forms the wall of the gingival crevice in health. It is continuous with the attached gingiva.

Gingival abscess A localized collection of pus confined to the gingival tissue.

Gingival assessment Evaluation of the gingiva for inflammation.

Gingival crevice A shallow opening between the free gingiva and the enamel or cementum. In gingival health it is called the gingival sulcus and in disease a pocket.

Gingival crevicular fluid Fluid originating in the gingival connective tissue that seeps through the sulcular and junctional epithelium. Flow increases in the presence of inflammation.

Gingival pocket (pseudopocket) See Pocket, gingival.

Gingival recession Apical migration of the marginal gingiva resulting in exposure of the root surface to the oral environment.

Gingival sulcus Space between the tooth and the marginal gingiva in gingival health. If bleeding is present, it is not a sulcus but a pocket.

Gingivitis Inflammation of the gingiva without involvement of the underlying bone or periodontal attachment. The following are gingival diseases listed in the new classification of periodontal diseases (American Academy of Periodontology, 1999):

> Drug-influenced gingivitis: Gingivitis or gingival enlargement caused by drugs (e.g., Ca channel blockers, phenytoin, cyclosporine, and oral contraceptives).

> Plaque-associated gingivitis: Gingivitis caused by dental plaque alone.

> Pregnancy-associated gingivitis: Hormonally influenced inflammation and enlargement of the gingiva during pregnancy.

> Puberty-associated gingivitis: Hormonally influenced inflammation of the gingiva during puberty.

Graft, osseous (bone)

> Allograft (allogenic graft): Bone taken from human beings (cadavers) other than the patient. Bone is bought from tissue banks. Three types: freeze-dried bone allograft (FDBA); demineralized freeze-dried bone allograft (DFDBA), and frozen.

> Alloplast (alloplastic graft): Synthetic or natural bone (inorganic) substitutes.

> Autograft: Tissue such as bone (osseous material; organic) taken from the patient's mouth or extraoral area such as the hip.

Graft, soft tissue

> Connective tissue graft: Connective tissue (donor) taken from underneath the epithelium and placed in a prepared recipient bed for the purposes of root coverage and increasing the amount of attached gingiva.

> Free gingival graft: Gingiva taken from an area in the patient's mouth, usually the palate (donor), and placed in a prepared recipient bed primarily to increase the amount of attached gingiva.

Grinding See Bruxism.

Growth factors A substance that affects the growth of a cell or an organism.

Guided bone regeneration (GBR) Bone regeneration (surgical) procedure using barrier membrane to regenerate bone.

Guided tissue regeneration (GTR) Periodontal procedures performed in an attempt at regeneration. Barrier techniques are used with materials that exclude the junctional epithelium from the wound site in an attempt to allow periodontal ligament cells to populate the wound site.

H

Halitosis Bad breath.

Hemostasis Control of and stopping bleeding.

Histopathogenesis Pathologic (disease) changes within the periodontal structures at a microscopic level.

Host Referring to the body or self.

Host cells Cells normally present in the body (e.g., polymorphonuclear leukocytes [PMNs] macrophages, fibroblasts).

Host-derived enzymes Enzymes produced and secreted by cells in the human body such as neutrophils (PMNs) or fibroblasts.

Host response How the body responds to an implanted device or material.

Humoral immunity Branch of the immune-system that depends on antibodies.

Hypertropy Increase in bulk of a part or organ not due to tumor formation.

I

Iatrogenic Factor situation caused by dental or medical treatment; abnormal condition induced by a clinician.

Immune response Mechanisms used by the body as protection against environmental agents that are foreign to the body.

Immune system Components include the lymph nodes, thymus, spleen, and bone marrow.

Immunity The organism's (or body's) capacity for successfully resisting the actions of harmful foreign substances or pathogenic (disease-producing) microorganisms such as bacteria or viruses.

Immunodeficiency A deficiency in the immune system caused by an upset in the number of lymphocytes.

Immunoglobulins Group of large glycoproteins that are secreted by plasma cells and function as antibodies in the immune system. (E.g. IgA, IgG, IgM)

Implant, endosseous Dental implant placed within bone.

Implementation Carrying out a plan for doing something (e.g. developing a treatment plan and treating a patient according to the treatment plan.)

Incidence The rate of new occurrence of the disease in a population over a given period of time.

Index (plural: Indices) A screening tool designed to quantify and simplify the disease assessment in population surveys. Examples include plaque, debris, calculus, and periodontal destruction.

Infection Pathogenic invasion of the body and the body's response to these organisms.

Infective endocarditis Inflammation of the inner lining of the heart caused by a microbial infection.

Inflammation Protective response elicited by injury or destruction of tissues that attempts to destroy or wall off the injurious agent and tissue. It is also the cellular and vascular tissue reaction that occurs when tissue is injured.

Inflammatory cells Cells involved in the inflammatory response of tissues to injury or infection (e.g., PMNs, macrophages, mast cells).

Inflammatory periodontal diseases A group of inflammatory diseases of the periodontium including gingivitis and periodontitis.

Inflammatory process A localized protective reaction of tissue to irritation, injection or injury.

Informed consent A written agreement by patients to voluntarily have treatment performed on them or to participate in a study.

Infrabony defect See Periodontal bony defects.

Interdental Between two adjacent teeth.

Interdental septum That part of the alveolar process extending between adjacent teeth.

Interproximal Pertaining to the area between two adjacent teeth. See Interdental.

Interradicular That part of the alveolar process between the roots of a multirooted tooth (e.g., molars, premolar).

Interview process a face-to-face meeting with the patient for questions and answers.

J

Junctional epithelium Epithelium that is located at the base of the gingival crevice.

K

Keratin A protein that is the main component of keratinized epithelium synthesized by keratinocytes.

Keratinocyte A cell found in the epithelium (a type of epithelial cell) that forms keratin.

L

Lamina dura A layer of compact bone forming the wall of a tooth alveolus (alveolar bone). In a radiograph, it appears as a thin radiopaque line separated from the tooth by the radiolucent image of the periodontal ligament space.

Lamina propria The gingival connective tissue layer under the epithelium.

Lipooligosaccharide Another name is endotoxin. A component of gram-negative bacteria which is released upon destruction of the bacterial cell, can cause tissue and bone destruction.

Load External mechanical force applied to a tooth, implant, or prosthesis.

Lymphadenopathy Lymph nodes that are abnormal in size, consistency, or number.

Lymph nodes Small, round, or oval organs containing lymphocytes. Found in groups or chains in certain regions, often associated with large blood vessels.

Lymphocyte A type of white blood cell involved in the immune response. There are two types of lymphocytes: T cells and B cells.

M

Macrophage A large tissue cell responsible for removing damaged tissue, cells, and bacteria through phagocytosis. Increase in number in chronic inflammation.

Malocclusion Deviation from the acceptable relationship of opposing teeth. See Angle's classification of malocclusion.

Marginal Pertaining to the margin or edge.

Marginal ridge A ridge or elevation of enamel that is on the border of the occlusal surface of a tooth.

Mast cell A large tissue cell that releases inflammatory substances or mediators when damaged.

Masticatory (mastication) The process of chewing food.

Microbiota See Biota, oral.

Microflora Bacteria living in a part of the body (e.g., the mouth, intestines, nose). See also Biota, oral.

Microorganisms Organisms of microscopic size (e.g. bacteria, yeasts, simple fungi).

Migration, pathologic The movement of a tooth out of its natural position, usually as a result of advanced periodontal disease.

Mobility, tooth The degree of looseness of a tooth beyond physiologic movement. Tooth movement away from its normal position in a buccal/lingual or apical direction when slight pressure is applied.

Monitoring The act of listening or watching.

Mucogingival involvement (defect) A discrepancy in the relationship between the gingival margin and the mucogingival junction. Usually, there is minimal to no attached gingiva.

Mucogingival junction Demarcation between the attached gingiva and alveolar mucosa.

Mucosa A mucous membrane.

> Alveolar mucosa: Mucosa covering part of the alveolar process and continuing into the vestibule and floor of the mouth. It is movable and loosely attached to the underlying periosteum.
>
> Masticatory mucosa: Mucosa of the gingiva and hard palate.

Murmur A sound produced within the heart at one of its orifices.

N

National Health and Nutrition Examination Survey (NHANES I) A national survey of adults from 1960 to 1962.

National Health and Nutrition Examination Survey (NHANES III) This is the seventh in a series, beginning in 1960, of national examination surveys of the U.S. population conducted by the National Center for Health Statistics in collaboration with the National Institute for Dental Research (NIDR). The survey was designed to collect data representative of the total U.S. civilian, non-institutionalized population age 12 months and older.

National Institute of Dental Research (NIDR) Survey A national survey of employed adults between 18 and 64 years of age conducted by the National Institute of Dental Research. It was named the National Survey of Oral Health of U.S. Adults 1985–1986. More than 15,000 people were examined, representing over 100 million working adults in the United States.

Necrotizing periodontal diseases Formerly known as acute necrotizing ulcerative gingivitis (ANUG). Since acute is a clinical descriptive term, it should not be used as a diagnostic classification. Thus the correct term is necrotizing ulcerative gingivitis. In the new classification, NUG is a type of necrotizing periodontal disease. It is an inflammation of the gingiva characterized by necrosis of the gingival margin and interdental papillae. Included in this classification is necrotizing ulcerative periodontitis (NUP), which is characterized by necrosis of gingival tissues, periodontal ligament, and alveolar bone.

Necrotizing ulcerative gingivitis An infection of the gingiva characterized by punched ont or cratered papillae, with bleeding and pain.

Necrotizing ulcerative periodontitis An infection characterized by necrosis of the gingival periodontal ligament and alveolar bone.

Neutrophil See Polymorphonuclear leukocyte.

Nitrogenous Compounds or substance containing nitrogen.

Nonmetallic materials Non-stainless steel e.g., plastic.

Non-nitrogenous compounds or substances that do not contain nitrogen.

O

Objective Based on facts; not affected by personal feelings.

Objective data Signs or observations made by the clinician that can be verified by another person.

Obligate Able to survive only in a specific environment (e.g., an obligate anaerobe is only able to live in a nonoxygen environment).

Occlusal adjustment (also called selective grinding or occlusal equilibration) Reshaping the occlusal or incisal surfaces of teeth by grinding to create harmonious contact relationships between the upper and lower teeth.

Occlusal therapy A treatment to establish and maintain a stable, comfortable and functional occlusion.

Occlusal trauma Injury to the attachment apparatus as a result of excessive occlusal forces.

> Primary occlusal trauma: Excessive occlusal forces placed on a healthy periodontium that produces changes in the periodontal tissues. Examples include placement of a "high" restoration and orthodontic movement of teeth.

> Secondary occlusal trauma: Normal forces of mastication on a periodontium with bone loss (periodontitis) that produce changes in the periodontal tissues.

Occlusion Contact of opposing teeth (maxillary and mandibular teeth); centric occlusion: maximum intercuspation of maxillary and mandibular teeth.

Open bite Anterior or posterior teeth do not occlude with the opposing teeth.

Operculum gingival flap overlying the crown of an erupting tooth.

Opsonins a molecule that acts as a binding enhancer for phagocytosis (e.g. complement).

Oral biofilms See biofilms.

Oral cancer a cancer in the oral cavity, on lips and the oropharynx (part of throat at back of the mouth)

Oral epitheluim Epithelium covering oral mucous membranes.

Oral hygiene self-care Removal of dental plaque with brushes, dental floss, and other oral aids.

Oral prophylaxis See Prophylaxis.

Osseointegration The biologic phenomenon by which bone grows up to and contacts the surface of implants, thereby anchoring them to the jaw bone.

Osseous Referring to bone.

Ostectomy Surgical removal of supporting bone.

Osteoblast A cell that forms bone.

Osteoclast A cell that resorbs bone.

Osteoconduction Bone growth by laying down of form from the surrounding bone. Bone material acts as a scaffolding along which bone will be laid down.

Osteointegration New bone growth from osteoprogenitor cells.

Osteonecrosis of the jaw (ONJ) A severe bone disease causing necrosis of the jaws, especially the mandible. Usually associated with bisphosphonate usage.

Osteoplasty Surgical reshaping or removal of nonsupporting bone.

Outcome measure The recording of activity or effort that can be expressed in a quantitative or qualitative manner (assessing therapy completed). (e.g. the outcome measure of initial therapy is periodontal probing and oral hygiene assessment.

Overbite Vertical overlap of the upper incisor teeth over the lower incisor teeth.

Overdenture A removable partial or complete denture that is supported by implants or implant/tissue.

Overjet Horizontal projection of the upper teeth beyond the lower teeth.

P

Panoramic film A type of conventional radiograph showing the entire area of the mandible and maxilla.

Papillary Pertaining to the interdental papillae.

Parafunctional habit A habit characterized by abnormal (out of the normal range) function (e.g., bruxism, pencil chewing, nail biting).

Paralleling technique A technique in intra-oral radiographs in which the film is positioned parallel to the long axis of the teeth.

Passive eruption Physiologic process with recession of the gingiva from the enamel apically toward the cementoenamel junction.

Pathogenic Disease-producing.

Pathologic mobility Horizontal or vertical displacement of a tooth beyond its physiologic movement.

Patient adherence Term used to describe how well a patient is sticking to their hygiene program; compliance.

Patient education The process of informing a patient about a health (dental) matter.

Periapical film A type of conventional radiograph that shows the entire tooth, including the area around the root apex.

Periapical pathology Disease occurring around the apex of a tooth.

Pericoronitis (also termed pericoronal abscess) Inflammation of the operculum or tissue flap over a partially eurupted tooth, especially a third molar.

Peri-implant Around a dental implant.

Peri-implant disease A descriptive term used to describe non-specific inflammation around the dental implant. There are two types of peri-implant disease: Peri-implantitis which is inflammation with loss of bone surrounding a functioning implant. Peri-implantitis may show the following symptoms; bleeding on probing, increased probing pocket depth, mobility, suppuration and pain. Peri-implant mucositis which is inflammation localized to the soft tissues and not involving bone is reversible with treatment.

Peri-implantitis Inflammation of the gingival tissues around an implant and bone loss.

Perimucosal seal Tissue tension provided by the circular fibers between the gingiva and the implant.

Periocoronal abscess See pericoronitis.

Periodontal Occurring around a tooth.

Periodontal abscess

    Abscess, periodontal (also called lateral periodontal abscess) Localized accumulation of pus in periodontal tissues formed by the disintegration of tissue.

Periodontal assessment Steps followed to evaluate periodontal tissues.

Periodontal bony defects A deviation from the normal form or contour of bone due to periodontal disease.

    Crater (interproximal crater): A two-wall infrabony defect (facial and lingual bony walls remain).

    Hemiseptum defect: The remaining interdental bone septum where the mesial or distal part has been destroyed, with one bony wall remaining (half of a septum).

    Infrabony defect: A general term to describe any periodontal bony defect associated with vertical (angular) bone loss. These defects are named according to the number of bony walls remaining in the interproximal area that surround the pocket (e.g., one-wall, two-wall, and three-wall).

    Intrabony defect: A type of three-wall defect with three bony walls remaining. The defect may or may not be totally lined by cortical bone and may have cancellous bone behind. Not all three-wall defects are intrabony.

Periodontal debridement The removal of a foreign material (e.g., plaque, calculus) or dead tissue from the crown, root surface, pocket space, pocket wall, and bone surface.

Periodontal diseases A bacterial infection affecting the gingiva (gingivitis) and attaching fibers and bone (periodontitis)

Periodontal disease activity (PDA) The ongoing loss of connective tissue attachment and bone at a particular point in time (e.g., at the clinical examination appointment). It is difficult to determine disease activity. A 2 to 3 mm change in clinical attachment level must occur before a site can be labeled disease-active.

Periodontal disease severity The total periodontal destruction and healing that occur prior to the clinical examination. Disease severity is determined after the periodontal assessment (visual, periodontal probing, radiographs) is completed. Severity can be classified as mild, moderate, or severe.

Periodontal ligament (fibers) The connective tissue that surrounds the root surface of the tooth and attaches it to the alveolar bone.

Periodontal maintenance Also referred to as recare, or continuing care. An extension of periodontal therapy.

Procedures performed at selected intervals to assist the periodontal patient in maintaining oral health.

Periodontal pathogens   Bacteria that cause periodontal disease.

Periodontal pocket   See Pocket, periodontal.

Periodontal probing   Measures the location where physical resistance of the probe is met by the junctional epithelial attachment to the tooth.

Periodontal regeneration   Restoring lost supporting tissue around the tooth, including new Alveolar bone, cementum, and periodontal ligament fibers.

Periodontal therapy   Treatment of the periodontal lesion.

Periodontics   The specialty of dentistry dealing with the prevention, diagnosis, and treatment of diseases of the tissues that surround the teeth.

Periodontist   A dental practitioner who practices periodontics.

Periodontitis   Inflammation of the supporting tissues of teeth where there is connective tissue attachment loss and alveolar and supporting bone loss. The following is a classification system developed by the American Academy of Periodontology (1999):

Aggressive periodontitis: Formerly known as early-onset periodontitis (e.g., juvenile periodontitis, prepubertal periodontitis, and rapidly progressive periodontitis). Except for the presence of periodontitis, patients are otherwise clinically healthy. There is rapid attachment loss and bone destruction. Patients have defects in host defense. Includes prepubesent children who have periodontal destruction without any modifying systemic conditions. The following specific features are identified:

Generalized aggressive periodontitis: Formerly known as generalized juvenile periodontitis. Usually affects persons under 30 years of age, but patients may be older. Generalized interproximal attachment loss affecting at least three permanent teeth other than first molars and incisors.

Localized aggressive periodontitis: Formerly known as localized juvenile periodontitis (LJP). Circumpubertal onset. Primarily affects the first permanent incisors and first molars. Attachment loss may progress at a rate three to five times faster than chronic periodontitis. These patients are characterized by a lack of clinical signs of inflammation, harbor Actinobacillus actinomycetecomitans in their microflora, and display an altered immune response.

Chronic periodontitis: Formerly known as adult periodontitis. A form of periodontitis that usually is prevalent in adults but can occur in children and adolescents (formerly known as prepubertal periodontitis). The amount of periodontal destruction is consistent with the presence of local factors. Bone resorption usually progresses slowly.

Necrotizing periodontal diseases: Replaces necrotizing ulcerative gingivitis (NUG) and necrotizing ulcerative periodontitis (NUP). A form of periodontitis seen in the HIV/AIDS patient. (See necrotized periodontal diseases)

Refractory periodontitis: Patients who do not respond to conventional periodontal therapy treatment. It is not considered a single disease entity because it can occur in all forms of periodontitis.

Periodontium   Comprises the periodontal tissues that support and surround the teeth, including the gingiva, cementum, periodontal ligament, and alveolar and supporting bone.

Periodontology   The scientific study of the periodontal structures in health and disease.

Periosteum   Connective tissue covering the outer surface of bone.

Phagocytosis   The process of destroying bacteria by devouring and digesting them by phagocytic cells such as polymorphonuclear leukocytes and macrophages.

Pharmacokinetics   What the body does to a drug (e.g., absorption, distribution, metabolism, and elimination).

Phase-contrast microscopy   A method of using a microscope through which the shape, size, and mobility of bacteria can be viewed.

Phenytoin   An anticonvulsant drug that can cause gingival enlargement.

Plaque-Associated gingivitis   See Gingivitis.

Pocket

Gingival pocket: A deepening of the gingival crevice due to the coronal migration of the gingival margin without apical migration of the junctional epithelium (loss of attachment) and bone loss. Examples: drug-influenced gingival enlargement, inflammation of the gingiva. Also called a pseudopocket.

Periodontal pocket: A pathologic deepening of the gingival sulcus characterized by apical migration of the junctional epithelium and alveolar bone loss. Two types of periodontal pockets: infrabony and suprabony.

Infrabony pocket: A periodontal pocket that extends apical to the adjacent alveolar crest or into an infrabony defect (a defect with a vertical pattern of bone loss). There is apical migration of the junctional epithelium and bone loss; the base of the pocket is apical to the crest of alveolar bone.

Suprabony pocket: A periodontal pocket that extends coronal to the alveolar crest or into a suprabony defect with a horizontal pattern of bone loss. The base of the pocket is coronal to the crest of alveolar bone.

Polishing The removal of acquired pellicle, bacterial plaque, and stain from the external tooth surface through mechanical means and an abrasive agent.

Polymorponuclear leukocyte (PMN) The major mobile phagocytic white blood cell involved in engulfing, killing, and digesting microorganisms. The first cell to migrate to the acute inflammatory site. Impairment in their function is related to the pathogenesis of aggressive periodontitis.

Population survey A statistical term used to evaluate representative samples of individuals within a study population to assess the true risk for disease and quantify how many individuals are or will be affected by disease.

Prevalence The proportion of individuals in a population having periodontal disease or the number of individuals expected to have periodontal disease in a specific time.

Primary herpetic gingivostomatitis An initial oral infection caused by herpes simplex type 1 in young children. They are at risk for developing extensive oropharyngeal vesicular eruptions when first infected with the virus.

Primary occlusal trauma See Occlusal trauma, primary.

Primary prevention Action performed to preclude or prevent the development of a disease. (e.g., use of fluorides to prevent caries)

Probing See Periodontal probing.

Probing depth The distance from the soft tissue (gingiva or alveolar mucosa) margin to the tip of the periodontal probe. The health of the attachment apparatus can affect the measurement.

Problem-based in reference to learning. Learning that is driven by a question or problem and uses various methods of inquiry research to address the question or problem.

Prognosis A prediction or forecast of the course and outcome of a disease.

Prophylaxis Prevention of disease.

Antibiotic prophylaxis: Antibiotic coverage necessary before invasive dental procedures that cause bleeding to prevent a bacteremia that ultimately could cause infective endocarditis or serious infections.

Oral prophylaxis: The removal of plaque, calculus, and stains from the exposed and unexposed surfaces of the teeth by scaling and polishing as a preventive measure for the control of local irritational factors.

Proximal Surface of a tooth next to another tooth.

Pseudocleft Slit or fissure of the gingiva associated with severe gingival inflammation or certain medications causing the papillae to enlarge and approach each other and not due to pocket formation.

Pseudopocket See Pocket, gingival or Pocket, pseudo.

Pus See Suppuration.

R

Radicular Pertaining to the root.

Recession See Gingival recession.

Recurrent When signs of disease return.

Reevaluation Pertaining to evaluating the results of therapy a second time (e.g., evaluating the results of initial or surgical therapy).

Regeneration, periodontal Formation of new alveolar and supporting bone, cementum, and periodontal ligament on a previously diseased root surface.

Resistance, antibiotic An antimicrobial agent no longer is effective in killing or inhibiting growth of microorganisms.

Rete pegs See Epithelial ridges.

Retreatment (chap 28) After active periodontal therapy more treatment is needed to get the disease under control.

Rheumatic heart disease A disease of the heart resulting from rheumatic fever, chiefly manifested by abnormalities of the valves.

Risk assessment Pertaining to periodontal risk assessment. Is a test tool to help you understand whether you are at a risk for developing a periodontal disease.

Risk factors Characteristics that have been shown to directly cause periodontal disease (e.g., dental plaque, diabetes mellitus, tobacco smoking).

Risk indicators Behavioral and socioeconomic characteristics that are associated with periodontal diseases but are not considered to cause the disease (e.g., aging). Risk factors are not causal – just puts an individual more at risk.

Root planing A treatment procedure designed to remove cementum or surface dentin that is rough, impregnated with calculus, or contaminated with toxins or microorganisms.

S

Saccharolytic Bacteria that can break down a sugar molecule.

Scaler A periodontal instrument that is designed to scale primarily supragingival tooth surfaces.

  Sonic: Produces mechanical vibrations by means of air pressure rather than electrical energy. The operating frequency is between 3,000 and 8,000 cycles per second.

  Ultrasonic: Devices operating at frequencies between 18,000 and 50,000 cycles per second. They use electrical energy to produce mechanical vibrations that will remove calculus.

  Magnetostrictive ultrasonic: Produces mechanical movement using a low-voltage magnetic signal. The operating frequency is between 18,000 and 45,000 cycles per second. The handpiece contains coils that activate the interchangeable inserts, causing them to vibrate. The working ends can be used on all sides, providing better adaptation to the tooth surfaces.

  Piezoelectric ultrasonic: Produces mechanical movement using a high-voltage magnetic signal. The operating frequency is between 25,000 and 50,000 cycles per second. Only two sides of the working end are adapted to the tooth surface.

Scaling The removal of dental plaque, calculus, and stains from the crown and root surfaces.

Screening A single examination to separate periodontally healthy from diseased patients and to determine the patient's dental needs. It does not make a specific dental hygiene diagnosis or tell the type of treatment to be given. It simply requires probing depth measurements and conventional radiographs.

Secondary occlusal trauma See Occlusal trauma, secondary.

Secondary prevention Activities are aimed at early disease detection, thereby increasing opportunities for interventions to prevent progression of the disease and development of symptoms (e.g., removal of all calculus and dental biofilms while performing root debridement).

Selective grinding See Occlusal adjustment.

Severity Degree of disease involvement, quantifying the amount of attachment loss or probing depth. May be expressed as mild or slight, moderate, and severe.

Sign Any abnormality indicative of disease, discoverable by the clinician at the evaluation of a patient.

Single-stage implant An implant placed in a one-stage surgery.

Smoking cessation A means to quit smoking.

Soft tissue healing Natural process by which the body repairs itself after periodontal debridement or surgery.

Sonic See Scaler, sonic.

Stem cells Cells from which all the blood cells "stem" or come.

Stillman's toothbrushing method See toothbrushing methods.

Stippling The "orange peel" appearance (depressions) on the attached gingiva. Stippling is not present on the free gingiva.

Subgingival (submarginal) Beneath the gingiva or gingival margin; into the crevice.

Subgingival debridement Other term: subgingival scaling. Removal of plaque and calculus apical to the gingival margin.

Subjective As described in an individual's words or opinions rather than facts.

Subjective data Those facts that are observable and measurable by the clinician. Personal feeling entering into the testing method or result analysis (e.g., patient's description of pain).

Substantivity Ability of a substance to absorb or bind to a surface such as the tooth root, tissues, bacterial plaque, or enamel and slowly released over time in its active form.

Sulcular epithelium Epithelium that lines the gingival crevice.

Sulcus See Gingival sulcus.

Supporting bone See Bone, supporting.

Suppuration The formation of pus. An inflammatory or purulent exudate formed within the tissues. It consists of neutrophils, bacteria, degenerated and liquefied cells, and tissue fluids that form within the tissues in disease and escape through the ulcerated pocket epithelium into the oral cavity.

Supragingival Coronal (above) to the free gingival margin.

Supragingival debridement Other term: supragingival scaling. Removal of plaque and calculus coronal to the gingival margin.

Surface texture The tactile quality of a material or tissue; the arrangement of parts of the tissue as it affects the appearance or feel of the surface.

Surgery The act and art of treating injuries or disease by manual operations.

   Mucogingival surgery: Periodontal surgery involving the soft tissue (gingival) aspects such as root coverage or increasing the height and width of the alveolar ridge.

   Osseous surgery: Periodontal surgery involving the addition or resection (removal) of bone.

Symptom A departure from the normal in function, appearance, or sensation experienced by a patient. A subjective sign.

Syndrome The aggregate of signs and symptoms associated with any morbid process and constituting together the picture of the disease.

Systemic Affecting or pertaining to the whole body.

Systemic disease A disease that affects the entire body instead of a specific organ.

Systemic drug delivery Administration of a drug by mouth (oral) or parenterally (e.g., intravenous, intramuscular, subcutaneous).

T

Temporomandibular joint The connecting sliding hinge mechanism between the mandible (lower jaw) and the base of the skull (temporal bone).

Therapeutic levels (of a drug) Concentration of a drug in body fluids that causes a pharmacologic effect.

Toothbrushing methods

   Bass bristles of toothbrush are placed at a 45-degree angle into the gingival sulcus and a vibratory motion in used. When using a modified version the bristles are moved down toward the occlusal/incisal part of the tooth. The occlusal surfaces of the teeth are brushed with a back and forth motion.

   Charters' bristles of toothbrush are placed parallel to the long axis of the tooth and pointed incisally. The bristles are placed at a 45-degree angle and the brush is shimmied back and forth until the bristles engage the gingival tissues and interproximal area.

Stillman The brush is placed against the buccal or lingual aspects of the tooth with the bristles pointing toward the gingival margin. The sides of the bristles should extend about 3 to 4 mm onto the attached gingival but should not extend beyond the mucogingival junction. The bristles are placed at a 45-degree angle and the brush is shimmied in a mesiodistal direction while moving it toward the occlusal/incisal edge.

Tooth mobility Referring to pathologic mobility. Loosening of a tooth or teeth. Mobility is an important diagnostic sign.

Tooth wear Loss of tooth structure (e.g., abrasion, erosion, attrition).

Topical delivery Referring to the administration of a drug or agent as a rinse or into the gingival crevice.

Toxin Substance that is harmful to the body (e.g., endotoxin).

Treatment plan List of treatment that the patient needs.

Treatment planning The act of making a list of treatment that the patient needs.

Trifurcation Anatomic area where roots diverge in a three-rooted tooth.

U

Ultrasonic See Scaler, ultrasonic.

V

Vascular Refers to blood.

W

Wear facet A flattened, highly polished worn spot on the occlusal or incisal surface of a tooth (usually seen on the side of a cusp). It may be a clinical sign of attrition.

World Health Organization A specialized agency of the United Nations with primary responsibility for international health matters and public health.

X

Xerostomia Dryness of the mouth due to inadequate salivary secretion as a result of aging, salivary gland conditions, or medications.

Answers to Self-Quiz Questions

Chapter 1

1. c
2. c
3. c
4. c
5. b
6. c
7. a
8. a
9. d
10. d

Chapter 2

1. b
2. b
3. c
4. b
5. c
6. a
7. c
8. a
9. b
10. a

Chapter 3

1. d
2. a
3. b
4. a
5. c
6. a
7. c
8. b
9. d
10. c

Chapter 4

1. c
2. c
3. a
4. a
5. a
6. a
7. c
8. b
9. d
10. d

Chapter 5

1. b
2. d
3. a
4. c
5. c

Chapter 6

1. b
2. c
3. c
4. a
5. b
6. e
7. b
8. d
9. c
10. a

Chapter 7

1. c
2. c
3. a
4. b
5. c
6. a
7. a
8. c
9. b
10. a

Chapter 8

1. d
2. a
3. d
4. d
5. d
6. c
7. d
8. a
9. d
10. c

Chapter 9

1. c
2. a
3. b
4. a
5. b
6. d
7. b
8. a
9. b
10. c

Chapter 10

1. c
2. b
3. d
4. a
5. c
6. b
7. a
8. b
9. b
10. d

Chapter 11

1. a
2. b
3. b
4. b
5. c

Chapter 12

1. b
2. c
3. a
4. d
5. b

Chapter 13

1. a
2. d
3. c
4. a
5. d

Chapter 14

1. b
2. a
3. b
4. c
5. e

Chapter 15

1. d
2. a
3. a
4. c
5. e
6. c
7. a
8. b
9. a
10. b

Chapter 16

1. b
2. b

3. a
4. c
5. c
6. c
7. c
8. b
9. a
10. a

Chapter 17

1. a
2. c
3. d
4. c
5. c
6. b
7. a
8. c
9. a
10. c

Chapter 18

1. b
2. d
3. b
4. d
5. b
6. b
7. c
8. b
9. c
10. c

Chapter 19

1. a
2. c
3. b
4. e
5. a
6. c
7. a
8. b
9. a
10. a

Chapter 20

1. c
2. b

3. c
4. d
5. c
6. a
7. b
8. e
9. c
10. c

Chapter 21

1. d
2. c
3. c
4. c
5. a

Chapter 22

1. d
2. c
3. b
4. b
5. c
6. a
7. b
8. c
9. a
10. b

Chapter 23

1. c
2. d
3. c
4. d
5. a

Chapter 24

1. a
2. c
3. b
4. e
5. d
6. b
7. d
8. a
9. d
10. e

Chapter 25

1. b
2. a
3. a
4. a
5. b
6. c
7. b
8. b
9. b
10. a

Chapter 26

1. b
2. c
3. b
4. a
5. a
6. c
7. b
8. c
9. d
10. e

Chapter 27

1. c
2. c
3. b
4. a
5. c

Chapter 28

1. d
2. a
3. a
4. c
5. d
6. b
7. d
8. c
9. c
10. c

Case I

1. d
2. c
3. a

4. b
5. a
6. b
7. e
8. a
9. d
10. b

Case II

1. a
2. a
3. d
4. d
5. d
6. c
7. b
8. a
9. c
10. b

Case III

1. b
2. a
3. b
4. c
5. a
6. b
7. b
8. c
9. d
10. a

Case IV

1. d
2. a
3. c
4. a
5. a
6. a
7. c
8. a
9. b
10. a

Index

*Page numbers with f indicate figures;
those with t indicate tables.*

Abrasives, 301
Abscesses
    defined, 439
    differences between types of, 174t
    gingival, 171
    periapical, 172–73, 173f
    pericoronal, 173, 175, 175f
Abscesses, periodontal, 170–75
    acute *vs.* chronic, 172, 172f
    differential diagnosis, 172–73, 173f
    features, 171, 171f, 172f
    microbiology, 171–72
    radiographically detectable, 243
    treatment, 173
Absorbable sutures, 387
Absorbed controlled (sustained)-release
        devices, 340–42
    chlorhexidine gluconate chip, 340–41
    doxycycline hyclate gel, 341
    minocycline hydrochloride micros-
        pheres, 341–42
Acidophilus tablets, 339
Acquired pellicle, 55–56
Actisite, 340
Acute periodontal abscess, 172, 172f
ADA Guide to Dental Therapeutics
        (ADA), 333, 449–50
Adhesins, 56
Adjunctive systemic antibiotics, 336
Adjunctive treatment, 280–81
Adopted Names Council of United
        States, 333
Advanced lesions, 129
Adverse drug events, 336
    systemic antimicrobial agents, clas-
        sification of, 337t
Adverse drug reaction (ADR), 336
Adverse pregnancy outcomes, 103–4
Advice, patient, 308–10
Age
    changes with periodontium physiol-
        ogy, 22–23
    implantology and, 414
    as risk factor, 95

Aggressive periodontitis (AgP), 44,
        137, 141–42, 279
AIDS, 77, 99
Alcohol, 101
Alcohol-free mouthrinses, 324–25
    antimicrobials, selective, 325
Alloderm, 385–86
Allogeneic grafts, 396–97
Allografts, 396–97
Alloplastic grafts, 397–98
Alloplasts, 397–98
Alveolar bone crest, 21, 21f
Alveolar mucosa, 7, 11
Alveolar process, 19–21
    alveolar bone crest, 21, 21f
    anatomy, variations in, 21, 22f
    bone composition, 21
    metabolism, 21
    morphology, 20–21, 20f
    parts of, 19–20, 19f, 20f
Alzheimer's disease, 104
Amalgam tattoo, 203
American Academy of Periodontology
        (AAP), 150, 259, 325, 340
    classification recommendations,
        117
    publications, 461
    on steroids, 101–2
    term *periodontal maintenance*
        adopted by, 446
American Dental Association (ADA),
        321, 333, 449–50
American Dental Hygienist's Associa-
        tion (ADHA), 349
American Heart Association (AHA),
        184
American National Standards Insti-
        tute (ANSI), 235
Amoxicillin, 338
Anatomic factors, 85–86
    implant-tissue interface, 423–25
    keratinized gingiva, 425–26
    root morphology, 85, 86–87f
    teeth *vs.* dental implants, 423–26
    tooth position, 87, 87f
Anesthetics, 352
Antibiotic prophylaxis, 467–68

Antibiotics, 333–34
    chemotherapeutic agents, 333
    classification of, 336
    defined, 333, 339
    periodontal pathogens, 333
    resistance to, 340
Antibodies, 76–77
Anticalculus dentifrices, 304
Anticollagenase feature, 336–37
Antigens, 74–75, 75f
Antimicrobials, 280–81
Antiplaque/antigingivitis agents, 321–25
Antiseptics, 321, 333
Aphthous stomatitis, 443
Apically positioned flap, 370–73
    contraindications, 371
    healing, 372
    indications, 371
    objectives, 370
    periodontal dressing, 372
    techniques, 371–72
Appliances, intraoral, 166, 166f, 192
Arestin, 340, 341–42
Arm and Hammer Toothpaste, 291, 304
Aspartate aminotransferase (AST), 252
Aspirin for toothache, 90
Assessment phase of therapy, 179
Atridox, 340, 341, 342
Attached gingiva, 5–6, 5f
Attachment apparatus, 3f, 16f
    alveolar process, 19–21
    cementum, 18–19
    periodontal ligament, 15–18
Attachment level, 15
Attachment of dental calculus, types of,
        85
Attrition, 162–63, 163f
Augmentin, 338
Autografts, 396
Azalides, 339
Azithromycin dihydrate, 339

Bacteria. *See also* Microorganisms
    causing respiratory diseases, 104
    combined mechanisms, 62
    in dental biofilms, 53
    in dental plaque, 52

Bacteria (*cont.*)
  direct effect, 61
  health and disease associated characteristics, 54
  host response (*See* Host response to bacteria)
  indirect effect, 62
  mechanisms of bacterial action, 61
  morphology/types of, 53–55, 54t, 55t
  nutrients, 59
  saccharolytic/asaccharolytic, 53
  tissue invasion, 59–60
Bacteriology, 426–27
Bad breath. *See* Halitosis
Baking soda, 303–4
BANA (benzoyldi-arginine-2-naphthylamide), 254
Barrier membranes, types of, 405–7
  bioabsorbable membranes, 405–7, 407t
  nonabsorbable membranes, 405
Basal lamina, 13
Bass method, 305
Beagle model, 159
Behavior, 286
Benzocaine, 352
Beta-lactamases, 338
Bioabsorbable membranes, 405–7
Bioactive glass, 397–98
Biofilms, dental, 334. *See also* Plaque, dental
  formation, 56–58
  microorganisms of, 55–59
  subgingival plaque, 58–59
  supragingival plaque, 55–58
Biologic environment, 426t
Biologics, 398–99
Biologic width, 14, 15f
Bio-Oss, 398
Biotene, 305
Bisbiguanides, 322–23
Bisecting technique, 235–36, 236f
Bisphosphonate-related osteonecrosis of the jaw (BRONJ), 97–99, 98f
Bisphosphonates, 97–99, 98f, 98t
Bitewing radiographs, 237, 237f
Black-line stain, 193
Bland-type implants, 415
Bleeding, gingival, 205–6
  case study, 475–80
Bleeding on probing (BOP), 205, 217–18, 428, 449
Blood dyscrasias, gingivitis associated with, 123
Blood supply, 426
B-lymphocytes, 75–77, 75f, 76f
Bone composition, 21

Bone grafts, 399–400
  allogeneic grafts, 396–97
  allografts, 396–97
  alloplastic grafts, 397–98
  alloplasts, 397–98
  autografts, 396
  common, 399–400t
  defined, 396
  types of, 397t
  xenografts, 398
Bone loss, 129
  determining (*See* Bone loss, radiographic determination of)
  horizontal, 134, 135f
  infrabony defects, 135
  one-wall bony defect, 136, 136f
  patterns of, 133–36, 133f, 134f
  patterns of, factors related to, 136–37, 137f
  and pocket formation, relationship of, 133
  three-wall bony defect, 136, 136f
  two-wall bony defect, 136, 136f
  vertical or angular, 134–35, 135f, 136f
Bone loss, radiographic determination of, 239–41, 241f
  interpretation of, 239–41
  patterns of, 240, 240f
  severity, 240–41
Bone morphogenic proteins (BMPs), 398
Bone quality, 418t
Bone-replacement materials
  classification of, 396–98
  objectives of, 398
  types of, 397
Bone resorbing factors, 132–33
Bone substitute materials, 396, 399–400, 399–400t
Bony defects, response to, 396t
Bránemark implant system, 423
Braun Oral-B Interclean, 299
Braun Oral-B Plaque Remover, 294
Breath odor, 290t
BreathRx, 291
Bruxism, 157–58, 191–92, 191f
Buccal cortical plate, 20
Bundle bone, 19–20
Bupropion HCl, 452
Buttressing bone, 21

Calcium channel blockers, 123
Calculus, 82–85, 83f
  clinical significance of, 82–85
  defined, 84
  in radiographs, 241, 241f
  removal, 352
  structure of, 85
  subgingival, 84–85

  supragingival, 84
  types of attachment, 85
Calculus indices, 40
Cancellous bone, 20
Cannabis (marijuana) smoking, 101
Cardiovascular disease, 102–3
Caries, 189
  dental evaluation for, 189
  root, 189, 189f, 391
  root-surface, 189
Cases
  bleeding gums, 475–80
  loose teeth, 487–93
  periodontal disease, 481–86
  spaces between teeth, 469–74
Cautions, 328–29
  irrigation *vs.* toothbrushing, 328–29
Cell renewal, 8
Cells involved in regeneration, 400–404
Cell-to-cell tissue junction, 13
Cellular immunity, 75, 77–78
Cellular turnover, 11
Cementoenamel junction (CEJ), 4, 203, 357
Cementum, 18–19
  abnormalities, 19
  and enamel, relationship of, 18, 18f
  physiologic features, 19
  removal, 353
  types of, 18
Centric occlusion (CO), 154, 165
Centric relation (CR), 154
Cepacol, 323
Cephalosporins, 338
Cervical enamel projections (CEPs), 85, 86f, 227–28
Cetylpyridinium chloride, 323
Chairside desensitizing products, 313t
Charters method, 308
Chemical agents, use of, 328
Chemical injury, 90, 90f
Chemotaxis, 73
Chemotherapeutic agents, 321, 333
Chemotherapy, 333
Chewing gum, 291
Chew sticks, 293
Chief complaint (CC), 183–84
Chlorhexidine, discoloration due to, 195
Chlorhexidine gluconate, 281, 322
Chlorhexidine gluconate chip, 340–41
Chondroitin sulfatase, 62
Chromic gut, 387
Chronic periodontal abscess, 172, 172f
Chronic periodontitis, 139–41, 139t, 279
Cigarette smoking, 100–101, 381, 450–52. *See also* Smoking cessation
Ciprofloxacin, 339

Clefts, gingival, 203
Clindamycin HCI, 339
Clinical applications, 254
Clinical attachment level (CAL), 212, 218–19, 218f, 357
Clinical connective tissue attachment loss, 66
Clinical examination, 187–96
  dental evaluation, 188–92
  dentinal hypersensitivity, 195–96
  extraoral/intraoral examination, 188
  gingival assessment, 198–206
  periodontal assessment, 209–28
  tooth stain evaluation, 192–95
Clinician skill, 354–55
COE-pak, 389
Col, 7
Colgate Total, 291
Collagen, 11
Collagenase, 13, 62, 252
Collagen organization, 12
Color, assessment of, 199
Compact bone, 20
Complement system, 74
Computed tomography (CT scanning), 244, 245–46, 245f
  cone beam, 245–46
  traditional, 245, 245f, 246f
Computer technology, 179
Cone beam computed tomography (CBCT), 245–46
Connective attachment loss, 212
Connective tissue attachment, 12, 16–17, 16f
Connective tissue interface, 11, 13
Contact relationships, malpositioning and proximal, 190–92
Continuing care, 272
Continuous sutures, 388
Contour, assessment of, 203
Contraindications, 366
  apically positioned flap, 371
  modified Wildman flap (MWF), 369
Contributory, defined, 82
Controlled force probe, 213–16, 214–15f
Controlled (sustained)-release drug delivery, 334, 340–43
Conventional radiographs, 234, 236–38
  benefits and limitations of, 237
  bitewing radiographs, 237, 237f
  panoramic radiology, 237–38
  periapical radiographs, 237
  selection criteria for, 236t
Conventional tomograms, 245–46
Cooling water spray, 421
Cool Mint Listerine, 323
Coronary artery calcification (CAC), 103
Coronary heart disease (CHD), 102–3

Cortical bone, 418
C-reactive protein (CRP), 103
Crowding of teeth, 190, 190f
Crown-lengthening procedures, 377
C-terminal cross-linked telopetide (CTx), 99
Culture techniques, 252–53, 254
Curets, 433
Curettage, 350
Cyclosporine, 123
Cytokines, 74
Cytotoxic agents, 61
Cytotoxic T-cells, 77

Debris indices, 27, 40
Deep scaling, 349
Delayed passive eruption, 223, 223f
Delivery systems. See Local drug delivery systems; Systematic drug delivery system
Demineralized freeze-dried bone (DFDBA), 397–98
Dental calculus. See Calculus
Dental evaluation, 188–92. See also Periodontal visit
  caries, 189
  components of, 188
  dental implants, 189–90
  intraoral appliances, 192
  malpositioning and proximal contact relationships, 190–92
  number of teeth, evaluating, 188
  restorative status, 189
Dental examination, 446. See also Periodontal visit
Dental floss, 296–98
Dental history, 185
Dental hygiene, 178–81
  assessment, 179
  diagnosis, 180
  evaluation, 180–81
  implementation, 180
  social, economic, and cultural decisions in assessment, 180
  technology and documentation, 179
  treatment plan, 180
Dental implants
  compounds of, 414
  evaluation of, 189–90, 450
  home care, 305–7
  implant-supported overdentures, 423
  implant-tissue interface, 423–25
  instruments for, appropriate, 432–33
  maintenance program (See Dental implants, maintenance program)
  material, 397
  overloading of, 429–30

perimucosal seal, 423
site, preservation/development of, 421–23
teeth vs., 423–26
Dental implants, maintenance program, 427–33
  clinical parameters, evaluation of, 427–28
  hard tissue, evaluation of, 429
  in-office irrigation, 433
  instruments for implants, appropriate, 432–33
  mobility, 429
  overloading of implants, 429–30
  peri-implant disease, stages of, 430
  problem implant, identification of, 429
  success, criteria for, 429
  superstructure removal, 430–32
Dental implants, types of, 414–17
  endodontic implants, 417
  endosseous implants, 415–16
  subperiosteal implants, 416
  transosteal implants, 416
Dental/medical history, 183. See also Patient history
Dental tape, 296–98
Dentifrices, 300–305
  components of, 301–2
  defined, 300
  fluoride, 302–3
  other categories of, 304–5
  patient-applied treatment, 311–12
  sodium bicarbonate/hydrogen peroxide, 303–4
  stannous fluoride, 303
  tartar-control, 304
  with therapeutic benefits, 302t
  triclosan-containing, 303
  zinc citrate-containing, 304
DentinBloc, 391
Dentogingival unit, 13–15
  formation of, 14–15
Dentomycin, 343
Deplaquing, 349
Desensitization, assessment of patients' need, 311
Devices, 325–28, 398–99
  in-office irrigation, 326–28
Diabetes mellitus, 95–96, 96f, 102
Diabetes mellitus-associated gingivitis, 122–23
Diagnosis phase of therapy, 180
Diagnostic tests, supplemental, 250. See also Periodontal diseases, detecting and monitoring
Direct digital radiography, 243–44, 244f
Disastemas, 191, 191f

Diseased periodontal unit, 355
Disease progression, 44–45
Disulfiram, 338–39
DMDx Test, 253
DNA probe analysis, 253
Doctor West's Miracle Toothbrush, 296
Documentation, 179
Double papillae flap, 381
Doxycycline, 337–38, 343
Doxycycline hyclate gel, 341
Drifted teeth, 190, 190f
Drug-induced gingival diseases, 278
Drug Information Handbook for Dentistry (Lexi-Comp, Inc.), 333
Drug use, 100–102
  alcohol, 101
  gingival overgrowth due to, 101–2, 102f, 205, 205f
  information resources, selected, 333
  tobacco products, 100–101
  xerostomia due to, 101

Early/immediate loading, 420
Early-onset periodontitis, 137, 141–42, 279
Education, patient, 286–87
Efficacy, 326
Elastases, 62
Electric interdental cleaning devices, 299
Elyzol, 342
Enamel and cementum, relationship of, 18, 18f
Endocrine system, 95–99, 117, 122–23
  bisphosphonates, 97–99, 98f, 98t
  diabetes mellitus, 95–96, 96f, 102, 122–23
  diabetes mellitus-associated gingivitis, 122–23
  hormones, 96–97
  menstrual-cycle gingivitis, 122
  pregnancy gingivitis, 122
  puberty gingivitis, 117, 122
Endodontic implants, 417
Endodontic lesions, 142, 143f
Endodontics, 378
Endodontic stabilizers, 417
Endogenous stains, 193
Endosseous implants, 415–16
End-tuft brush, 298
Enlargement. *See* Gingival enlargement
Enzyme-based assays, 254
Enzyme-linked immunosorbent assay (ELIZA), 253–54
Enzymes, 61
  common, 62
  host-derived, 61, 252

Enzyme-suppression therapy, 343–44
  matrix metalloproteinases, 343
  subantimicrobial-dose doxycycline (SDD), 343–44
Epidemiology
  defined, 26
  future trends, 47
  incidence and disease progression, 44–45
  indices, 26–41
  introduction and definitions, 26
  methodology, accuracy of, 41
  prevalence, 42–44
  treatment needs, 47
  variables, 45–47
Epithelial cell-to-cell attachment, 13
Epithelial rests of Malassez, 18
Epithelium, 365, 400
Epithelium interface, 11
Epithelium-tooth surface, 13
Erosion, 192, 192f
Erythromycin, 339
Established lesion (few B cells/plasma cells), 115–16
Ethanol, 324
Evaluation
  clinical parameters of, 427–28
  hard tissue, 429
  phase of therapy, 180–81
Exaggerated inflammatory response, 122
Exercise, 166
Exodontics, 88
Extraoral halitophobia, patient with, 292
Extraoral/intraoral examination, 188
Extrinsic stains, 193, 195

Factitious disease, 89, 89f
Family history, 185
Fetal exposures to periodontal pathogens, 104
Fibroblasts, 13
Film type in radiographs, 235
Flap, defined, 368
Flap classification, 368–69
Flap surgery, 264
Floss cords, 305
Floss holder, 297
Floss threader, 297
Fluoride dentifrices, 302–3
Fluorides
  in-office treatments, 313–14
  oral rinses, 324
  patient-applied treatment, 312
Food and Drug Administration (FDA), 340, 389
Food impaction, 89–90, 90f
Free (marginal) gingiva, 4–5, 203
Free gingival graph (FGG), 381–82

Free gingival groove, 4
Fremitus, 162, 162f, 224
Frenum attachment, 7
Fresh Burst Listerine, 323
Full-mouth survey, 234
Functional occlusion, 154
  ideal or normal, 154
  malocclusion, 154, 155f
  overbite, 155
Fungal diseases, 124
Furcations, 225–28, 225f
  cervical enamel projections, 227–28
  classification of, 226–27, 226t, 227f
  locating, 227, 227f
  periodontal maintenance therapy and, 449
  and root anatomy, 354

Gas chromatography, 288
Gel-Kam, 324
Gender as risk factor, 95
Generalized aggressive periodontitis (GAP), 141
Genetic assays, 254
Genetics, 94–95, 254
Genotype PST™ Plus, 254
Genuine halitosis, 288
Geriatric patients, 281
  plaque control, 281
  treatment considerations, 281
  xerostomia, 281
Gingiva, 3, 3f
  attached, 5–6, 5f
  exaggerated inflammatory response, 122
  free (marginal), 4–5
  free gingival groove, 4
  gingival crevice, 4
  gingival crevicular fluid (GCF), 4
  interdental, 6–7, 6f
  overgrowth due to drugs, 101–2, 102f
  recession of, root caries and, 189, 189f
  stippling, 5–6, 5f, 6f
Gingival abscess
  defined, 171, 439
  treatment steps for, 439t
Gingival assessment, 198–206
  changes seen in health and gingivitis, 200–202t
  color, 199
  consistency, 203–4
  contour, 203
  drug-influenced gingival enlargement, 205, 205f
  gingival bleeding, 205–6
  hormonal-influenced gingivitis, 204–5
  objectives of, 199

periodontal maintenance therapy, 446–47
of risk factors for gingival diseases, 199
size (gingival enlargement), 204
surface texture, 204
Gingival connective tissue, 11–13, 11f
cellular and vascular elements, 13
collagen organization, 12
components of, 11–12
connective tissue attachment, 12
connective tissue/epithelium interface, 11
gingival fibers, 12, 12t, 13f
Gingival crevice, 4
Gingival crevicular fluid (GCF), 4, 69, 103, 337
Gingival crevicular fluid (GCF) assays, 250–52, 251f, 251t
host-derived enzymes, 252
prostaglandin E₂, 252
Gingival diseases, 112–24
clinical features of, 122
common, 118–20t
dental plaque-induced, 117, 122–24, 278
drug-induced gingival diseases, 278
of fungal origin, 124
histopathogenesis of gingivitis, 113–16
lesions of genetic origin, 124
manifestations of systemic conditions, 124
modified by medications, 123–24, 278
modified by systemic factors, 117–24
non-plaque-induced, 124, 278
periodontal diseases, classification of, 117–24
risk factors for, assessment of, 199
of specific bacteria origin, 124
of viral origin, 124
Gingival embrasures, types of, 295–99
dental floss, 296–98
dental tape, 296–98
electric interdental cleaning devices, 299
interdental brushes, 298
interdental cleaning devices, clinical features of, 296t
rubber-tip stimulator, 298
single-tuft brushes, 298
toothpicks, wooden, 298–99
Gingival enlargement
assessment of, 204
drug-influenced, 123–24, 205, 205f, 278

Gingival epithelium, 7–11, 8f
cell renewal, 8
elements of, 7, 9f
junctional epithelium, 10–11
keratinization process, 8
lamina propria, 7, 8f
layers of, 7, 9f
oral epithelium, 8–10
sulcular epithelium, 10
Gingival fibers, 12, 12t, 13f
of gingival connective tissue, 12, 12t, 13f
of periodontal ligament, 16–17, 17t
principal, 16, 16f
Sharpey's, 19
Gingival fibroblasts, 322
Gingival flap, 441
Gingival indices, 40–41
Gingival overgrowth, 278
Gingival pocket, 116, 116f
Gingival recession
classification of, 380–81
clinical significance of, 221
etiology of, 219–21, 220–21f
hypersensitivity and, 311
measuring, 219
pathogenesis of, 221
periodontal maintenance therapy, 448–49
surgical procedures, 391
Gingival unit, clinical anatomy of
lining mucosa, 7
masticatory mucosa, 4–7 (See also Gingiva)
specialized mucosa, 7
Gingival unit, microscopic anatomy of
alveolar mucosa, 11
cell-to-cell tissue junction, 13
dentogingival unit, 13–15
gingival connective tissue, 11–13
gingival epithelium, 7–11, 8f
Gingivectomy/gingivoplasty, 363, 366–68
contraindications, 366
defined, 366
healing, 366–68
indications, 366
surgical care procedures, 267–368t
technique, 366
Gingivitis, 66. See also Gingival diseases
associated with blood dyscrasias, 123
associated with dental plaque, 117
associated with endocrine system, 117, 122–23, 204–5
changes seen in, assessment of, 200–202t
defined, 113
healing after debridement, 355–56

histopathogenesis of (See Gingivitis, histopathogenesis of)
hormonal-influenced, 204–5
leukemia-associated, 123
nonsurgical treatment of, 261t
pathogenesis of (See Gingivitis, pathogenesis of)
periodontal changes, radiographically detectable, 242
pregnancy, 96, 96f
treatment phases, 273
Gingivitis, histopathogenesis of, 113–16
established lesion (few B cells/plasma cells), 115–16
initial lesion (PMN dominated), 115
stages in, 113–15, 114f
Gingivitis, pathogenesis of, 116–17
gingival pocket, 116, 116f
host response to gingival inflammation, 116–17
Gore-Tex Regenerative Membrane Titanium Reinforced, 405
Green stain, 193, 195
Grinding/clenching of teeth, 157–58, 191–92, 191f
selective grinding, 165–66
Group function, 154, 156f
Growth factors, 398
Guided bone regeneration, 395, 405, 421
Guided tissue regeneration (GTR), 400–407
barrier membranes, types of, 405–7
cells involved in, 400–404
defined, 239, 402, 405–7, 421
surgical procedure, 404–5
Guided tissue regeneration (GTR) for root coverage, 385–86
Guidelines for the Management of Patients with Periodontal Diseases (American Academy of Periodontology), 267

Halimeter, 288
Halitophobia, 288
Halitosis, 287
bad breath, oral conditions that cause, 288
causes to consider in patient with, 288
classification of patients with, 287–92
corresponding treatment needs, 289t
defined, 287
extraoral halitophobia, patient with, 292
genuine, 288
oral malodor (See Oral malodor)
over-the-counter (OTC) products, 292
pathologic, 288

Halitosis (*cont.*)
pseudo-halitosis, management of patients with, 292
treatment needs for breath odor, 290t
Hard tissue evaluation, 429
Healing
apically positioned flap, 372
following periodontal surgery, 365
gingivectomy/gingivoplasty, 366–68
modified Wildman flap (MWF), 370
of periodontal unit, 355
postoperative instructions, general, 365
types of, 365
Healing response and outcome of therapy, 355–57
diseased periodontal unit, 355
gingivitis, 355–56
healing periodontal unit, 355
periodontitis, 356–57
Helper T-cells, 77
Hematologic system, 99
Hemidesmosome, 13, 14f
Hemiseptal defect, 375
Hemostasis, 388
Herbal-based dentifrices, 304
Herpes virus (HSV 1), 442
Hertwig's epithelial root sheath (HERS), 399
Heterografts, 398
Histopathogenesis
defined, 113
of gingivitis, 113–16
Page and Schroeder's histopathologic periodontal lesions, 129, 129f, 130t
of periodontitis, 129–30
Home oral irrigation, 325, 327t
Hormonal-influenced gingivitis, 204–5
Hormones, 96–97, 96f
Host-derived enzymes, 61–62, 252
Host response to bacteria, 65–78
bacteria-host challenge, 68–69
bacterial components, 68–69
immune response, 74–77
inflammatory response, 69–74
oral defense mechanisms, 69
periodontal disease activity, 65–69
Host response to gingival inflammation, 116–17
Host response to periodontal disease, 69–77
immune response, 74–77
inflammatory response, 70–74
Human immunodeficiency virus (HIV), 77, 99, 99f, 279
necrotizing ulcerative gingivitis as sign of, 148–50

Humectants, 302
Humoral immunity, 75–77
Hyaluronidase, 62
Hydrogen peroxide, 324
Hypersensitivity, dentinal, 195–96, 310–14, 391
after surgical procedures, 391
desensitization, assessment of patients' need, 311
etiology of, 195–96
identification, 196
in-office treatment, 312–13
patient-applied treatment, 311–12
sensitivity analysis, 254

Iatrogenic factors, 87–88
exodontics, 88
orthodontics, 88, 88f
restorative dentistry, 87–88, 88f
Immediate implant placement in extraction sockets, 421
Immune response, 74f
activation of, 74–75, 74f
cellular immunity, 77–78
humoral immunity, 75–77
key elements in, 75
lymphocytes in, 75–77, 75f, 76f, 77f
Immunoglobulins (Ig), 76
Immunologic assays, 253–54
Immunopathologic mechanisms, 62
Immunosuppression, 149–50
Implantology, 413–33. *See also* Dental implants
age, 414
bacteriology, 426–27
radiographs (*See* Implantology, radiographs in)
social factors, 414
surgical procedure (*See* Implantology, surgical procedure)
systemic diseases, 414
Implantology, radiographs in, 244–46
conventional tomograms, 245–46
pantomograms (panoramic films), 244–45
periapical/occlusal films, 244
postoperative implant evaluation, 246
Implantology, surgical procedure
bone, quality of, 418t
dental implant site, preservation/development, 421–23
immediate implant placement in extraction sockets, 421
prostheses, 423
single-stage, 419–20
single-tooth replacements, 420–21
two-stage, 418–19
Implementation phase of therapy, 180

Incidence
defined, 26
and disease progression, 44–45
Indications, 328, 334–36
gingivectomy/gingivoplasty, 366
modified Wildman flap (MWF), 369
nitroimadazoles, 338
periodontal plastic surgery, 378–80
selection, 336
Indices, 26–41
calculus, 40
criteria for, 27
defined, 26
gingival, 40–41
historically important and commonly used, 28–39
of periodontal destruction, 41
plaque and debris, 27, 40
significance of, 26–27
Inflammatory lesion, 426
Inflammatory periodontal disease, 129, 199, 350
Inflammatory process, 69
Inflammatory response, 70–74
acute *vs.* chronic, 72t
elements of inflammatory system, 70–71
inflammatory process, 71–74, 71f, 71t
key elements in, 70
Informed consent, 273
defined, 273
Infrabony defect, 374, 396
Initial lesion (PMN dominated), 115
In-office irrigation, 326–28, 433
chemical agents, use of, 328
efficacy, 326
periodontal pathogens, 327
In-office treatment, 312–13
chairside desensitizing products, 313t
for dentinal hypersensitivity, 312–13
fluorides, 313–14
oxalate salts, 312–13
restorative materials/restorations, 314
Interdental brushes, 298
Interdental care, 295–99
gingival embrasures, types of, 295–99
Interdental cleaning devices
clinical features of, 296t
improper use of, 310
Interdental gingiva, 6–7, 6f
Interdental papillae, 6–7, 6f, 203
Interdental septum, 238–39, 239f
Interleukin-1 (IL-1), 74, 94, 254
Internal bevel incision, 368
International Workshop for a Classification of Periodontal Diseases and Conditions the American Academy of Periodontology, 117

Interproximal bone, 429
Interview process, 183. *See also* Patient history
Intraosseous defects, 374
Inverse beval incision, 368–69
Iodine, 324

Junctional epithelium, 10–11, 355, 357
    cells in, 10–11
    cellular turnover, 11
    layers of, 10
    semipermiable structure, 10
Juvenile periodontitis, 279

Keratinization process, 8
Keratinized gingiva, 425–26, 428
Keratinocytes, 9
Keyes technique, 303–4
Kilovoltage, 234

Lamina propria, 7, 8f, 11–12, 13
Langerhans cells, 10
Lasers, 368
Lateral abscess, 439–41
Laterally positioned flap, 381
Lectins, 56
Lesions
    advanced, 129
    endodontic, 142, 143f
    established (few B cells/plasma cells), 115–16
    gingival, of genetic origin, 124
    inflammatory, 426
    initial (PMN dominated), 115
    Page and Schroeder's histopathologic periodontal, 113–15, 113t, 114f, 129, 129f, 130t
    traumatic, 124
Leukemia-associated gingivitis, 123
Lincomycins, 339
Lingual cortical plate, 20
Lining mucosa, 7
    alveolar mucosa, 7
    frenum attachment, 7
Lipooligosaccharide (LOS), 61
Listerine, 307, 323, 325
Literature, periodontal, 464–65
Local contributory risk factors, 81–91
    anatomic factors, 85–86
    contributory, defined, 82
    dental calculus, 82–85
    iatrogenic factors, 87–88
    traumatic factors, 89–91
Local drug delivery systems
    absorbed controlled (sustained)-release devices, 340–42

controlled (sustained)-release drug delivery, 340–43
    other products, 342–43
Localized aggressive periodontitis (LAP), 141
Loose teeth, 487–93
Low-birth-weight, premature births (PLBW), 103
Lymphadenopathy, 441
Lymphocytes, 10, 13, 75–77, 75f, 76f, 77f
Lymphokines, 77

Macrolides, 339
    adverse effects, 339
    azalides, 339
    drug-drug interactions, 339
    drug-food interactions, 339
    second-generation drugs, 339
Macrophages, 13, 73–74, 73f, 141
Maintenance care, 272
Malocclusion, 154, 155f
Malpositioning contact relationships, 190–92
Mandibular staple implants, 416
Manual toothbrushes, design of, 292–93
Marginal gingiva, 203
Marijuana smoking, 101
Mast cells, 13
Masticatory mucosa. *See* Gingiva
Material floss, 297
Matrix metalloproteinases (MMPs), 69, 343
Mattress sutures, 388
Mechanical plaque control, 292
    evaluation of, 292
    oral biofilms, 292
Mechanism of action
    nitroimadazoles, 338
    powered toothbrushes, 294
Medical history, 184–85
Medications
    associated with gingival enlargements, 123–24
    gingival diseases modified by, 123–24
    over-the-counter (OTC) products, 292
    penicillin (beta-lactams), 338
    second-generation drugs, 339
Melanocytes, 9–10
Menopause, 97
Menstrual-cycle gingivitis, 122
Merkel cells, 10
Methacrylate resins, 314
Microbial tests, 252–53
    culture techniques, 252–53
    microscopic techniques, 253
    nucleic acid (DNA) probe analysis, 253

Microbiology of periodontal diseases, 51–62
Micro-IDent Plus, 253
Microorganisms, 52
    of dental biofilms, 55–59
    of dental implants, 60
Microscopic techniques, 253
Miller classification, 380–81
Milliamperage, 235
Minocycline hydrochloride microspheres, 341–42
Mobility, 429
Moderate chronic periodontitis, 275
Moderate periodontitis, 242, 242f
Modified Wildman flap (MWF), 369–70
    contraindications, 369
    healing, 370
    indications, 369
    objectives, 369
    technique, 369–70
Motivation, 286
Mouthrinses, 291
Mucogingival junction (MGJ), 5
    defects, 363
    delayed passive eruption, 223, 223f
    examination, 222–23, 223f
    procedures, 380
Muscle/temporomandibular joint, 163

National Cancer Institute (NCI), 322, 451
National Institute of Dental and Craniofacial Research Survey of Oral Health of Adults in the United State, 95
Natural Citrus Listerine, 323
Natural dentifrices, 304
Necrotizing periodontal diseases, 147–50
    common features of, 149t
    necrotizing ulcerative gingivitis, 148–50, 149f
    necrotizing ulcerative periodontitis, 150, 150f
    as periodontal emergency, 441–42
    treatment planning, 279
Necrotizing ulcerative gingivitis (NUG), 99, 148–50, 149f, 279, 338, 441, 442t
Necrotizing ulcerative periodontitis (NUP), 99, 150, 150f, 279, 441
Needles, 388
Neutrophils, 10, 73
Nitrogenous, 97
Nitroimadazoles, 338–39
    adverse effects, 338–39
    drug-drug interactions, 338–39
    indications, 338
    mechanism of action, 338

Nonabsorbable membranes, 405
Nonabsorbable sutures, 387
Nonkeratinized epithelium, 8
Nonmetallic materials, 433
Nonnitrogenous, 97
Non-plaque-induced gingival diseases, 124, 278
Nonspecific plaque hypothesis, 259
Nonsurgical/initial preparation, 271
Nonsurgical periodontal therapy, healing after, 348–58
    defined, 349–50
    outcome of, healing response and, 355–57
    periodontal debridement, 350–55
    prophylaxis, 349
    reevaluation of intentional, 357–58
    root planning, 349
    scaling, 349–50
Nucleic acid (DNA) probe analysis, 253
Number of teeth, evaluating, 188
Nutritional status, 100
Nylon toothbrush, 296

Objective data, 179
Occlusal force, 156–57
Occlusal therapy, 165–67
    approaches to, common, 165
    orthodontics, 166
    parafunctional habits, control of, 166
    restorative procedures, 166
    selective grinding, 165–66
    splinting, 166–67, 167f
Occlusal trauma, 153–67
    animal studies, 159
    beagle model, 159
    classification of, 160, 160t
    clinical findings (See Occlusal trauma, clinical findings in)
    defined, 156
    human studies, 159
    occlusal force, 156–57
    parafunctional habits, 157–58
    pathogenesis of, 159–60
    premature occlusal contact, 157, 157f
    primary, 160–61, 161f
    radiographic findings in, 163–64, 164f
    role of, in periodontal disease, 158–59
    secondary, 161, 161f
    therapy (See Occlusal therapy)
    treatment outcomes, 164–65
Occlusal trauma, clinical findings in, 161–63
    attrition, 162–63, 163f
    fremitus, 162, 162f
    muscle/temporomandibular joint, 163
    tooth migration, 162

    tooth mobility, 161–62
    tooth structure, 163
Occlusion, 90–91, 154–56
    centric, 154, 165
    functional, 154
    group function, 154, 156f
    ideal or normal, 154
    malocclusion, 154, 155f
    overbite, 155
    protrusive, 154–55
One-wall bony defect, 136
Open flap debridement (OFD), 396
Operculum, 441
Opsonins, 74
Opsonization, 74
Oral biofilms, 292, 334
Oral contraceptives, 96
Oral epithelium, 8–10, 69
    cells in, 9–10
Oral Health Information Suite, 266
Oral home care, 305–8, 306–7t. See also Oral hygiene self-care
    implant home care, 305–7
    orthodontic home care, 307–8
    post-periodontal surgical home care, 305
Oral hygiene devices, improper use of, 310
    interdental devices, 310
    toothbrushing, 310
Oral hygiene evaluation, 450
Oral hygiene for periodontal patient, 285–314
    advice, patient, 308–10
    dentinal hypersensitivity, 310–14
    instructions, 390
    oral hygiene devices, effects of improper use of, 310
    periodontal disease, oral home care for patients with, 305–8
    periodontal disease control, 286–87
    preventive measures, 287–92
Oral hygiene self-care, 292–305
    behavior, 286
    defined, 286
    dentifrices, 300–305
    interdental care, 295–99
    methods, 292–305
    motivation, 286
    powered toothbrushes, 294
    tongue cleansing, 299–300
    toothbrushes, 292–94
Oral irrigation, 325–29
    cautions, 328–29
    devices, 325–28
    home, 325
    indications, 328

Oral malodor
    defined, 287
    diagnosis and assessment of, 288–90
    examination of patient, instructions before, 290
    gas chromatography, 288
    Halimeter, 288
    organoleptic measurement, 290
    organoleptic scoring scale, 291
    psychological assessment, 290
    self-assessment, 288
    simple determination of, 290
    tongue sulfide probe, 290
Oral malodor, treatment of, 291–92
    chewing gum, 291
    mouthrinses, 291
    oral hygiene, 291
    periodontal/restorative dental treatment, 292
    tongue cleaning, 291
    toothpastes, 291
    xerostomia, 292
Oral physiotherapy. See Oral hygiene self-care
Oral piercings, 91, 91f
Oral rinses, 321
    alcohol-free mouthrinses, 324–25
    bisbiguanides, 322–23
    classification of, 321–25
    fluorides, 324
    oxygenating agents, 324
    phenolic compounds, 323
    povidone-iodine, 324
    prebrushing rinses, 324
    quaternary ammonium compounds, 323–24
    substantivity, 321
Oral rinses, classification of, 321–25
Oral-systemic disease connection, 93–104. See also Systemic diseases
    periodontal diseases as risk factors for systemic conditions, 102–4
    systemic risk factors for periodontal diseases, 94–102
Oraquix, 352
Organoleptic, 291
Organoleptic measurement, 290
Orthodontics, 88, 88f, 166
    home care, 307–8
Osectomy, 375–77
Osseointegration, 416
Osseous defects
    classification of, 374–75
    crown-lengthening procedures, 377
    periodontal flap surgery with osseous resection, 374–77

root resection, 377–78
treatment procedures, 374–78
Osseous recontouring, 375
Osseous resective surgery, 375–76
Osteoblasts, 21
Osteoclasts, 21
Osteocytes, 21
Osteograf/N, 398
Osteonecrosis of the jaw (ONJ), 97–99, 98f
Osteoplasty, 375–77
Osteoporosis, 97
Overbite, 155
Overloading of implants, 429–30
Over-the-counter (OTC) products, 292
Oxalate salts, 312–13
Oxygenating agents, 324

Page and Schroeder's histopathologic periodontal lesions, 113–15, 113t, 114f, 129, 129f, 130t
Palatogingival groove, 228
Panoramic radiology, 237–38
Pantomograms (panoramic films), 244–45
Papillae, interdental, 6–7, 6f, 203
Parafunctional habits, 157–58, 166
Parakeratinized epithelium, 8
Paralleling technique, 235–36, 236f
Parameters of Care (American Academy of Periodontology), 259
Partial flap, 368
Partial-thickness flap, 368
Pathogenesis. *See also* Histopathogenesis
of gingival recession, 221
of occlusal trauma, 159–60
of periodontitis lesion, 131–37
Pathologic halitosis, 288
Pathologic tooth migration, 224, 225f
Patient adherence to therapy, 455, 456
Patient-applied treatment, 311–12
dentifrices, 311–12
for dentinal hypersensitivity, 311–12
fluorides, 312
Patient education, 286–87
Patient history, 182–85
chief complaint, 183–84
dental history, 185
family history, 185
medical history, 184–85
personal profile, 183
of present illness, 184
social history, 183
Pedicle graft, 381
Penicillin (beta-lactams), 338
Periapical abscess, 172–73, 173f
Periapical/occlusal films, 244
Periapical radiographs, 237

Pericoronal abscess, 173, 175, 175f, 441
Peri-implant disease, 143, 143f
defined, 430
stages of, 430
Peri-implantitis, 279
pathogens associated with, 427
Peri-implant mucositis, 430
Peri-implant sulcus, 431
Perimucosal seal, 423
PerioChip, 340–41
Periocline, 343
Periocoronitis, 441
Periodontal abscess, 439–41
defined, 439
treatment steps for, 439t
Periodontal assessment, 209–28, 448–49
changes (*See* Periodontal changes, radiographically detectable)
examination techniques, 216–28
fremitus, 224
furcation involvement, 225–28, 225f
mucogingival considerations, 222–23
palatogingival groove, 228
pathologic tooth migration, 224, 225f
periodontal probing depths (*See* Probing depths)
periodontal screening and recording, 216
rationale for, 210–11
structure (*See* Periodontal structures identified by radiographs)
suppuration, 223, 224f
tooth mobility, 223–24
Periodontal changes, radiographically detectable, 242–43
gingivitis, 242
moderate periodontitis, 242, 242f
periodontal abscess, 243
severe periodontitis, 242, 243f
slight (mild) periodontitis, 242, 242f
Periodontal debridement, 349, 350–55, 352–53
adverse effects of, 353
defined, 349
deplaquing, 349
gingivitis, healing after, 355–56
inflammatory periodontal disease, 350
limitations of (*See* Periodontal debridement, limitations)
outcomes of (*See* Periodontal debridement, outcomes)
periodontitis, healing after, 356–57
personal debridement, 350
procedures, 352–53
professional debridement, 350
rationale and indications for, 350–51
subgingival debridement, 349, 352–53
supragingival debridement, 349

supragingival scaling, 349
treatment sequence, 351–52
Periodontal debridement, limitations, 353–55
clinician skill, 354–55
furcations, 354
pocket depth, 353–54
root anatomy, 354
time spent, 354–55
Periodontal debridement, outcomes, 351
probing, bleeding on, 351
probing depths/clinical attachment level, 351
subgingival microbiota, 351
tissue consistency, 351
Periodontal destruction, indices of, 41
Periodontal disease activity (PDA)
defined, 66
gingivitis progressing into periodontitis, 67
models of disease activity, 65–67
Periodontal diseases, 138t
activity, detecting (*See* Periodontal diseases, detecting and monitoring)
case study, 481–86
classification of, 117–24
control, 286–87
defined, 26
dental plaque-induced gingival diseases, 117–24
education, patient, 286–87
extent of, 26
humoral immunity and, 75–77
inflammatory, 129, 199
microbiology of, 51–62
non-plaque-induced gingival diseases, 124
in occlusal trauma, 158–59
oral home care for patients with, 305–8, 306–7t
recurrent, 446, 452, 454
refractory, 446
risk assessment for, 264–67
risk factors and indicators, 53
as risk factors for systemic conditions, 102–4 (*See also* Systemic diseases)
social factors contributing to, 94
systemic risk factors for, 94–102 (*See also* Systemic diseases)
treatment phases, 268–71
Periodontal diseases, detecting and monitoring, 249–54
clinical applications, 254
enzyme-based assays, 254
genetics assays, 254
gingival crevicular fluid assays, 250–52, 251f, 251t

Periodontal diseases, detecting and monitoring (*cont.*)
  immunologic assays, 253–54
  microbial tests, 252–53
  supplemental diagnostic tests, 250
Periodontal dressing, 389
Periodontal emergencies, 438–43
  gingival abscess, 439
  necrotizing periodontal diseases, 441–42
  pericoronal abscess, 441
  periodontal abscess, 439–41
  primary herpetic gingivostomatitis, 442–43
Periodontal flap surgery, 368–73
  apically positioned flap, 370–73
  flap classification, 368–69
  modified Wildman flap, 369–70
  osseous defects, classification of, 374–75
  with osseous resection, 374–77
  ostectomy, 375–77
  osteoplasty, 375–77
Periodontal health, 273–78
  treatment, phases of, 272
Periodontal information resources, 461
Periodontal ligament, 15–18
  abnormalities, 17–18
  connective tissue attachment, 16–17, 16f
  fiber groups of, 16–17, 17t
  space, 17, 239
Periodontal maintenance therapy, 445–56
  chemotherapeutics, 454
  components of periodontal visit (*See* Periodontal visit)
  dentist-periodontist relationship, 456
  frequency of intervals, 454–56
  indications for, 446
  objectives of, 446
  patient adherence, 455, 456
  refractory/recurrent periodontal diseases, 446, 452, 454
  smoking and, 450–52
  treatment, 452–54
Periodontal pathogens, 252, 327, 333
Periodontal plastic surgery, 378–86
  gingival recession, classification of, 380–81
  indications, 378–80
  soft tissue graphs, types of, 381–86
Periodontal pocket, 129, 131–32
  bone loss related to, 133
  formation of, 129, 131–32, 132t
  types of, 132, 132t
Periodontal probing depths. *See* Probing depths
Periodontal problem list, 265–66t

Periodontal regeneration, 395. *See also* Regenerative periodontal surgery
Periodontal/restorative dental treatment, 292
Periodontal risk calculator (PCR), 266
Periodontal screening and recording (PSR), 216
Periodontal structures identified by radiographs, 238–39, 238f
  interdental septum, 238–39, 239f
  periodontal ligament space, 239
Periodontal surgery, 271–72, 362–91. *See also* Nonsurgical periodontal therapy, healing after; Regenerative periodontal surgery
  contradictions to, 363–64
  defined, 363
  gingivectomy, 363
  healing following, 365
  indications of, 363
  limitations of, 364
  mucogingival defects, 363
  objectives of, 363
  osseous defects, procedures for treating, 374–78
  periodontal dressing, 389
  periodontal plastic surgery, 378–86
  pocket reduction/elimination, procedures for, 366–73
  preoperative preparation, 364
  requirements for, 364
  surgical and postoperative care, 389–91
  surgical procedures, effects of, 391
  sutures, 387–89
  types of, 364–65
Periodontal therapy
  goals of, 259
  ongoing care, 259–64
  subgingival debridement, 353
Periodontal tissue regeneration, 395
Periodontal treatment phases, 272
Periodontal visit, 446–50
  components of, 448
  dental examination, 446
  dental implants, 450
  extraoral/intraoral examination, 446
  gingival assessment, 446–47
  medical and dental update, 446
  oral hygiene evaluation, 450
  periodontal assessment, 448–49
  plaque-control regimen, 450
  radiographic review, 449–50
Periodontist, referral to. *See* Referral to periodontist

Periodontitis, 66, 137–43, 279
  aggressive, 137, 141, 279
  associated with endodontic lesions, 142
  chronic, 139–41, 139t, 279
  common features of, 140t
  defined, 129
  diagnosis of, 260–61t
  etiology of, 141–42
  healing response and outcome of therapy, 356–57
  histopathogenesis of, 129–30
  lesions (*See* Periodontitis lesion, pathogenesis of)
  as manifestation of systemic diseases, 142–43
  nonsurgical treatment of, 261t
  prevalence of, 43–44
  recurrent, 142
  refractory, 137, 139, 142
  as risk factor for systemic conditions, 143
  treatment of, 144
Periodontitis lesion, pathogenesis of, 131–37
  see also bone loss
  bone resorbing factors, 132–33
  pocket formation, 129, 131–32, 132t
  site specificity, 133
Periodontium
  abscesses of (*See* Abscesses, periodontal)
  aging and changes with, 22–23
  defined, 3, 3f
  physiology of, 21–22, 22f
Personal debridement, 350
Personal digital assistants (PDAs), 333
Personal profile, 183
Petrolatum, 390
Phagocytic cell, 73
Phagocytosis, 73, 74
Phenolic compounds, 323
Phenytoin, 123
The Physician's Desk Reference (PDR), 333
Pik Pocket, 326
Plaque, dental. *See also* Biofilms, dental
  cells, 60
  control, 281
  control regimen, 450
  defined, 334
  dental plaque-induced gingivitis, 278
  formation of, 58f
  gingivitis associated with, 117
  supragingival, 55–58
Plaque and debris indices, 27, 40
Plaque-associated gingivitis, 117
Pocket depth, 353–54

Pocket reduction/elimination, procedures for, 366–73
    gingivectomy/gingivoplasty, 366–68
    periodontal flap surgery, 368–73
Polishing, 349–50
Polymorphonuclear leukocytes (PMNs)
    in aggressive periodontitis, 141–42
    in inflammatory process, 73–75, 73f
    in necrotizing ulcerative gingivitis, 149
    in oral epithelium, 10–11
    in periodontal disease activity, 66
Polytetrafluoroethylene (e-PTFE), 405
Population surveys, 26
Postoperative care
    complications, 390
    implant evaluation, 246
    instructions, general, 365
    regenerative periodontal surgery, 407–8
    visit management, 390–91
Post-periodontal surgical home care, 305
Povidone-iodine, 324
Powered toothbrushes, 294
    effectiveness of, 294
    mechanism of action, 294
    recommending, 294
Prebrushing rinses, 324
Pregnancy gingivitis, 96, 96f, 122
Pregnancy tumor, 204
Preoperative preparation, 364
Present illness, history of, 184
Prevalence, 42–44
    of aggressive periodontitis, 44
    defined, 26
    of gingivitis, 42–43
    of periodontitis, 43–44
Preventive measures, 287–92
    halitosis (See Halitosis)
    mechanical plaque control, 292
    primary prevention, 287
    secondary prevention, 287
Primary herpetic gingivostomatitis, 442–43
    defined, 442
Primary occlusal trauma, 160–61, 161f
Primary prevention, 287, 446
Probes, 212–13
    controlled force, 213–16, 214–15f
Probing, bleeding on, 351
Probing depths, 211–13
    bleeding on probing (BOP), 449
    bleeding sites, 217–18
    clinical attachment level, 212, 218–19, 218f
    connective attachment loss, 212
    debridement outcomes, 351
    disease progression, 212

examination techniques, 216–19, 216f, 217f, 218f
of gingival recession (See Gingival recession)
limitations of probing, 211–12
monitoring of, in periodontal maintenance therapy, 449
screening method, 211–12
soft tissue evaluation, 427–28
Problem-based learning (PBL) approach, 259–64
    defined, 259
    gingivitis, nonsurgical treatment of, 261t
    periodontal therapy, 259–64
    periodontitis, 260–61t
    surgical periodontal therapy, selected procedures, 262–64t
Problem/evidence-based treatment planning, 258–81
    adjunctive treatment, 280–81
    geriatric patients, 281
    informed consent, 273
    periodontist, referral to, 267–73
    problem-based learning (PBL) approach, 259–64
    problem list, 264–67
    treatment guidelines, 273–80
Problem implant, identification of, 429
Problem list, 264–67
    periodontal, 265–66t
    periodontal diseases, risk assessment for, 264–67
    treatment planning, 267
Professional debridement, 350
Prognosis, 279–80
    defined, 279
    determining, common clinical factors used in, 280
    teeth, prognostic classification for individual, 280
Prophylaxis, 349
Prostaglandins (PGs), 71–72, 72f
Prostaglandins of the E series (PGE_2), 77, 252
Prostheses, 423
Proteases, 62
Proteoglycans, 12
Protrusive occlusion, 154–55
Proximal contact relationships, 190–92
Pseudo-halitosis, management of patients with, 292
Pseudomembranous colitis, 339
Pseudopocket, 116, 116f
Psychological assessment, 290
Puberty, 96–97
Puberty gingivitis, 117, 122
Pulpal etiology, 440

Pursestring arrangement, 425
Purulent exudate, 223, 224f
Pus, 223, 224f
Pyorrhea alveolaris, 364
Pyrophosphates, 304

Quality assessment, 281
Quaternary ammonium compounds, 323–24
Quinolones, 339

Race as risk factor, 95
Radicular bone, 20
Radiographic assessment, 233–46
    conventional (See Conventional radiographs)
    digital imaging, 243–44
    digital subtraction radiology, 244
    frequency of radiographs, 243
    in implantology, 244–46
    intraoral technique (See Radiographs, intraoral)
    of periodontal changes, 242–43
    periodontal interpretation (See Radiographs, in periodontal interpretation)
    of periodontal structures, 238–39
    periodontal visit, 449–50
Radiographs, in periodontal interpretation, 239–42
    anatomic configurations, 241–42
    bone loss (See Bone loss, radiographic determination of)
    calculus, 241, 241f
Radiographs, intraoral, 234–36
    exposure time, 234
    film type, 235
    kilovoltage, 234
    milliamperage, 235
    paralleling vs. bisecting technique, 235–36, 236f
    parameters, 234–35, 235f
Rapidly progressive periodontitis, 279
Rationale
    periodontal debridement and indications for, 350–51
    for use of antibiotics, 333–34
Reattachment, 365
Recall, 272
Recurrent periodontal diseases, 142, 446, 452, 454
Reevaluation of initial therapy, 357–58
    measurements of, 357
    tissue response, 357–58
    ultrasonic vs. hand-activated instrumentation, 358

Referral to periodontist, 267–73
  gingivitis, 273
  guidelines for co-management and, 267–73
  moderate chronic periodontitis, 275
  periodontal diseases, 268–71
  periodontal health, 272
  periodontal treatment, phases of, 272
  refractory periodontitis (nonresponsive cases), 277
  severe chronic periodontitis, 276–77
  slight (mild) chronic periodontitis, 274
  treatment, phases of, 271–73
Refractory periodontal diseases, 137, 139, 142, 277, 446
Regenerative periodontal surgery, 394–409
  biologics, 398–99
  bone grafts, 396–98, 399–400
  bone-replacement materials, objectives of, 398
  bone substitutes, 396–98, 399–400
  bony defects, response to, 396t
  complications following, 409t
  defined, 409
  devices, 398–99
  guided tissue regeneration, 400–407
  objectives of, 395–96
  open flap debridement, 396
  periodontal tissue regeneration, 395
  postoperative care, 407–8, 408t
  procedures used to enhance, 395
  root surface treatment, 408–9
  therapy, risk factors for, 409
Regenerative therapy, risk factors for, 409
Respiratory diseases, 104
Restorations, 314
Restorative care, 272
Restorative dentistry, 87–88, 88f, 272
  evaluation for, 189
  procedures, 166
Restorative materials, 314
Retreatment, 449
Risk assessment
  defined, 264
  for periodontal diseases, 264–67
Risk-determinants, 264
Risk factors, 26, 46–47. See also Systemic diseases
  for gingival diseases, identifying, 199
Risk indicators, 45–46, 264
Root anatomy, 354
Root canal therapy, 378
Root caries, 189, 189f, 391
Root debridement, 264
Root morphology, 85, 86–87f
Root planning, 349

Root resection, 377–78
Root sensitivity, 311
Root surface, 132
  caries, 189
  characteristics, 352–53
  treatment, 408–9
Rubber-tip stimulator, 298

Saliva, 69
Scalers, 433
Scaling, 349–50
Scar formation, 365
Scope Original, 323
Seal and Protect, 314, 391
Secondary occlusal trauma, 161, 161f
Secondary prevention, 287, 446
Second-generation drugs, 339
Selection, 336
Selective grinding, 165–66
Self-assessment, 288
Semipermiable structure, 10
Sensitivity analysis, 254
Severe periodontitis, 242, 243f, 276–77
Severity, defined, 26
Silk, 387
Single-stage surgical procedure, 419–20
Single-tooth replacements, 420–21
Single-tuft brushes, 298
Sinus grafts, 421–23
Slight (mild) periodontitis, 242, 242f, 274
Sling sutures, 388
Smokeless tobacco, 101
Smoking, 381, 450–52
Smoking, Tobacco, and Cancer Program of the National Cancer Institute, 451
Smoking cessation
  pharmacologic therapy, 452, 453–54t
  program, 451
Social history, 183
Sodium bicarbonate/hydrogen peroxide dentifrices, 303–4
Sodium fluoride, 313
Sodium valproate, 123
Soft tissue evaluation, 428
Soft tissue graphs, types of, 381–86
  double papillae flap, 381
  free gingival, 381–82
  guided tissue regeneration (GTR) for root coverage, 385–86
  laterally positioned flap, 381
  pedicle graft, 381
  subepithelial connective tissue graft, 382–85
Sonicare, 294
Spaces between teeth, 469–74
Specialized mucosa, 7

Specially denatured (SD) alcohol, 324
Splinting, 166–67, 167f
Split-thickness flap, 368
Stains, tooth. See also Tooth stain evaluation
  black-line, 193
  common, classification of, 194–95t
  endogenous, 193
  green, 193, 195
  significance of, 195
  tobacco, 193
Stanimax, 324
Stannous fluoride, 303, 313, 324
Steroids, 101–2
Stippling, 5–6, 5f, 6f
Subantimicrobial-dose doxycycline (SDD), 343–44
Subepithelial connective tissue graft, 382–85
Subgingival bacteria, 325
Subgingival biofilm, 334
Subgingival debridement, 352–53
  calculus removal, 352
  cementum removal, 353
  periodontal debridement, 349
  periodontal debridement procedures, 352–53
  periodontal therapy, 353
  root surface characteristics, 352–53
Subgingival dental calculus, 84–85
Subgingival microbiota, 351
Subgingival plaque, 58–59
Subjective data, 179
Subperiosteal implants, 416
Sulcular epithelium, 10
Superstructure removal and replacement, 430–33
Suppuration, 223, 224f
Suprabony pocket, 374
Supragingival bacteria, 325
Supragingival debridement, 349
Supragingival dental calculus, 84
Supragingival environment, 69
Supragingival plaque, 55–58, 69
Supragingival scaling, 349
Surface texture, assessment of, 204
Surgical and postoperative care, 389–91
  oral hygiene instructions, 390
  postoperative complications, 390
  postoperative visit management, 390–91
  procedures, 267–368t
  surgical complications, 389–90
Surgical complications, 389–90
Surgical gut, 387
Surgical periodontal therapy, selected procedures, 262–64t

Surgical procedures
 barrier membranes, 404–5
 effects of, 391
 for guided tissue regeneration,
  404–5
Sustained-release device, 340
Sutures, 387–89
 absorbable, 387
 materials used in periodontics, 387t
 needles, 388
 nonabsorbable, 387
 synthetic, 387
 techniques, 388–89
Systematic and local drug delivery systems, 332–44. *See also* Local
  drug delivery systems; Systematic drug delivery system
 antibiotics, rationale for use of,
  333–34
 biofilm, dental plaque as, 334
 delivery systems, 334
 drug actions, 334
 drug information resources, selected,
  333
 enzyme-suppression therapy, 343–44
 precautions/contraindications, 343
Systematic drug delivery system,
  334–40
 adverse drug events, 336
 antibiotic resistance, 340
 defined, 334
 indications, 334–36
 main features of, 335t
 systemic antibiotics, 336–39
Systemic antibiotics, 336–39
 cephalosporins, 338
 lincomycins, 339
 macrolides, 339
 nitroimadazoles, 338–39
 penicillin (beta-lactams), 338
 quinolones, 339
 tetracyclines, 336–38
Systemic antimicrobial agents, classification of, 337t
Systemic diseases
 adverse pregnancy outcomes, 103–4
 age, gender, and race, 95
 Alzheimer's disease, 104
 cardiovascular disease, 102–3
 drug use status (*See* Drug use)
 endocrine system (*See* Endocrine
  system)
 genetics, 94–95
 hematologic system, 99
 HIV/AIDS, 99, 99f
 nutritional status, 100
 respiratory diseases, 104
 stress, 95

Tartar. *See* Calculus
Tartar-control dentifrices, 304
Teeth *vs.* dental implants, 423–26
 anatomy, 423–26
 biologic environment, 426t
 blood supply, 426
 inflammatory lesion, 426
TefGen-FD, 405
TefGen-RE, 405
Teflon, 433
Temporomandibular joint (TMJ),
  163
Tetracyclines, 336–38
 adverse effects, 337–38
 anticollagenase feature, 336–37
 drug-drug interactions, 337–38
 drug-food interactions, 337–38
 gingival crevicular fluid (GCF), con-
  centration in, 337
Therapeutic benefits of dentifrices, 302t
Three-dimensional computed tomogra-
  phy (CT) imaging, 245, 245f,
  246f
Three-wall bony defect, 135
Thumb sucking, 158
Time spent, 354–55
Tipped teeth, 190, 190f
Tissue consistency, 351
Tissue peeling, 304
Tissue response, 357–58
Tissue sloughing, 304
Titanium, 416
T-lymphocytes, 75–77, 75f, 76f, 77f
Tobacco. *See also* Smoking cessation
 products, 100–101
 stains, 193
Tomograms, 245–46
Tongue cleansing/brushing, 291,
  299–300
Tongue coating, 291
Tongue print, 291
Tongue sulfide probe, 290
Tongue thrusting, 158
Tooth-accumulated materials (TAMs),
  61–62
Toothbrushes, 292–94
Toothbrushing
 frequency of, 293–94
 improper use of, 310
Toothbrush trauma, 89
Tooth migration, 162
Tooth mobility, 161–62, 223–24
 measurement of, 224
 surgical procedures, 391
Toothpastes, 291
Toothpicks, wooden,
  298–99
Tooth position, 87, 87f

Tooth stain evaluation, 192–95. *See
  also* Stains, tooth
 development of, 192–93
 endogenous stains, 193
 extrinsic stains, 193, 195
 significance of evaluation, 192–93
Tooth structure, 163
Tooth wear, conditions of, 191–92,
  191f
Topical drug delivery systems, 320–29
 antiplaque/antigingivitis agents,
  321–25
 chemotherapeutic agents, 321
 oral irrigation, 325–29
 oral rinses, 321
 topical delivery, 321
Transosteal implants, 416
Traumatic factors, 89–91
 chemical injury, 90, 90f
 factitious disease, 89, 89f
 food impaction, 89–90, 90f
 occlusion, 90–91
 oral piercings, 91, 91f
 toothbrush trauma, 89
Traumatic lesions, 124
Traumatic overbite, 155
Treatment, phases of, 271–73
 gingivitis, 273
 maintenance care, 272
 moderate chronic periodontitis, 275
 nonsurgical/initial preparation, 271
 periodontal diseases, 268–71
 periodontal health, 272
 periodontal surgery, 271–72
 periodontal treatment, 272
 refractory periodontitis (nonresponsive cases), 277
 restorative care, 272
 severe chronic periodontitis, 276–77
 slight (mild) chronic periodontitis,
  274
 treatment planning, 271
Treatment guidelines, 273–80
 gingival diseases, 278–78
 necrotizing periodontal diseases, 279
 peri-implantitis, 279
 periodontal health, 273–78
 periodontitis, 279
 prognosis, 279–80
Treatment plan, 180
Trench mouth. *See* Necrotizing periodontal diseases
Triclosan-containing dentifrices, 303
Trimus, 441
Tuft dental floss, 297
Tumor necrosis factor (TNF), 74
Two-stage surgical procedure, 418–19
Two-wall bony defect, 136

Ultrasonic *vs.* hand-activated instrumentation, 358

Variables, 45–47
  risk factors, 46–47
  risk indicators, 45–46

Vaseline, 389
Vertical releasing incision, 377
Viadent Advanced Care, 304, 323
Vitamin deficiencies, 100

Water Pik, 326
White blood cells, 10

Xenografts, 398
Xerostomia (dry mouth), 101, 281, 292

Zinc citrate-containing dentifrices, 304